Managing Health Services Organizations

Managing Health Services Organizations

Third Edition

by

Jonathon S. Rakich, Ph.D.
The University of Akron

Beaufort B. Longest, Jr., Ph.D., FACHE
The University of Pittsburgh

Kurt Darr, J.D., Sc.D., FACHE
The George Washington University

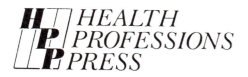
**HEALTH
PROFESSIONS
PRESS**

Baltimore • London • Toronto • Sydney

Health Professions Press, Inc.
P.O. Box 10624
Baltimore, Maryland 21285-0624

Typeset by Brushwood Graphics, Inc., Baltimore, Maryland.
Manufactured in the United States of America by
Rose Printing Company, Inc., Tallahassee, Florida.

First printing, August 1992.
Second printing, December 1992.
Third printing, August 1993.
Fourth printing, August 1994.

The *Instructor's Manual for Managing Health Services Organizations,* by Jonathon S. Rakich, Beaufort B. Longest, Jr., and Kurt Darr, is also available from Health Professions Press, P.O. Box 10624, Baltimore, Maryland 21285-0624.

Library of Congress Cataloging-in-Publication Data

Rakich, Jonathon S.
    Managing health services organizations/Jonathon S. Rakich, Beaufort B. Longest, Jr., Kurt Darr.—3rd ed.
        p.   cm.
    Includes bibliographical references and indexes.
    ISBN 1-878812-09-2
    1. Health facilities—Administration.   I. Longest, Beaufort B., Jr.   II. Darr, Kurt.   III. Title.
[DNLM: 1. Health Facilities—organization & administration—United States. 2. Hospital Administration—United States. WX 150 R162n]
RA971.R26   1992
362.1′1′068—dc20
DNLM/DLC
for Library of Congress   92-1466
                                                                                                      CIP

Contents

About the Authors

Jonathon S. Rakich, Ph.D., College of Business Administration, The University of Akron, Akron, Ohio 44325

Jonathon S. Rakich is Distinguished Professor of Management and Health Services Administration in the College of Business Administration, and Distinguished Professor of Biomedical Engineering in the College of Engineering at The University of Akron. Professor Rakich received his Ph.D. from Saint Louis University and his MBA from The University of Michigan. He specializes in strategic planning and health care policy and is coordinator of The University of Akron's Master of Science in Management—Health Services Administration option program. During his 25-year teaching career, he has written or coauthored 3 books (in 9 editions), 30 journal articles (including those in *Health Care Financing Review, Health Care Management Review, Hospital & Health Services Administration,* and *Hospital Topics*), and more than 30 conference proceedings and professional papers.

Professor Rakich has been awarded a postdoctoral fellowship with the Department of Health and Human Services, and he has served on the boards of trustees of a health systems agency and a home health agency. While on sabbatical in 1979, Professor Rakich served an administrative residency at Akron City Hospital. During his sabbatical in 1989, he participated in on-site research of the Canadian health care system. Professor Rakich is a member of the Academy of Management, the Canadian Operational Research Society, and the Decision Sciences Institute. He is a faculty affiliate of the American College of Healthcare Executives.

Beaufort B. Longest, Jr., Ph.D., FACHE, Graduate School of Public Health, University of Pittsburgh, Pittsburgh, Pennsylvania 15261

Beaufort B. Longest, Jr. is Professor of Health Services Administration in the Graduate School of Public Health, and Professor of Business Administration in the Joseph M. Katz Graduate School of Business at the University of Pittsburgh. He is also Director of the University of Pittsburgh's Health Policy Institute. Previously, he was a member of the faculty of the W.K. Kellogg Graduate School of Management at Northwestern University. He also served as Director of the University of Pittsburgh's Health Administration Program during the period when it was reorganized from a program located exclusively in the Graduate School of Public Health to its current arrangement as an interschool program of the business and public health schools. Professor Longest completed his undergraduate work at Davidson College and received his Master of Health Administration and Ph.D. degrees from Georgia State University. He is a Fellow of the American College of Healthcare Executives.

Professor Longest's research in the fields of health management and policy has been supported by federal grants and grants from a number of foundations. He contributes frequently to the literature in health management and health policy; Professor Longest is the author or coauthor of 5 books, 12 book chapters, and numerous articles. He has been a board member of six health and human services organizations and consults with provider organizations, associations, and government agencies in the health field. His professional expertise is in the areas of strategic management in the health sector and health policy.

Kurt Darr, J.D., Sc.D., FACHE, Department of Health Services Management and Policy, The George Washington University, Washington, D.C. 20052

Kurt Darr is Professor of Hospital Administration in the Department of Health Services Management and Policy, School of Business and Public Management, and Professor of Health Care Sciences in the School of Medicine and Health Sciences at The George Washington University. He holds the Doctor of Science degree from The Johns Hopkins University School of Hygiene and Public Health, and a Master of Hospital Administration and Juris Doctor degree from the University of Minnesota.

Professor Darr completed his administrative residency at Rochester Methodist Hospital in Minnesota, and subsequently served as an Administrative Associate at the Mayo Clinic and Assistant Chief of Operating Services Division at St. Albans Naval Hospital. He completed postdoctoral fellowships with the Department of Health and Human Services, the World Health Organization, and the Accrediting Commission on Education for Health Services Administration. Professor Darr is a Fellow of the American College of Healthcare Executives. He is a member of the District of Columbia and Minnesota Bars, and he serves as an arbitrator and mediator for the American Arbitration Assocation.

Professor Darr regularly presents seminars on health services ethics, hospital organization and management, quality improvement, and applying the Deming method in the health field. Professor Darr is the author and editor of several books used in graduate health services administration programs and numerous articles on health services topics.

The authors have collaborated extensively. Other books by the authors are: *Cases in Health Services Management* (2nd ed.) (edited by J. Rakich, B. Longest, Jr., & K. Darr), Baltimore: Health Professions Press, 1987; *Hospital Organization and Management: Text and Readings* (4th ed.) (edited by K. Darr & J. Rakich), Baltimore: Health Professions Press, 1989; *Ethics for Health Services Management: Case Studies in Health Administration* (edited by K. Darr), Chicago: American College of Healthcare Executives, 1985; *Ethics in Health Services Management* (2nd ed.) (K. Darr), Baltimore: Health Professions Press, 1991; *Principles of Hospital Business Office Management* (B. Longest, Jr.), Chicago: Hospital Financial Management Association, 1975; *Hospital Cost Containment Programs: A Policy Analysis* (B. Longest, Jr. & Colleagues), Cambridge: Ballinger Publishing Co., 1978; and *Management Practices for the Health Professional,* (4th ed.) (B. Longest, Jr.), Norwalk, CT: Appleton & Lange, 1990.

Preface

The epigram introducing the first chapter of this book states: "The beginning of the 21st century beckons both with challenge and opportunity for improved health of Americans." From now until then, and most likely well beyond, health services managers will be confronted with change—a constant that will challenge them to improve the organization, delivery, and financing of health services. Our purpose in preparing this book is to help managers meet these demands and seize the opportunities; by doing so they will make a major contribution to improving health.

This book is most beneficial for two types of users: 1) students engaged in the formal study of health services management, and 2) current managers who wish to supplement their experience and refresh their knowledge of applied management theory. It is about managing organizations that deliver health services. Historically, hospitals and nursing facilities have been the most prominent health services organizations (HSOs). Others that have become important more recently include managed care organizations (including HMOs and PPOs), multiorganizational systems, ambulatory care organizations, home health agencies, birth centers, and hospices. All face new environments—a mosaic of external forces including new rules and technologies; changing demography; increased competition, public scrutiny, and expectations; greater accountability; and more constraints on resources. Managerial excellence makes a difference in the efficient and effective delivery of health services. HSO managers must be prepared if they are to respond to these and other challenges. We hope this book will aid in their preparation.

Pedagogically, our objective is to present management theory in a way that demonstrates its generic applicability to all types of HSOs. This is accomplished by using a process orientation that focuses on how managers manage. It examines management functions, concepts, and principles as well as managerial roles within the context of HSOs and their external environment. For nascent managers, we seek to introduce new terminology and concepts to provide a foundation for professional development. For experienced managers, we seek to reinforce present skills and experience while providing and applying new theory, as well as traditional theory and concepts in new ways. For both, we seek to assist them in their task of meeting the challenges ahead. It is clear that health services management is exceptionally dynamic and HSOs' environments are turbulent. As a result, there are both risks and opportunities. Prepared and innovative managers who have vision lead rather than follow, and those who seize opportunities will make a difference to their HSOs and the improvement of health care.

The chapters of this third edition, similar to the first and second editions, are grouped into seven parts. The one chapter in Part I, "A Framework of Management in Health Services Organizations," develops an input-conversion-output management model for HSOs. This model incorporates managerial functions and roles, as well as the dimensions of organizational culture, values, and stakeholders, and it is linked to the external environment. The management model is a framework for all succeeding parts and chapters.

Part II, "The Health Services Environment," describes and analyzes the setting and context in which HSO managers work. The first of the four chapters in this part presents a comprehensive summary and overview of the health care delivery system in the United States, including extensive data about providers, institutional provider associations, health personnel, licensure and accreditation, and health care financing and expenditures. It also includes comparative data on international health care expenditures, a description of the Canadian universal-comprehensive health care system, and an analysis of policy differences between the United States and Canada. The remaining three chapters are devoted to ethical, legal, and technological considerations in health care. Issues are identified and the implications for HSO managers are addressed in these chapters. Managers must have a clear understanding of the relationship between their HSOs and the broader scheme of health care.

The two chapters in Part III, "Structuring Health Services Organizations," address organizational theory and HSO structure. The first chapter presents the classic concepts of organization design and analyzes contemporary perspectives on these concepts. The second chapter describes how various types of HSOs: acute care hospitals, nursing facilities, managed care organizations, home health agencies, birth centers, and hospices are organized. The history, functions, numbers, management structure, governance, and professional staff organization (PSO) are described for each. Managers can manage only in a formal setting, and HSOs are among the most complex organizations. Understanding the management, governance, and PSO dimensions of HSOs and their interaction is vital for managers.

Part IV, "Strategic Planning and Interorganizational Linkages for Health Services Organizations," has two chapters. The first chapter presents objective and strategy formulation including a comprehensive strategic planning model that incorporates marketing as a contextual variable for external environment assessment and interaction. Objectives provide the focus for all organization activity. The companion chapter details new HSO arrangements and interorganizational linkages. In sum, the chapters consider the array of strategies from integration to diversification that HSOs may use to accomplish their objectives. Uncertainty results from change and HSOs are no longer insulated from it. Their managers must understand these forces as they develop responses to them.

Part V, "Problem Solving, Quality Improvement, and Control in Health Services Organizations," has three chapters. The first of these chapters treats managerial problem solving and decision making. The second chapter focuses on continuous quality improvement (CQI) in HSOs, including the dimensions of quality and the philosophy and models of CQI. The tenets of quality experts W. Edwards Deming, Joseph M. Juran, and Philip B. Crosby are presented, and CQI is linked to productivity improvement. As organizational leaders, managers are stewards of the HSO's culture and philosophy. It is their responsibility to ensure that quality pervades both. The third chapter in this section includes a number of interrelated topics: control, risk management and quality assessment/improvement, and resource allocation. Each topic applies models and methods to HSOs. The greatest challenge facing HSO managers is continuous improvement of the quality of services produced by their organizations. Efforts to improve quality will result in judicious use of the resources entrusted to them. Meeting these challenges will leave an admirable legacy—improved health for society.

Part VI, "Managing People in Health Services Organizations," includes four chapters that cover the behavioral dimension of managing HSOs. A central theme throughout the book, but especially in these chapters, is that managers accomplish objectives through human and other resources. Skills in motivation, leadership, and communication are requisite to effective management, as is awareness of the complexity of organizational dynamics and change. Chapters that include contemporary theories are devoted to each of these subjects.

Part VII, "Human Resources Management in Health Services Organizations," has two chapters. Personnel and human resources management—the acquisition and retention of human resources—as well as labor relations are a primary responsibility of senior management. It is important, therefore, that all HSO managers understand the dimensions of managing human resources and the legal environment affecting them. Human resources are the HSO's most important resource—they are an asset worthy of major investment. They are critical to accomplishing the HSO's objectives.

The epigraph to the last chapter suggests that managers and employees must be partners. Managerial effectiveness and the work of managers will be judged by how well they develop staff. It is only through employee empowerment that the full potential of the organization to provide excellence and affordability in health services will be realized. It is the partnership of managers and staff that will enable HSOs to meet the challenges of the 21st century.

Acknowledgments

Professor Rakich gratefully acknowledges the support of his wife, Tana. Russell J. Petersen, Ph.D., Dean, College of Business Administration, and Alan G. Krigline, Ph.D., Head, Department of Management, The College of Business Administration, The University of Akron, provided assistance and encouragement in numerous ways. Special thanks are owed to Linda Peavy, my graduate assistant, and to Norma Pearson, Professor of Bibliography.

Professor Longest gratefully acknowledges the support of his wife, Carolyn. Donald R. Mattison, M.D., Dean, Graduate School of Public Health, and H.J. Zoffer, Ph.D., Dean, Joseph M. Katz Graduate School of Business, provided assistance and encouragement in numerous ways. Edgar N. Duncan, Ph.D., Associate Dean, Graduate School of Public Health, was kind enough to allow me to use his extensive personal library of management literature. Special thanks are also owed to my administrative assistants, Lily Maskew and Elly Poster.

Professor Darr gratefully acknowledges the support of his wife, Anne. Ben Burdetsky, Ph.D., Dean, School of Business and Public Management, and Richard F. Southby, Ph.D., Chairman, Department of Health Services Management and Policy, provided assistance and encouragement in numerous ways. Special thanks are owed to Corrie Perelmutter, my teaching assistant.

The authors received valuable assistance in revising Chapter 17, "Personnel/Human Resources Management," from Robert S. Peel, Vice President of Human Resources, St. Lawrence Hospital, Lansing, Michigan, and Kathryn Comer Peel, Director, Corporate Office of Human Resource Services, Mercy Health Services, Farmington, Michigan.

Numerous members of the staff at Health Professions Press are owed a special debt: Barbara Karni, our efficient managing editor; Megan Westerfeld, copyeditor extraordinaire; Roslyn Udris, effective production manager; and Tania Bourdon, responsive production coordinator.

The authors also wish to thank the several publishers and authors who granted permission to reprint materials to which they hold copyright. Last, but certainly not least, the authors are grateful to the many users of the second edition whose comments and critiques aided us in preparing this third edition.

To our parents—

Eva and John
Mary Teachey and Beaufort
Emma and Johannes Kurt

Managing Health Services Organizations

I / A Framework of Management in Health Services Organizations

1 / The Management Process and Managerial Roles

*The beginning of the twenty-first century
beckons both with challenge and opportunity for
improved health of Americans.*

Healthy People 2000[1]

Health services organization (HSO) managers—those appointed to positions of authority, who enable others to do their work effectively, who have responsibility for resource utilization, and who are accountable for work results—can be proud of their organizations and what they do. They are part of a distinct profession with the unique obligation of providing health services to and contributing to the health of the general populace.

As the year 2000 approaches, HSOs and their managers will be confronted with change—a constant that will affect both the organization and delivery and the financing of health services. HSO managers confronted and responded to change in the 1980s[2] and this will occur in the 1990s and into the 21st century, but at an accelerated pace. As reported in the United States Department of Health and Human Services's publication, *Healthy People 2000,* "the year 2000 connotes change."[3] The year 2000 will inaugurate a new century and a new millennium in which momentous issues concerning the vitality and health of the people will emerge. Issues during this period will include an aging population, miraculous but costly technologies to diagnose and treat disease, and efforts to modify lifestyles and emphasize wellness and prevention. Concern about health care costs will continue, as will the debate about access to health care; however, fundamental changes in national health policy are unlikely.

Instead, the health services system will change incrementally[4] in detail, but not substance.[5] During this time, increased expectations by consumers and payors of health care will affect providers. HSOs and their managers will be scrutinized regarding the costs and quality of the care they provide. There will be "demands for greater efficiency in the delivery of services and for greater evidence of the effectiveness of care."[6] Both quality of outcomes and continuous improvement in the process of providing health care will be emphasized.[7] The challenges for HSOs and their managers will be great; the opportunities will be even greater. Managerial excellence makes the difference in efficient and effective delivery of health services, and HSO managers will seize the opportunities and accept and respond to the challenges.

This book is about managing HSOs, and this chapter provides the conceptual framework. The introduction distinguishes between health care and health services delivery and provides the focus. Management in HSOs is presented next, including discussion of types of managers and the management process and descriptions of management functions, activities characteristic of senior managers, and managerial roles. A section on organizational culture and philosophy follows. Included are philosophies about customers and continuous quality improvement, about employees, and about stakeholders—those with a vested interest in the HSO and who seek to influence it. A management model for HSOs is developed using an input-conversion-output perspective, and each component is described. Using a systems perspective, the external environment affecting the HSO and its managers is presented. Finally, the framework and structure derived from the management model and used in succeeding parts of this book are described.

3

Health Care and Health Services

Health care—the total societal effort, organized or not, whether private or public, that attempts to guarantee, provide, finance, and promote health—changed markedly during the 20th century. It is moving toward the ideal of wellness and prevention of disease and disability, in comparison with acute restorative care, and public policy initiatives have been more interventionist. Health services are the delivery component of health care. They are provided by practitioners and organizations and have undergone significant change—smoothly at times, turbulently at others.

Health Services Organizations

Delivery of health services involves the organized public or private efforts that assist individuals primarily in regaining health, but also in preventing disease and disability. Delivery of service to patients occurs in a variety of organizational settings. (For ease of reading, the term "patient" is used to describe anyone served by an HSO.) All HSOs can be classified by ownership and profit motive. In addition, they can be classified by whether the patient is admitted as an inpatient or outpatient and, for an inpatient, by the average length of stay. These categories and classifications are developed in Chapter 2, "The Health Care Delivery System," and in Chapter 7, "How HSOs Are Organized."

Historically, hospitals and nursing facilities have been the most common and dominant HSOs engaged in delivery of health services. They remain prominent in the contemporary health services system, but other HSOs have achieved stature. Among them are outpatient clinics, imaging centers, free-standing urgent care and surgical centers, large group practices, and home health agencies. Multiorganizational systems, both vertically and horizontally integrated, are widespread. Health maintenance organizations (HMOs), preferred provider organizations (PPOs), and managed care systems are financial and delivery arrangements that became prominent in the 1980s.[8] These various HSOs and others face new environments containing a wide range of external pressures, including new rules and technologies, changed demography, accountability to multiple constituents, and constraints on resources. As a result, HSO managers must work smarter, not just harder, and they must allocate and use resources more effectively and strive for continuous quality improvement and continued excellence in an increasingly restrictive environment.

Focus of the Book

The book presents the subject of management in a way that demonstrates its generic applicability to all types of HSOs, yet offers illustrations pertinent to certain of them. The text has a process orientation and provides an overview of management—what managers do and how they go about managing—rather than a narrow and organization-specific presentation. A process orientation examines functions, activities,[9] and events involved in accomplishing something, as well as their relationships to each other in the context of a broad setting. By nature, the view must be more general and present managerial functions, roles, practices, concepts, and techniques that transcend levels of the organizational hierarchy and are generic to various HSOs.

Conversely, a narrow orientation focuses on specifics in a limited fashion, without linkage to a broader and more important foundation and without generic applicability to a wide range of HSOs. Generally, the book does not address detailed, organization-specific subjects, such as the structure of housekeeping, nursing, or clinical services, or business office practices, or the design of a patient information system. Specifics are used to accomplish the primary purpose—a presentation of the general subject of management. By embracing a process orientation, this text examines how HSO managers manage, the functions they perform, and to a lesser degree, their roles. Primarily, the focus is on senior and middle-level management, rather than supervisory levels. All organizations are treated generically, but, as the dominant and most complex type of HSO, acute care hospitals are a common example.

This study of management provides readers with knowledge and reinforces, in an orderly fashion, that which they may already know. It is meant to widen the perspective of persons with diverse, perhaps technical backgrounds. Most readers will attain middle-level management positions. Some material presented, such as strategic planning, will enable these readers to understand early in their careers the functions and roles of senior managers and the decisions they make. Many readers will attain senior management positions and will have years of experience to hone their skills and supplement their knowledge. Regardless of the reader's professional level, the conceptual framework of management establishes a knowledge base that can grow and evolve as individuals mesh it with past and future experience.

MANAGEMENT IN HSOs

Types of Managers

HSO managers are defined as *persons appointed to positions of authority who enable others to do their work effectively, who have responsibility for resource utilization, and who are accountable for work results.* This broad definition includes persons with titles such as nurse team leader; maintenance foreman; dietary, surgery, or medical records supervisor; director of pharmacy, laboratory, outpatient clinic, social services, or business office; medical director; or president or vice president.

Traditional classification of managers is by level in the organization hierarchy; common nomenclature is top or senior management, middle-level management, and supervisory or first-line management.[10] Other common terms for these classifications are policy level, administrative or coordinative level, and operations level.[11] Regardless of title or level, managers have several common attributes; they are: 1) formally appointed to positions of authority, 2) charged with directing and enabling others (subordinates and nonsubordinates) to do their work effectively, 3) responsible for utilizing resources, and 4) accountable to superiors for results. The primary distinction between managers and others in the organization is that nonmanagers have some responsibility for resources used in their jobs and are accountable to superiors, but nonmanagers are not formally appointed to positions of authority to direct the work of others.

The primary differences between levels of managers are the degree of authority and the scope of responsibility and organizational activity at each level. For example, senior managers, such as hospital chief executive officers (CEOs), skilled nursing facility administrators, or public health commissioners, have authority over and are responsible for the entire organization—all employees, resources, and individual and organizational results. They are accountable to the governing body. Unlike managers in industry, HSO senior managers, especially hospital CEOs, have a unique responsibility in that they must also be responsive to and gain the cooperation of non-employees—physicians—whose influence on the HSO is substantial.[12] Reporting to senior managers are vice presidents and numerous middle-level managers, each of whom is responsible for smaller segments of the organization. Middle-level managers, such as department heads and heads of services, have authority over and are responsible for a specific segment, in contrast to the organization as a whole. Finally, first-line managers, who generally report to middle-level managers, have authority over and are responsible for overseeing specific work and a particular group of workers.

Managers can also be differentiated by the extent to which they use certain skills: human relations, conceptual, and technical.[13] All managers use human relations skills because they accomplish work through people. Human relations skills include motivation, leadership, and communication skills. The degree to which each is used varies with the nature of the position, scope of responsibility, work activity, and number, types, and skills of subordinates. Senior managers use disproportionately more conceptual skills in their jobs than do middle-level or first-line managers.

These include recognizing and evaluating multiple complex issues and understanding their relationships, engaging in planning and problem solving that profoundly affect the HSO, and thinking globally about the organization and its environment.[14] In contrast, first-line managers tend to use job-related technical skills, or skills that involve specialized knowledge, more than either middle-level or senior managers. Figure 1.1 shows the relationship of these skills, degree of authority, and scope of responsibility and activities for each management level.

The Management Process

Management has been defined in ways that appear to be different but that have a strong underlying similarity. Some regard management as getting things done through people;[15] others consider it the process of reaching organization goals by working with and through people.[16] Management is defined here as *the process, composed of interrelated social and technical functions and activities (including roles), occurring in a formal organizational setting for the purpose of accomplishing predetermined objectives through the utilization of human and other resources.*[17] Health services administration is defined similarly by the Commission on Education for Health Services Administration:

> Health services administration [management] is planning, organizing, directing, controlling, and coordinating the resources and procedures by which needs and demands for health and medical care and a healthful environment are fulfilled by the provision of specific services to individual clients, organizations, and communities.[18]

Management has four main elements:

1. It is a process—a set of interactive and interrelated ongoing functions and activities.
2. It involves accomplishing organizational goals or objectives.
3. It involves achieving these objectives through people and the utilization of other resources.
4. It occurs in a formal organizational setting.

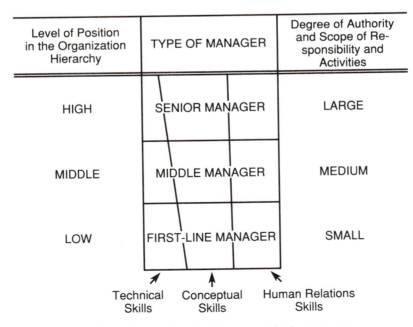

Figure 1.1. Skills used by different types of health services organization managers.

The set of primary social and technical functions characteristic of the management process includes planning, organizing, staffing, directing, controlling, and decision making. These functions are the logical grouping of generic management activities. Other activities inherent in management are integration, coordination, change, and sometimes representation. All health services managers perform these functions and activities to some degree regardless of hierarchical level. The intensity and focus of their efforts depend on authority and the scope of responsibility and work. Interrelationships of the primary social/technical management functions are presented in Figure 1.2.

Management Functions

The traditional classification of management functions describes how managers do what they do (the activities they perform) to accomplish objectives (achieve work results) through people and utilization of other resources.

Planning   Planning is a technical managerial function that enables HSOs to deal with the present and anticipate the future. It involves deciding what to do as well as when and how to do it. Planning may be long term or short term. It is also primary because the organizing, staffing, directing, and controlling management functions are predicated on forecasts, objectives, strategies, and operational programs developed through planning.

When planning, senior managers assess the HSO's external environment and how it will affect them, develop or redefine overall organizational and component objectives, determine specific means or strategies to accomplish objectives, and design operational plans and establish policy. When predetermined courses of action are developed, needed resources can be identified and acquired, and allocation can be made to give order and focus to organization efforts. In short, the manager predetermines the organizational arrangement for accomplishing objectives so that haphazard activities are minimized or do not occur.

Senior HSO managers are typically concerned with the planning function activities of external environment assessment and objective and strategy formulation for the organization, but middle-level and first-line managers also plan. Objectives that are consistent with and support those established for the organization as a whole are set by middle-level and first-line managers for their areas of responsibility. Planning done by these managers focuses on program and operations design as well as implementation procedures and work scheduling.

Organizing   The management function of organizing is technical; it means establishing authority and responsibility relationships, and formal structure and reporting relationships. Organizing focuses on grouping activities and resources in a logical manner, including the division of work and job design, work methods and processes, coordination among units, and use of infor-

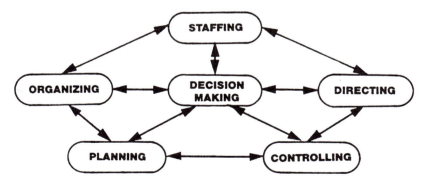

Figure 1.2.   Interrelationships of the management process functions.

mation and feedback systems. Organizing establishes the formal setting for individual and group activities. Elements of such activities are structure, tasks/technology, and people relationships, with an awareness of how each affects the other. Senior managers are concerned with broad aspects of organizing, such as authority and responsibility relationships, departmentation of the organization, and coordination of its components. Middle-level and first-line managers are concerned with specific tasks related to job design, work process flow, and work methods and procedures.

Staffing   The function of staffing is acquiring and retaining human resources, and staffing has both technical and social aspects. Technical aspects are human resource planning, job analysis, recruitment, testing, selection, performance appraisal, compensation and benefits administration, employee assistance, and safety and health. Social aspects are activities that influence the behavior and performance of organization members: training and development, promotions, counseling, and discipline. All managers engage in staffing function activities, such as appraising subordinate performance, determining compensation changes and promotions, and participating in corrective counseling. However, unlike other functions, most staffing activities are centralized in a human resource department that is responsible for human resource acquisition and retention for the organization, as well as labor relations and collective bargaining.

Directing   The directing function is social-behavioral in nature and focuses on initiating action in the organization—it is people oriented. Principal directing function activities include motivating, leading, and communicating, as well as other activities that influence employee behavior. Examples include conflict resolution, behavior modification, and integrating people with structure and tasks. Managers at all levels direct subordinates, and all organized work is accomplished through people. Figure 1.1 shows that managers at all levels use human relations and behavioral skills. All managers motivate, lead, and communicate, yet their approaches, styles, and methods differ because of the nature and scope of their responsibilities and the number and types of subordinates reporting to them.

Controlling   The controlling function is technical and focuses on monitoring, adjusting, and improving performance. Controlling means establishing performance standards to measure results, as well as the techniques and systems to monitor and intervene. Control for senior managers focuses on overall results produced, such as quality of care, expenditures compared to revenues, and resource utilization. First-line managers focus on control in their areas of responsibility—for example, number of lab tests performed per employee per day, number of meals served, and time between dictation and transcription of medical records. The control function monitors outputs (work results) and inputs (resources used), but it must also monitor process, or how the work is done. Continuous quality improvement requires that all processes be systematically monitored, evaluated, and changed to improve quality and ensure that the needs of customers are met.

Decision Making   Decision making is a technical management function that is a part of all other management functions, as shown in Figure 1.2. Managers are decision makers. HSO managers make decisions when they monitor and control work; when they plan, establish, or change organizational arrangements and work process and content; when they acquire and assign personnel; and when they direct efforts of others.

Decision making means choosing. It is a function all managers perform. However, its scope and nature, the techniques used, and the importance of decisions concerning structure, tasks/technology, and people relationships and their integration vary with the manager's position, degree of authority, and scope of responsibility. Senior managers make policy decisions affecting the organization and allocating resources among departments; first-line managers make decisions about allocating and utilizing resources provided by senior management.

Senior Management Activities

Empiricism is a methodology used to describe and understand management; it presumes that the work of managers can be understood by observing them. Research supported by the Association of University Programs in Health Administration involving 149 hospital CEOs and 42 executive directors of prepaid group practice health plans identified three clusters of activities generic to senior managers: internal management, environmental surveillance, and external relations.[19]

Internal management involves managing and maintaining internal HSO operations. Environmental surveillance monitors and surveys the organization's external environment to identify and assess the effects of changes. Finally, external relations are those in which "executives engage for the general purpose of maintaining contact with people or organizations that are pertinent to the [health services] organization's present or future operations."[20] The primary activities of senior managers reported by the study are grouped by function in Figure 1.3.

Senior management activities, as described in Figure 1.3, focus on policy and are concerned with overall scope and broad direction for the HSO. For example, senior management sets policy on staffing, and middle-level managers operationalize and implement the policy. Similarly, senior management sets policy on new services—a planning function activity—and middle-level managers are involved in the specifics of design and implementation of those services.[21]

Managerial Roles

All HSO managers engage in planning, organizing, staffing, directing, controlling, and decision making to some degree. In addition, they perform other activities related to accomplishing work and organizational objectives that do not readily fall within the functional classification. For example, a hospital CEO or other senior managers may serve on an areawide mental health task force; an HMO president may testify before a legislative body; the administrator of a nursing facility may serve on a state licensing board; the vice president of nursing at an academic medical center may teach in a nursing baccalaureate program; and a Department of Veterans Affairs hospital CEO may lobby members of Congress.

Researchers have studied roles as a way to describe management that goes beyond the functional groupings of planning, organizing, staffing, directing, controlling, and decision making. These roles are defined as the behavior or activities associated with a management position because of its authority and status. Mintzberg's classification identifies interpersonal, informational, and decisional roles.[22] These roles and their subclassifications are shown in Figure 1.4.

Interpersonal Roles The three interpersonal roles presented in Figure 1.4 are figurehead, liaison, and influencer. All managers, but especially senior managers, are figureheads because they engage in ceremonial and symbolic activities such as presiding over an event honoring long-service employees, speaking at retirement dinners, and ribbon-cutting for a new building wing.

Liaison involves formal and informal internal and external contacts. Internally, these contacts extend beyond the chain of command and are analogous to coordination among work units. External liaison is more extensive than coordination and means cultivating informal contacts and acquaintance-familiarity with other HSO managers to develop personal relationships that facilitate cooperation. It can also involve formal and informal liaison with the HSO's external stakeholders.

The influencer (leader) role includes activities inherent in the directing function, the purpose of which is to motivate and lead. However, it is more extensive because managers influence by example and by reason of position, and subordinates tend to emulate this behavior and adopt the values it represents.

PLANNING (INTERNAL MANAGEMENT)

- Defining the general course and goal priorities for the organization
- Determining matters for the governing board or owner(s) to consider
- Determining new diagnostic, treatment, and nonprofessional services to be added, and new construction

PLANNING (ENVIRONMENTAL SURVEILLANCE)

- Determining and establishing priorities for new services
- Determining what other organizations in the service area are doing and what services they are offering
- Interpreting how legislative and regulation trends might affect the organization
- Interpreting how health services delivery and financing trends might affect the organization

ORGANIZING (INTERNAL MANAGEMENT)

- Determining how authority and responsibility are divided among individuals and departments
- Determining formal communication patterns (and reporting relationships) within the organization

STAFFING (INTERNAL MANAGEMENT)

- Determining departmental staffing levels
- Determining salary scales and fringe benefits for management personnel
- Evaluation, training, and development of management personnel

DIRECTING (INTERNAL MANAGEMENT)

- Motivating, advising, and counseling management personnel

CONTROLLING (INTERNAL MANAGEMENT)

- Developing and improving management information systems and procedures to be fed back to operations
- Containing costs of professional services to patients and improving efficiency and productivity in nonprofessional departments
- Developing and improving accounting and budgeting practices
- Improving the accessibility of the organization's patient care services and monitoring patient opinions about the care received

EXTERNAL RELATIONS

- Informing the community-at-large about the organization
- Dealing with community leaders on matters about the organization
- Influencing legislation and regulations
- Dealing with government licensing agencies

Figure 1.3. Senior management activities. (Adapted from Kuhl, Ingrid K. *The executive role in health services delivery organizations.* Washington, D.C.: Office of Applied Research, Association of University Programs in Health Administration, 1977.)

Informational Roles   The three informational roles of a manager are monitor, disseminator, and spokesperson. Mintzberg asserts that, by virtue of the manager's interpersonal contacts with subordinates and their network of contacts, the manager emerges as the nerve center of that unit.[23] Managers continuously gather information from internal network contacts, external liaison contacts, and formal organization sources such as superiors and subordinates. They filter, evaluate, and choose to act on or react to that information, including deciding whether to disseminate

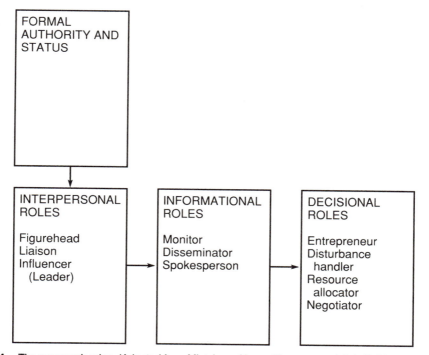

Figure 1.4. The manager's roles. (Adapted from Mintzberg, Henry. The manager's job: Folklore and fact. *Harvard Business Review* 53 [July–August 1975]: 55. Reprinted by permission of *Harvard Business Review*. Copyright © 1975 by the President and Fellows of Harvard College; all rights reserved.) See also Henry Mintzberg. *Mintzberg on management: Inside our strange world of organizations.* New York: The Free Press, 1989, p. 6.

all or parts of it to their contacts, including subordinates and superiors. For example, a manager may choose not to disseminate information critical of an employee or may inform subordinates of a potential organization change before rumors begin.

The informational role is readily observed in senior managers. They speak to outside groups, represent their organization to others, and testify before legislative and regulatory bodies. In addition, to some degree all managers seek to inform influential internal or external persons who can affect their organizational unit. At times, according to Mintzberg, this involves presenting the best side of the situation or withholding disadvantageous information.[24]

Decisional Roles The four decisional roles of a manager are entrepreneur, disturbance handler, resource allocator, and negotiator. Mintzberg uses the term "entrepreneur," but "change agent" is more descriptive of the role. HSOs are internally dynamic and continuously affected by their environment. Managers must seek to improve, modify, and rearrange work through planned, conscious, and controlled change. Managers must decide how services should be provided in the future, and must incorporate the impact of work change on people and of people on work design into such decisions.

Mintzberg states that

> no organization can be so well run, so standardized that it has considered every contingency in the uncertain environment in advance. Disturbances arise not only because poor managers ignore situations until they reach crisis proportions, but also because good managers cannot possibly anticipate all the consequences of the actions they take.[25]

When disturbances arise, managers are decision makers with regard to services, structure, work processes, external forces, and interpersonal conflict, for example. At the senior management level, pressures from professional staff, subordinates, the external public, patients/customers, competitors, regulators, legislators, and accreditors can cause a loss of equilibrium. In response, the manager makes accommodation or change decisions. At the operational level, a snowstorm or a 10% budget reduction affects work, causes disruption, and requires that the manager make decisions.

Resource allocator is another role of managers—they decide who gets what. Senior managers allocate people, equipment, and supplies. In turn, middle-level managers allocate resources among their units. First-line managers allocate (assign) people, material, and equipment to specific jobs. According to decision theory, implicit in resource allocation is the fact that once allocations are made, there are fewer resources for other needs. Consequently, priorities are a critical ingredient in decision making, and negotiating for resources is an essential managerial activity—and a vital skill.

The negotiator role involves interacting with superiors, persons in other departments, and subordinates. Negotiation affects resource allocation, resolution of disturbances, implementation of change, and interpersonal behavior. For example, resolving conflict among subordinates or organizational units includes deciding which points to negotiate.

Role Characteristics   The interpersonal, informational, and decisional roles suggest the variety of managerial activities. Some are easily grouped within planning, organizing, staffing, directing, controlling, and decision making: resource allocation in decision making, internal liaison in organizing, and leading and disseminating information in directing. However, activities such as figurehead and spokesperson do not fit this classification scheme, nor do all managers perform them.

The combination of roles managers adopt is partly predicated on the manager's level and the attributes of the organization.[26] For example, senior managers often engage in figurehead and spokesperson activities, whereas middle-level or first-line managers may not. Intensity, or the degree to which one role and its elements become more important than another, is affected by the same variables. First-level managers may spend a great deal of time on resource allocation, such as job assignments, and little time on negotiation. Finally, roles are not mutually exclusive; they flow together and are linked. For example, a manager without liaison contacts lacks information, and this affects the decision-making role.

ORGANIZATIONAL CULTURE AND PHILOSOPHY

The process of management occurs in a formal setting known as an organization. All organizations have distinct and identifiable cultures,[27] and HSOs are no exception.[28] In fact, HSOs have a culture that is very different from the typical business enterprise because they provide a service unique in society and because they are humanitarian in nature. HSO managers manage in the special context of the HSO's culture.

An HSO's culture is its ingrained pattern of shared beliefs, values, behaviors, and assumptions, with associated symbols and rituals, that are acquired over time by members.[29] It is the historically developed sense of the "institution's legacy"[30]—what it is and what it stands for—that permeates the entire organization and is known to all who work in it. Examples of shared beliefs are the commitment to patients and to meeting their needs and respecting them as individuals, with the unshakable belief that they are the primary reason for the HSO's existence. Important values are duty, respect, trust, integrity, honesty, equity, and fairness.[31] These values and beliefs shape organizational objectives and prescribe acceptable behavior for members—managers and employees—as well as acceptable relationships between the HSO and its external constituents. By adhering to these values and beliefs, HSOs retain their unique character and the privileges society has accorded them.[32]

An organization's philosophy is its explicit and implied view of itself and what it is. Generally expressed in mission statements,[33] the philosophy is directly linked to and rooted in the organization's cultural beliefs and values. The philosophy and culture of an organization should be compatible. Among other things, philosophy depicts the desired nature of the relationships between the HSO and its customers, employees, and external constituents.

Philosophy About Customers and Continuous Quality Improvement

Customer service must be the overriding commitment of HSOs, and it must be integral to the culture. To remain competitive—indeed, to survive—HSOs must meet the needs and expectations of all customers.[34] A philosophy that reflects this commitment to customer service and quality patient care is continuous quality improvement (CQI). Based on the tenets of Philip B. Crosby, W. Edwards Deming, Joseph M. Juran, and others, CQI focuses on improving processes in the organization. Because of improved processes, the quality of outcomes and level of patient satisfaction will rise.[35] In CQI the concept of customer is very broad and includes internal users of goods and services produced by the HSO, such as patients, physicians, and staff, as well as external stakeholders such as third-party payors.

The philosophy of CQI has been embraced by the Joint Commission on Accreditation of Healthcare Organizations in its "Agenda for Change,"[36] and this has important implications for HSO accreditation as well as resource allocation and utilization, and competitive position.[37] One major attribute of the CQI philosophy is that it is continuous.[38] Improvement of quality is ongoing and occurs throughout the HSO. Outcomes are important, but the primary focus is on process analysis and improvement. Methods include continuous evaluation of work processes and systems; design of and methods for work; analysis of structure, tasks/technology, and people relationships; training and skills enhancement of human resources; and how managers manage. A second attribute of CQI is that it is pervasive and requires a commitment to quality at all levels from senior management to workers.[39] To be effective, CQI must become part of the shared beliefs and values of all organization members. Management's role is to establish and perpetuate an environment in which the philosophy of quality is integral to the work of all employees.[40] The philosophy of CQI is the primary subject of Chapter 11, "Quality and Productivity Improvement," and the theme of CQI is continued in Chapter 12, "Control, Risk Management, Quality Assessment/Improvement, and Resource Allocation."

Philosophy About Employees—The Human Resource Perspective

Managing HSOs can only be done through people. An organization's philosophy about employees is rooted in its cultural beliefs and values and directly affects the HSO's ability to achieve objectives, meet customer expectations, and implement and sustain initiatives such as CQI. This philosophy includes concepts such as respect for employees as individuals,[41] whether they are viewed as the principal component in accomplishing organizational objectives, the extent of their involvement and participation in decision making about work and work systems design, and the way management oversees their work.[42] In Chapter 17, "Personnel/Human Resources Management," the philosophy termed the "human resource perspective" is presented in detail, and this theme continues in Chapter 18, "Labor Relations." This perspective includes the premise that employees are the HSO's most important resource, that employers and employees have reciprocal obligations to each other, that shared goals increase employee identification and involvement, and that there is a climate of mutual respect.[43] Labor relations is committed to making employees partners, not adversaries.

Philosophy About Stakeholders

Stakeholders are constituents with a vested interest in the affairs and actions of the HSO. They are individuals, groups, or organizations affected by the HSO and who may seek to influence it.[44] A well-thought-out and implemented philosophy about stakeholders is prerequisite to an HSO's strategic planning, resource allocation and utilization, customer service, and ability to cope with the external environment. Fottler and co-workers classify stakeholders into three groups. Internal stakeholders "operate entirely within the bounds of the organization and typically include management and professional and nonprofessional staff."[45] Interface stakeholders "function both internally and externally to the organization"[46] and include medical staff, the governing body, and stockholders in the case of for-profit HSOs. External stakeholders such as suppliers, patients, and third-party payors, including government, provide resources. The HSO needs them to survive. Other external stakeholders are competitors, special-interest groups, local communities, labor organizations, and regulatory and accrediting agencies.

HSOs must assess stakeholders to determine which are relevant, which are a potential threat, and which have the potential to cooperate.[47] Such assessment suggests appropriate HSO behavior toward them, ranging from ignoring to negotiating to co-opting and cooperating, and also suggests which of the conflicting priorities, needs, demands, and pressures they present should be addressed by the HSO.[48] Balancing the demands of multiple stakeholders with different interests is a major challenge.[49] Levey and Hill suggest that the need for HSO managers to balance demands can pose "moral dilemmas arising from responsibilities to patients, governing boards, [professional] staff, and community."[50] It is the CEO's responsibility to balance demands based on the HSO's cultural beliefs and values. Balancing maintains ethical values and social responsibility and prevents inappropriate demands made by single-interest stakeholders from predominating.[51]

A stakeholder philosophy is consistent with CQI. "For example, patients as consumers were passive stakeholders until this decade."[52] Now they are major stakeholders, as are third-party payors, who aggressively seek to influence HSOs. External stakeholders are a fact of life, and responding to their legitimate interests while minimizing the effects of inappropriate demands is a necessity. Stakeholder influence is treated extensively in Chapter 8, "Strategic Planning and Marketing."

Senior Management and Culture

Managers, especially those who are senior, are important in maintaining the HSO's culture. They "have a critical role as the conscience of the enterprise like it or not, for good or ill."[53] Attentiveness to symbols and rituals is important, and managers must nurture and reinforce the shared beliefs and values of organization members. When introducing change, managers must recognize how beliefs and values are affected and that it may be necessary to consciously change beliefs and values if they are incompatible with or pose barriers to meritorious change.[54] More importantly, the conduct of managers[55] conveys to employees and other stakeholders the HSO's beliefs, values, and philosophies about customer service and CQI, about employees, and about stakeholder relations. As Zuckerman observes,

> the CEO must lead the organization in adapting to the external environment and in managing the internal organization. The CEO also plays an overarching role, however, in providing strategic direction and vision to the organization, serving as the keeper of the corporate values, and assuring that the organization achieves its mission.[56]

A MANAGEMENT MODEL FOR HSOs

Earlier in this chapter, management was defined as the process, composed of interrelated social and technical functions and activities (including roles), occurring within a formal organizational setting for the purpose of accomplishing predetermined objectives through the utilization of human and other resources. It was suggested that all HSO managers engage in the management functions of planning, organizing, staffing, directing, controlling, and decision making. These interrelated functions describe how managers accomplish objectives through people and the utilization of other resources in a formal setting. Managerial roles, which are the various behaviors or activities associated with certain management positions, were described, as was the impact of culture and stakeholders on the HSO and how it is managed.

In this section, a management model for HSOs is presented and described. It has an input-conversion-output perspective that integrates systems theory. The model serves as the framework and structure for the remainder of the book.

Input-Conversion-Output Perspective

HSOs are settings in which *inputs* (resources) are *converted* to *outputs* (work results and objective accomplishment). Management is the catalyst. Figure 1.5 presents this input-conversion-output perspective and depicts the following relationships:

The HSO is the formal setting where outputs are produced (objectives accomplished) through utilization (conversion) of inputs (resources).

Managers are the catalyst that converts inputs to outputs through managing. Managers manage in the context of the organization's culture, which is composed of shared beliefs and values and derived philosophy. Internal and interface stakeholders influence the management process.

The HSO (and its managers) interact with, are affected by, and affect the HSO's external environment, which is composed of outside forces and influences, including stakeholders.

Inputs are obtained from the external environment and outputs go into it.

The HSO management model that is the structure and framework of this book is presented in Figure 1.6. It incorporates the input-conversion-output perspective presented in Figure 1.5, but is significantly more detailed. The discussion that follows references the major components of the model by the numbers in brackets.

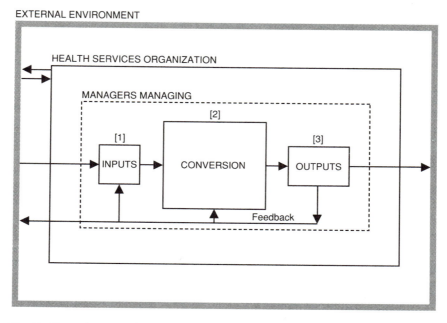

Figure 1.5. Health services organizational model.

Inputs (Resources)   The "inputs" component [1] in Figure 1.6 shows that resources are acquired and used to generate "outputs" [3]. Objectives are accomplished by the work of individuals and the organization. Inputs include human resources, material/supplies, technology/equipment, information, capital resources, and patients/customers.

Human resources in HSOs include managers, physicians, dentists, nurses, technologists, pharmacists, dietitians, social workers, and clerical and housekeeping personnel. Material inputs (resources) are supplies of all types, such as x-ray film, food, linen, drugs, and instruments. Technological resources include equipment, such as magnetic resonance imaging scanners, heart catheterization equipment, and fetal monitors, as well as knowledge of the HSO's staff.

Internal information sources include diverse areas such as patient data, reports, schedules, and budgets. External information includes government policy, legislation, stakeholder views, economic data and forecasts, and the HSO's more immediate environment—the health care system—which includes regulation, accreditation, competition, and third-party payers. Capital resources are physical plant and funds. Finally, patients are an input resource that may be viewed as the primary raw material that is converted; disease is prevented or care is provided to restore health or minimize disability.

These inputs are necessary for the HSO to function. Eliminating or restricting any of them may compromise the effectiveness of the whole organization. For example, a rapid rise in supply costs could affect an output such as the cost of care or provision of a service; or high interest rates may prevent capital expansion. Obsolete equipment may detract from providing better care, or a lack of human resources may mean some services are unavailable.

Outputs (Objectives)   The "output" component [3] of the model shows that individual and organizational work results [3a] are produced by conversion [2] of inputs. Output for HSOs is presented at two levels: specific individual and organizational work results [3a] at all levels, which, if appropriate and desirable [4], lead to achieving objectives [3b], which are why the organization exists. Objectives [3b] include patient care and customer services; quality of care and CQI; delivering care at appropriate costs; growth, but certainly survival and fiscal integrity; meeting responsibilities to stakeholders and society; participating in medical education, training, and research; and maintaining the HSO's reputation and image.

The governing body establishes or changes overall objectives. Middle-level and first-line managers set consistent subsidiary objectives. This results in multiple organizational objectives of greater and lesser importance that change over time. Quality of care is a primary component. Other objectives depend on the type of HSO. For example, the home health agency seeks primarily to provide quality patient care services at appropriate costs to its clients, and secondarily to grow in size. By comparison, a nongovernmental acute care hospital has the primary objective of providing a range of diagnostic and restorative services of different intensity to the community, and it also has the objective of training medical residents. A Department of Veterans Affairs hospital may have the primary objective of caring for veterans; a community health center provides care to an indigent population; a family planning center has the objective of providing counseling and referral services; and a public health department seeks to improve general health through preventive measures. In contrast, a university-based hospital may have several equally important objectives, such as providing patient care; providing specialized treatment, which requires different inputs, combinations of sophisticated equipment, and medical specialists; training health care personnel; and research.

Conversion (Integration)   Conversion of inputs to outputs occurs in a formal setting that conceptually includes the "conversion" component [2] of Figure 1.6. Elements of conversion are [2a] structure, tasks/technology, and people. Conversion occurs when managers [5] integrate structure, tasks/technology, and people [2b] in the context of the organizational culture [7] and in response to meeting the needs of internal, interface, and external stakeholders.

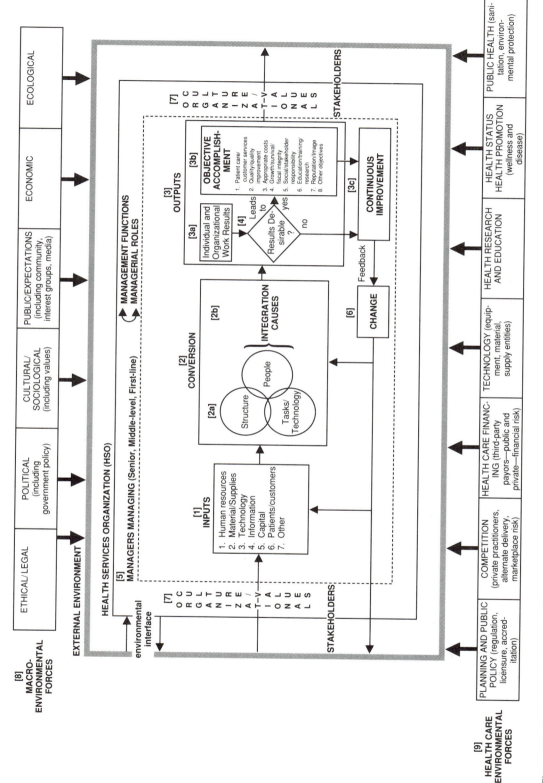

Figure 1.6. Management model for HSOs.

17

The "structure" element of setting [2a] in Figure 1.6 conceptualizes formally designed arrangements characteristic of the HSO, such as authority and responsibility and superior and subordinate relationships; grouping work activities; and coordination, communication, information, and control mechanisms. The "tasks/technology" element of setting [2a] represents work specialization: job design; work processes, methods, and procedures; and logistical, material, and work flows. It also represents technological characteristics of the setting, such as equipment, human and machine relationships, and to some degree information and knowledge used by managers and staff to perform their duties (tasks).

Work occurs only through people, and managers accomplish it by integrating [2b] structure, tasks/technology, *and* people. To do so managers must contend with shared beliefs and values of the organization's culture, with the dynamics of formal and informal organization, and with positive and negative individual behavior, including roles, perceptions, expectations, and values. These subjects are presented in Chapter 13, "Motivation," Chapter 14, "Leadership," Chapter 15, "Communication," and Chapter 16, "Organizational Change."

Linkage, Change, and Continuous Improvement

When performing interrelated management functions and activities, including managerial roles [5], managers determine the nature of the model's components and link and integrate them. Figure 1.6 shows this with the dashed boundary line that surrounds the components in the HSO: inputs [1], conversion [2], outputs [3], and change [6]. For example, when *planning,* managers determine the individual and organizational work that will lead to accomplishing the HSO's objectives. Once determined, human and other input resources [1] can be identified, acquired, and allocated.

When managers *organize,* they shape the setting where conversion occurs—the structure, tasks/technology, and people relationships. *Staffing* is the acquisition and retention of human resources. *Directing* is initiating work activity through people by motivating, leading, and communicating. To direct, managers integrate structure, tasks/technology, and people, often through activities characteristic of interpersonal, informational, and decision-making managerial roles, and cause individual and organizational work results to occur.

Finally, *controlling* means that managers monitor individual and organizational work results [3a] and compare them with standards and expectations to determine if objectives [3b] are being achieved. If results are inconsistent with standards and/or expectations [4], managers make changes [6] through a feedback loop. For example, if utilization review or medical care assessment determines that care is substandard, managers change the conversion setting (the structure, tasks/technology, and people components) and/or change input resources. Even if objectives are being met [3b], a philosophy of CQI requires that assessment of HSO activity be continuous [3c]. The implication of CQI is that HSOs can improve outcomes by evaluating, changing [6], and improving processes used in conversion [2] and/or the inputs used [1].

EXTERNAL ENVIRONMENT (A SYSTEMS PERSPECTIVE)

HSOs evolve constantly, as does their management. The model in Figure 1.6 shows a continuous, circular flow of inputs [1], conversion [2], outputs [3], improvement [3c], and change [6]. The model is not a closed sequence of events, however. HSOs are not isolated from their external environment. The gray boundary in Figure 1.6 denotes the environment external to the HSO. There are two components of the external environment: the macroenvironment [8] and the health care environment [9]. There are two implications inherent in the interfacing of HSOs with the external environment. First, HSOs are affected by the external environment—the inputs they use come from it. Second, HSOs also affect the external environment—the outputs they produce go into it. HSO managers seek to influence, modify, and change the external environment. This is denoted by the change loop arrow [6] in Figure 1.6 that extends to the environment. Advocacy and lobbying with external stakeholders are indeed responsibilities of senior management. Initiatives to influence, among other things, general economic conditions, health status, and public policy are legitimate. Zuckerman states that

> the linkage between environment and organization should be a two-way interaction. . . . In essence, the CEO has a role as an advocate for the organization, for the constituents that it represents, and for the population that it serves. CEOs should and do seek to influence the formulation and implementation of public policy.[57]

Systems theory allows relationships between an HSO and its environment to be conceptualized. A system is a set of interrelated and interdependent parts. A subsystem is part of a system; a suprasystem is a set of systems. The HSO may be viewed as a system composed of subsystems: structure, tasks/technology, people, and management subsystems; or patient care, ancillary services, professional staff, and financial, informational, physical, and administrative subsystems. As an entity, the HSO may also be viewed as a subsystem of the health care system [9], which is, in turn, part of a macrosocietal suprasystem [8].

Macroenvironment

Adopting a systems perspective implies that a suprasystem, its systems, and their subsystems are interrelated, are interdependent, and simultaneously affect one another at all levels. Using this perspective, the macroenvironment [8] would be a societal suprasystem (see Figure 1.6) composed of systems that include ethical/legal, political, cultural/sociological, public (i.e., external stakeholders such as the community at large, interest groups, and media), economic, ecological, and health care systems [9]. All affect one another; for example, the political and economic systems affect the health care system and each reaches down to multiple subsystems—one of which is the HSO.

Health Care Environment

More proximate to and having a more direct effect on the HSO (subsystem) is the health care environment (system). The forces and influences in the health care environment affecting the HSO, its managers, and how they manage are presented in Figure 1.6 [9]. Interface stakeholders such as professional staff are important and profoundly affect the HSO. Equally important are external stakeholders such as patients, third-party payors, and government, as well as special interest groups, local communities, and licensure, regulatory, and accrediting agencies. Other forces include competition by other HSOs, numbers and skills of practitioners, public and private financing of health care, and resource entities for technology, equipment, and materials. A final, more remote group of health care environmental forces that affect HSOs include: health research and education; health status, wellness, prevalence of disease, and health promotion and awareness; and the status of public health, general sanitation, and protection from hazardous substances and injurious working conditions.

Needless to say, managing HSOs is difficult, demanding, and frustrating. Conflict, resource constraints, demanding stakeholders, new rules, greater accountabilities, and an increasingly hostile environment confront HSO managers. As the year 2000 approaches the challenges will be great. Managerial excellence will make a difference.

FRAMEWORK AND STRUCTURE OF THE BOOK

The management model presented in Figure 1.6 is the basis for the framework and structure of this book. The following material presents an overview of the remaining parts of the book, in which various aspects of the model are examined in greater detail.

About Part II: The Health Services Environment

The four chapters in Part II detail the HSO environment and the forces that have an impact on it. Chapter 2, "The Health Care Delivery System," describes the system, types of organizations, the environment, expenditures and trends, and health services personnel. The universal and comprehensive health care system in Canada is presented; differences between it and the system in the United States are highlighted.

Chapter 3, "Ethical Considerations," provides a framework that managers can use to understand, analyze, and solve ethical problems. Specific administrative and biomedical ethical issues are included. An introduction to the law and the legal aspects of managing HSOs is provided in Chapter 4, "Legal Considerations." Especially useful is material on how managers can effectively interact with the legal system and legal counsel. Chapter 5, "Health Services Technology," provides an understanding of health care technology, including its effects, assessment, and how it is managed.

About Part III: Structuring Health Services Organizations

The two chapters in Part III cover organization design and theory and HSO structure. Chapter 6, "Concepts of Organization Design," presents general organization theory and concepts, including classical principles and contemporary concepts as related to organizations, and the dynamics of informal organization. Chapter 7, "How HSOs Are Organized," details the backgrounds, structures, and functions of various HSOs including acute care hospitals, nursing facilities, ambulatory health services, hospice, managed care, birth centers, and home health agencies.

About Part IV: Strategic Planning and Interorganizational Linkages for Health Services Organizations

Part IV contains two chapters. Chapter 8, "Strategic Planning and Marketing," examines planning from an output-input perspective. There is emphasis on strategic planning, which is composed of objective and strategy formulation. The chapter highlights a strategic planning model with special attention to marketing and stakeholder assessment. Chapter 9, "Interorganizational Relationships," details new HSO organizational forms and relationships. Included are corporate reorganization, diversification, joint ventures, and multiorganizational systems.

About Part V: Problem Solving, Quality Improvement, and Control in Health Services Organizations

In Chapter 10, "Managerial Problem Solving and Decision Making," the decision-making function is examined, particularly as it relates to problem solving. Factors that influence problem solving and decision making are presented in the context of a problem-solving model. The relationship between problem solving and CQI is explored. The principal themes of Chapter 11, "Quality and Productivity Improvement," are CQI and productivity improvement. The need for both is addressed. The philosophy of CQI is developed. Two models of CQI and the principles of quality experts W. Edwards Deming, Joseph M. Juran, and Philip B. Crosby are presented. CQI and its relationship to process improvement as well as methods to improve productivity through better work methods, flows, job design, facilities layout, and scheduling are discussed.

Chapter 12, "Control, Risk Management, Quality Assessment/Improvement, and Resource Allocation," completes Part V and focuses on controlling individual and organizational work results (outputs) through techniques such as management information systems, management and operations auditing, and budgeting. Control of medical care quality through risk management and quality assessment and improvement is discussed. The chapter concludes with applications of quantitative techniques useful in resource allocation, such as volume analysis, capital budgeting, cost-benefit analysis, and simulation.

About Part VI: Managing People in Health Services Organizations

The four chapters in Part VI are the "people" element of the conversion process in Figure 1.6. As managers manage, they achieve work results through people. The directing function (motivate, lead, and communicate) integrates structure, tasks/technology, and people.

Chapter 13, "Motivation," presents the concept of motivation, models and defines it, and reviews the literature on content and process theories of motivation. The final section in this chapter integrates the theories of motivation. Chapter 14, "Leadership," differentiates transactional and transformational leadership and models and defines leadership. The extensive literature on leader behavior and situational theories of leadership is reviewed. The final section integrates the theories of leadership.

Chapter 15, "Communication," examines the third activity traditionally included in the directing function—communication. Interpersonal and organizational communication channels, models, and barriers are described, as well as stakeholder communications. Finally, Chapter 16, "Organizational Change," examines the pressures for change, typologies and the process of organizational change, and the role of managers as change agents. HSOs are dynamic, and managing change and understanding its impact on human resources are critical to the conversion process.

About Part VII: Human Resource Management in Health Services Organizations

The two chapters in Part VII describe the essence of the staffing function. Chapter 17, "Personnel/ Human Resources Management," focuses on human resource acquisition and retention, including recruitment, selection, training and development, and compensation and benefits administration, along with legislation relevant to each. Chapter 18, "Labor Relations," is devoted solely to labor relations and collective bargaining. The history of unionization and legislation pertinent to HSOs is presented.

SUMMARY

This chapter on the management process and managerial roles establishes the book's foundation. HSO managers are defined as persons appointed to positions of authority who enable others to do their work effectively, who have responsibility for resource utilization, and who are accountable for work results. A classification scheme for senior, middle-level, and first-line managers and skills characteristic of each are presented.

The focus is a process orientation, and the chapter provides an overview of generic functions and activities characteristic of managers, regardless of the type of HSO. Management is defined as the process, composed of interrelated social and technical functions and activities (including roles), occurring within a formal organizational setting for the purpose of accomplishing predetermined objectives through the utilization of human and other resources. The primary management functions presented are planning, organizing, staffing, directing, controlling, and decision making. Senior HSO managerial activities are described within this functional classification, as are the interpersonal, informational, and decisional managerial roles. Organizational culture, with derivative philosophies about customers, employees, and stakeholders, provides a context for managing.

The management model for HSOs has an input-conversion-output perspective (Figure 1.6). It provides the book's conceptual framework. The input and output components of the model are described. Extensive discussion of the conversion component demonstrates that, when managers manage, they integrate the HSO's structure–tasks/technology–people elements to achieve individual and organizational work results.

Integrating general systems theory with the management model emphasizes the importance of the external environment for HSOs. Primarily, this environment consists of the health care system and the macroenvironmental suprasystem, and these affect managers as well as organizations and how they are managed. Increasingly important is the effect HSOs have on these environments.

DISCUSSION QUESTIONS

1. What is the distinction between *health care* and *health services delivery?* Discuss.
2. Define the term "manager." Discuss.
3. Define "management" and include the basic ingredients of the definition. Why is management a process?
4. How are managers at various levels in HSOs classified and differentiated?
5. Figure 1.4 shows various managerial roles. Relate these roles to the management function classification. What managerial roles are not presented in Figure 1.4? Discuss.
6. What relationship do managers have to the input-conversion-output perspective of HSOs?
7. Carefully examine Figure 1.6. Describe and discuss: 1) its components and how they flow and link, and 2) the way in which management functions and managerial roles interrelate with the components.
8. Figure 1.6 shows that outputs are composed of individual and organizational work results that accomplish objectives. How do individual and organizational work results fulfill objectives? Choose an HSO with which you are familiar and identify its objectives.
9. Figure 1.6 shows two external environments and the forces that affect HSOs. How do these forces affect HSOs? Are there others?
10. Identify an HSO. Group internal, interface, and external stakeholders. For stakeholders in each group indicate if the stakeholder is: 1) important; 2) influential; 3) a positive influence or threat; and 4) whether the HSO must cooperate with or co-opt, or ignore the stakeholder.
11. Identify and list beliefs and values as well as symbols and rituals characteristic of the culture of a college or university (or an HSO).

CASE STUDY 1:   THE CEO's DAY

Terry Blaze, the 45-year-old president and CEO of Midvale Community Hospital, rose early on Monday morning. A busy schedule of meetings and several major issues that would require full attention and careful decisions lay ahead. While getting dressed, Blaze thought about what to say to two county commissioners at a breakfast meeting in a local restaurant at 6:30 A.M. The county coroner had called Blaze the previous Wednesday asking if Midvale Community Hospital would permit the coroner's office to use some of the hospital's facilities. As a 500-bed teaching hospital with 1,600 employees and a medical staff of 150 physicians, Midvale was the largest of the four hospitals located in the metropolitan area, which has a population of about 350,000. Recent budget reductions to the coroner's office by the county commissioners had prompted the inquiry; consequently, the coroner was searching for ways to run his office on a reduced budget by drawing on the goodwill and resources of other community organizations.

Blaze had scheduled the meeting with the commissioners to see if they were aware of the coroner's request. Blaze was relatively open-minded about the situation, wanted to maintain the existing good relations between the commissioners and the hospital, and wanted to respond to the needs of the community provided that the hospital's basic objectives were not jeopardized or its resources inappropriately used. However, getting caught in the middle of the county's political problems could be disastrous.

At 7:30 A.M. Blaze attended a campaign fund-raiser breakfast for the state senator who represented the district in which Midvale was located. Blaze spoke to the senator about how the state's recently announced Medicaid payment reductions would affect Midvale and asked that the senator use his influence to try to have funding restored. After circulating among the other guests,

Blaze went to the hospital. As soon as Blaze arrived at the office at 8:15 A.M., the executive secretary, Billie, mentioned that Dr. Smith, president of the professional staff organization (PSO), composed of physicians, dentists, podiatrists, and clinical psychologists having privileges at Midvale, insisted on speaking privately with Blaze about a problem involving a staff physician before the scheduled 9:00 A.M. meeting of the PSO executive committee. Blaze immediately called Dr. Smith, and at the end of the conversation wondered whether it had been a correct decision to tell Dr. Smith to handle the problem as he thought appropriate. Relations between administration and the PSO are always delicate, but this time it seemed best to let Dr. Smith handle the situation and keep Blaze informed.

At 8:30 A.M., the vice president for operations arrived and accompanied Blaze to the hospital's conference room. All department heads were present. Because of a recent decision by Blaze and the board to establish a satellite facility in an adjacent county, most departments would be expanded, work loads would be increased, and coordination mechanisms between the hospital and satellite facility would have to be developed. Blaze explained the reasons for the decision, described the planning that had occurred before the decision was made, indicated how Midvale would work with the state planning agency in obtaining a certificate of need, and described how it would affect Midvale and its patients, as well as other area hospitals. Blaze asked the department heads to inform their subordinates before the official announcement was made to the press on Wednesday. A question-and-answer session followed.

Behind schedule, Blaze arrived at the 9:00 A.M. PSO executive committee meeting 10 minutes late and found that it had been postponed until the next day. Since the next meeting on the day's schedule was not until 10:00 A.M., Blaze returned to the office and asked Billie to hold all calls. Blaze had given considerable thought over several months to the board's directive that options be evaluated for expanding the scope of the hospital's services, particularly in light of the government's attitude favoring competition among health services organizations and especially the actions of other area hospitals and the area's newly formed HMO. Mindful of the hospital's limited resources, rising costs, changing patient mix, and the changes in Medicare and Medicaid reimbursement, Blaze was concerned about accomplishing the hospital's objectives during the next 5 years in this changing environment. Of particular concern was the restlessness of some members of the PSO, who wanted the addition of new services and an on-site medical office building.

Blaze recalled the discussions that had occurred at past board and management executive staff meetings. After weighing the options, Blaze realized that the hospital would need three feasibility studies to be performed by external hospital consultants. Blaze dictated a memo to the vice president for operations and the assistant vice president for planning, instructing them to begin studies for the addition of an open heart surgery unit and a construction program to add 34 psychiatric beds and a physicians' office building adjacent to the hospital. Blaze did not approve a study for a regional burn unit because this service, although desirable, would contribute less to the hospital's objectives than the others, and limited resources meant some projects could not be undertaken.

At 10:00 A.M. Blaze met with the chair of psychiatry. Blaze informed him of the feasibility study, but the meeting continued negotiations about making the position of psychiatry department chair salaried. This would be the first such salaried PSO position and would set a precedent with long-term implications.

At 10:30 A.M. Blaze interviewed a finalist for the position of director of marketing. At 11:00 A.M. Dr. Loren, who had requested clinical privileges, arrived for a meeting. It was a long-standing policy for the president of the PSO and the CEO to interview all those seeking privileges.

At 11:30 A.M., Blaze returned phone calls that required immediate attention. The first was to a board member whose daughter was being admitted for minor surgery. The second was to a former patient with a complaint about his bill. Billie told Blaze that the former patient had already spoken to patient accounts, but he was still dissatisfied. Blaze spoke briefly with him and gave assurances that the matter would be rectified. The last phone call was to the director of human resources. They decided that the human resources director should accept the mayor's invitation to serve on the health department's personnel evaluation task force. This would require approximately 8 hours per week for 6 months, but they agreed it would help the hospital and community.

As was customary, Blaze had lunch in the hospital cafeteria and circulated among the employees before and after eating. It was a simple yet effective way to stay in touch with the staff.

Two major meetings were scheduled in the afternoon. From 1:00 to 3:00 P.M. the budget committee reviewed next year's operations and capital expenditures budgets. The executive staff and comptroller had prepared options for review. Among those Blaze approved for presentation to the board was an increase in the number of nursing service employees, a reduction in the equipment budget, and the annual pay increase for nonprofessional personnel that had been discussed previously. Blaze had positive relations with the board and told the executive administrative staff that the recommendations would likely be approved. However, a source of displeasure was last month's adverse overtime budget variance and the cost overrun on supplies. Both were unacceptable because census and patient days were below expectations. Blaze firmly told the senior managers to monitor their areas closely and report variations weekly.

The second meeting that afternoon was with the board task force on diversification. Near the end of the meeting Blaze told them about ordering the physicians' office building feasibility study and told them they should be thinking about incorporating a for-profit subsidiary to own and manage the office building. The major consideration was how reimbursement would be affected by allocating overhead to either the not-for-profit hospital or the for-profit subsidiary. The board task force asked Blaze to include these revenue–cost implications in the feasibility study.

On returning to the office at 4:00 P.M., Blaze approved the agenda for Friday's weekly senior management staff meeting, gave Billie several items for the agenda of the next board meeting, and returned phone calls. At 5:00 P.M. Blaze left the hospital to attend a 5:30 P.M. area hospital executive's council quarterly meeting. The meeting featured a presentation by the new dean of the medical school located in Midvale about how her plans would affect teaching hospitals and their medical education and residency programs. During the half-hour drive to and from the medical school, Blaze dictated several letters and memos and took a call on the car phone. Blaze went to a restaurant at 7:00 P.M. for dinner and left at 8:00 P.M. to attend a United Way trustees board meeting. At 10:00 P.M. Blaze returned home and did paperwork for an hour before retiring.

Questions

1. Terry Blaze engaged in activities related to the functions of management and roles of managers. Identify which of Blaze's activities relate to the management functions and managerial roles presented in the chapter.
2. Use the environmental portion of the management model in Figure 1.6 to: 1) identify internal, interface, and external stakeholders with whom Blaze interacted; and 2) identify other environmental forces that affected Blaze as well as Blaze's actions that affected the environment.
3. Identify other HSOs and discuss how the same activities of a CEO apply to them.

CASE STUDY 2:   AMERICAN HOSPITAL ASSOCIATION
ROLE AND FUNCTIONS OF EXECUTIVE MANAGEMENT[58]

The American Hospital Association (AHA), in its statement on the "Role and Functions of Hospital Executive Management," identified the following as responsibilities of senior management:

1. *Executive management should initiate and monitor organizational mechanisms to ensure that the hospital has effective organizational structures and processes.* Executive manage-

ment should develop and recommend to the governing board an effective organizational plan that takes into consideration the interdependent leadership roles of executive management, the governing board, and the medical staff, and that clearly assigns responsibilities for specific organizational programs and services to specific components and individuals. The organizational plan should clearly define relationships between the board's broad policy responsibility, the medical staff's shared responsibility for quality of care, and executive management's responsibility for overall operations.

2. *Executive management is expected to infuse the mission and philosophy of the institution into the entire organization.* This function requires an understanding by executive management of the relationships between the philosophy of the hospital as a center for community health and the goal of improving the health status of the community. It also requires a system for communicating the hospital's philosophy to the community. . . .

3. *Executive management should assume primary responsibility for ensuring that members of the hospital organization are kept informed about public policy and environmental issues and their effects on the hospital.* Executive management is responsible for establishing mechanisms for identifying and obtaining information about public policy issues and decisions affecting the hospital and, when necessary, for developing an appropriate organizational response. Executive management should take the initiative to work with other community organizations on public policy issues and decisions affecting the health status of the community.

4. *Executive management should take the initiative in ensuring that the hospital has a broadly based strategic planning program.* Strategic planning provides the hospital with a powerful management tool to help determine its goals and objectives in relationship to changes in the environment and the needs of its community, to establish its priorities, to choose the most appropriate organizational structure to achieve its goals and objectives, and to provide benchmarks for evaluating the achievements of its goals and objectives.

5. *Executive management should assume responsibility for the cost-effective management of the hospital's resources.* This responsibility requires a commitment to provide the most economical and highest quality services possible in keeping with available resources and to communicate this commitment to the entire organization and the community. This commitment implies a willingness to assume leadership, along with the governing board and the medical staff, in introducing new patient care technologies and programs that are of high quality, are medically necessary and appropriate, and are efficiently, yet compassionately, provided. It implies a responsibility to engage the medical staff in a cooperative effort to eliminate obsolete technologies and programs, and a willingness to introduce new management techniques and practices to improve the utilization of human and financial resources. It also implies a willingness to experiment with and make the community aware of alternatives to traditional means of health care delivery and financing, such as health maintenance organizations, independent practice associations, consumer choice health plans, and others. Finally, it implies the existence of an effective system for financial and management reporting that enhances the monitoring and evaluation of organizational performance.

6. *Executive management should provide a work atmosphere that recognizes the vital importance of human resources to the health care organization.* The provision of a positive work atmosphere implies a moral and ethical commitment to the needs of people, a concern for their health and status and quality of life, and a commitment to fostering respect and satisfaction for all.

Questions

1. For each statement (1, 2, 3, 4, 5, and 6), identify the explicit or implicit managerial functions involved.

2. For each statement (1, 2, 3, 4, 5, and 6), identify the explicit or implicit senior managerial roles involved.

CASE STUDY 3: A MANAGEMENT FUNCTION QUESTIONNAIRE

For each of the following items, circle the response that most accurately depicts the HSO for which you currently work or one where you previously worked. Support your rating with examples. If you have no experience in an HSO, use any organization as a frame of reference.

		High			Low
1.	*Culture:* how well the values and beliefs are communicated and understood by organization members.	1	2	3	4
2.	*Objectives:* how well organizational objectives are articulated by senior management and understood by members.	1	2	3	4
3.	*Planning:* how well management anticipates the future and plans for future activities.	1	2	3	4
4.	*Organizing:* whether organizational arrangements are rational and the extent of coordination and cooperation among units.	1	2	3	4
5.	*Staffing:* whether there are adequate personnel with appropriate skills.	1	2	3	4
6.	*Directing:* whether managers give guidance and clear instructions to employees.	1	2	3	4
7.	*Motivating:* whether managers positively influence subordinates and facilitate effective behavior.	1	2	3	4
8.	*Communicating:* whether the content and flow of communication keeps employees informed.	1	2	3	4
9.	*Controlling:* whether control methods and systems are in place and operating properly.	1	2	3	4
10.	*Decision making:* whether major decisions by senior management are reasonable and well thought out.	1	2	3	4

NOTES

1. U.S. Department of Health and Human Services. *Healthy people 2000,* 1. Publ. no. (PHS) 91-50213. Washington, D.C.: U.S. Government Printing Office, 1990.
2. Stevens, Rosemary. The hospital as a social institution, new-fashioned for the 1990s. *Hospital & Health Services Administration* 36 (Summer 1991): 165; Wesbury, Stuart A. Meeting the challenge: The health care executive's role. *Hospital & Health Services Administration* 33 (Fall 1988): 276–278.
3. U.S. Department of Health and Human Services, *Healthy people,* 1.
4. Levey, Samuel, and James Hill. National health insurance—the triumph of equivocation. *New England Journal of Medicine* 321 (December 21, 1989): 1751.
5. Longest, Beaufort B., Jr. American health policy in the year 2000. *Hospital & Health Services Administration* 33 (Winter 1988): 420.
6. Joint Commission on Accreditation of Healthcare Organizations. *The Joint Commission's agenda for change: Stimulating continual improvement in the quality of care,* 1. Oakbrook Terrace, IL, 1990.
7. McLaughlin, Curtis P., and Arnold D. Kaluzny. Total quality management in health: Making it work. *Health Care Management Review* 15 (Summer 1990): 7.
8. Meyers, Eugene D. Managed care and vertical integration: Implications for the hospital industry. *Hospital & Health Services Administration* 32 (August 1987): 320.
9. In his study of HSO managers, Kovner used the term "episodes of work"; see Kovner, Anthony R. The work of effective CEOs in four large health organizations. *Hospital & Health Services Administration* 32 (August 1987): 286–287; *and* Kovner, Anthony R. *Reality managing: The work of effective CEOs in large health organizations,* 143–144. Ann Arbor, MI: Health Administration Press, 1988.
10. Aldag, Ramon J., and Timothy M. Stearns. *Management,* 15–16. Cincinnati, OH: South-Western Publishing Co., 1991; Van Fleet, David, D. *Contemporary management,* 2d ed., 11. Boston: Houghton Mifflin Company, 1991.
11. Bateman, Thomas S., and Carl P. Zeithaml. *Management Function and Strategy,* 25. Homewood, IL: Irwin, 1990.
12. Johnson, Everett A., and Richard L. Johnson. *Hospitals in transition,* 75. Rockville, MD: Aspen Systems Corporation, 1982.
13. Hodgetts, Richard M., and Dorothy M. Cascio. *Modern health care administration,* 38. New York: Academic Press, 1983.
14. Bateman and Zeithaml, *Management function,* 22–23.

15. Higgins, James M. *The management challenge,* 6–7. New York: Macmillan Publishing Company, 1991; Liebler, Joan Gratto, Ruth Ellen Levine, and Hyman Leo Dervitz. *Management principles for health professionals,* 1. Rockville, MD: Aspen Publishers, Inc., 1984; McConnell, Charles R. *The effective health care supervisor,* 17. Rockville, MD: Aspen Systems Corporation, 1982.

16. Charns, Martin P., and Marguerite J. Schaefer. *Health care organizations: A model for management,* 11–12. Englewood Cliffs, NJ: Prentice Hall, Inc., 1983; Hodgetts and Cascio, *Modern health care,* 26; Ivancevich, John M., James H. Donnelly, Jr., and James L. Gibson. *Management principles and function,* 4th ed., 5. Homewood, IL: Irwin, 1989; Longest, Beaufort B., Jr. *Management practices for the health professional,* 4th ed., 35. Norwalk, CT: Appleton and Lange, 1990; Pearce, John A., II, and Richard B. Robinson, Jr. *Management,* 4. New York: Random House, 1989; Van Fleet, *Contemporary management,* 8.

17. A classical article defining management and management theories is Koontz, Harold. The management theory jungle. *Academy of Management Journal* 4 (December 1961): 174–188.

18. Commission on Education for Health Administration. *Education for health administration,* 15. Ann Arbor: Health Administration Press, 1975; see also Austin, Charles J. What is health administration? *Hospital Administration* 19 (Summer 1974): 27; and Munson, Fred C., and Howard S. Zuckerman. The managerial role. In *Health care management: A text in organization theory and behavior,* 2d ed., edited by Stephen M. Shortell and Arnold D. Kaluzny, 44–45. New York: John Wiley & Sons, 1988.

19. Kuhl, Ingrid K. *The executive role in health services delivery organizations,* 4–13. Washington, D.C.: Association of University Programs in Health Administration, 1977.

20. Kuhl, *Executive role,* 13.

21. Other studies of HSO CEO activities are reported in American College of Hospital Administrators. *The evolving role of the hospital chief executive officer,* 13–14, chpt. 3. Chicago: The Foundation of the American College of Hospital Administrators (now the American College of Healthcare Executives), 1984; activities of CEOs in multi-institutional systems in Kleiner, Stanley G. 1984. The role of hospital administrators in multihospital systems. *Hospital & Health Services Administration* 29 (March 1984): 33–41; and activities of physician-managers in Kindig, David A., and Santiago Lastiri-Quiros. The changing managerial role of physician executives. *The Journal of Health Administration Education* 7 (Winter 1989): 38–39.

22. Mintzberg, Henry. The manager's job: Folklore and fact. *Harvard Business Review* 53 (July–August 1975): 54–59. Mintzberg, Henry. *Mintzberg on management: Inside our strange world of organizations,* 16. New York: The Free Press, 1989. Munson and Zuckerman provided an excellent review of the managerial role literature, including other role classifications (Munson and Zuckerman, Managerial role, 38–76). For applications of roles for physician-executives, see Alpander, Guven G., and Robert A. Strong. A perceptual study of the role of the president of the medical staff. *Hospital & Health Services Administration* 36 (Summer 1991): 273–275; Ruelas, Enrique, and Peggy Leatt. The roles of physician executives: A framework for management education.

The Journal of Health Administration Education 2 (Part 1) (Spring 1984): 154–155; *and* Schneller, Eugene S. The leadership and executive potential of physicians in an era of managed care systems. *Hospital & Health Services Administration* 36 (Spring 1991): 48–50.

23. Mintzberg, *Mintzberg on management,* 17.

24. Mintzberg, *Mintzberg on management,* 19

25. Mintzberg, *Mintzberg on management,* 20.

26. Munson and Zuckerman, The managerial role, 72.

27. Deal, Terrence E., Allan K. Kennedy, and Arthur H. Spiegel, III. How to create an outstanding hospital culture. *Hospital Forum* 26 (January/February 1983): 22.

28. Darr, Kurt. Importance and relevance of the organizational philosophy. *Hospital Topics* 65 (July/August 1987): 9.

29. Conner, Daryl. Corporate culture: Healthcare's change master. *Healthcare Executive* 5 (March/April 1990): 28.

30. Deal, Terrence E. Healthcare executives as symbolic leaders. *Healthcare Executive* 5 (March/April 1990): 25.

31. Brozovich, John P., and Stephen M. Shortell. How to create more humane and productive health care environments. *Health Care Management Review* 9 (Fall 1984): 47.

32. Friedman, Emily. Ethics and corporate culture: Finding a fit. *Healthcare Executive* 5 (March/April 1990): 18.

33. Gibson, C. Kendrick, David J. Newton, and Daniel S. Cochran. 1990. An empirical investigation of hospital mission statements. *Health Care Management Review* 15 (Summer 1990): 35–36.

34. Albert, Michael. Developing a service-oriented health care culture. *Hospital & Health Services Administration* 34 (Summer 1989): 167.

35. Crosby, Philip B. *Quality is free: The art of making quality certain.* New York: McGraw-Hill Book Company, 1979; Crosby, Philip B. *Quality without tears: The art of hassle-free management.* New York: McGraw-Hill Book Company, 1984; Darr, Kurt. Applying the Deming method in hospitals: Part 1. *Hospital Topics* 67 (November/December 1989): 4–5; Darr, Kurt. Applying the Deming method in hospitals: Part 2. *Hospital Topics* 68 (Winter 1990): 4–6; Deming, W. Edwards. *Out of the crisis.* Boston: Massachusetts Institute of Technology, 1986; James, Brent C. *Quality management for health care delivery.* Chicago: The Hospital Research and Educational Trust, 1989; Juran, Joseph M. *Managerial breakthrough: A new concept of the manager's job.* New York: McGraw-Hill Book Company, 1964; Juran, Joseph M. *Juran on planning for quality.* New York: The Free Press, 1988; Lowe, Ted A., and Joseph M. Mazzeo. Crosby, Deming, Juran: Three preachers, one religion. *Quality* 25 (September 25, 1986): 22–25; Neuhauser, Duncan. The quality of medical care and the 14 points of Edwards Deming. *Health Matrix* 6 (Summer 1988): 7–10; Walton, Mary. *The Deming management method.* New York: Perigee Books, 1986.

36. O'Leary, Dennis S. CQI—a step beyond QA. *Joint Commission Perspectives* 10 (March/April 1990): 2.

37. Labovitz, George H. Beyond the total quality management mystique. *Healthcare Executive* 6 (April 1991): 15.

38. Lynn, Monty, and David P. Osborn. Deming's quality principles: A health care application. *Hospital & Health Services Administration* 36 (Spring 1991): 114–117.

39. Casalou, Robert F. Total quality management in health care. *Hospital & Health Services Administration* 36 (Spring 1991): 135.

40. Darr, Applying the Deming method, Part 1, 4.

41. Bettinger, Cass. Use of corporate culture to trigger high

performance. *The Journal of Business Strategy* 10 (March/April 1989): 40.

42. Metzger, Norman. The changing health care workplace: A challenge for management development. *Journal of Management Development* (Special Issue on Health Care) 10 (1991): 55.

43. Robbins, Stephen A., and Jonathon S. Rakich. Hospital personnel management in the late 1980s: A direction for the future. *Hospital & Health Services Administration* 31 (July/August 1986): 19–20.

44. Fottler, Myron D., John D. Blair, Carlton J. Whitehead, Michael D. Laus, and Grant T. Savage. Assessing key stakeholders: Who matters to hospitals and why? *Hospital & Health Services Administration* 34 (Winter 1989): 526.

45. Fottler, Blair, Whitehead, Laus, and Savage, Assessing key stakeholders, 527.

46. Fottler, Blair, Whitehead, Laus, and Savage, Assessing key stakeholders, 527.

47. Blair, John D., Grant T. Savage, and Carlton J. Whitehead. A strategic approach to negotiating with hospital stakeholders. *Health Care Management Review* 14 (Winter 1989): 15.

48. Blair, John D., and Carlton J. Whitehead. Too many on the seesaw: Stakeholder diagnosis and management for hospitals. *Hospital & Health Services Administration* 33 (Summer 1988): 154.

49. Zuckerman, Howard S. Redefining the role of the CEO: Challenges and conflicts. *Hospital & Health Services Administration* 34 (Spring 1989): 37.

50. Levey, Samuel, and James Hill. Between survival and social responsibility: In search of an ethical balance. *The Journal of Health Administration Education* 4 (Spring 1986): 227.

51. Levey and Hill, Between survival, 226.

52. Blair and Whitehead, Too many, 154.

53. Stevens, Hospital as a social, 172.

54. Pointer, Dennis D. Responding to the challenges of the new healthcare marketplace. *Hospital & Health Services Administration* 30 (November/December 1985): 16.

55. Deal, Healthcare executives, 26.

56. Zuckerman, Redefining the role, 35–36.

57. Zuckerman, Redefining the role, 27.

58. Excerpted from American Hospital Association, Institutional Practices Committee. *Role and functions of hospital executive management: Management advisory*, 1–4. Chicago: American Hospital Association, 1990. Reprinted with permission of the American Hospital Association, copyright 1990.

BIBLIOGRAPHY

Albert, Michael. Developing a service-oriented health care culture. *Hospital & Health Services Administration* 34 (Summer 1989): 167–183.

Aldag, Ramon J., and Timothy M. Stearns. *Management.* Cincinnati, OH: South-Western Publishing Co., 1991.

American College of Hospital Administrators. *The evolving role of the hospital chief executive officer.* Chicago: The Foundation of the American College of Hospital Administrators (now the American College of Healthcare Executives), 1984.

Austin, Charles J. What is health administration? *Hospital Administration* 19 (Summer 1974): 14–29.

Blair, John D., and Carlton J. Whitehead. Too many on the seesaw: Stakeholder diagnosis and management for hospitals. *Hospital & Health Service Administration* 33 (Summer 1988): 153–166.

Brozovich, John P., and Stephen M. Shortell. How to create more humane and productive health care environments. *Health Care Management Review* 9 (Fall 1984): 43–53.

Casalou, Robert F. Total quality management in health care *Hospital & Health Services Administration* 36 (Spring 1991): 134–146.

Crosby, Philip B. *Quality is free: The art of making quality certain.* New York: McGraw-Hill Book Company, 1979.

Crosby, Philip B. *Quality without tears: The art of hassle-free management.* New York: McGraw-Hill Book Company, 1984.

Darr, Kurt. Importance and relevance of the organizational philosophy. *Hospital Topics* 65 (July/August 1987): 9

Darr, Kurt, Content of an organizational philosophy. *Hospital Topics* 65 (November/December 1987): 8–9.

Darr, Kurt. Applying the Deming method in hospitals. Part 1. *Hospital Topics* 67 (November/December 1989): 4–5.

Darr, Kurt. Applying the Deming method in hospitals. Part 2. *Hospital Topics* 68 (Winter 1990): 4–6.

Deal, Terrence E., Allan K. Kennedy, and Arthur H. Spiegel, III. How to create an outstanding hospital culture. *Hospital Forum* 26 (January/February 1983): 21–34.

Deming, W. Edwards. *Out of the crisis.* Boston: Massachusetts Institute of Technology, 1986.

Fottler, Myron D., John D. Blair, Carlton J. Whitehead, Michael D. Laus, and Grant T. Savage. Assessing key stakeholders: Who matters to hospitals and why? *Hospital & Health Services Administration* 34 (Winter 1989): 525–546.

Gibson, C. Kendrick, David J. Newton, and Daniel S. Cochran. An empirical investigation of hospital mission statements. *Health Care Management Review* 15 (Summer 1990): 35–45.

Higgins, James M. *The management challenge.* New York: Macmillan Publishing Company, 1991.

Ivancevich, John M., James H. Donnelly, Jr., and James L. Gibson. *Management principles and function*, 4th ed. Homewood, IL: Irwin, 1989.

James, Brent C. *Quality management for health care delivery.* Chicago: The Hospital Research and Educational Trust, 1989.

Johnson, Everett A., and Richard L. Johnson. *Hospitals in transition.* Rockville, MD: Aspen Systems Corporation, 1982.

Juran, Joseph M. *Managerial breakthrough: A new concept of the manager's job.* New York: McGraw-Hill Book Company, 1964.

Juran, Joseph M. *Juran on planning for quality.* New York: The Free Press, 1988.

Koontz, Harold. The management theory jungle. *Academy of Management Journal* 4 (December 1961): 174–188.

Kuhl, Ingrid K. *The executive role in health services delivery organizations.* Washington, D.C.: Office of Applied Research, Association of University Programs in Health Administration, 1977.

Levey, Samuel, and James Hill. Between survival and social responsibility: In search of an ethical balance. *The Journal of Health Administration Education* 4 (Spring 1986): 225–231.

Longest, Beaufort B., Jr. American health policy in the year 2000. *Hospital & Health Services Administration* 33 (Winter 1988): 419–434.

Lowe, Ted A., and Joseph M. Mazzeo. Crosby, Deming, Juran: Three preachers, one religion. *Quality* 25 (September 25, 1986): 22–25.

Mintzberg, Henry. The manager's job: Folklore and fact. *Harvard Business Review* 53 (July–August 1975): 54–59.

Mintzberg, Henry. *Mintzberg on management: Inside our strange world of organizations.* New York: The Free Press, 1989.

Munson, Fred C., and Howard S. Zuckerman. The managerial role. In *Health care management: A text in organization the-ory and behavior,* 2d ed., edited by Stephen M. Shortell and Arnold D. Kaluzny. New York: John Wiley & Sons, 1988.

Pearce, John A., II, and Richard B. Robinson, Jr. *Management.* New York: Random House, 1989.

Stevens, Rosemary. The hospital as a social institution, new-fashioned for the 1990s. *Hospital & Health Services Administration* 36 (Summer 1991): 163–173.

Van Fleet, David D. *Contemporary management,* 2d ed. Boston: Houghton Mifflin Company, 1991.

Wesbury, Stewart A. Meeting the challenge: The health care executive's role. *Hospital & Health Services Administration* 33 (Fall 1988): 275–281.

Zuckerman, Howard S. Redefining the role of the CEO: Challenges and conflicts. *Hospital & Health Services Administration* 34 (Spring 1989): 25–38.

II / The Health Services Environment

2 / The Health Care Delivery System

*The health care system [functions] through
complex interactions among government, health
professionals, consumers, third party payors,
employers, and delivery systems. These groups
use competition, standards, and regulation to
pursue a balance in their respective health care
goals of access, finance, and quality. There is no
single source of governance or health policy, nor
is there a single set of shared values or goals
among these groups: the health care system is an
amalgamation of many different agendas.*
Healthy America: Practitioners for 2005[1]

This chapter describes the United States health care system—the macroenvironment in which the health services organization (HSO) manager works. In addition, a basic background for the Canadian health services system is provided.

United States national health expenditures are projected to exceed $800 billion (more than 13% of gross national product [GNP]) in 1992, with projections of $1,615 billion (more than 16% of GNP) by the year 2000. The amount is staggering, and it suggests the magnitude of the problems facing HSO managers. This chapter provides a conceptual framework and facts about health care resources that show historical development, nature, extent, and relationships. Resources include HSOs, programs, personnel, technology, and financing. Detailed information about several types of HSOs—including acute care hospitals, hospices, managed care organizations, nursing facilities, ambulatory care organizations, birth centers, and home health agencies—is provided in Chapter 7, "How HSOs are Organized."

Data here describe the manager's environment. Successful managers have a comprehensive and accurate understanding of the world beyond their HSO, and this includes a comprehensive understanding of trends and developments. The management model in Chapter 1, "The Management Process and Managerial Roles," describes this relationship and should be referred to as necessary (see Figure 1.6).

Data are drawn from numerous sources, with the federal government the most common; these data are supplemented by specialized data from private groups. Substantial reliance is placed on figures and tables. Readers should understand the individual presentations and their interactions, and consider the effects various segments of the system have on one another.

CONCEPTUAL FRAMEWORK OF HEALTH CARE

Health and System Goals

Chapter 1 distinguishes the health care system from the health services system. Blum's model, shown in Figure 2.1, provides a useful conceptualization of elements affecting health. It portrays medical care services (prevention, cure, care, rehabilitation) as much less important than the environment and somewhat less important than heredity and life-styles in affecting health (well-being). In discussing the model, Blum states that the "largest aggregate of forces resides in the

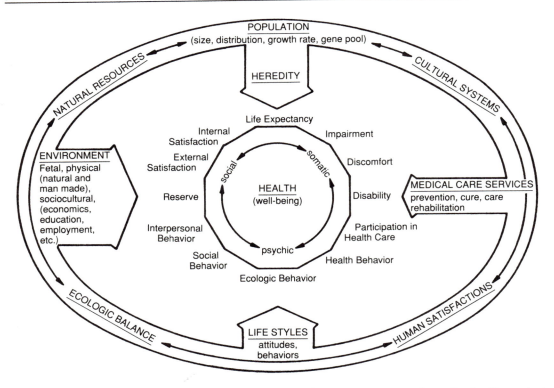

Figure 2.1. The force-field and well-being paradigms of health. (From Blum, Henrik K. *Expanding health care horizons: From a general systems concept of health to a national health policy,* 2d ed., 37. Oakland, CA: Third Party Publishing Company, 1983; reprinted by permission.)

person's environment. One's own behavior, in great part derived from one's experience with one's environment, is seen as the next largest force affecting health."[2] Managers must understand other influences on health status, both as factors leading to an episode of illness and their effect on recovery and long-term absence of illness and minimization of disability if the individual is subjected to them again. HSO managers must have a broad view of illness and health and must look beyond the organization. They must understand that, at best, the health services system has a limited effect and can provide only stopgap measures if negative influences on health undo what has been done.

Blum suggests goals for the health system:

—prolonging life and preventing premature death;
—minimizing departures from physiological or functional norms by focusing attention on precursors of illness;
—minimizing discomfort (illness);
—minimizing disability (incapacity);
—promoting high-level "wellness" or self-fulfillment;
—promoting high-level satisfaction with the environment;
—extending resistance to ill health and creating reserve capacity; and
—increasing opportunities for consumers to participate in health matters.[3]

These goals are part of the conceptual framework to be kept in mind in using this book.

Lack of Synchrony

There are wide geographic variations in the hospitalization rates and length of hospital stay by diagnosis. The variations are true differences that cannot be explained by understanding or estimating the effect of variables such as age, sex, and climate. In addition, there are significant differences in hospitalization rates and lengths of stay by diagnosis within geographic regions, as well as within individual hospitals. The most plausible explanation to account for these differences is variation in how physicians practice medicine—physician practice patterns. It is reasonable to posit that some rates of hospitalization and lengths of stay are more appropriate than others; that means these differences have significant implications for managers of HSOs, especially hospitals, as they strive to increase efficiency in their organizations.

Other data show significant differences between morbidity and mortality caused by various diseases and the amount of hospitalization for that disease. For example, heart disease accounts for 11.7% of patients discharged from hospitals, but accounts for 35.8% of deaths and 10.6% of conditions that limit activity; cerebrovascular disease accounts for 2.5% of patients discharged from hospitals, but accounts for 7.1% of deaths and 1.8% of conditions that limit activity; and diabetus mellitus accounts for 1.5% of patients discharged from hospitals, but accounts for 1.8% of deaths and 4.0% of conditions that limit activity.[4] The measures are out of synchrony. There are numerous reasons for this: hospitals are constrained by available technology; hospitalization may be inappropriate to treat the condition that causes death or limits activity; and some conditions require more attention to prevention. Such data should be viewed, however, as partially explanatory of the appropriate relationship between HSOs and health needs.

There are important distinctions between the need and the demand for health services. Need is measured by morbidity and mortality data, and by disability that limits activity. Need is more objective than demand. Demand occurs when need (or perceived need) is converted into delivery of services. As suggested, need and demand do not have a one-to-one relationship. Need may not become demand because persons lack knowledge about a disease or because mores dissuade them from seeking help. Demand may be less than need because persons lack financial resources or because there are no HSOs to provide services. Furthermore, some demand is very subjective; cosmetic surgery is a commonly cited example. Relationships between need and demand must be considered as health services are planned. Ethical dimensions of need and demand are addressed in Chapter 3, "Ethical Considerations."

A BRIEF HISTORY OF HEALTH SERVICES IN THE UNITED STATES

Technology

The importance of public health measures such as ensuring the availability of pure food and water was demonstrated during the "great sanitary awakening" in the mid-19th century, and this led to establishment of state and local health departments. At about the same time major contributions to medical knowledge resulted from the work of Pasteur, Lister, and Koch. Their efforts led to antisepsis and later asepsis, which, in addition to technology such as radiographs, inhalation anesthesia, blood typing, and improved clinical laboratories in the latter 19th century, permitted significant surgical interventions with greatly reduced morbidity and mortality. These developments required an organization, personnel, and systems to deliver the new wonders that medicine had to offer. Acute care hospitals were an obvious choice.

It was common for acute care hospitals to be sponsored by private, not-for-profit corporations that had been formed by concerned citizens and wealthy benefactors; local governments sponsored others. Many smaller hospitals were established as for-profit corporations, often by individual physicians who wanted a place to hospitalize patients. Long-term care facilities, often called nursing homes, were rare because extended families assisted their relatives. Persons with mental illness were warehoused and isolated from society in facilities owned almost exclusively by state governments. Effective, large-scale treatment for them did not occur until after World War II with the development of psychoactive drugs. Another type of HSO sponsored by local governments was public health departments.

Morbidity and Mortality

Changes in the causes of mortality since 1970 are shown in Table 2.1. Except for tuberculosis, which had declined rapidly by the end of the 19th century because of improved nutrition and housing, and leprosy, which was never a major medical problem in the United States, there were few chronic diseases before the 20th century. Primarily, persons died of acute gastrointestinal and respiratory tract infections that usually occurred before they developed a chronic disease. Health problems common at the middle of the 19th century were largely solved through preventive measures undertaken by public health departments. Pure food and water and improved sanitation were major contributors. Causes of mortality that replaced earlier problems have usually been much less amenable to easy prevention or inexpensive treatment. As a result, there has been greater emphasis on acute services, an emphasis that substantially increased costs. Table 2.1 shows declining mortality rates well into the 21st century. This suggests increased longevity and the likelihood of more chronic diseases. Figure 2.1 shows a link between life-style and medical problems. If prevention is to be effective, behavior must be modified. Such efforts raise questions of individual choice and liberty rights, and these are far more complex than purifying water and protecting food supplies. Two questions are: What should be the limits of society's efforts to force persons to live healthfully? What is society's obligation to aid persons whose illnesses result from unhealthy activities?

Social Welfare

A major shift in the locus of responsibility for social welfare occurred with the Social Security Act of 1935. Its passage resulted from the catastrophic economic and social problems of the Depression. Before 1935, local governments, as well as state governments, provided social welfare programs. City and county governments might own a "poor farm," for example, where needy persons could live and work. Since 1935 there has been a massive shift of perceived and actual responsibility for social welfare from state and local governments to the federal government. This accretion continued virtually uninterrupted until revenue sharing and other programs were developed in the 1970s and 1980s. Federally sponsored national health insurance programs were proposed and seriously considered at various times during the 20th century, most notably in the late 1940s and late 1960s. Such national programs were considered again in the early 1990s. At all three times their provisions covered the gamut from all-encompassing federal programs to modest interventions. They were, nonetheless, potentially very expensive programs. Before the decade of the 1990s, numerous factors caused these proposals to be defeated. The opposition of organized medicine has often been mentioned; however, its role is overstated. Historically, the primary reason has been a lack of voter interest: most persons had private hospitalization insurance, usually furnished by their employers. The momentum for a universal scheme dwindled further after Medicare and Medicaid were enacted in the mid-1960s and provided significant coverage for millions who had had inadequate access, and as it became clear how expensive such programs could be. The decade of the 1990s may see a different result, however, as the high costs of health insurance and concern about the uninsured increase interest in national health insurance once again.

In 1988, a program covering catastrophic health care was enacted as part of Medicare. It capped out-of-pocket payments and required a modest premium based on income. The need to pay a premium caused a great furor among a vocal minority of those covered, and the law was

Table 2.1. Trends in United States death rates

	1970	1975	1980	1985	1990[a]	2000[a]	2010[a]	2020[a]	2030[a]	2040[a]
Death rate (per 100,000 population)	1,041.8	934.0	878.0	830.0	791.7	722.8	667.8	633.2	601.9	573.2
Major causes of death										
Heart disease	413.2	361.3	335.9	303.3	265.2	214.4	183.6	164.8	148.2	133.2
Cancer	173.6	177.2	184.0	187.6	187.0	194.6	196.6	192.3	187.9	183.5
Vascular disease	162.3	134.6	103.4	82.5	66.9	42.4	33.6	29.4	25.7	22.5
Violence	83.9	74.7	70.7	60.1	57.4	47.4	43.1	41.5	40.0	38.6
Respiratory disease	60.8	55.6	57.0	65.4	65.0	66.3	66.7	65.4	64.0	62.7
Congenital malformations and diseases of early infancy	28.2	20.5	16.1	13.4	11.4	7.3	5.8	5.0	4.3	3.7
Digestive disease	23.2	19.1	19.7	18.9	17.8	16.1	15.2	14.5	13.9	13.3
Diabetes mellitus	20.7	17.3	15.4	14.7	13.7	10.9	9.7	9.0	8.5	7.9
Liver cirrhosis	15.7	15.0	13.5	11.0	9.7	8.0	7.4	7.2	7.0	6.8
AIDS	0.0	0.0	0.0	2.5[b]	22.8[b]	33.6	22.4	21.8	21.8	21.8
Other	60.1	58.6	62.3	70.5	74.8	81.8	83.9	82.4	80.7	79.1

Data for 1970–1985 are from the National Center for Health Statistics. *Vital Statistics of the U.S., Annual Report.* Washington, D.C., 1970, 1975, 1980, & 1985.
[a]Estimates are made by the Social Security Administration in unpublished data for 1991. Estimates are derived using alternative II assumptions that are based on past death rates trends and are derived through use of the least squares statistical estimation method. For those under 65, numerators are provided by the National Center for Health Statistics and denominators are from the Bureau of the Census. Numerators for those over 65 are from unpublished Medicare data and denominators are from the Bureau of the Census population estimates.
[b]AIDS data through 1990 are from the Centers for Disease Control; projections are from the Social Security Administration.

37

repealed before it became fully implemented. The experience disillusioned many in Congress. The question of catastrophic coverage will be an issue for a group that is increasing rapidly—the elderly. In 1990, 12.7% of the population was 65 or older; by 2030 it is projected this proportion will grow to 22.9%.[5] These data suggest there will be greatly increased demand for health services in geriatrics, chronic diseases, rehabilitation, and institutional long-term care. Unanswered is how these needs will be financed.

Other Systems

By comparison, Western Europe, notably Germany and England, had government involvement in financing health services much earlier. In 1883, Chancellor Otto von Bismarck achieved passage of a social insurance scheme, including a health services component, for certain working-class Germans. In 1911, England adopted a national health insurance program. In 1948, England (the United Kingdom) established the National Health Service (NHS), which included government ownership of the health services system. Western European and Canadian health services systems have much more governmental control and financing, generally, than do those in the United States. It is noteworthy that, despite greater government involvement in planning and financing, in the past many of these countries experienced inflation in health services costs similar to that in the United States. However, since about 1985, United States increases have been well ahead of those in all other countries.[6] Countries where budgetary allocations to health services are determined prospectively spend substantially less than the United States. For example, in 1989 the United Kingdom spent 5.8% of its gross domestic product on health, Canada spent 8.7%, and the United States consumed 11.8%.[7] An important reason for the difference is that far less is spent on high technology in the United Kingdom and Canada; for example, computed tomography scans and renal dialysis units are less available. Furthermore, elective procedures are less readily available and there are often long waiting periods, called queues.

The health services system of Canada has been suggested as offering lessons for Americans as they seek to improve access to health services, enhance delivery, and reduce costs. A final section in this chapter compares expenditures among various countries and describes the Canadian health services system and compares it to that in the United States.

Federal Initiatives

It was primarily not-for-profit acute care hospitals, including those operated by state and local governments, that benefited from early federal programs. From 1946 to 1981, the Hill-Burton Act (Hospital Survey and Construction Act of 1946 [PL 79-725]) provided more than $4 billion in grants, loans, and guaranteed loans in a federal-state matching program. Hill-Burton aided nearly 6,900 hospitals and other health care facilities in more than 4,000 communities. Initially, the funds were used to construct new inpatient (acute care hospital) facilities, and later they were used to remodel and construct outpatient facilities. The number of hospitals increased by more than 800 in this period. In return for Hill-Burton assistance, facilities agreed to provide a reasonable volume of services to persons unable to pay (uncompensated services) for periods of time that varied by the type of assistance. The annual dollar volume of uncompensated services is equal to the lesser of 3% of operating costs or 10% of the amount of federal assistance received, adjusted by inflation.[8]

Figure 2.2, with "reactions" and "results," shows trends in the United States health services system since 1945. It is noteworthy that the "escalation in health care costs" and the "emphasis on secondary and tertiary care and inadequate attention to other levels of care" effects have been very important in the "reactions" and "results" sections of the figure. Thoroughly studying Figure 2.2 will enable the reader to exploit the information it provides.

Other federal government programs provided additional resources. These included generous

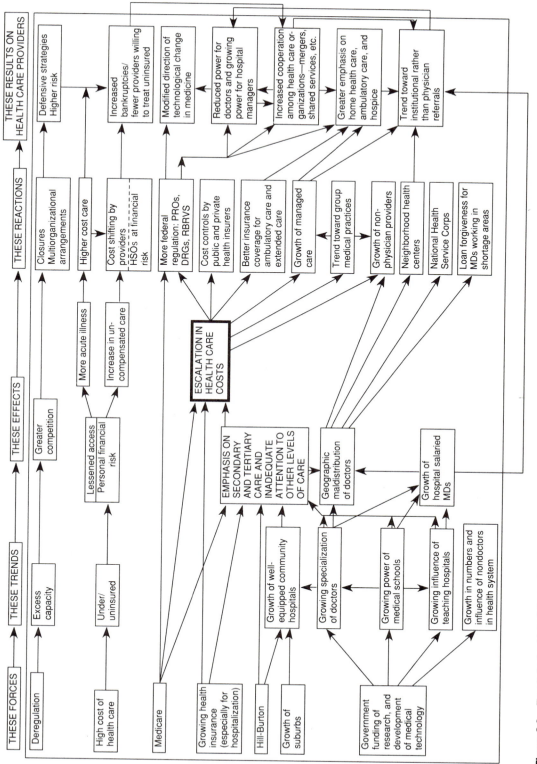

Figure 2.2. Trends in the United States health care system since 1945. (From Cambridge Research Institute. *Trends affecting the U.S. health care system*, 409. Health Planning Information Series, Human Resources Administration, Public Health Service, Department of Health, Education and Welfare. Washington, D.C.: U.S. Government Printing Office, 1976; revised and updated by authors, 1992.)

funding for research activities that became the National Institutes of Health (NIH). From early experimentation on cancer in the 1930s, the institutes grew in number and importance. Much of the research is done by contracting with universities and academic medical centers. In 1990, the NIH had a budget of $7.6 billion for 13 institutes and affiliated activities, compared with $3.4 billion for nine institutes and affiliated activities in 1980.[9]

Federal programs to educate more physicians, nurses, technicians, and managers were established and funded in the 1960s. Congress was convinced that the knowledge produced by NIH and the hospitals built by the Hill-Burton program could improve health status only if there were sufficient numbers of trained personnel.

During the same postwar period the federal government built large numbers of Veterans Administration (now Department of Veterans Affairs [DVA]) hospitals to deliver services to former military personnel. The DVA system is separate from services provided to other groups that have been special historically, such as American Indians, active duty and retired military personnel and their dependents in Army, Navy, and Air Force hospitals, and merchant seamen in Public Health Service hospitals.

In 1965, amendments to the Social Security Act of 1935 directed the federal government to pay for health services to two large groups. An exclusively federal program, Medicare, now pays for services rendered to people 65 and over and to people with severe and permanent disabilities. Medicaid, a state-federal cost-sharing program, pays for certain health services of persons who meet eligibility criteria based on income levels set by the states. These programs have become very large in terms of both the number of beneficiaries and expenditures.

Meanwhile, there were federal efforts to rationalize the health services system. The Comprehensive Health Planning and Public Health Service Amendments Act of 1966 (PL 89-749) was first. It built on existing voluntary planning and the modest planning requirements in the Hill-Burton Act and was designed to enhance use of planning processes and techniques in the health services system. This legislation was amplified and expanded with passage of the National Health Planning and Resources Development Act of 1974 (PL 93-641). This law was a major change that increased the control planning agencies had over expansion of hospitals and services—an attempt to regulate the supply side. An effort to monitor the utilization and quality of services provided under Medicare and Medicaid programs was enacted when the Social Security Amendments of 1972 (PL 92-603) established professional standards review organizations (PSROs). Political changes caused a reassessment of the usefulness of the planning and PSRO programs. Federal support of planning has ended. PSROs were replaced by professional review organizations, which are discussed later.

Such regulatory controls were considered essential to slow the rapid inflation of health care costs. Data for the period 1950–1989 show that, except for 1978–1979 and 1979–1980, the average annual percentage change for the "medical care component" of the consumer price index has led the increase for "all items," usually by wide margins.[10] Since 1980, the rate of inflation for "hospitals and related services" has been consistently much higher than in health services as a whole.[11]

The Tax Equity and Fiscal Responsibility Act of 1982 (PL 97-248) and the Social Security Amendments of 1983 (PL 98-21) established a prospective payment system to address the problem of cost increases in hospitals. The rate of reimbursement for Medicare would be determined prospectively and would be based on diagnosis-related groups, which tie the payment from federal government for Medicare patients to a hospital's case mix. Since the mid-1970s, state governments have also been concerned about rising health services costs. They focused on certificate of need and rate review. States control Medicaid expenditures by setting arbitrary limits on what they will pay; this typically causes providers to incur a deficit for Medicaid patients.

The effect of federal legislative initiatives is that hospitals have been forced to become more efficient. Improvements have occurred. Hospitals cannot control their environments, however. In addition, they may have to provide large amounts of uncompensated care. In such circumstances, the hospital can only survive if it finds other sources of revenue. Previously, unpaid costs were shifted to Blue Cross, commercial insurance companies, and private-pay patients. Increasingly, third-party carriers are objecting to this cost shifting. This leaves only private-pay patients—a group too small to make up the difference. In addition to the question of fairness, cost shifting is a major political issue, especially with regard to the uninsured and the costs of medical education. To protect themselves financially, hospitals are developing new organizational entities and relationships through corporate restructuring and joint ventures. The result is a mix of not-for-profit and for-profit organizations; for many hospitals this has resulted in an enhanced revenue stream to offset deficits elsewhere. These developments are discussed in Chapter 9, "Interorganizational Relationships."

PRESENT STRUCTURE OF THE HEALTH SERVICES SYSTEM

Various types of HSOs are found in both the private (owned by private individuals or groups) and public (owned by government) sectors. HSOs may be institutions, the most prominent of which are hospitals and nursing facilities, or they may be programs and agencies such as public health departments and visiting nurse associations. (Information about selected HSOs is found in Chapter 7.) All depend on their environments (see Figure 1.6). The range of health services delivery and various providers is shown in Figure 2.3. The two parts of preventive care, education and prevention, should be noted. Prevention can be divided into primary, secondary, and tertiary.

> *Primary* prevention involves prevention of the disease or injury itself. Improved highway design, school education programs concerning smoking and substance abuse, and immunization against poliomyelitis or measles are examples of primary prevention. *Secondary* prevention blocks progression of an injury or disease from an impairment to a disability. Use of the Papanicolaou smear to look for early cellular changes that are thought to be precursors of cancer is a good example of secondary prevention. An impairment has already occurred, but disability may be prevented through early intervention. Treatment of certain streptococcal infections with penicillin can prevent the occasional development of rheumatic fever and serious heart disease. Early detection of high blood pressure can reduce the probability of a heart attack or stroke. *Tertiary* prevention blocks or retards the progression of a disability to a state of dependency. The early detection and effective management of diabetes can prevent some of the dependencies associated with the disease, or at least slow their rate of progression. Prompt medical care followed by rehabilitation can limit the damage caused by a cerebrovascular accident (stroke) and the same is true for heart attacks. Good vehicular design can reduce the dependency which might otherwise occur as a result of a crash.[12]

HSOs such as state and local public health departments will have programs at all three levels. Hospitals and nursing facilities, for examples, are more likely to engage in secondary and tertiary prevention than in primary prevention.

Physician–patient interactions overwhelmingly occur in physician offices. In 1989, 59.6% of contacts occurred in physicians' offices; only 13.2% occurred through hospital inpatient and outpatient or emergency room contacts.[13] Despite a trend for more physicians to be employed by HSOs, most are likely to be self-employed entrepreneurs who share a receptionist and billing and perhaps diagnostic equipment, or they are in a partnership or are "employees" of a physician (professional) corporation such as a multispecialty group practice.

CLASSIFICATION AND TYPES OF HSOs

Profit or Not for Profit

HSOs may be classified by whether they seek to make a profit (for profit or investor owned) that is paid to owners (investors), or whether the profit (sometimes called excess of income over expense)

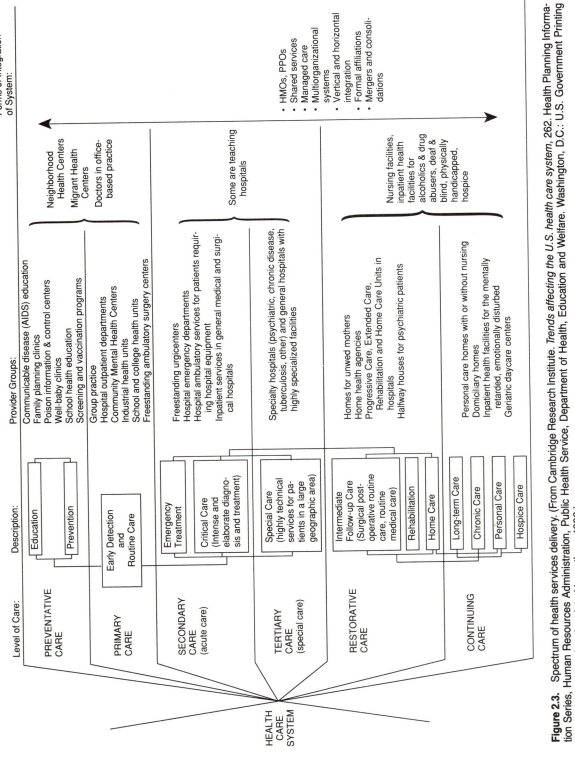

Figure 2.3. Spectrum of health services delivery. (From Cambridge Research Institute. *Trends affecting the U.S. health care system*, 262. Health Planning Information Series, Human Resources Administration, Public Health Service, Department of Health, Education and Welfare. Washington, D.C.: U.S. Government Printing Office, 1976; revised and updated by authors, 1992.)

is not available to any person or corporation (not for profit) and is used by the HSO to enhance the content or quality of health services or to reduce charges. Government-sponsored HSOs are not for profit, even though they are publicly owned, as compared with private ownership through either a for-profit or not-for-profit corporation.

Ownership

Another means of classifying HSOs is by ownership. In addition to private ownership, whether sectarian or nonsectarian, not for profit or investor owned, many HSOs are publicly owned. Cities or counties own (control) public health departments, as well as other types of providers such as hospitals. States establish special tax districts to finance HSOs, usually acute care hospitals. HSOs owned by state government include health departments, planning agencies, and facilities such as psychiatric hospitals or institutions for persons with mental retardation. Many states own university teaching hospitals to treat acute illness, conduct research, and educate health personnel.

Historically, the federal government has been involved in financing, and to a lesser extent, delivering health services—preventive, acute, and, more recently, long-term care for special groups. There are a number of examples. The United States Public Health Service (PHS) hospitals were established in the late 18th century to care for merchant mariners. PHS hospitals treating general acute care problems were operated until 1981, when the few remaining hospitals were closed or converted to other purposes. The Gillis W. Long Hanson's Disease Hospital in Carville, Louisiana, is the last PHS hospital and treats victims of leprosy. At the end of 1989, the Indian Health Service (part of the PHS, which is in the Department of Health and Human Services) operated 43 hospitals and 127 health centers, school health centers, and health stations.[14] In 1991, the DVA operated 172 hospitals, 126 nursing facilities, and 35 domiciliary residences for former military personnel with service-connected medical problems.[15] The DVA has made a significant contribution to medical education: more than one out of every two practicing physicians has received some training in a DVA medical center.[16] In 1989, DVA medical centers supported the training of approximately 12% of residents.[17] In addition, a large number of acute care hospitals and various types of clinics are operated by the United States Army, Navy, and Air Force to serve active duty and retired military personnel and their dependents.

Length of Patient Stay

A third way to classify HSOs is by the length of time a patient is in treatment. A general dichotomy divides them by whether services are delivered to inpatients, generally defined as patients whose treatment is 24 hours or longer, or to outpatients, whose treatment is less than 24 hours. In turn, inpatient HSOs are divided into short term (acute) and long term. The American Hospital Association (AHA) defines a short-term hospital as one in which the average length of stay is less than 30 days; a long-term hospital has patient stays that average 30 days or longer. Nursing facilities typically treat only inpatients, and lengths of stay are measured in months or years. HSOs such as home health agencies and physician group practices treat only outpatients. Some, such as hospices, have inpatients, but may also treat patients in their homes.

Role in Health Services System

A fourth way to classify HSOs is by their role in the health services system. Chapter 7 describes the history, numbers, functions, and organization of a variety of HSOs, of which there are many types, including acute care hospitals, hospices, managed care organizations, nursing facilities, ambulatory care organizations, birth centers, and home health agencies. Health services may be provided in public health department screening programs, in family planning and substance abuse treatment centers, or through sanitation efforts to protect food and water supplies. There are thousands of privately and publicly owned and operated emergency medical units such as rescue squads and ambulance services, often organized into emergency medical services systems. In addition, there are programs more oriented to social welfare activities; some only raise funds, others deliver specialized services. Depending on their activities, they may or may not be considered HSOs. The total number of HSOs ranges in the tens of thousands.

Unique Institutional Providers In addition to inpatient HSOs, such as hospitals and nursing facilities, there are many other types of inpatient facilities that provide health and health-related services. Regrettably, data collection about them has been sporadic. Such facilities include resident facilities or schools for special groups of people who are, for example, blind, deaf, emotionally disturbed, and physically disabled; persons with mental retardation; dependent children; unwed mothers; alcoholics; drug abusers; and people with multiple disorders.

The 1986 Inventory of Long Term Care Places, conducted by the National Center for Health Statistics, surveyed only two types of facilities: nursing and related care homes and facilities for mentally retarded persons. Nursing facilities are described in Chapter 7. In 1986, there were approximately 250,000 people with mental retardation in 14,639 facilities in the United States.[18] Of these facilities, 12,703 had fewer than 15 beds, 1,531 had 16 to 99 beds, and only 405 had 100 beds or more.[19] Approximately 1,900 were government owned and the remainder were divided between for-profit and not-for-profit ownership.[20]

Community services may reduce the need for long-term inpatient care. Examples of community services include diagnostic and evaluation clinics, day care centers, early childhood education facilities, rehabilitation programs, and summer camps and recreational facilities. All offer alternatives to institutional placement. Community-sponsored educational services are provided by local school districts under the direction of state special education programs. Developmental disability programs are operated at local levels with state funding.

Mental Health Mental health organizations are defined as HSOs that primarily provide mental health services to mentally ill or emotionally disturbed persons. Included are public or private psychiatric hospitals, psychiatric services in general hospitals, outpatient psychiatric clinics, and mental health day/night facilities. Since 1955, there have been significant changes as to where mental health services are delivered. In the mid-1950s, state and county mental hospitals accounted for 77% of inpatient services; 23% were outpatient. By 1975, a reversal had occurred and 76% of services were outpatient.[21] Inpatient treatment continues to be a major type of care, and in 1986, 1.3 million persons were admitted to inpatient psychiatric organizations.[22]

Teaching Hospitals There are approximately 1,300 hospitals involved in graduate medical education in the United States.[23] They fall under the general rubric of teaching hospital and offer a wide range of secondary and tertiary medical services. These 1,300, plus an unknown but large number of other hospitals, participate in training a wide variety of persons in health care occupations. Many teaching hospitals are part of a medical center complex that includes a medical school. Those without a medical school are almost always affiliated with one. Their prominence in medical education, added to activities in research and publishing in the medical and scientific literature, makes teaching hospitals very important in the health services field.

Membership as a teaching hospital in the Council of Teaching Hospitals (COTH), a division of the Association of American Medical Colleges, is limited to hospitals that sponsor, or significantly participate in, at least four approved, active residencies. At least two of these residency programs must be in medicine, surgery, obstetrics/gynecology, pediatrics, family practice, or psychiatry. In the case of specialty hospitals, such as children's, rehabilitation, and psychiatric institutions, exceptions to the residency requirement may be made.[24] In 1991, there were only 405 member hospitals of the COTH, but their influence is far greater than this number suggests. They train over 80% of the medical and surgical residents in the United States.[25] In 1987, there were 420 COTH members (6% of short-term nonfederal hospitals), but 21% of hospital beds, 23% of admissions, 28% of outpatient visits, 20% of emergency department visits, and 25% of births occurred in these hospitals.[26]

A unique HSO that may fit into more than one of the categories described above merits special attention. The premier institution among all HSOs is the academic medical center hospital, a subset of teaching hospitals. Academic medical center hospitals are those in which a majority of the chiefs of service at the hospital chair the academic departments in a medical school. In 1989, there were 123 academic medical center hospitals in the United States.[27]

HEALTH SERVICES WORKERS

In 1989, 9.1 million persons were employed at health services sites, a number that has more than doubled since 1970 and that has risen much faster than the total employed population.[28] The only larger group of employees in the United States is the number of persons employed by all levels of government. More than half (4.6 million) of the 9.1 million are employed in hospitals. The second largest site of employment is nursing and personal care facilities, which employed 1.5 million in 1989.[29] The remainder are employed in physician, dental, and chiropractic offices and other sites where health services are delivered. Table 2.2 shows numbers of employees and changes over the past 2 decades by health services sites of employment.

Table 2.3 shows various types of health services personnel in the United States for selected years from 1970 to 1988. The rapid growth is apparent; many categories doubled in 2 decades. Table 2.4 shows selected health services occupations employed in community hospitals for 1981 and 1988. Most changes are unremarkable. It is notable, however, that registered nurses employed in community hospitals have increased significantly in these 8 years—by more than 140,000—but the numbers of licensed practical nurses and ancillary nursing personnel have decreased substantially in the same period. This reflects an effort to upgrade staffing in these institutions. Table 2.5 shows historical data and projections for physicians for 1990 and 2000. Comparing the number of active physicians per 10,000 population establishes a ratio, which permits accurate comparisons over time. The projected doubling of this ratio from 1950 to the year 2000 has concerned health occupations planners. In the late 1970s, the Graduate Medical Education National Advisory Committee (GMENAC) projected a significant physician surplus by the 1990s. Studies by

Table 2.2. Persons employed in health service sites in the United States, selected years 1970–1989 (in thousands)[a]

Site of employment	Year				
	1970[b]	1975	1980	1985	1989
Total	4,246	5,945	7,339	7,910	9,110
Offices of physicians	477	618	777	894	1,039
Offices of dentists	222	331	415	480	560
Offices of chiropractors[c]	19	30	40	59	97
Hospitals	2,690	3,442	4,036	4,269	4,586
Nursing and personal care facilities	509	891	1,199	1,309	1,521
Other health service sites	330	634	872	899	1,325
	Percentage of employed civilians				
All health service sites	5.5	6.9	7.4	7.4	7.8

From National Center for Health Statistics, Public Health Service, U.S. Department of Health and Human Services. *Health United States 1990,* 160. Washington, D.C.: U.S. Government Printing Office, 1991.

[a]Data are based on household interviews of a sample of the civilian noninstitutionalized population.

[b]April 1, derived from decennial census; all other data years are annual averages from the Current Population Survey.

[c]Data for 1980 are from the American Chiropractic Association; data for all other years are from the U.S. Bureau of Labor Statistics.

Table 2.3. Active health personnel in the United States, selected years 1970–1988 (in thousands)

Occupation category	1970	1980	1988
Physicians (total)	290,862	427,028	539,228
Federal		17,548	21,746
Nonfederal		409,480	517,482
Doctors of medicine[a]	279,212	393,407	493,743[b]
Doctors of osteopathy	11,650	16,073	23,739
Dentists[c]	95,700	121,240	142,200
Optometrists	18,400	22,330	26,100
Pharmacists	112,570	142,780	157,800
Podiatrists	7,110	8,800	11,500
Registered nurses (total)	750,000	1,272,900	1,648,000
Associate and diploma		908,000	1,054,300[d]
Baccalaureate		297,300	468,860[d]
Masters and doctorate		67,300	103,810[d]
Veterinarians	25,900	36,000	47,500

From National Center for Health Statistics, Public Health Service, U.S. Department of Health and Human Services. *Health United States 1990*, 165. Washington, D.C.: U.S. Government Printing Office, 1991.

[a]Excludes physicians not classified according to activity status.

[b]Doctors of medicine data are as of January 1, 1988.

[c]Excludes dentists in military service.

[d]Data are for 1987.

the American Medical Association (AMA) and the Health Resources and Services Administration (part of the Department of Health and Human Services) published in 1988 supported the findings and projections of GMENAC. The AMA study agrees that supply will probably grow faster than demand, "but it disclaims the notion of a surplus or shortage because that would imply judgments

Table 2.4. Full-time equivalent employment in selected occupations for community hospitals: United States, 1981 and 1988

Occupation	1981	1988
All occupations[a]	3,069,955	3,231,745
Administrators and assistant administrators	26,734	35,715
Registered nurses	629,354	770,613
Licensed practical nurses	234,226	170,637
Ancillary nursing personnel	280,614	244,297
Medical record administrators and technicians	38,186	46,937
Licensed pharmacists and pharmacy technicians	47,053	58,759
Medical technologists and other laboratory personnel	147,451	148,635
Dietitians and dietetic technicians	40,192	35,126
Radiologic service personnel	90,738	101,098
Occupational therapists and recreational therapists	8,481	13,133
Physical therapists and physical therapy assistants and aides	27,675	32,680
Speech pathologists and audiologists	2,463	4,346
Respiratory therapists and respiratory therapy technicians	47,312	55,690
Medical social workers	13,915	18,685
Total trainee personnel[b]	66,906	67,587

From National Center for Health Statistics, Public Health Service, U.S. Department of Health and Human Services. *Health United States 1990*, 166. Washington, D.C.: U.S. Government Printing Office, 1991.

[a]Includes occupational categories not shown.

[b]This category is composed primarily of medical residents.

Table 2.5. Active physicians and number per 10,000: United States and outlying U.S. areas, selected 1950–1988 estimates and 1990 and 2000 projections[a]

Year	All active physicians[b]	Active physicians per 10,000 population
1950	219,900	14.1
1960	259,400	14.0
1970	326,500	15.6
1975	384,500	17.4
1980	457,500	19.7
1985	534,400	22.0
1988	573,600	23.3
	Projections	
1990	601,100	24.0
2000	721,600	26.9

From National Center for Health Statistics, Public Health Service, U.S. Department of Health and Human Services. *Health United States 1990,* 163. Washington, D.C.: U.S. Government Printing Office, 1991.

aNotes: Population estimates include residents in the United States, Puerto Rico, and other U.S. outlying areas; U.S. citizens in foreign countries; and the Armed Forces in the United States and abroad. For 1990 and 2000, the Series II projections of the total population from the U.S. Bureau of the Census are used. Estimation and projection methods are from the Bureau of Health Professions.

*b*The numbers for doctors of medicine differ from American Medical Association figures because physicians not classified by activity status and whose addresses are unknown are included in this table.

about the adequacy of current utilization rates by all segments of the population."[30] Other, contemporary analyses reached different conclusions, however. They concluded that the demand for physicians' services would increase as fast as the numbers of physicians increased.[31] A surplus would suggest the potential for various problems, while concomitantly creating opportunities for HSO managers. With or without a surplus, however, a more significant problem has been and will continue to be a maldistribution of physicians. This is especially true in rural areas.

Chapter 18, "Labor Relations," addresses health services labor relations. A brief comment here provides a context for the discussion of health services workers in later sections of this chapter. Most physicians and other licensed independent practitioners (LIPs) are self-employed private entrepreneurs. In contrast, almost all other caregivers are employed by LIPs in their practices or by a partnership or corporation such as a nursing facility or hospital. Physicians in residency programs are usually employed by the residency site. These relationships are part of the context for labor relations in HSOs.

EDUCATION OF MANAGERS

Hospital administration was identified as a distinct educational discipline when the University of Chicago established the first master's degree program in 1934. It followed by 1 year the founding of the American College of Hospital Administrators, now the American College of Healthcare Executives (ACHE), in 1933. These were milestones in the development of a professional identity. In 1991, 60 graduate programs were accredited by the Accrediting Commission on Education for Health Services Administration, which is composed of representatives from health services professional associations. Five of these programs are in Canada.[32] A number of graduate programs exist or are being developed in Latin America. United States master's degree programs have more than 25,000 graduates.

Consistent with changes in their environment, educational programs typically provide a generic education in health services, rather than hospital, management. Some offer specialty preparation in hospital, nursing facility, or ambulatory services management. Educational content varies and is best described as eclectic, with significant emphasis on business management skills.

The didactic portion for accredited programs is two academic years—four semesters. Most programs include field experiences of varying lengths. Many require a 1-year residency that allows application of the academic preparation under the guidance of an on-site preceptor.

The most common educational preparation for HSO managers is the master's degree. The basic curriculum in accredited health services management graduate programs covers eight areas:

Assessment and understanding of the health status of populations; determinants of health and illness; and factors influencing the use of health services.

Understanding of the organization, financing, and delivery of health services, drawing on the social science disciplines (broadly defined to include economics, law, political science, psychology, sociology, and related disciplines).

Understanding of, and development of skills in, economic, financial, policy, and quantitative analysis.

Understanding of the values and ethical issues associated with the practice of health services administration, and the development of skills in ethical analysis.

Understanding of, and development of skills in, positioning organizations favorably in the environment and managing these organizations for continued effectiveness.

Provision of opportunities for development of leadership potential including stimulating creativity, and interpersonal and communication skill development.

Understanding of, and development of skills in, the management of human, capital, and information resources.

Understanding of, and development of skills in, evaluation methods to assess organizational performance and, in particular, methods to assure the quality of services provided.[33]

As with the graduate programs, rapid growth in the number of undergraduate programs preparing health services management personnel occurred in the late 1960s and early 1970s. There are 32 undergraduate programs affiliated with the Association of University Programs in Health Administration.[34] However, there are probably more than 100 such programs in the United States. Foci of the two levels of education are different. Master's programs prepare graduates to become senior-level line or staff managers; baccalaureate programs train middle-level supervisors or department managers. A continuing problem is the articulation between graduate and undergraduate programs.

In 1991, no states licensed hospital administrators, while all states licensed nursing facility administrators. Managers in other types of HSOs are unlikely to be licensed. A state's regulatory arm is exercised when problems suggest that a profession's self-regulation and self-discipline are ineffective and the state must act to protect the public.

LICENSURE, CERTIFICATION, AND REGISTRATION OF CAREGIVERS

Except for managers, licensing of health services personnel is ubiquitous. In 1990, every state and the District of Columbia licensed 14 of 44 health care occupations studied by the AHA. Five states regulated 30 or more of these 44 health care occupations. The trend is toward more regulation of health personnel—the Omnibus Budget Reconciliation Act of 1987 requires states to register nursing aides, for example.[35]

There are important distinctions among licensure, registration, and certification.

Licensure: a process performed by government that allows someone to engage in an occupation after finding that the applicant has achieved a certain minimum competency. Physicians and dentists are always licensed, for example.

Registration: qualified individuals are listed on an official roster maintained by a governmental or nongovernmental body. The registered nurse is an early example. States may require registration for someone to engage in a health occupation, thus giving registration the effect of licensure. Persons who are registered may use that designation (e.g., registered dietitian).

Certification: a process by which a *nongovernmental* agency or association grants recognition to someone who meets its qualifications. States may require certification for someone to engage in a health occupation, thus giving certification the effect of licensure. Nurse-midwives are certified, for example.

Physicians (MD [medical doctor]) or osteopaths (DO [doctor of osteopathy]) are the only LIPs with unlimited licenses. State licensing authorities may put limits on a physician's license, but this is rare since disciplinary actions against physicians are uncommon. For all intents and purposes physicians and osteopaths are equivalent and are called physicians in this discussion.

Generally, nonphysician health services workers may be divided into two groups: those licensed to treat patients independently (also called LIPs) and those who may or may not be licensed, but who are dependent on the orders of a physician or nonphysician LIP to allow them to deliver health services. Nonphysician LIPs have state licenses that limit their practice to certain parts of the body or specific medical problems; optometrists, podiatrists, dentists, and chiropractors are examples. In many states, nurse-midwives and some types of nurse-practitioners are LIPs, too. Some states allow registered nurses without specialty training to perform certain examinations and procedures. Applying this general principle is complicated because many types of HSOs, but always acute care hospitals, further limit the scope of practice of health services workers (even of physicians) to activities in which they have demonstrated competence. Similarly, HSOs may limit further even the limited license of nonphysician LIPs to activities that are ordered or supervised by physicians.

Dependent caregivers may or may not be licensed, but they undertake delivery of services only on receiving an order from an LIP. Dependent caregivers include medical technologists, pharmacists, radiographers, licensed practical nurses, and nursing assistants. The caregivers may be licensed, registered, or certified. Licensing is a state function under the police power. Distinctions beyond this are blurred. Registered nurses and pharmacists use "registered" as a synonym for licensure. Dietitians are registered by a private association and are licensed in a number of states.

Certification is a process of approval involving a professional association and oftentimes the AMA. Certificates are issued after passing an examination, the eligibility for which requires certain academic preparation. A confusing aspect of the process is that sometimes the certificate is issued by a body that uses the title "registry." Often the specialty group of physicians also certifies. For example, the American Society of Clinical Pathologists certifies laboratory technologists. Persons unable to meet the private certifying group's standards are likely to be unemployable in an HSO, and this means certification has the effect of licensure. Concomitantly, if the person who is certified does not continue to meet the group's standards and loses certification, employment is likely to be forfeited.

Physicians

Medicine is one of the learned professions and, historically, physicians have been held in high regard. The most important modern effort to improve medical education occurred in 1910 when Abraham Flexner's study of medical education in the United States showed its weaknesses. The science curriculum was enhanced, the didactic portion was lengthened, and the clinical component was strengthened. Weak schools failed when they could not meet the more stringent standards.

The beginning of the 20th century marked the emergence of allopathic medicine as the dominant theory of treating disease. Allopathy holds that interruptions of the body's normal functioning must be treated with massive and dramatic intervention to restore health. Development of the germ theory of disease causation and increasingly efficacious surgery at the turn of the century gave allopathy a clear scientific basis, which secured its place and dominance in western medical practice. Increasingly common and effective chemical therapies in the early 20th century also added to its stature. Major competing theories in the mid- to late-19th century were naturopathy, osteopathy, homeopathy, and chiropractic. Osteopaths are educated in osteopathic medical schools, but in virtually all other respects are the same as allopaths. Many osteopaths enter allopathic residency training programs. Holistic medicine is a contemporary theory of disease causation emphasizing health promotion and prevention. It is increasingly considered complementary to allopathy.

In 1950, there were 79 United States medical schools; by 1970 there were 103. In 1990, there were 126 accredited medical schools with 65,016 students.[36] In 1989, 16,781 MDs were graduated. It is projected that the number of medical school graduates will decline to 15,774 by the year 2000.[37] Medical schools are accredited by the Liaison Committee on Medical Education, which is composed of representatives of professional associations in medicine and medical education. Osteopathic physicians are educated at 15 colleges of osteopathic medicine, which graduated more than 1,617 DOs in 1989.[38] In 1988, there were more than 23,000 DOs in the United States.[39] In 1991, Canada had 16 accredited medical schools, none of them osteopathic, which graduated 1,708 MDs in 1990.[40]

Two major studies in the late 1970s reported that more medical schools and greater numbers of students would cause a physician surplus by the late 1980s. This led to a decrease in state and federal support. The end of federal capitation grants to medical schools (a fixed payment per student) meant that tuition or subsidies from other sources had to be increased. Some medical schools have financial problems and may close. Others are reducing admissions. The extent of public support in the past is shown by the fact that in 1979 medical student tuition and fees paid only a little over 5% of the cost; 55% was paid directly by government. Income from hospitals and clinics, nongovernmental grants and contracts, and endowment and philanthropy covered the difference.[41] Tuition and fees continued to contribute only 4.3% of revenues in 1989–1990. The largest contributions during this time came from practice plans (29.8%), state and local governments (14.1%), and federally funded research (13.0%).[42] Out-of-state tuition at some public medical schools and tuition at some private (nongovernmental) medical schools was almost $25,000 per year in 1991.

Following graduation from medical school, which is either a 4-year postbaccalaureate education or sometimes part of a 6- or 7-year combined baccalaureate-medical doctor (MD) degree, the new physician begins a residency.* Intern is a title no longer used to describe new medical school graduates who engage in full-time postgraduate clinical training. The generic concept used is postgraduate year. Each postgraduate year (the years following graduation from medical school) is numbered. A PG-II has had 1 year of clinical experience after medical school and is in the second. Such experience is also termed a residency; those in residencies are called residents. Each medical specialty determines the number of postgraduate years and the specific clinical content of those years so that the program may be accredited and consequently be the basis for eligibility to be certified in that specialty. For example, anesthesiology requires 1 year of general residency and 3 years of residency in anesthesiology; family practice requires 3 years of residency in family practice; neurological surgery requires 1 year of general residency and 5 years of neurological surgery residency.[44] Residents are supervised in their clinical activities by more senior residents and by teaching faculty (physicians) who are active staff at the hospital. Residencies are accredited by the Accreditation Council for Graduate Medical Education (successor to the Liaison

---

*In the early 1980s some medical schools implemented admissions policies designed to reverse a trend toward goal-oriented training in premedical education. For example, the Johns Hopkins University School of Medicine Flexible Medical Admissions Program offered ensured deferred admission to accepted undergraduate juniors and seniors. This relieves much of the pressure associated with gaining entrance to medical school and encourages students to pursue broader studies.[43]

Committee on Graduate Medical Education), which is composed of professional associations in the medical field. Each specialty has a residency review committee that sets standards for specialty training and accredits the program.

Physicians are licensed in most states after passing an examination and completing 1 year of residency. Some states require 2 years of residency. The license granted by the state is unlimited in terms of activities a physician may undertake. Thus, physicians may legally prescribe all medications (except some narcotics and experimental drugs) and perform all medical and surgical activities. It is only in the HSO that the scope of this otherwise unlimited right to practice medicine is modified. Limiting practice activities to those consistent with demonstrated current competence is especially important in acute care hospitals because of the acuity of illnesses and the significant treatments provided there. However, protecting the patient by ensuring the competence of physicians and other LIPs, such as podiatrists and dentists, is vital in all HSOs. This is done through the credentialing process, which includes a review of didactic and clinical experience, licensure, specialty certification, and health status, among other aspects. Periodic review of clinical performance in the HSO is part of the recredentialing process that is necessary for the practitioner to continue to have privileges in that HSO. Credentialing and recredentialing is detailed in Chapter 7, "How HSOs Are Organized." In the early 1990s, state medical boards came under significant criticism for failing to be sufficiently aggressive in disciplining physicians with problems related to their professional activities.[45]

Nonphysician Caregivers

Nowhere is there greater fragmentation and specialization of work than in HSOs. Each new technology seems to require another type of technical expertise. In the early years of modern medicine, physicians usually worked independently of other caregivers. As support became necessary, some physician activities were performed by technicians. Nursing is the earliest example, and sonographers are among the most recent.

These changes will continue as old technologies evolve and others are introduced. The use of roentgen rays (the x-ray), which were discovered by Wilhelm Roentgen in 1895, is an instructive example. Roentgenology became radiology. In turn, it bifurcated into diagnostic radiology and therapeutic radiology. Diagnostic radiology has added computers, analysis of cellular emissions, and use of sound waves, and has become known as diagnostic imaging. Similarly, therapeutic radiology now includes linear accelerators added to x-ray equipment, and the use of radioactive sources has spawned the specialty of nuclear medicine. Organization and specialization are needed to deliver state-of-the-art medicine, but such services are available only at considerable economic and organizational cost.

Dentists Dentists are LIPs who typically provide services in an office or clinic. They may be employed or be on an HSO's attending staff. In either case, they should be subject to a credentialing process; it is required in hospitals.

Dentistry is the art and science of healing concerned with the oral region of the human body. Dentists are educated in 56 dental schools in the United States and 10 in Canada.[46] These dental schools graduated 4,233 and 457 dentists, respectively, in 1990.[47] To become a doctor of dental surgery (DDS) or doctor of dental medicine (DMD) in the United States requires a minimum of 6 years beyond high school, including at least 2 years of predental education.[48] The dental school curriculum concentrates on basic sciences, applying health sciences to delivery of oral health services, and applying basic biomedical and dental sciences to the practice of dentistry. About 10% of dentists are specialists. Specialization requires a minimum of 2 years of advanced study and practice at the postdoctoral level. Specialty areas include dental public health, endodontics, oral pathology, oral and maxillofacial surgery, pedodontics, periodontics, and prosthodontics.[49] In 1990, 15 states issued specialty licenses in most of these specialty areas.[50] The issuance of specialty licenses distinguishes dentistry from medicine. Certification by the medical specialty boards, albeit by private organizations, has a similar effect. Table 2.3 shows 142,200 dentists in the United States civilian sector in 1988.

Podiatrists   Podiatrists are LIPs who typically provide services in an office or clinic. They may be employed or be on an HSO's attending staff. In either case, they should be subject to a credentialing process; it is required in hospitals.

Podiatry is the branch of the healing arts and sciences that treats the foot and its related or governing structures by medical, surgical, or other means. Three years of undergraduate education are required for admission to one of the seven colleges of podiatric medicine in the United States. The first 2 years of instruction emphasize basic medical sciences, such as anatomy, physiology, microbiology, biochemistry, pharmacology, and pathology. The last 2 years emphasize clinical sciences, including general diagnosis, therapeutics, surgery, anesthesia, and operative podiatric medicine. Graduates are awarded the degree of doctor of podiatric medicine (DPM). Most graduates take a residency of from 1 to 3 years. Podiatrists are licensed throughout the United States. The American Podiatric Medical Association has approved specialty boards in podiatric orthopedics, podiatric surgery, and podiatric public health.[51]

Nurses   Early recognition and increased stature of nursing were achieved largely through the efforts of Florence Nightingale, an Englishwoman who worked in the mid-19th century. Until then, secular nursing had a poor reputation. Dorothea Dix was an early nursing leader in the United States. As education and professional standards improved and licensing was introduced in the United States, registered nurses (RNs) became second only to physicians on the patient care team. Nurse licensing began in the early 1900s and initially concentrated on state registration. In March 1903, North Carolina nurses were the first to succeed in establishing state registration, and only persons found qualified by a board of examiners could be listed as registered nurses. Successful applicants were allowed to use the initials RN and were listed in a county registry. In 1923, all states and the District of Columbia and Hawaii had *voluntary* nurse licensure.[52] In 1991, all states and the District of Columbia had mandatory licensing statutes.[53] RNs are licensed, but with rare exceptions are not LIPs.

It is estimated that 1.6 million of the 2 million licensed RNs in the United States (80%) are working as nurses.[54] Contributing to the nursing shortage that began in the mid-1980s have been changes in hospital staffing patterns (focus on primary nursing [all-RN staff]); decreasing use of other types of nursing personnel, which are described below; demand for RNs outside the acute care hospital; and failure of beginning RN salaries to keep pace with inflation.[55] In 1989, significant percentages of RN positions in various types of HSOs were vacant: hospitals (12.7%), nursing facilities (18.9%), home health agencies (12.9%), and health maintenance organizations (10.5%).[56] The early 1990s experienced a resurgence of interest in nursing, and this augurs well for the health services field.[57] HSO managers will be challenged to recruit and retain RNs, as well as use RN resources effectively. (Productivity is addressed in Chapter 11, "Quality and Productivity Improvement"; employee recruitment and retention are discussed in Chapter 17, "Personnel/Human Resources Management."

RNs are educated in programs of varying length located in different educational settings: associate (2 years), diploma (hospital based, 3 years), or baccalaureate (college or university based, 4 years). Organized nursing developed a strong preference for baccalaureate-trained nurses, which led to a rapid decline in the number of diploma programs in the late 1960s and early 1970s. This caused major dislocations in the health services field and directly contributed to the RN shortage in the 1970s and indirectly to that in the 1980s. Nursing as a profession has yet to clearly define its role and relationship to the physician.

In 1991, the National League for Nursing (NLN) accredited 1,109 of the 1,470 basic RN programs in the United States. Total basic RN programs included 489 baccalaureate programs (47 not accredited), 829 associate degree programs (313 not accredited), and 152 diploma programs (1 not accredited).[58]

In addition to RNs, there are licensed practical nurses (LPNs), who are sometimes called licensed vocational nurses (LVNs). Nurse aides (sometimes called nursing assistants) are another common category of nursing personnel. Practical nurses and nurse aides are clinically and usually administratively subordinate to the RN.

In the late 1970s, the American Nurses Association (ANA) undertook an RN certification program. In 1991, there were 20 clinical and 2 administrative areas for certification, such as community health nurse, gerontological nurse, clinical specialist in medical-surgical nursing, and nursing administration. Each has different requirements, but all include clinical experience and passing an examination, as well as current licensure.[59] In 1982, almost 11,000 RNs were certified by the ANA.[60] By 1991, there were more than 77,000.[61]

Most states have categories of personnel who were RNs first and then obtained preparation in a specialty. Examples are nurse-clinicians and nurse-practitioners. A few are certified by private associations (e.g., certified registered nurse-anesthetists and certified nurse-midwives). Certified nurse-midwives, for example, are licensed as RNs, certified by the American College of Nurse-Midwives, and licensed in almost one half of the states as nurse-midwives. Such persons are LIPs.

Pharmacists   A type of nonphysician caregiver commonly found in HSOs is the pharmacist. Professional pharmacists emerged later than professional nurses and their role in the spectrum of care is narrower than that of nurses. Pharmacists are educated in 74 colleges and schools of pharmacy in the United States. Pharmacists may earn a baccalaureate in pharmacy in a 5-year program or a doctorate in pharmacy in a 6-year program. Licensure requires graduation from an accredited program, completion of an internship, and passing a state board licensing examination. Most states participate in a national licensing examination administered by the National Association of Boards of Pharmacy. Pharmacists are not LIPs and respond to orders written by LIPs such as physicians, podiatrists, and clinical psychologists. Table 2.3 shows that there were 157,800 pharmacists in the United States in 1988.

Dietitians   A type of nonphysician caregiver always found in hospitals and nursing facilities is the dietitian. Dietitians may do nutritional counseling in health maintenance organizations and other HSOs, as well. Like pharmacists, dietitians emerged later than nurses and their role in the spectrum of care is narrower than that of professional nursing. Historically, dietitians were registered by a professional society, the American Dietetic Association. Beginning in the mid-1980s they began to be licensed or certified in a number of states. In 1991, dietitians were licensed in 16 states, certified in 9, and registered in 1.[62] Dietitians are educated in 4-year programs that include a majority of didactic education, but with a significant component of clinical experience that is 1 year or longer.

Technologists   Radiologic technologists include radiographers, radiation therapists, nuclear medicine technologists, and diagnostic medical sonographers. The titles reflect the extent of specialization. As an example, radiographers are trained in a 2-year program that may be based in a junior college or hospital. There are 4-year programs leading to a bachelor of science in radiologic technology. Most of the training is scientific and clinical. Radiographers are certified by the American Registry of Radiologic Technologists.[63]

Medical technologists are usually trained in a 4-year curriculum, although some programs are shorter; a significant portion is clinical. They perform various tests in chemistry, immunology, bacteriology, and hematology. Training programs are usually found in a university affiliated with a hospital laboratory. They are certified by the AMA and the American Society of Clinical Pathologists. In 1991, about one half of the states had licensing or certification laws for medical technologists. Both radiologic technicians and medical technologists are dependent nonphysician caregivers in that they act only in response to the order of an LIP and have no independent access to the patient.

Physician Assistants   Another type of dependent caregiver commonly found in HSOs is the physician assistant (PA). PAs are not licensed and need not be RNs. PAs are trained in a 24-month program, approximately half of which is devoted to clinical rotations in which students work in medical settings under close supervision of a physician. A number of programs award baccalaureate degrees; some award master's degrees.[64] In their practice PAs work under the direction or supervision of a physician. The National Commission on Certification of Physician Assistants certifies PAs, and this certification is used by the states in regulating PAs.[65] In 1991, 20,000 PAs were practicing in 48 states.[66] "Hospitals are the fastest-growing areas of PA employment. Although approximately 10% of all PAs were employed by hospitals in 1976, more than one third were working in hospitals by 1987."[67]

Shortages of Personnel

A survey in 1988 identified the number of hospitals that had difficulty recruiting and retaining physical therapists (48%), pharmacists (31%), radiologic technologists (25%), medical technologists (22%), and respiratory therapists (7%). It was also reported that 88% of hospitals had difficulty recruiting RNs and 85% reported difficulty retaining them.[68] These findings have limited generalizability beyond hospitals, but they do suggest the types of shortages nonhospital HSOs may face in recruiting and retaining important categories of allied health personnel now and in the future.

Projections about the growth in demand to the year 2000 for various types of health services personnel do not include RNs and pharmacists among those with the greatest increase. The personnel with the top nine percentages of projected growth include physical therapists (87%), medical records technicians (75%), radiologic technologists (65%), occupational therapists (52%), speech pathologists/audiologists (34%), respiratory therapists (34%), dietitians/nutritionists (34%), lab technologists/technicians (24%), and emergency medicine technicians (15%). Such data suggest significant potential problems for HSO managers.[69]

STATE AND FEDERAL REGULATION OF HSOs

When the states delegated certain powers to a federal government and ratified the United States Constitution, they retained a wide range of authority traditionally held by the sovereign. In sum, these are known as the police power, which is defined as the power to protect the health, safety, public order, and welfare of the public. Consistent with the police power, states have enacted legislation to regulate and license a wide variety of HSOs. Licensure as it applies to various types of HSOs is described in Chapter 7. Suffice it to say here that HSOs required to obtain and retain a license must submit to inspections and other regulation.

Inspections

Inspections by state and local authorities concentrate on the physical plant and safety. The Life Safety Code, which is published by the National Fire Protection Association, a private voluntary association, is a prominent source for standards. Unless a problem is being investigated, however, the authorities pay little attention to quality of care. City and county ordinances also apply to HSOs (because some state powers have been delegated to local government), but these tend to address matters such as radiation safety, sanitation of food and water, and disposal of wastes.

Planning and Rate Regulation

Much of what happens in the states is stimulated by federal government. As noted, the Hill-Burton Act of 1946 encouraged statewide planning for hospital services. In 1966, the Comprehensive Health Planning Act encouraged use of planning methodologies to allocate resources and improve access in the health services field more appropriately and contain costs. States were expected to develop health planning agencies known as "a" and "b" agencies to assist in health planning.

In the late 1960s, states began enacting laws to control the problems of increasing health services costs. They were especially concerned about cost increases in Medicaid, which affected them directly. These initiatives sought to control capital expenditures and the costs of health services through rate review. States such as New York and Maryland were among the first to enact capital expenditure review laws. Others were prompted by the Social Security Amendments of 1972 (PL 92-603). This law included two provisions important to HSOs. One established professional standards review organizations (PSROs) to review the quantity and quality of care provided for Medicare patients in hospitals. PSROs complemented the planning legislation by seeking to control use of health services, thus reducing costs. In addition, section 1122 of the law required capital expenditure review, which enhanced planning agency control. Because of the disproportionately large amount of money consumed by hospitals as compared with other types of HSOs (more than 40% of the total), a great deal of attention has been and is being directed at them.

The National Health Planning and Resources Development Act of 1974 (PL 93-641) mandated that each state have a health planning and development agency and a network of health systems agencies (HSAs). The HSAs superseded the scattered areawide health planning agencies ("b" agencies) established in the 1966 law and made recommendations to the state health planning and development agency or the state health coordinating council, which applied state certificate-of-need (CON) laws and gave final approval. Planning laws sought to control costs by focusing on the supply of services.

CON laws required HSOs to obtain approval for adding a new service or for construction or renovation projects exceeding a certain cost, usually several hundred thousand dollars. The purpose was to rationalize the supply of health services by controlling capital expenditures and preventing unneeded expansion. Critics of CON argued that this artificial limitation on the supply of services caused inflation. In 1983, 49 states had CON laws.[70]

In the late 1970s criticism about the usefulness of mandated planning grew. The antiregulatory mood in health services fit with the movement toward deregulation elsewhere in the economy. On January 1, 1987, the National Health Planning and Resources Development Act of 1974 was repealed.[71] In the years since, states have scaled back their involvement in planning. By 1989, 11 states had repealed CON review programs and 5 others had deregulated hospitals and other acute care services.[72] In 1991, 39 states continued to have some type of CON program.[73] "Most states, have taken a . . . moderate approach, streamlining programs, deregulating services and providers—particularly those perceived as not contributing to long-term health cost increases—and raising expenditure threshold levels to exempt all but the most costly projects."[74]

As of 1983, mandatory health services rate review (cost review) programs had been enacted in six states.[75] In addition, there were more than 20 voluntary programs. By regulating what HSOs charged or were paid, the states began to treat them as public utilities. States with rates of increase in health services costs below the national average were exempt from the federal diagnosis-related group (prospective payment) system for Medicare patients. In the mid-1980s exempt states included New York, New Jersey, Maryland, and Massachusetts.[76] By 1991, only Maryland was exempt. Since 1971, Maryland has had a highly regulated, all-payor system to pay for hospital-based in- and outpatient care. For 15 consecutive years, hospital costs in Maryland rose at rates below the national average. In 1990 for example, hospital cost increases were 8.7% compared with a national average of 8.96%, an estimated saving of $5.3 million to Marylanders.[77] Hospital costs are increased an average of about 7% to pay the costs of uncompensated care.[78] The success of the Maryland system may provide a model for other states.

UR, PSROs, and PROs[79]

Utilization review (UR) was a mandated part of hospital participation in the original Medicare law. Hospitals were required to certify the necessity of admission, continued stay, and professional services rendered to Medicare beneficiaries. Review was totally delegated to hospitals.

Rapid Medicare cost increases in the late 1960s suggested that hospital-based UR programs were ineffective. PSROs were established by the Social Security Amendments of 1972 (PL 92-603) as federally funded physician organizations responsible to assure the appropriateness, medical necessity, and quality of care furnished to Medicare beneficiaries. As with UR, emphasis in the PSRO program was on hospital review. PSRO hospital review had three related functions:

Admission and continued stay review. Criteria were used to determine which cases needed physician peer review; such review was performed on either a concurrent or a retrospective basis. Initially 100%, review was decreased to focused review.

Quality assurance. These activities were directed toward identifying deficiency areas to improve quality of care.

Profile analysis. PSROs had a data system to profile patients, practitioners, and providers; compare current and previous patterns of care; and identify utilization patterns that deviated from locally established norms.

Ten years later PSROs had not proved cost effective, nor had they proved to have a significant effect on quality. To remedy these problems, Congress established professional review organizations (PROs) as part of the Tax Equity and Fiscal Responsibility Act of 1982. The law required that PROs be outcome oriented (rather than process and structure oriented) and that outcomes be measured against performance standards. Provisions include:

Hospitals must have an agreement with a PRO to perform review in order to participate in Medicare.

PROs may be for-profit or not-for-profit organizations either comprising physicians, osteopaths, and dentists actively practicing medicine in the PRO area or having available at least one physician in every generally recognized specialty for physician review purposes. Preference is given to physician-sponsored organizations.

PRO areas are generally statewide; there were 53 in 1991.

PROs contract with the federal government.

PROs perform utilization and quality review and take corrective action, as necessary. Required activities include validation of diagnosis-related groups and admission, transfer, and outlier review. Other types of review have been added. For example, the Consolidated Omnibus Budget Reconciliation Act of 1985 added a requirement for second opinions for surgery and denial of payment for care that is substandard; the Omnibus Budget Reconciliation Act of 1986 added review of ambulatory surgery and quality review of health maintenance organizations and competitive medical plans; the Omnibus Budget Reconciliation Act of 1987 added a requirement that allows 20 days for providers and physicians to discuss tentative PRO findings and requires a survey of health maintenance organization enrollees to assess issues.

The core of PRO activities is that they are to deny Medicare payment for medically unnecessary care or care rendered in an inappropriate setting, or if it is determined that the quality of care was substandard. In addition, they are to educate problem providers; review 100% of problem cases; exert peer pressure; and, where correction is not achieved or where a gross and flagrant quality problem occurs, recommend that the provider be excluded from participating in the Medicare program.

A clear emphasis over the years has been to expand the scope of work for PROs to include all federal payments for medical services. Part of this trend will be to include care in physicians' offices. A major initiative for the early 1990s is implementation of a uniform clinical data set to enhance the ability of PROs to consistently select cases that require review. This data base will allow epidemiological studies and inter-PRO comparisons. The future will likely emphasize quality rather than utilization.

PROs have had their critics, however. Criticism has focused on the fact that few physicians and hospitals have been disciplined by PROs. From 1986 to early 1990, a total of fewer than 100 sanctions had been issued by PROs. Some PROs have never issued a sanction. Another measure of PRO effectiveness is the percentage of denied payments for what were deemed to be inappropriate hospital admissions. Between 1986 and 1988, 2.1% of all hospital admissions were deemed inappropriate by PROs. By comparison, the inspector general of the Department of Health and Human Services found 10% of admissions were inappropriate; a further random sample of Medicare patients found 12% inappropriate.[80] Clearly, much work remains.

Diagnosis-Related Groups

By the early 1980s a more direct means of cost control was undertaken when the Tax Equity and Fiscal Responsibility Act of 1982 and the Social Security Amendments of 1983 mandated a prospective payment system (PPS) for Medicare through diagnosis-related groups (DRGs). The Health Care Financing Administration (HCFA), which is the component of the Department of Health and Human Services (DHHS) responsible for administering Medicare and Medicaid, established fixed rates for each Medicare inpatient admission by diagnosis. In 1990, there were 490 DRGs.[81] Hospitals that can provide services at lower costs may retain the difference. Those exceeding the DRG rate must make up the difference from other sources.

The change from cost-based reimbursement to payment according to rates prospectively determined by HCFA has had and will continue to have major effects on hospitals. One is that they were inspired to unbundle subacute, recuperative, and rehabilitative care from a patient's acute-episode hospital stay. For example, hospital-based nursing facility beds were established to provide transitional care. Previously, reimbursement was based on costs and there were few incentives for efficiency. Under prospective payment, hospitals must be certain that their average costs per DRG do not exceed HCFA rates. Managers and physicians will have to collaborate to eliminate unnecessary tests and procedures and reduce length of stay, and, in general, hospitals will have to become more efficient. The DRG payment system initially applied only to Medicare patients, but state Medicaid programs, Blue Cross, and other third-party payors increasingly use it for inpatient services. Moreover, DRG-like methodologies will be used for outpatient clinics and nursing facilities in the future.

Resource Utilization Groups

Diagnosis-related groups are applied to hospitalized Medicare beneficiaries. Long-term care is developing its own classification system in which nursing facility residents who have similar resource consumption are put into groups. Initially, these groups were based on the ability of nursing facility residents to engage in activities of daily living (ADL), which are major explanatory factors in resource use. Since the mid-1980s, resource utilization groups (RUGs) have undergone significant derivation and validation and have evolved to RUG-II.

> A classification based on ADLs would clinically be relatively barren and thus would likely not find clinical acceptance. The RUG-II system utilizes a clinical hierarchy of five types of residents (heavy rehabilitation, special care, clinically complex, severe behavioral problems, and reduced physical functions). A second component is a summarization of the ADLs into an index based on toileting, eating, and transfer. Together, these produce a system of 16 relatively homogeneous groups of nursing [facility] residents.[82]

In 1991, RUG-II was in use to determine nursing facility payment for Medicaid in New York and Texas, and there were plans to implement it in at least six other states.[83] It is a concept that is likely to spread, and the ongoing development of RUG-III is further evidence of the continuing interest in this concept.

Ambulatory Patient Groups

Other points of service delivery have drawn the attention of regulators and lawmakers. It is likely that a DRG-like payment system will be used for hospital outpatient services in the near future.[84] Research in the late 1980s led to development of ambulatory patient groups (APGs). APGs are designed to explain the amount and type of resources used in an ambulatory visit. Patients in each APG are assumed to have similar clinical characteristics, similar resource use, and similar costs.[85] There are differences between DRGs and APGs, however. The hospital inpatient DRG system assigns each patient to a single DRG. Under the APG system, patients are described by a list of APGs that correspond to each service provided. Diversity of outpatient service settings, wide variation in why outpatient care is required, and the high percentage of costs associated with ancillary services necessitate a classification scheme that can reflect the diversity of services rendered.[86]

The incentives in such payment systems may lead to underutilization of services and consequently to inappropriate treatment of patients. The DRG system of payment is apparently causing patients to be discharged from hospitals more rapidly. A Rand Corporation study reported in 1990 found that mortality rates of Medicare patients have been unchanged by DRGs, but it also showed that more patients have been released from hospitals in an unstable state since DRGs began.[87] This finding has significant implications for home health agencies, nursing facilities, and of course, for hospitals. Continued surveillance and caution are needed.

Resource-Based Relative Value Scale

In 1992, HCFA began implementing a fee schedule for physicians who participate in Part B of Medicare, a change mandated by the Omnibus Budget Reconciliation Act of 1989 (PL 101-239). Previously, physician payment under Part B was based on usual, customary, and reasonable charges. Among the most important results of the previous method of payment was that procedure-based specialties such as surgery were more highly paid than specialties based on cognitive skills (e.g., evaluation and management), such as internal medicine. The new schedule uses a resource-based relative value scale (RBRVS)[88] and results in dramatic changes in physician payment patterns. The prospectively set reimbursement is a function of the resources used to produce physician services and is divided into three components: physician work, practice expenses, and malpractice insurance.[89] Nonphysician practitioners whose services are paid under Part B of Medicare continue to have their fees tied to those of the physician, and their fees move in the same direction as those of the physician. Thus, the greater the proportion of a nonphysician practitioner's time devoted to evaluation and management services, the greater the likelihood that Medicare income will rise.[90]

The RBRVS system increases reimbursement for family and general practice physicians by about 15%; payments to ophthalmologists and anesthesiologists decline the most, about 35%, but those to other procedure-based specialists such as surgeons decrease as well.[91] Publication in mid-1991 of a proposed physician fee schedule that projected a 16% decrease in payments to all physicians by 1996 caused a storm of controversy.[92] To prevent physicians who have not signed a Medicare participation agreement (accepting Medicare as full payment for services [sometimes called assignment]) from balance-billing patients, the Omnibus Budget Reconciliation Act imposes a cap on the amount a nonparticipating physician may balance-bill a Medicare beneficiary.[93] The federal application of RBRVS is only to Medicare. However, RBRVS is very likely to be used by other third-party payors—as they have used DRGs. The effect will be a major change in how physicians are paid. Other likely effects are that physicians employed in high-technology practices will generate less income for their employers; physicians will try to unbundle services and move more of them out of hospitals to their offices; physicians may seek to have lost income made up by hospitals; physicians may limit their willingness to care for Medicare beneficiaries; and adjustments in how physicians are paid in rural compared with urban areas will make it easier for rural hospitals to attract physicians, thus increasing access by rural beneficiaries while potentially decreasing it for urban beneficiaries.[94]

Other Regulators

In addition to the DHHS, which affects reimbursement through HCFA, a multitude of federal regulators affect management of HSOs. These activities are based on authority in the federal Constitution to regulate interstate commerce and to provide for the general welfare. Regulators include independent agencies such as the Securities and Exchange Commission and various other executive branch departments and bureaus. The Department of Justice and Federal Trade Commission enforce the Sherman Antitrust Act (1890) and the Clayton Act (1914) and their various amendments prohibiting anticompetitive practices. The National Labor Relations Board applies provisions of the National Labor Relations Act (1935) and its amendments to the process of union organizing and collective bargaining. The Occupational Safety and Health Administration enforces provisions of the Occupational Safety and Health Act (1974) to safeguard the work environment. The Food and Drug Administration enforces provisions of the Food, Drug, and Cosmetic Act of 1906 and its amendments and regulates drugs and medical devices. The Securities and Exchange Commission enforces the Securities Exchange Act of 1934, as amended, and affects how investor-owned HSOs market, sell, and trade stock. The Nuclear Regulatory Commission enforces provisions of the Atomic Energy Act (1954) and regulates and licenses the nuclear industry, thus regulating hazards arising from storage, handling, and transportation of nuclear materials. The Equal Employment Opportunity Commission enforces the Equal Pay Act of 1963, Title VII of the Civil Rights Act of 1964, and the Age Discrimination in Employment Act of 1967, among others, and investigates complaints about treatment of employees. The Bureau of Alcohol, Tobacco, and Firearms of the Treasury Department enforces the alcohol and tobacco tax provisions of the Internal Revenue Code and the Alcohol Administration Act of 1935 and regulates use of tax-free alcohol.

It should be noted that many federal regulatory, review, and control activities have been applied to HSOs only since the early 1970s. This resulted in significant dislocation and some paranoia on the part of HSO managers. Too many changes occurred too rapidly; there was too little time to adjust and assimilate.

JOINT COMMISSION ON ACCREDITATION OF HEALTHCARE ORGANIZATIONS

No voluntary, private organization has affected HSOs, especially hospitals, as has the Joint Commission on Accreditation of Healthcare Organizations (Joint Commission), which until 1986 was known as the Joint Commission on Accreditation of Hospitals (JCAH). The Joint Commission traces its lineage to the Hospital Standardization program established by the American College of Surgeons (ACS), which began surveying hospitals in 1918. Until 1951, the ACS single-handedly worked to improve hospital-based medical practice. Its director during most of this highly formative period was Malcolm T. MacEachern, a physician who was an early leader in the hospital field. In 1951, the Joint Commission was formed by the ACS, the AMA, the AHA, the American College of Physicians, and the Canadian Medical Association, which later left the Joint Commission and assisted in establishing the Canadian Council on Health Facilities Accreditation. The new

Joint Commission began accrediting hospitals in 1953. In addition to commissioners sent by the founding organizations, one is sent by the American Dental Association and there are 3 public commissioners, for a total of 24 commissioners on the Joint Commission's governing body.[95]

Use of the word "hospitals" in its title had become a misnomer because the Joint Commission accredited several types of HSOs long before its name was changed. The accreditation program for hospitals is its largest, but there are also programs for mental health care, home care, ambulatory care, and long-term care. Each has its own standards, but duplication for multiprogram HSOs is eliminated by combining visits from various accreditation activities. This means HSOs with two or more types of health services programs accredited by the Joint Commission will not have different surveyors reviewing compliance with common standards, such as physical plant, licensure, and corporate bylaws.

Standards for various services and facilities are developed by professional and technical advisory committees (PTACs) established by the Joint Commission. PTACs are composed of experts who often also represent health services professional and trade associations. In this sense, the Joint Commission leads the various components of the health services system that it accredits, but at the same time it reflects their level of development. Being too far ahead of the field makes standards overly demanding and difficult to meet, but merely reflecting the state of development limits progress.

The importance of a hospital being accredited by the Joint Commission was greatly enhanced in 1965 with passage of Medicare, which specified that Joint Commission–accredited facilities were in "deemed status" (eligible) for purposes of Medicare reimbursement. In 1966, "conditions of participation" and applicable procedures were distributed to hospitals by the Department of Health, Education, and Welfare, now DHHS. The conditions of participation corresponded to the Joint Commission's 1965 standards and focused on minimum levels of performance. By 1970 the Joint Commission's *Accreditation Manual for Hospitals* emphasized optimum achievable rather than minimal standards and had grown from 10 pages in 1965 to 152 pages.[96] Legislation in 1972 mandated federal oversight of Joint Commission accreditation: the secretary of the DHHS was authorized to develop conditions of participation more stringent than Joint Commission standards and to review accredited hospitals on the basis of random sampling or complaints. The conditions of participation emphasized physical plant (Life Safety Code) and safety and minimized the content and processes of clinical practice and organization; Joint Commission emphases were the opposite. Revised conditions of participation became effective in 1986. The two programs have evolved toward each other; if they become substantially alike, the Joint Commission may become redundant.

The Joint Commission lists several benefits that result from accreditation:

> Identification of strengths and weaknesses with particular attention to areas in which performance
>   may be improved;
> On-site education and consultation;
> Increased staff morale and enhanced ability to recruit professional staff;
> Public recognition of the organization's commitment to quality;
> Eligibility for reimbursement by many third-party payers;
> Immediate eligibility to participate in the Medicare program; and
> Recognition, in most states, of compliance with state licensure requirements.[97]

In 1989, the Joint Commission implemented its "Agenda for Change," a program to evaluate the clinical and organizational performance of hospitals. The Joint Commission is in the process of developing clinical indicators—quantitative measures to evaluate patient care that do not directly measure quality but instead flag areas that require further review.[98] The indicators will allow interhospital comparisons of performance.

The Joint Commission will continue to be a major force in developing performance expectations for HSOs. Even those that choose not to be accredited by the Joint Commission will benefit from considering its standards in developing and managing their programs. The Joint Commission's emphasis in the 1990s will be continuous quality improvement, the theory and application of which are described in Chapter 12, "Control, Risk Management, Quality Assessment/Improvement, and Resource Allocation."

ASSOCIATIONS FOR PERSONS AND ORGANIZATIONS

The health services field has many professional and trade associations that represent personal and institutional providers, both in generic groups and in an increasingly large number of subsets.

Personal Professional Associations

Managers   The premier professional association for HSO managers is the American College of Healthcare Executives (ACHE), formerly the American College of Hospital Administrators (ACHA), which was established in 1933. It has more than 22,000 affiliates. Membership includes those in managerial positions running the gamut of HSOs. The important categories of affiliation are nominee, member, and fellow. Each is separated by time and achievement requirements, which include number of years in the category, passing an examination, or submitting case studies. ACHE offers a variety of continuing educational activities and publishes and enforces a code of ethics.

Examples of other professional groups include specialized managerial personnel in HSOs: the Academy of Medical Group Management, the American College of Mental Health Administrators, the American College of Health Care Administrators (nursing facilities), and the American College of Osteopathic Hospital Administrators. Some have levels of affiliation and advancement requirements. All provide a forum and educational activities to improve the content and quality of professional practice. The American Public Health Association does not focus on managers but has a broad membership of those in public health and other HSOs.

Physicians   Preeminent among physician groups is the American Medical Association (AMA). It was formed in 1847; in 1991 it had 288,275 members, including physicians, medical students, and residents.[99] The AMA is synonymous with "organized medicine," and it has been both a conservative and a progressive force in health care. Its conservatism is exemplified by historical opposition to national health insurance and resistance to salaried physician arrangements as well as to innovations such as health maintenance organizations, which were seen as infringing on professional independence and total commitment to the patient. The AMA has been a progressive force by embracing programs such as Medicare once enacted, and by encouraging federal expenditures for basic and applied research and medical and paramedical education. Its involvement in establishing standards for medical education and licensure have contributed significantly to the unequalled standards of American medicine and medical practice. The AMA publishes and enforces a code of ethics.

Other Physician Affiliations   There are many other associations for physicians. The National Medical Association represents about 16,000 African-American physicians and has goals similar to those of the AMA. In addition, there are associations, usually termed "colleges" or "academies," whose membership is based on medical specialties. Among the most prominent are the American College of Physicians and the American College of Surgeons. The titles fellow or diplomate are used to refer to affiliates. As with the ACHE, these associations represent the interests of affiliates and assist them in continuing education.

Nonphysician Affiliations   The list of other associations of individuals in health services is almost endless. Each new type of provider sees the need for a professional association to focus common interests. Some are not so recent; the American Nurses Association was established in 1896.[100] Other examples of nonphysician providers include the American Dental Association, the

American Podiatry Association, the American Psychological Association, the Association of Operating Room Nurses, the National Association of Social Workers, the American Pharmaceutical Association (pharmacists), the National Federation of Licensed Practical Nurses, and the American Academy of Physician Assistants. The hundreds of professional associations for organizational and personal providers and managers in the health services field are a measure of its specialization and fragmentation.

Organizational Professional Associations

American Hospital Association (AHA)   With 4,850 institutional members having 978,615 beds, the AHA is the most prominent association for hospitals.[101] Founded in 1898, the AHA educates and represents its members. Increasingly, it is the focal point for hospitals' efforts to participate in the political process. In 1991, the AHA's executive offices were moved to Washington, D.C., while its other activities remained in Chicago. In many respects the AHA is an umbrella organization—members are likely to belong to other institutional associations with more specialized orientations. Examples are described below. Representing hospitals with divergent goals and objectives make the AHA's role difficult.

Federation of American Health Systems (Federation)   The Federation is the investor-owned counterpart to the AHA. It was established in 1966 and in 1990 had a membership of almost 1,400 institutions in the United States, Puerto Rico, and 11 foreign nations. The Federation's chief function is to serve as the investor-owned hospital industry's advocate to Congress, the executive branch, the media, academia, and the public. In addition, it is the clearinghouse from which members and others can obtain information on health care issues and industry positions, policies, and statistics.[102]

American Osteopathic Hospital Association (AOHA)   The AOHA is the trade association for osteopathic hospitals. In 1991, it had 98 members. There are approximately 200 osteopathic hospitals in the United States.[103] Osteopathic hospitals were established to provide treatment based on the theory that the body is capable of making its own remedies against disease when it is in its normal structural relationship and has a favorable environment and nutrition. These hospitals still emphasize the importance of normal body mechanics and manipulative methods of detecting and correcting structural problems. However, they also utilize generally accepted conventional medical and surgical treatment, and osteopathic medical training is very much like that for allopathic physicians. Osteopathic hospitals may be accredited by the American Osteopathic Association (AOA), as well as by the Joint Commission. In 1991, the AOA accredited 138 osteopathic hospitals, with 22,437 beds.[104]

Other Hospital Associations   The Catholic Health Association and Protestant Hospital Association represent subsets of hospitals with sectarian ownership and interests. The former is much larger and more influential. In addition, there are regional and state hospital associations that link affiliation to geographical or state communities of interest. As states have become more involved in regulatory and control processes, state hospital associations have increasingly undertaken lobbying.

American Health Care Association (AHCA)   The AHCA, founded in 1949, is the largest trade association for long-term care providers in the United States. In 1991, its membership included 10,000 not-for-profit (25%) and for-profit (75%) facilities, with 1 million residents.[105] AHCA promotes professional standards in delivery of long-term care. It is active in the federal political process as an advocate for its members.

American Association of Homes for the Aging (AAHA)   The AAHA is the trade association for voluntary and public not-for-profit homes for the aging, health-related facilities, and homes and community services. Its member organizations serve more than 500,000 persons. The AAHA has established group insurance and purchasing programs for its members. In addition, it is active in lobbying at the federal level.[106]

Group Health Association of America (GHAA) The GHAA is the trade association for all types of health maintenance organizations (HMOs). It assists in organizing new plans and expanding existing plans through consultation, public relations, and research. It is active in legislative affairs that promote the interests of group practice. In 1991, it had 290 member plans, which was about one half of the HMOs in the United States.[107]

Medical Group Management Association (MGMA) The MGMA was established in 1926 and seeks to improve the management of medical group practice (ambulatory care) by enhancing the professionalism of group managers; providing education programs and material; engaging in research; establishing liaison with consumers, providers, and others involved in health care; and being active in government relations. In 1991, MGMA had 11,800 members.[108]

EDUCATIONAL ACCREDITORS

The quality of the didactic and clinical programs in which health service workers are educated must be reviewed. Monitoring groups are organized similarly to the Joint Commission. Various accreditors have boards (policy-making bodies) composed of representatives from important professional groups in their fields. Accrediting committees, commissions, and groups have greater importance if they are recognized by the Office of Postsecondary Education of the Department of Education. Accreditation by a recognized accreditor is one of eight criteria that make a program eligible for federal support. There are, however, alternatives to accreditation acceptable to the Department of Education.

Managers

Programs for graduate education of health services managers are accredited by the Accrediting Commission on Education for Health Services Administration (ACEHSA). ACEHSA's board is composed of representatives from various professional and institutional associations in the health field, as well as public members. They include the ACHE, the AHA, the Association of University Programs in Health Administration (the programs' trade association), the American College of Health Care Administrators, the American College of Medical Group Administrators, the Association of Mental Health Administrators, the American Public Health Association, and a joint seat occupied by the Canadian Hospital Association and the Canadian College of Health Service Executives.[109] The accreditation process is similar to that of the Joint Commission. In 1991, ACEHSA accredited 60 graduate programs in the United States and Canada.

The Council on Education for Public Health (CEPH) accredits schools of public health and certain graduate public health programs offered in educational settings other than schools of public health. Schools of public health often have management emphases in their curricula. CEPH is composed of representatives from the American Public Health Association, the Association of Schools of Public Health, and graduate program and public representatives. In 1991, CEPH accredited 24 schools of public health, 9 graduate programs in community health education, and 12 graduate programs in community health/preventive medicine.[110]

Accreditors cooperate with one another when health services management education is sited in schools or programs that are accredited by more than one of them. For example, the American Assembly of Collegiate Schools of Business (AACSB) accredits graduate (and undergraduate) business programs. If health services management graduate education and business graduate education are found in the same unit, accreditation activities are coordinated. In addition, when there is overlap, efforts are made to make standards and reporting formats compatible.[111]

Physicians

Figure 2.4 shows the relationships among various medical groups and accreditors of medical education at different levels. At the far left, the Council for Medical Affairs provides policy development and review activities. The Liaison Committee on Medical Education, the Accreditation

PARENT ORGANIZATIONS OF THE CFMA, LCME, ACGME, AND ACCME
PARENT ORGANIZATIONS ESTABLISH POLICY

ABMS AMA AHA AAMC CMSS

COUNCIL FOR MEDICAL AFFAIRS

FUNCTION:
Forum for discussion of issues relevant to medical education

REPRESENTATIVES

Two senior elected officers and the Chief Executive Officer of:
ABMS
AMA
AHA
AAMC
CMSS

CFMA Secretary
P.O. Box 7586
Chicago, IL 60680

AMA   AAMC

LIAISON COMMITTEE ON MEDICAL EDUCATION

FUNCTION:
Accrediting M.D. programs

REPRESENTATIVES

AMA (6)
AAMC (6)
CACMS (1)
Public (2)
Participants (non-voting):
   Students (2)
   Federal (1)

LCME Secretary
(odd years)
515 N. State St.
Chicago, IL 60610

(even years)
1 Dupont Circle N.W.
Washington, D.C. 20036

ABMS AMA AHA AAMC CMSS

ACCREDITATION COUNCIL FOR GRADUATE MEDICAL EDUCATION

FUNCTION:
Accrediting GME Programs

REPRESENTATIVES

ABMS (4)
AMA (4)
AHA (4)
AAMC (4)
CMSS (4)
Resident Physicians
   Section AMA (1)
Public (1)
Federal (non-voting) (1)

ACGME Secretary
515 N. State St.
Chicago, IL 60610

ABMS AMA AHA AAMC CMSS AHME FSMB

ACCREDITATION COUNCIL FOR CONTINUING MEDICAL EDUCATION

FUNCTION:
Accrediting CME Providers

REPRESENTATIVES

ABMS (3)
AMA (3)
AHA (3)
AAMC (3)
CMSS (3)
AHME (1)
FSMB (1)
Public (1)
Federal (non-voting) (1)

ACCME Secretary
Box 245
Lake Bluff, IL 60044

AAMC	Association of American Medical Colleges	
ABMS	American Board of Medical Specialties	
AHA	American Hospital Association	
AHME	Association For Hospital Medical Education	
AMA	American Medical Association	
CACMS	Committee on Accreditation of Canadian Medical Schools	
CMSS	Council of Medical Specialty Societies	
FSMB	Federation of State Medical Boards	

Figure 2.4. Relationships among various medical groups and accreditors of medical education at different levels. (From American Board of Medical Specialties Research & Education Foundation. *Annual report & reference handbook—1991*, 49. Evanston, IL, 1991; reprinted by permission.)

Council for Graduate Medical Education, and the Accreditation Council for Continuing Medical Education accredit various levels of medical education. The importance of continuing medical education as part of a lifelong learning experience is apparent.

Nurses

The National League for Nursing (NLN) accredits schools of nursing. The NLN supports and accredits nursing education in all settings: baccalaureate (4-year, university–based, leading to a bachelor of science in nursing [BSN]), diploma (3-year, hospital–based, leading to a diploma in nursing), and associate (2-year, junior college–based, leading to an associate of arts [AA]). In this sense it has been at odds with the nurse professional association, the American Nurses Association, which supports BSN preparation. The NLN is composed of individuals, educational institutions, and nursing service agencies.[112]

Medical Specialty Boards

In 1991, there were 23 specialty boards in various branches of medicine and surgery. Recognition of specialization came late in the development of medicine in the United States, and undoubtedly gained impetus from the tremendous expansion of medical technology that occurred early in the 20th century. The American Board of Ophthalmology was the first formed, in 1917; the most recent, Emergency Medicine, was formed in 1976. Each board offers a general certification of specialization. In addition, most boards recognize subspecialization by offering certificates of special qualifications and certificates of added qualifications.[113]

Boards play a vital role by certifying training and monitoring continued competence of physicians who claim special expertise and skills. Through their association, the American Board of Medical Specialties (ABMS), the boards play a significant role in undergraduate, postgraduate, and continuing medical education. Figure 2.4 shows these relationships. It is notable that the various specialty boards are themselves composed of representatives of associations organized around the particular specialty.

Although the Accreditation Council accredits residencies, the content of residency education is largely determined by the residency review committees—much as the professional and technical advisory committees do for the Joint Commission. The importance of continuing medical education is evidenced in that several specialty boards require a minimum number of hours of such education during a specific period of time. In addition, several have instituted recertification policies, which means specialists must demonstrate continuing competence to remain certified. The trend is to increase these requirements.

Managers and members of professional staff organizations must be increasingly vigilant regarding board certification. In 1989, there were 105 *self-designated* medical specialty boards that had no ABMS recognition.[114] The proliferation of boards dilutes a major reason for specialty certification: allowing the public to identify practitioners who have earned formal recognition of skill in a specialty. The problem is especially significant outside the HSO, where there are few controls. Some states are beginning to regulate use of the terms "board certification" and "board certified."[115]

Board certification alone does not entitle any physician to clinical privileges in an HSO. Similarly, neither does state licensure. Licensure is more basic, and lawful medical practice is impossible without it; specialty certification is only one indicator of competence. The HSO has an independent moral and legal duty to determine competence initially and then to continually monitor the care delivered in it by LIPs, board certified or not. The credentialing process is detailed in Chapter 7, "How HSOs Are Organized."

FINANCING HEALTH SERVICES

Expenditure Trends

For almost 3 decades, the percentage of gross national product (GNP) devoted to health services has increased. Table 2.6 provides a wealth of information about aggregate and per capita national health expenditures, as well as percentage distribution and average annual percentage growth by source of funds. These expenditures are shown in current dollars (unadjusted for inflation). Table 2.6 shows that in 1989 health services consumed 11.6% of the GNP, or $604.1 billion. National health expenditures continue to increase rapidly, and it is projected that they will consume 14.7% of GNP ($1,072.7 billion) by 1995 and 16.4% of GNP ($1,615.9 billion) by the year 2000. The period of rapid inflation occurred soon after passage of Medicare and Medicaid in 1965; this demand-push stimulation was undoubtedly instrumental in the initial and continuing cost increases. These increases have been a major factor in state and federal efforts to control health services costs, or at least limit what they will pay. Table 2.7 shows national health care expenditures as aggregate amounts and by type of expenditures for selected years from 1965 through 2000.

Because such a large percentage of expenditures is consumed by hospitals (see Figure 2.5), most state and federal cost control has been directed at them. It is alleged that hospitals have been inefficiently managed and that excessive use of high technology, expensive tests, and treatments have been major causes of cost increases.

Sources and Uses of Funds in Health Care

This section describes sources and consumption of funds in various parts of the United States health care system. Figure 2.5 shows sources of funds for national personal health expenditures and how they were used from 1960 to 1980 and projections for their use for 1990 and 2000. Private sources, which were more than 75% in 1960, continued their decline from 1960 on, although less dramatically. After a very large increase between 1970 and 1980, the share borne by federal government increased much more slowly between 1980 and 1990; a significant increase is projected between 1990 and 2000, however. The portion paid by state and local government declined between 1960 and 1980, but an increase is projected between 1980 and 2000. In terms of national personal health spending, the large share consumed by hospitals is obvious. Nursing home (nursing facility) care expenditures increased 20% between 1970 and 1980, but stabilized by 1990. Expenditures for drugs and other medical nondurables declined more than 25% between 1970 and 1980. "Other professional services" increased steadily between 1970 and 1990, with increases of about 50% in each decade from a small base. Total expenditures in Figure 2.5 do not include program administration and net costs of private health insurance, government public health activities, and research and construction. These account for the difference in total expenditures between it and Table 2.6.

Tables 2.8 and 2.9 show annual percentage increases for various items on the consumer price index (CPI) for selected years since 1950. Table 2.8 shows all items and selected components on the CPI compared with the medical care component. With few exceptions, the percentage increase of the medical care component has consistently been greater than that of all other items. In several years energy had greater increases than medical care, but in one year it had a larger decrease and in several years very small increases. Medical care has maintained steady, significant increases year after year.

Table 2.9 shows the average annual percentage change for all items and various components of medical care. Hospital and related services had double-digit increases in the 20 years following enactment of Medicare. Increases slowed somewhat after 1985. The contribution of physicians' services to medical care services has also been significant but is considerably less than hospital

Table 2.6. National health expenditures aggregate and per capita amounts, percent distribution, and average annual percentage growth, by source of funds: selected years 1965–2000[a]

Item	1965	1975	1980	1985	1989	1990	Projected[b] 1991	1992	1995	2000
						Amount in billions				
National health expenditures	$41.6	$132.9	$249.1	$420.1	$604.1	$670.9	$738.2	$809.0	$1,072.7	$1,615.9
Private	31.3	77.8	143.9	245.0	350.9	388.7	419.8	455.5	586.8	842.1
Public	10.3	55.1	105.2	175.1	253.3	282.2	318.4	353.6	485.8	773.7
Federal	4.8	36.4	72.0	123.6	174.4	192.8	217.0	240.8	330.1	534.9
State and local	5.5	18.7	33.2	51.5	78.8	89.4	101.4	112.8	155.7	238.8
						Number in millions				
U.S. population[c]	204.0	224.7	235.3	247.2	257.0	259.6	262.1	264.6	272.0	282.9
						Amount in billions				
Gross national product	$705	$1,598	$2,732	$4,015	$5,201	$5,463	$5,650	$6,045	$7,284	$9,865
						Per capita amount				
National health expenditures	$204	$592	$1,059	$1,699	$2,351	$2,585	$2,817	$3,057	$3,944	$5,712
Private	154	346	612	991	1,365	1,498	1,602	1,721	2,158	2,977
Public	50	245	447	708	985	1,087	1,215	1,336	1,786	2,735
Federal	24	162	306	500	679	743	828	910	1,214	1,891
State and local	27	83	141	208	307	344	387	426	572	844

(continued)

Table 2.6. *(continued)*

Item	1965	1975	1980	1985	1989	1990	1991	Projected[b]		
								1992	1995	2000
Percentage distribution										
National health expenditures	100.0	100.0	100.0	100.0	100.0	100.0	100.0	100.0	100.0	100.0
Private	75.3	58.5	57.8	58.3	58.1	57.9	56.9	56.3	54.7	52.1
Public	24.7	41.5	42.2	41.7	41.9	42.1	43.1	43.7	45.3	47.9
Federal	11.6	27.4	28.9	29.4	28.9	28.7	29.4	29.8	30.8	33.1
State and local	13.2	14.1	13.3	12.3	13.1	13.3	13.7	13.9	14.5	14.8
Percentage of gross national product										
National health expenditures	5.9	8.3	9.1	10.5	11.6	12.3	13.1	13.4	14.7	16.4
Average annual percentage growth from previous year shown										
National health expenditures	—	12.3	13.4	11.0	9.5	11.1	10.0	9.6	9.9	8.5
Private	—	9.5	13.1	11.2	9.4	10.8	8.0	8.5	8.8	7.5
Public	—	18.3	13.8	10.7	9.7	11.4	12.8	11.0	11.2	9.8
Federal	—	22.4	14.6	11.4	9.0	10.6	12.5	11.0	11.1	10.1
State and local	—	13.1	12.1	9.2	11.3	13.3	13.4	11.3	11.3	8.9
U.S. population[c]	—	1.0	0.9	1.0	1.0	1.0	1.0	1.0	0.9	0.8
Gross national product	—	8.5	11.3	8.0	6.7	5.0	3.4	7.0	6.4	6.3

From Sonnefeld, Sally T., Daniel R. Waldo, Jeffrey A. Lemieux, and David R. McKusick. Projections of national health expenditures through the year 2000. *Health Care Financing Review* 13 (Fall 1991):16.

Note: Columns may not add up to totals because of rounding. Data source: Health Care Financing Administration, Office of the Actuary: Data from the Office of National Health Statistics.

[a]*Note:* Columns may not add up to totals because of rounding.

[b]1990 and later data revised by supplement of November, 1991, to the Sonnefeld et al. paper.

[c]July 1 Social Security area population estimates.

68

Table 2.7. National health expenditures as aggregate amounts and by type of expenditure (billions of dollars): United States, selected years 1965–2000[a]

Type of expenditure	1965	1975	1980	1985	1989	1990	1991	Projected		
								1992	1995	2000
National health expenditures	41.6	132.9	249.1	420.1	604.1	670.9	738.2	809.0	1,072.7	1,615.9
Health services and supplies	38.2	124.7	237.8	404.7	583.5	648.6	714.4	783.8	1,043.1	1,576.1
Personal health care	35.6	116.6	218.3	367.2	530.7	589.3	651.1	716.7	956.5	1,456.0
Hospital care	14.0	52.4	102.4	167.9	232.8	257.7	285.4	313.9	425.4	654.2
Physician services	8.2	23.3	41.9	74.0	117.6	132.7	148.5	165.5	225.6	360.5
Dental services	2.8	8.2	14.4	23.3	31.4	33.8	36.1	38.6	47.1	63.1
Other professional services	0.9	3.5	8.7	16.6	27.0	30.7	34.5	38.7	51.6	75.4
Home health care	0.1	0.4	1.3	3.8	5.4	6.5	7.5	8.5	12.1	18.8
Drugs and other medical nondurables	5.9	13.0	20.1	32.3	44.6	48.5	51.8	55.5	67.7	91.0
Vision products and other medical durables	1.2	3.1	5.0	8.4	13.5	14.3	14.9	16.1	20.0	28.4
Nursing home care	1.7	9.9	20.0	34.1	47.9	53.6	59.1	64.9	85.8	130.8
Other personal health care	0.8	2.7	4.6	6.8	10.5	11.5	13.3	14.9	21.3	33.9
Program administration and net cost of private health insurance	1.9	5.1	12.2	25.2	35.3	40.5	43.3	45.9	60.8	85.3
Government public health activities	0.6	3.0	7.2	12.3	17.5	18.8	20.0	21.2	25.8	34.8
Research and construction	3.5	8.3	11.3	15.4	20.6	22.3	23.8	25.2	29.6	39.8
Research[b]	1.5	3.3	5.4	7.8	11.0	11.7	12.5	13.3	16.1	22.3
Construction	1.9	5.0	5.8	7.6	9.6	10.6	11.3	11.9	13.5	17.5

From Sonnefeld, Sally T., Daniel R. Waldo, Jeffrey A. Lemieux, and David R. McKusick. Projections of national health expenditures through the year 2000. *Health Care Financing Review* 13 (Fall 1991): 17.

[a]Data source: Health Care Financing Administration, Office of the Actuary: Data from the Office of National Health Statistics. *Note:* Columns may not add up to totals because of rounding.

[b]Research and development expenditures of drug companies and other manufacturers and providers of medical equipment and supplies are excluded from research expenditures, but they are included in the expenditure class in which the product falls.

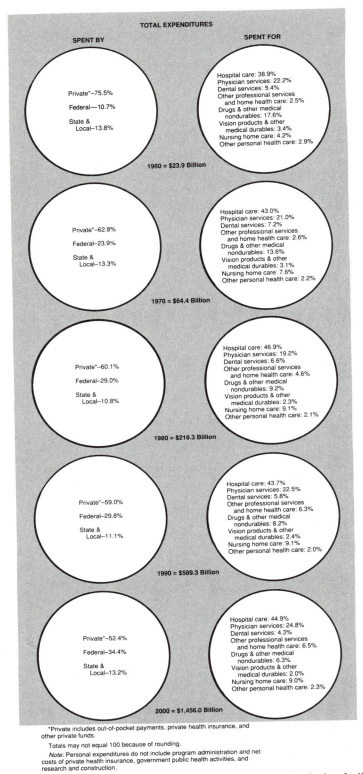

TOTAL EXPENDITURES

SPENT BY

SPENT FOR

Private*–75.5%
Federal—10.7%
State & Local–13.8%

Hospital care: 38.9%
Physician services: 22.2%
Dental services: 9.4%
Other professional services and home health care: 2.5%
Drugs & other medical nondurables: 17.6%
Vision products & other medical durables: 3.4%
Nursing home care: 4.2%
Other personal health care: 2.9%

1960 = $23.9 Billion

Private*–62.8%
Federal–23.9%
State & Local–13.3%

Hospital care: 43.0%
Physician services: 21.0%
Dental services: 7.2%
Other professional services and home health care: 2.6%
Drugs & other medical nondurables: 13.6%
Vision products & other medical durables: 3.1%
Nursing home care: 7.6%
Other personal health care: 2.2%

1970 = $64.4 Billion

Private*–60.1%
Federal–29.0%
State & Local–10.8%

Hospital care: 46.9%
Physician services: 19.2%
Dental services: 6.6%
Other professional services and home health care: 4.6%
Drugs & other medical nondurables: 9.2%
Vision products & other medical durables: 2.3%
Nursing home care: 9.1%
Other personal health care: 2.1%

1980 = $218.3 Billion

Private*–59.0%
Federal–29.8%
State & Local–11.1%

Hospital care: 43.7%
Physician services: 22.5%
Dental services: 5.8%
Other professional services and home health care: 6.3%
Drugs & other medical nondurables: 8.2%
Vision products & other medical durables: 2.4%
Nursing home care: 9.1%
Other personal health care: 2.0%

1990 = $589.3 Billion

Private*–52.4%
Federal–34.4%
State & Local–13.2%

Hospital care: 44.9%
Physician services: 24.8%
Dental services: 4.3%
Other professional services and home health care: 6.5%
Drugs & other medical nondurables: 6.3%
Vision products & other medical durables: 2.0%
Nursing home care: 9.0%
Other personal health care: 2.3%

2000 = $1,456.0 Billion

*Private includes out-of-pocket payments, private health insurance, and other private funds.

Totals may not equal 100 because of rounding.

Note: Personal expenditures do not include program administration and net costs of private health insurance, government public health activities, and research and construction.

Figure 2.5. Sources and uses of personal health expenditures, 1960, 1970, and 1980, and projections for 1990 and 2000. (Data for 1960 and 1970 from Levit, Katharine R., Helen C. Lazenby, Cathy A. Cowan, and Suzanne W. Letsch. National health expenditures, 1990. *Health Care Financing Review* 13 [Fall 1991]: 45–46. Data for 1980 and projections for 1990 and 2000 from Sonnefeld, Sally T., Daniel R. Waldo, Jeffrey A. Lemieux, and David R. McKusick. Projections of national health expenditures through the year 2000. *Health Care Financing Review* 13 [Fall 1991]: 18, 20, 24.)

Table 2.8. Average annual percentage change in Consumer Price Index for all items and selected items: United States, selected years 1950–1989[a]

Year	All items	Medical care	Food	Apparel and upkeep	Housing	Energy	Personal care
1950–55	2.1	3.8	1.8	1.3	—	—	2.7
1955–60	2.0	4.1	1.5	1.3	—	—	3.0
1960–65	1.3	2.5	1.4	0.9	—	0.4	1.1
1965–70	4.3	6.2	4.0	4.4	—	2.2	3.5
1970–75	6.8	6.9	8.8	4.1	6.9	10.5	5.9
1975–80	8.9	9.5	7.7	4.6	9.9	15.4	7.2
1975–76	5.8	9.5	3.0	3.7	6.1	7.1	6.6
1976–77	6.5	9.6	6.3	4.5	6.7	9.5	6.5
1977–78	7.6	8.4	9.9	3.6	8.7	6.3	6.4
1978–79	11.3	9.2	11.0	4.3	12.3	25.1	7.6
1979–80	13.5	11.0	8.6	7.1	15.7	30.9	8.9
1980–85[b]	5.5	8.7	4.0	2.9	5.8	3.4	5.7
1980–81	10.3	10.7	7.8	4.8	11.5	13.6	8.8
1981–82	6.2	11.6	4.1	2.6	7.2	1.5	7.1
1982–83	3.2	8.8	2.1	2.5	2.7	0.7	5.1
1983–84	4.3	6.2	3.8	1.9	4.1	1.0	4.0
1984–85	3.6	6.3	2.3	2.8	4.0	0.7	3.8
1985–86	1.9	7.5	3.2	0.9	3.0	−13.2	3.3
1986–87	3.6	6.6	4.1	4.4	3.0	0.5	2.9
1987–88	4.1	6.5	4.1	4.3	3.8	0.8	3.7
1988–89	4.8	7.7	5.8	2.8	3.8	5.6	4.7

From National Center for Health Statistics, Public Health Service, U.S. Department of Health and Human Services. *Health United States 1990,* 188. Washington, D.C.: U.S. Government Printing Office, 1991.

[a]Data source: Bureau of Labor Statistics, U.S. Department of Labor: Consumer Price Index, various releases. (Data are based on reporting by samples of providers and other retail outlets.)

[b]1982–84 = 100.

and related services. Data such as these have caught the attention of federal policy makers. DRGs and RBRVs have been their response.

Much of the cost of health services is borne by employers, and many have been instrumental in forming coalitions to find ways to control them. Coalitions bring together hospitals, physicians, employers, labor, insurers, and sometimes government to collect and exchange data and discuss how to finance and deliver health services in a community. In 1988, there were approximately 150 coalitions in the United States, and most cities over 100,000 population have one.[116] Despite these and other efforts, total employer health plan costs almost doubled between 1985 and 1990, increasing from $1,724 to $3,217 per employee.[117]

Private Payment Under the Insurance Principle The first insurer to write "sickness" insurance did so in 1847, but the insurance industry, which was to become a giant of American business during the mid-1900s, paid little attention to health insurance until after World War II. Contributing to this lack of interest was a perception that sickness, and consequently paying for its treatment, was too unpredictable to fit into existing actuarial concepts.

It was not until 1929 that Blue Cross showed it could be done. Blue Cross began when a group of school teachers made an agreement with Baylor Hospital in Dallas, Texas, that it would provide room and board and certain diagnostic services for a specified monthly fee. In 1932, the first citywide plan was established with a group of hospitals in Sacramento, California. The comparable plan for physicians' services became known as Blue Shield and was established in California in 1939. Hospitals fostered development of Blue Cross to enhance their patients' abilities to

Table 2.9. Average annual percentage change in Consumer Price Index for all items and medical care components: United States, selected years 1950–1989[a]

Item and medical care component	1950–1960	1960–1965	1965–1970	1970–1975	1975–1980	1980–1985[b]	1985–1987	1987–1988	1988–1989
CPI, all items	2.1	1.3	4.3	6.8	8.9	5.5	2.8	4.1	4.8
Less medical care	—	1.2	4.1	6.7	8.8	5.3	2.5	3.9	4.6
CPI, all services	3.6	2.0	5.6	6.5	10.2	7.1	4.6	4.6	4.9
All medical care	4.0	2.5	6.2	6.9	9.5	8.7	7.1	6.5	7.7
Medical care services	4.3	3.1	7.3	7.6	9.9	8.6	7.2	6.4	7.7
Professional medical services	—	—	—	6.5	8.9	7.8	6.5	6.8	6.5
Physicians' services	3.4	2.8	6.6	6.9	9.7	8.2	7.3	7.2	7.4
Dental services	2.5	2.3	5.3	6.3	8.2	7.7	6.2	6.8	6.3
Eye care[c]	—	—	—	—	—	—	—	5.0	3.4
Services by other medical professionals[c]	—	—	—	—	—	—	—	5.8	5.4
Hospital and related services	6.6	5.8	13.9	10.2	12.2	10.9	6.5	9.3	11.5
Hospital rooms	—	—	—	—	—	11.2	6.6	9.3	10.3
Other inpatient services[c]	—	—	—	—	—	—	—	9.7	13.1
Outpatient services[c]	—	—	—	—	—	—	—	8.9	10.8
Medical care commodities	1.7	-0.8	0.7	2.8	7.2	8.8	6.6	6.8	7.8
Prescription drugs	2.2	-2.4	-0.2	1.6	7.2	10.6	8.3	8.0	8.7
Nonprescription drugs and medical supplies[c]	—	—	—	—	—	—	5.1	4.8	6.0
Internal and respiratory over-the-counter drugs	—	—	1.6	4.1	7.7	8.4	4.5	5.6	6.1
Nonprescription medical equipment and supplies	—	—	—	—	—	6.7	—	3.6	5.8

From National Center for Health Statistics, Public Health Service, U.S. Department of Health and Human Services. *Health United States 1990*, 189. Washington, D.C.: U.S. Government Printing Office, 1991.

[a] Data source: Bureau of Labor Statistics, U.S. Department of Labor: Consumer Price Index (CPI), various releases. (Data are based on reporting by samples of providers and other retail outlets.)

[b] 1981–1984 = 100, except where noted.

[c] December 1986 = 100.

pay the costs of hospitalization. By 1991, most Blue Cross and Blue Shield plans in the United States had merged into 55 combined plans; 20 Blue Cross or Blue Shield plans remained independent.[118]

Private health insurance coverage grew rapidly during the 1940s and 1950s. It received a boost during World War II when wages and salaries were subjected to federal controls but fringe benefits were not. Commercial carriers began writing health insurance in substantial amounts, and by 1955 they had more insureds than Blue Cross. By 1981, over 1,000 commercial insurance companies were writing health insurance in the United States.[119] Table 2.10 shows key health insurance statistics for 1985–1990. Overwhelmingly, private insurance coverage comes through the employment relationship. Table 2.10 shows that 189 million Americans had private health insurance coverage in 1989—76.2% of the population. The percentage increases to 87.4% when public programs are included. What is not known from these data is the extent of coverage and its adequacy to meet health needs of insureds. Table 2.11 shows the number of enrollees by type of plan and type of private health insurance carrier. In the late 1980s, the estimates of those without health insurance were between 31.3 (Table 2.10) and 37 million.[120] Some uninsureds are self-pay; most are medically indigent. These estimates do not show, however, the number who actually are unable to get care.

Historically, Blue Cross has been a service plan. Service plans pay providers directly, pursuant to a contract with them. More recently some Blue Cross plans have offered other types of coverage to be more competitive. In contrast to service plans, under indemnity plans—the type usually written by commercial insurers—the insured is indemnified (paid) by the company. There are dollar limits for each diagnosis or treatment. Assignment is a variation of indemnification. The insured assigns the right to payment to the provider, who receives payment directly. Blue Cross policies have limits, but they are expressed in days of care and services covered. Under Blue Shield, payment is made to the physician according to a fee schedule. Participating physicians accept payment under the fee schedule as payment in full (they have in effect accepted assignment); nonparticipating physicians bill the patient, who is reimbursed per the schedule. Another difference between Blue Cross (and Blue Shield) and commercial carriers is that the former are organized as not-for-profit corporations that pride themselves on low overhead costs in plan administration.

The percentage of expenditures paid directly by the consumer varies by type of service. Table 2.12 shows payments for hospital care, nursing home (nursing facility) care, and physician services from various sources. The decline in out-of-pocket payments for all three types of services is the most striking aspect of these data. The growth in importance of Medicare as a source of payment is noteworthy.

Government Programs   As noted, until 1965 the federal government concentrated on providing the wherewithal to support the private delivery of services. It financed little care. Direct services are provided to groups such as veterans, military personnel, and American Indians. State governments provide services for special health problems such as mental illness, tuberculosis, and mental retardation. States also operate general acute care teaching hospitals in connection with state medical schools. Other public HSOs, typically general acute care hospitals, are owned by local governments.

Figure 2.5 and Table 2.12 show the increases in public expenditures for health services. The federal government has sought to control the increase in expenditures through programs such as PROs, DRGs, and RBRVS. The states have sought to slow the growth in Medicaid expenditures by hospital preadmission screening, limiting hospital days available to any beneficiary, reducing what is paid for each day of care or each service, paying months or years after bills are submitted by the HSO, requiring patients to pay larger co-payments for optional services, increasing eligi-

Table 2.10.   Key health insurance statistics

	1985	1986	1987	1988	1989	1990	Percentage change, 1988–1989	Percentage change, 1990–1991
Persons with and without health care coverage[a] (millions)								
Total population	235.5	238.2	240.5	243.1	247.9	NA	0.7	NA
Persons with public and private coverage	204.2	204.7	208.7	211.6	216.6	NA	0.9	NA
Private health insurance	180.1	180.1	181.1	188.4	189.0	NA	0.3	NA
Employer-related	147.1	145.8	146.7	153.3	153.8	NA	0.3	NA
Persons without coverage	31.3	33.5	31.8	31.5	31.3	NA	−0.6	NA
Private health insurance claims payments[b] (billions)								
Total[c]	$117.6	$128.5	$151.7	$171.1	$185.3	NA	8.3	NA
Insurance companies	59.9	64.3	72.5	83.0	89.4	NA	7.7	NA
Blue Cross-Blue Shield	37.5	40.6	44.5	48.2	50.7	NA	5.2	NA
Other plans[c]	32.5	36.8	56.5	62.8	99.8	NA	27.1	NA
Private health insurance payment by category of service[d] (billions)								
Total	$134.1	$143.5	$156.3	$174.4	$196.4	$216.8	12.6	10.4
Hospital care	59.5	63.8	69.5	75.4	83.2	89.4	10.3	7.5
Physicians' services	33.7	38.3	43.9	49.1	52.8	58.2	7.5	10.2
Dentists' services	9.1	9.9	11.0	12.4	13.5	15.1	8.9	11.9
Other professional services[e]	5.2	6.1	7.5	8.9	10.6	12.8	19.1	20.8
Drugs and medical nondurables	5.2	5.5	6.0	6.5	7.3	8.3	12.3	13.7
Vision products and other medical durables	0.7	0.8	0.9	1.0	1.2	1.3	20.0	8.3
Home health care	0.3	0.3	0.3	0.3	0.4	0.5	33.3	25.0
Nursing home care	0.3	0.3	0.4	0.5	0.5	0.6	0.0	20.0
Program administration and cost of private health insurance	20.0	18.2	16.9	20.3	26.8	30.7	32.0	14.6

From *Source book of health insurance data,* 7. Washington, D.C.: Health Insurance Association of America, 1991.

[a]Source: U.S. Bureau of the Census, Current Population Survey.

[b]Source: Health Insurance Association of America, Source Book Survey.

[c]Other plans include self-insured plans, self-administered plans, plans employing third-party administrators, and health maintenance organizations.

[d]Source: Health Care Financing Administration, National Health Expenditure Accounts.

[e]Other professional services include fees for chiropractors, podiatrists, psychologists, therapists, audiologists, optometrists, portable X-ray suppliers, ambulance service suppliers, and free-standing ESRD facilities.

bility standards, and decreasing the range of services in the program. For many services Medicaid may pay only half of what it costs the HSO to provide them. Reducing what Medicaid pays has several implications. Other payors must make up the difference or the HSO goes bankrupt. Government programs do not pay charges, nor does Blue Cross. Commercial insurers are increasingly reluctant to pay charges, and the indemnity plans have always paid only a fixed fee regardless of what the beneficiary is charged. It is only self-pay patients who must pay charges, which reflect

Table 2.11. People with private insurance protection by type of insurer (millions)[a]

End of year	All insurers[b]	Insurance companies			Blue Cross-Blue Shield	Other plans[c]
		Total[b]	Group	Individual/family		
1940	12.0	3.7	2.5	1.2	6.0	2.3
1945	32.0	10.5	7.8	2.7	18.9	2.7
1950	76.6	37.0	22.3	17.3	38.8	4.4
1955	101.4	53.5	38.6	19.9	50.7	6.5
1960	122.5	69.2	54.4	22.2	58.1	6.0
1961	125.8	70.4	56.1	22.4	58.7	7.1
1962	129.4	72.2	58.1	23.1	60.1	6.9
1963	133.5	74.5	61.5	23.5	61.0	7.2
1964	136.3	75.8	63.1	34.0	62.1	6.8
1965	138.7	77.6	65.4	24.4	63.3	7.0
1966	142.4	80.4	67.8	24.9	65.3	6.6
1967	146.4	82.6	71.5	24.6	67.2	7.1
1968	151.9	85.7	74.1	25.3	70.1	7.3
1969	155.0	88.8	77.9	25.9	72.7	7.7
1970	158.8	89.7	80.5	26.7	75.1	8.1
1971	161.8	91.5	80.6	27.8	76.5	8.5
1972	164.1	93.7	81.5	29.1	78.2	8.1
1973	168.5	94.5	83.6	27.5	81.3	9.6
1974	173.1	97.0	85.4	28.8	83.8	11.1
1975	178.2	99.5	87.2	30.1	86.4	13.1
1976	176.9	97.0	86.8	27.0	86.6	14.9
1977	179.9	100.4	89.2	28.7	86.0	18.1
1978	185.7	106.0	92.6	36.1	85.8	21.5[f]
1979	185.7	104.1	94.1	34.4	86.1	25.5[f]
1980	187.4	105.5	97.4	33.8	86.7	33.2[f]
1981	186.2	105.9	103.0	25.3	85.8[f]	40.3[f]
1982	188.3	109.6	103.9	29.4	82.0[f]	48.2[f]
1983	186.6	105.9	104.6	22.2	79.6[f]	53.6[f]
1984	184.4	103.1	103.0	20.4	79.4[f]	54.4[g]
1985	181.3	100.4	99.5	21.2	78.7[f]	55.1[g]
1986	180.9	92.5	95.2[e]	11.7[e]	78.0[f]	64.9[g]
1987[d]	179.7	91.0	94.7[e]	10.0[e]	76.9[f]	66.9[g]
1988[d]	182.3	93.3	96.8[e]	10.7[e]	74.0[f]	71.3[g]
1989[d]	185.6	91.7	95.7[e]	9.7[e]	72.5[f]	77.1[g]

From *Source Book of Health Insurance Data,* 24. Washington, D.C.: Health Insurance Association of America, 1991. Reprinted by permission of Health Insurance Association of America.

[a]Data sources: Health Insurance Association of America, Blue Cross and Blue Shield Association, U.S. Department of Health and Human Services, Group Health Association of America, and Foster Higgins. *Note:* Some data were revised from previous editions. Data for 1978 and later have been adjusted downward due to new data on average family size. For 1975 and later, data include the number of persons covered in Puerto Rico and U.S. territories and possessions. Persons covered under insurance company ASO agreements and MPPs are included in the categories total insurance companies and group policies.

[b]The data in these columns refer to the net total of persons protected by more than one kind of insuring organization or more than one insurance company policy providing the same type of coverage, duplication.

[c]Other plans include self-insured plans, self-administered plans, plans employing third-party administrators, and health maintenance organizations.

[d]Data for 1987 and 1988 reflect the revised HIAA survey form and 1989 data reflect a change in the methodology.

[e]Excludes hospital indemnity coverage, which had been included in prior years. For 1989, group hospital indemnity coverage was 6.3 million individuals and individual hospital indemnity was 8.9 million individuals.

[f]Estimate.

[g]For 1984 and later, estimates of persons covered by "other plans" have been developed by HIAA in the absence of other available data.

Table 2.12. Expenditures on hospital care, nursing home care, and physician services and percentage distribution, according to source of funds: United States, selected years, 1960–1988[a]

Service and year	Total in billions	Out-of-pocket payments	Private health insurance	Other private funds	Government Total[b]	Government Medicaid	Government Medicare
			Percent distribution				
Hospital care							
1960	$9.3	20.7	35.6	1.2	42.5	—	—
1965	14.0	19.6	40.9	1.9	37.6	—	—
1970	27.9	9.0	34.4	3.2	53.4	8.1	18.8
1975	52.4	8.4	34.4	2.8	54.5	8.8	21.9
1980	102.4	5.2	36.6	4.9	53.3	9.4	25.8
1983	147.2	5.2	36.6	4.9	53.3	9.0	27.9
1984	157.2	5.1	36.2	4.6	54.0	9.1	28.8
1985	167.9	5.2	35.4	4.9	54.4	9.2	28.9
1986	179.3	4.8	35.4	4.8	55.0	9.2	28.5
1987	193.7	4.5	35.8	4.9	54.8	9.5	27.9
1988	211.8	5.3	35.4	4.9	54.4	9.5	27.5
Nursing home care							
1960	1.0	80.0	0.0	6.4	13.6	—	—
1965	1.7	64.5	0.1	5.8	29.5	—	—
1970	4.9	48.2	0.3	4.9	46.6	28.0	5.0
1975	9.9	42.1	0.7	4.8	52.3	47.5	2.9
1980	20.0	43.3	0.9	3.1	52.7	48.6	2.1
1983	28.9	47.1	1.0	2.3	49.5	45.7	1.8
1984	31.2	47.9	1.1	2.1	48.9	44.9	1.8
1985	34.1	48.6	1.0	1.9	48.5	44.6	1.7
1986	36.7	49.0	1.0	1.9	48.1	44.1	1.6
1987	39.7	47.8	1.0	1.9	49.2	45.2	1.6
1988	43.1	48.4	1.1	1.9	48.6	44.4	1.9
Physician services							
1960	5.3	62.7	30.2	0.1	7.1	—	—
1965	8.2	60.6	32.5	0.1	6.8	—	—
1970	13.6	42.8	35.2	0.1	21.9	4.6	11.8
1975	23.3	32.8	39.3	0.1	27.9	7.1	14.6
1980	41.9	26.9	42.9	0.1	30.2	5.1	19.0
1983	60.6	24.0	43.9	0.0	32.0	4.0	22.0
1984	67.1	23.3	45.3	0.0	31.4	3.8	21.5
1985	74.0	21.8	45.6	0.0	32.6	3.9	22.4
1986	82.1	19.9	46.7	0.0	33.3	3.9	23.1
1987	93.0	19.2	47.3	0.0	33.5	3.8	23.5
1988	105.1	18.9	47.6	0.0	33.4	3.6	23.6

From National Center for Health Statistics, Public Health Service, U.S. Department of Health and Human Services. *Health United States 1990*, 195. Washington, D.C.: U.S. Government Printing Office, 1991.

[a]Source: Office of National Cost Estimates, Office of the Actuary: National health expenditures, 1988. *Health Care Financing Review*. Vol. 11, No. 4. HCFA Pub. No. 03298. Health Care Financing Administration. Washington, D.C.: U.S. Government Printing Office, Summer 1990. (Data are compiled by the Health Care Financing Administration.) *Notes:* These data include extensive revisions back to 1960 and differ from previous editions of *Health, United States*. See Appendix I. The category out-of-pocket payments replaced direct payment. Other private funds replaced philanthropy and industry.

[b]Includes other government expenditures for these health care services, for example, care funded by the Department of Veterans Affairs and state and locally financed subsidies to hospitals.

the amounts third-party payors do not pay. The small number of self-payors makes this increasingly infeasible. *Cost shifting* raises basic questions of fairness.

Should any payor pay less than costs for services? Medicare is a case more politically difficult than Medicaid. This is because Medicare is exclusively a federal program and Congress has been unwilling to cut benefits, although it has increased co-payments and deductibles (Medicare, Part A, hospitalization) and the insurance premium (Medicare, Part B, physicians' treatment) several times in the past 25 years. Medicare has been termed an uncontrollable program. This is true because Congress has been unwilling to put limits on it. Once a beneficiary is eligible, all benefits are available. If any meaningful cost savings are to occur, benefit levels must be controlled. This is politically unpalatable.

TRENDS AND DEVELOPMENTS IN THE SYSTEM

This section describes some of the changes occurring in health services and how they will affect HSO managers. The discussion extrapolates from data and information in this chapter and identifies and describes the effect of *de novo* developments in the field.

Efforts to control what state and federal governments pay for health services programs will continue. The large component of fixed and semivariable costs in HSOs will limit the savings they can achieve. Because institutions, especially hospitals, consume such a large percentage of national health care expenditures, they will receive the most attention. Case-mix cost control through DRGs will subtly pressure hospitals to treat patients with the most remunerative diagnoses. There will be economic pressure to discharge patients as quickly as possible, perhaps earlier than clinically warranted. In addition, treating the less ill with alternative regimens and in HSOs such as ambulatory services leaves only the most ill in acute care hospitals, with the result that costs per patient day will increase. Unless hospitals close beds, discontinue services, and eliminate employees, the cost of hospitalization will rise. Using alternate sources of care is likely only to shift where payment is made, not reduce the total. There is evidence that total costs increase proportionately to the number of alternate sources of care.

Regulation was the watchword of the late 1960s and early 1970s. In the late 1970s and the early 1980s, a competitive environment emerged. Competition continued into the late 1980s, but a dramatic shift occurred as DRGs put major financial pressure on hospitals. These pressures have increased, and public and private payors of medical services have become less and less willing to set payment levels high enough to save the inefficient. The 1980s witnessed large numbers of bankruptcies, mergers, and joint activities among HSOs, especially hospitals. This trend will continue. Predictions in the early 1980s that by the end of the decade there would be a few national hospital systems, some major unaffiliated facilities, and few, if any, small freestanding hospitals proved incorrect. The advantages available to hospitals by joining alliances include shared services, group purchasing, and access to capital without merger or acquisition. Such advantages will enable effectively and efficiently managed HSOs to survive.

Corporate restructuring gained wide acceptance in the early 1980s. The concept has to do with protecting and enhancing the organization's assets and reimbursement, as well as expanding its range of activities. This area is very complex and results from state and federal efforts to control the HSO's income and expenses, as well as its freedom to establish services and facilities. Restructuring has applied almost exclusively to hospitals and is addressed in Chapter 9, "Interorganizational Relationships."

Fragmentation and ultraspecialization of HSO personnel is likely to continue. As a result, the problems of acquiring, retaining, and managing human resources and their appropriate role in HSOs will be exacerbated. These issues are addressed in Chapter 17, "Personnel/Human Resources Management."

INTERNATIONAL COMPARISONS[121]

So far this chapter has presented the conceptual framework for understanding the United States health care system, its historical development, information about health services workers, the HSO's environment, including regulation and accreditation, and the financing of health services. This section provides an international dimension that compares the United States health care system with other countries. First, aggregate health care expenditures among 24 countries are compared. Second, public satisfaction with health care is compared in 10 nations. Then, the Canadian health care system is described and compared with the United States system.

International Health Care Expenditures

Few sources present international health care expenditures in a comparable form. The most comprehensive data set is published by the Organization for Economic Cooperation and Development (OECD), based in Paris, France.[122] The OECD is composed of 24 member countries in western and southern Europe, North America, and selected Pacific rim countries. Member countries are listed in Tables 2.13, 2.14, and 2.15, and health care expenditure information provides a baseline for comparing them.

The OECD data use aggregate public and private expenditures for all health care sectors in each member country and are based on health expenditure and investment information reported as

Table 2.13. OECD (international) total health expenditures as a percentage of gross domestic product, 1970–1989

	1970	1975	1980	1985	1986	1987	1988	1989
Australia	4.9%	5.5%	6.5%	7.0%	7.1%	7.1%	6.9%	7.0%
Austria	5.4	7.3	7.9	7.6	8.3	8.4	8.3	8.2
Belgium	4.1	5.9	6.3	6.9	7.2	7.3	7.3	7.2
Canada	7.1	7.2	7.4	8.5	8.8	8.8	8.6	8.7
Denmark	6.1	6.5	6.8	6.3	6.0	6.3	6.4	6.3
Finland	5.7	6.3	6.5	7.2	7.4	7.4	7.2	7.1
France	5.8	7.0	7.6	8.5	8.5	8.5	8.6	8.7
Germany (West)	5.9	8.2	8.5	8.6	8.5	8.6	8.9	8.2
Greece	4.0	4.1	4.3	4.9	5.4	5.2	5.1	5.1
Iceland	5.2	6.2	6.5	7.4	7.8	7.9	8.5	8.6
Ireland	5.6	7.6	9.0	8.3	8.3	8.0	7.9	7.3
Italy	5.2	6.1	6.8	7.0	6.9	7.3	7.6	7.6
Japan	4.4	5.5	6.4	6.5	6.7	6.8	6.7	6.7
Luxembourg	4.1	5.6	6.8	6.8	6.7	7.2	7.3	7.4
Netherlands	6.0	7.7	8.2	8.2	8.1	8.5	8.4	8.3
New Zealand	5.2	6.7	7.2	6.6	6.9	7.3	7.4	7.1
Norway	5.0	6.7	6.6	6.4	7.1	7.5	7.4	7.6
Portugal	—	6.4	5.9	7.0	6.6	6.4	6.5	6.3
Spain	3.7	4.8	5.6	5.7	5.6	5.7	6.0	6.3
Sweden	7.2	7.9	9.5	9.3	9.0	9.0	9.0	8.8
Switzerland	5.2	7.0	7.3	7.6	7.6	7.9	8.0	7.8
Turkey	—	3.5	4.1	—	—	3.5	—	—
United Kingdom	4.5	5.5	5.8	6.0	6.0	5.9	5.9	5.8
United States	7.4	8.4	9.3	10.6	10.8	11.1	11.3	11.8
Mean[a]	5.4	6.5	7.1	7.4	7.4	7.6	7.6	7.6

From Schieber, George A., and Jean-Pierre Poullier. International health care spending: Issues and trends. *Health Affairs* 10 (Spring 1991): 109; reprinted by permission.

Source: *Health OECD, Facts and Trends* (Paris: OECD, forthcoming).

[a]Mean excluding Turkey.

Table 2.14. OECD (international) public health expenditures as a percentage of total health expenditure, 1960–1987

	1960	1965	1970	1975	1980	1985	1986	1987
Australia	52.6%	57.2%	52.6%	63.9%	61.7%	71.7%	72.1%	71.8%
Austria	66.7	66.5	63.0	69.6	68.8	66.9	67.6	67.6
Belgium	61.6	75.3	87.0	79.6	81.5	76.9	76.9	76.9
Canada	42.7	50.4	70.2	76.5	75.0	75.9	74.5	74.8
Denmark	88.7	85.9	86.3	91.9	85.2	84.5	85.7	85.5
Finland	54.1	66.0	73.8	78.7	79.0	78.5	78.5	78.5
France	57.8	68.1	76.4	76.9	81.6	80.1	79.1	78.3
Germany (West)	67.5	70.9	74.2	80.2	79.4	78.0	78.1	77.0
Greece	58.6	62.5	53.4	60.2	82.2	81.0	75.2	75.3
Iceland	—	—	89.5	89.2	88.8	87.6	87.8	88.6
Ireland	76.0	76.2	77.8	82.5	92.0	88.8	88.1	87.0
Italy	83.1	87.8	86.4	86.1	82.4	79.6	78.0	78.0
Japan	60.4	61.4	69.8	72.0	70.8	72.3	72.6	73.2
Luxembourg	—	—	—	91.8	92.8	89.2	89.5	91.6
Netherlands	33.3	68.7	84.3	76.5	78.8	78.9	77.0	77.8
New Zealand	80.6	83.8	80.3	83.9	83.6	85.2	86.3	82.5
Norway	77.8	80.9	91.6	96.2	98.4	96.3	96.4	97.6
Portugal	—	—	—	58.9	72.4	56.8	59.0	60.7
Spain	52.1	52.6	54.7	70.4	73.5	71.5	71.5	71.5
Sweden	72.6	79.5	86.0	90.2	92.1	91.1	90.9	90.6
Switzerland	61.3	60.8	63.9	68.9	67.5	68.4	68.2	68.2
Turkey	—	—	—	—	—	—	37.5	41.3
United Kingdom	85.3	85.8	87.0	91.1	89.6	86.9	86.9	86.6
United States	24.7	26.2	37.0	42.5	42.4	41.8	41.5	41.4
Mean	62.9	68.3	73.6	77.3	79.1	77.7	75.8	75.9
							(77.5)[a]	(77.4)[a]

From Schieber, George A., and Jean-Pierre Poullier. International health care expenditure trends: 1987. *Health Affairs* 8 (Fall 1989): 171; reprinted by permission.

Source: OECD, Health Data Bank.

[a]Mean excluding Turkey.

part of the national income and product accounts of the OECD.[123] Disaggregation of expenditures into sectors (e.g., hospital and physician services, long-term care, public health) is difficult because there is no consistent data base providing sufficient detail[124] and because sector components have no standard definitions. For example, in Germany (West), the Scandinavian countries, and the United Kingdom (UK), hospital-based physician salaries are included in hospital sector expenditures. In the United States and Canada (where most hospital-based physicians are paid a fee for service) those expenditures are reported in the physician services sector.[125] Similarly, there is no consistency in the sector reporting of long-term care (LTC) expenditures. Denmark does not classify "resident beds" as inpatient medical care, whereas Sweden does;[126] in the United States, LTC expenditures are included not in the hospital sector but in the LTC sector. Canada mixes them, and LTC expenditures are reported in both sectors, depending on the type of facility. Consequently, the most reliable indicators of health care expenditures by country are aggregates, not sectors, and the most meaningful comparisons among countries index aggregate expenditures to gross domestic product (GDP) and per capita measures.

Health Care Expenditures as a Percentage of GDP   The OECD's basic convention presents total aggregate health care expenditures as a percentage of societal wealth or productivity. The unit of measure is GDP, in contrast to gross national product (GNP). GDP:

is the value of all final goods and services produced in a country by the factors of production *located* in the country. GNP is the same for the factors of production *owned* by the citizens of the country. For most countries, GNP and GDP are quite close[127] (emphasis added).

Indexing expenditures to GDP permits comparisons among countries of the proportion expended for health care by eliminating the problems of differing units of currency and fluctuating exchange rates.

Table 2.13 presents aggregate health care expenditures as a percentage of GDP for the 24 OECD countries for selected years from 1970 through 1989. It can be noted that in most years the United States allocated more resources to health care than any other country. In 1989, the mean percentage of aggregate health care expenditures relative to GDP for all OECD countries was 7.6%. The United States was highest at 11.8%.

Public and Private Health Care Expenditures   OECD data in Table 2.14 show the proportion of aggregate health care expenditures purchased by public (government) versus private funds. In 1987, the mean public percentage was 75.9 and all but two countries had more than 60% of health care expenditures paid by public sources. The exceptions were the United States (41.4%) and Turkey (41.3%). Luxembourg, Norway, and Sweden were highest, with public funding in excess of 90%.

Per Capita Health Care Expenditures in United States Dollars   Per capita expenditures provide a third index to compare aggregate health care expenditures among OECD countries. For comparability, the OECD denominates each country's aggregate per capita health care expenditures in United States dollars using purchasing power parities (PPPs). "PPPs are price indexes that represent the average prices in specific countries relative to the average international

Table 2.15.   OECD (international) per capita health spending in U.S. dollars, 1970–1989

	1970	1975	1980	1985	1986	1987	1988	1989
Australia	176	321	528	846	895	955	986	1,032
Austria	149	336	618	821	922	983	1,041	1,093
Belgium	123	286	513	749	801	853	924	980
Canada	274	478	806	1,315	1,427	1,507	1,581	1,683
Denmark	209	335	571	770	778	839	870	912
Finland	163	305	513	826	876	943	998	1,067
France	192	365	656	991	1,036	1,088	1,173	1,274
Germany (West)	199	422	749	1,046	1,082	1,139	1,250	1,232
Greece	62	110	196	292	334	333	347	371
Iceland	152	321	638	964	1,115	1,252	1,350	1,353
Ireland	99	225	448	577	585	607	639	658
Italy	147	270	541	761	792	889	982	1,050
Japan	126	252	515	785	828	907	978	1,035
Luxembourg	150	319	616	879	921	1,053	1,146	1,193
Netherlands	207	418	707	931	954	1,033	1,076	1,135
New Zealand	174	354	523	667	722	796	811	820
Norway	154	350	624	900	1,046	1,147	1,214	1,234
Portugal	—	158	252	385	385	405	438	464
Spain	82	186	322	437	454	500	571	644
Sweden	274	475	864	1,187	1,192	1,266	1,328	1,361
Switzerland	247	477	734	1,104	1,143	1,244	1,323	1,376
Turkey	—	58	103	—	—	144	—	—
United Kingdom	146	272	454	658	697	747	793	836
United States	346	592	1,059	1,700	1,813	1,955	2,140	2,354
Mean[a]	175	332	585	852	904	976	1,042	1,094

From Schieber, George A., and Jean-Pierre Poullier. International health care spending: Issues and trends. *Health Affairs* 10 (Spring 1991): 113; reprinted by permission.

Source: *Health OECD, Facts and Trends* (Paris: OECD, forthcoming).

[a]Mean excluding Turkey.

prices for an entire group of countries for purchasing the same market basket of goods and services.[128] Table 2.15 shows that the mean per capita OECD expenditure in 1989 was $1,094. Greece had the lowest ($371); that of the United States was highest ($2,354).

Observations on Expenditures The data in Tables 2.13, 2.14, and 2.15 suggest several conclusions. First, since 1970 the United States has allocated a greater proportion of GDP to health care than all but one of the 24 OECD countries—Sweden in 1980, where aggregate health care expenditures were 9.5% (United States expenditures were 9.2%). Second, except for Turkey, the United States had the lowest proportion of aggregate expenditures paid by public versus private sources; 1987 United States public funding was 41.4%, compared to a mean of 75.9% for OECD countries. Finally, 1989 per capita expenditures (Table 2.15) are substantially higher in the United States than in all other OECD countries and exceed the second ranked country, Canada, by 39.8%.

International Satisfaction with Health Care Systems

The public's perception of and satisfaction with its health care system are variables of interest, particularly when related to the country's aggregate health care expenditures as a percentage of GDP and per capita. Survey results from 10 OECD countries reported by Blendon et al.[129] are presented in Table 2.16. Surveys were conducted in 1989 in Canada, the United Kingdom, and the United States, and in 1990 in Australia, France, Italy, Japan, the Netherlands, Sweden, and Germany (West), by Louis Harris and Associates. The sampling allowed a "95% confidence (level) that the error due to sampling could be approximately ± 3 or 4 percent for each question."[130]

Respondents considered the statement that, "On the whole, the health care system works pretty well, and only minor changes are necessary to make it work better," as an overall indicator of their satisfaction. Table 2.16 shows that positive responses exceeded 40% in 4 of 10 countries; Canada, the Netherlands, Germany (West), and France have a relatively high level of satisfaction.

Two questions gauged public perceptions of whether "fundamental changes are needed" or whether there is "the need to completely rebuild the system." Of the 10 nations, Italy (40%) and the United States (29%) had the highest percentage who responded that their systems should be completely rebuilt.

The researchers concluded that national health programs are no guarantee of public satisfaction. "The United States and Italy, the countries with the highest level of public disenchantment,

Table 2.16. The public's view of their health care system in 10 nations, 1990

	Minor changes needed[a]	Fundamental changes needed[b]	Completely rebuild system[c]
Canada	56%	38%	5%
Netherlands	47	46	5
West Germany	41	35	13
France	41	42	10
Australia	34	43	17
Sweden	32	58	6
Japan	29	47	6
United Kingdom	27	52	17
Italy	12	46	40
United States	10	60	29

From Blendon, R.J., R. Leitman, I. Morrison, and K. Donelan. Satisfaction with health systems in ten nations. *Health Affairs* 9 (Summer 1990): 188; reprinted by permission.

Source: Harvard-Harris-ITF, 1990 Ten-Nation Survey.

[a]On the survey, the question was worded as follows: "On the whole, the health care system works pretty well, and only minor changes are necessary to make it work better."

[b]"There are some good things in our health care system, but fundamental changes are needed to make it work better."

[c]"Our health care system has so much wrong with it that we need to completely rebuild it."

could not differ more in their health care arrangements."[131] Italy has a national health service and the United States does not. Data not included in Table 2.16 show that in five of nine countries with national health plans—Australia, Sweden, Japan, Great Britain, and Italy—a majority of respondents desired fundamental change in their systems.[132]

More insight into the United States public's concern about its system is obtained from surveys conducted by the Health Insurance Association of America (HIAA). Surveys in 1989 and 1990 using face-to-face interviews found that the public was not as dissatisfied with its health insurance as indicated in the Blendon et al. study presented in Table 2.16. Some 83% of respondents were pleased (i.e., very satisfied or somewhat satisfied) with their health insurance coverage, and these results were similar to HIAA survey results for the decade 1977–1987.[133] A more recent HIAA survey found that 44% of respondents believed fundamental changes are needed but only 25% believed that the system had to be completely rebuilt.[134] Lower percentages from this study compared with those reported in Table 2.16 are thought to be related to the context and ordering of questions. Regardless of the differences, there is clearly an expression of concern by the U.S. public with regard to the high cost of health care, including insurance premiums, and access to health care, particularly for the uninsured or the many who fear losing job-related insurance as a result of becoming unemployed.[135]

The responses of persons surveyed in the United States by HIAA showed that there is support for change in the health care system and that "public support is greater for reforms not involving direct government operation of the health insurance system than for government-run approaches such as Medicare."[136] A majority think a government-run national health insurance program would restrict choice of providers and that care would be less personal. Only 16% believe that such a system would increase quality of care; 39% indicated it would be more costly.[137] Figure 2.6 shows preferences for policy options for the uninsured. They range from increased availability of private insurance to expanding federal programs such as Medicare to those under 65. Ninety percent would address the problem through the private sector.

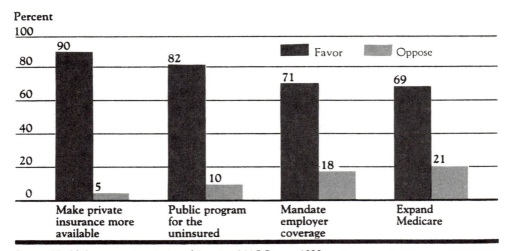

Source: Health Insurance Association of America, MAP Survey, 1990.

Figure 2.6. Public support for policy options for those without health care coverage. (From Jajich-Toth, Cindy, and Burns W. Roper. Americans' views on health care: A study in contradictions. *Health Affairs* 9 [Winter 1990]: 152; reprinted by permission.)

CANADA'S UNIVERSAL, COMPREHENSIVE HEALTH CARE SYSTEM[138]

Researchers and policymakers have shown considerable interest in the Canadian health care system and its applicability to the United States. This section describes the Canadian experience, compares it to the United States system, and identifies major policy differences between the two. It focuses on the hospital and physician services sectors.

The fundamental difference between the two privately delivered systems is the method of financing health care for inpatient and outpatient hospital and physician services.[139] This directly affects consumer access, cost of care, and resource distribution, as well as hospital and physician sector delivery arrangements and incentives. Comparing these systems may assist the United States, as consumers and government and other payors seek to contain rising costs. Lessons from the Canadian experience may shape United States national health policy during the 1990s.[140]

Similar to the United States, Canada is a developed and democratic Western nation. Canada has 10 provinces and 2 territories. With a population of 25.9 million, it has fewer people than California. Canada's health care system is similar to that of the United States. Its services are delivered privately; yet, Canada's universal health insurance and public financing more closely resemble those of countries in Western Europe. Culturally, the population is receptive to promoting the collective good, granting power to government, and accepting high tax burdens to have broad-based, government-sponsored social programs. Among them, Canadian "Medicare" is viewed as their "social jewel."[141]

The Canadian System

Canadian "Medicare" is the term used to refer to provincial- and territorial-based health insurance programs. Constitutionally, health care is a provincial responsibility,[142] and each province/territory has a health insurance plan that meets the minimum federal criteria specified in the federal Canada Health Act of 1984. These criteria are:

> *Universal*—insured persons entitled to covered services;
> *Comprehensive*—insured covered for medically necessary inpatient and outpatient hospital and physician services;
> *Portable*—coverage for residents who move to a different province or territory until new residency requirements are met;
> *Publicly administered*—plan managed on not-for-profit basis by public authority responsible to provincial government; and
> *Accessible*—availability unimpeded by charges, or otherwise.[143]

Canada does not have a single national health insurance system. Instead, provincial- and territorial-based plans provide universal, comprehensive coverage for medically necessary hospital and physician services.[144] The insurance system is publicly funded, but there is private delivery of care.[145] Patients may choose their providers, and the Canada Health Act eliminated all financial access barriers such as physician extra billing and hospital user charges.[146] By law, private insurance is limited to services not covered by provincial plans.

With some exceptions, such as quarantine, the operation of marine hospitals, and provision for the health needs of the armed forces and native peoples (Indians and Inuit), the federal role is to facilitate and support rather than to implement. The support consists primarily of providing transfer and cash payments to provincial- and territorial-based health insurance plans that meet Canada Health Act criteria.[147] Table 2.17 shows Canada's major federal health insurance legislation and indicates the extent of the federal government's fiscal responsibility for health care costs.

The evolution of Canada's health care insurance system was largely driven by the provinces, four of which had hospital insurance plans by 1950, long before the federal Hospital Insurance and

Table 2.17. Major Canadian federal health insurance legislation

Hospital Insurance and Diagnostic Services Act (HIDSA) of 1957	Inpatient initial (outpatient later) hospital services. Took effect July 1958. Five provinces joined in 1958; the last, Quebec, joined January 1, 1961.
	Federal fiscal responsibility was composed of 25% of national per capita costs plus 25% of provincial per capita costs times the number of insured persons.
Medical Care Act (MCA) of 1966	Physician services. Took effect July 1968. Three provinces were initial entrants; Northwest Territories was the last to join, April 1, 1971.
	Federal fiscal responsibility was composed of 50% of national per capita costs times the number of insured persons.
Federal-Provincial Fiscal Arrangements and Federal Post-Secondary Education and Health Contributions Act (EPF) of 1977	Relative to health care, the EPF changed the 25% + 25% (HIDSA) and 50% (MCA) federal fiscal responsibility amounts to 25% of 1975–1976 expenditures tied to GNP growth; block grant transfer payments and assignment of income tax and corporate tax points from the federal government to the provinces.
	Capped federal responsibility and tied it to GNP growth; changed provincial incentives/disincentives and transferred political consequences for no-cost control; ended discrimination between high/low spending provinces.
The Canada Health Act (CHA) of 1984	Repealed HIDSA and MCA, consolidated features under CHA, and amended EPF.
	Minimum criteria for provincial health insurance plan: —Public administration —Comprehensive (hospital inpatient and outpatient and physician services) —Universal (100% of the population) —Portable between provinces —Accessibility (banned user charges and extra billing through funding penalties)

Sources: Crichton, Anne, David Hsu, and Stella Tsang. *Canada's health care system: Its funding and organization*, 29–39. Ottawa, Ontario, Canada: Canadian Hospital Association, 1990; Deber, Risa B., and Eugene Vayda. The environment of health policy implementation: The Ontario, Canada example. In *Oxford textbook of public health*, edited by W. Holland, vol. III, 444. Oxford, England: Oxford University Press, 1985; Health and Welfare Canada. *Hospital Insurance and Diagnostic Services Act, annual report, 1977*. Ottawa, Ontario, Canada: Department of National Health and Welfare, 1977; Health and Welfare Canada. *Medical Care Act, annual report, 1977*. Ottawa, Ontario, Canada: Department of National Health and Welfare, 1977; Health and Welfare Canada. *Canada Health Act, annual report, 1986–87*, 7–8. Ottawa, Ontario, Canada: Department of National Health and Welfare, 1986/87; Iglehart, John K. Canada's health care system (part 1). *New England Journal of Medicine* 315 (July 17, 1986): 207; Statistics Canada. *Canada year book 1990*, part 3, 8–11. Ottawa, Ontario, Canada: Ministry of Supplies and Services, 1989; Taylor, Malcolm G. *Health insurance and Canadian public policy*, 2nd ed., 442. Montreal, Quebec, Canada: The Institute of Public Administration in Canada and McGill-Queens University Press, 1987; Taylor, Malcolm G. The Canadian health care system 1974–1984. In *Medicare at maturity*, edited by R.G. Evans and G.L. Stoddart, 5–16. Calgary, Alberta, Canada: The University of Calgary Press, 1989.

Diagnostic Services Act of 1957 and the Medicare and Medicaid programs in the United States. Similarly, Saskatchewan was first to enact a physician services insurance plan in 1961, 5 years before the federal Medical Care Act of 1966.[148] By 1971, all provinces and territories had hospital and physician services insurance plans covering the total population.[149]

A Comparison with the United States

A useful perspective is gained by comparing the Canadian health insurance and delivery system with that of the United States. Table 2.18 indicates that both countries have privately delivered health care. The primary difference lies in funding hospital and physician services. Canada has public funding; United States funding, except for Medicare and Medicaid, is largely private. This difference affects level of insurance coverage, extent of financial access barriers, and control of health care costs and system capacity.

Canada has approximately one tenth the population and economic activity of the United States. In 1988, Canada's population of 25.9 million[150] was just under one tenth of the United States popu-

Table 2.18. Canadian and United States health care system attributes

Attribute	Canada	United States
Delivery	Private	Private
Coverage	Universal, comprehensive	Mixed; Medicare, Medicaid, private; 37 million uninsured
Access	No financial barriers	Financial barriers
Role of private insurance	Small	Large
Funding	Public Simple Federal/provincial taxes (premiums in two provinces)	Largely private Complex Premiums and taxes for Medicare and Medicaid; private otherwise
Payor model	Single payor	Multiple payors
Locus of control	Centralized	Fragmented
Cost control	High and centralized	Low and fragmented
System capacity	High degree of control	Low degree of control
Hospitals	Prospective global budgets Not volume driven Low competition	Unit of service or DRG Volume driven High competition
Physicians	Fee-for-service Negotiated schedules Indirect volume control	Fee-for-service Medicare RBRVS No volume control

lation.[151] In 1987, Canada's GDP was $544 billion Canadian dollars; for the United States it was $4,473 billion United States dollars.[152] Canada had 55,275 physicians; the United States had 570,000.[153] In 1989, there were 1,238 Canadian hospitals with 177,000 beds and a bed: 1,000 population ratio of 7.0.[154] The United States had 6,800 hospitals with 1,248,000 beds and a bed: 1,000 population ratio of 5.2.[155]

Canada's estimated fiscal 1990 aggregate health care expenditures for all sectors were $50 billion ($41.5 billion U.S. dollars).[156] Estimated United States expenditures in calendar year 1990 were $670 billion. In 1989, Canada's aggregate health care expenditures as a percentage of GDP were 8.7%, substantially lower than the 11.8% for the United States. Similarly, per capita aggregate health care expenditures in United States dollars were $1,683 for Canada; United States expenditures of $2,354 exceeded Canada's by almost 40%.[157] Of all 1987 Canadian expenditures for health care, 74.8% were paid by public funds. In the United States, only 41.4% of health care expenditures—predominately Medicare and Medicaid—were paid by government.[158] Approximately 25% of Canadian expenditures were paid privately for services not covered by provincial health insurance plans. Examples of services not covered in Ontario (Canada's largest province, with 36% of the population) are cosmetic surgery, private duty nursing, preferred hospital accommodations (the additional cost of private or semiprivate rooms), nonhospital stay prescriptions, eyeglasses, routine dental care, and medical examinations required for employment or life insurance.[159] The mix between public and private expenditures for long-term care varies by province. In Ontario, patients occupying a chronic care bed in a hospital for more than 60 days or those in a licensed extended care facility in which skilled nursing care is required pay a room and board charge based on the amount of their old age security pension.[160] These charges are included in the private component of Canadian health care expenditures.

The most recent data comparing sectors are from 1987. They show that 39.2% of aggregate Canadian health care expenditures were for hospital care versus 39.5% in the United States. Physician services sector expenditures were 16.0% of the total in Canada and 20.5% in the United States.[161] Approximately one fourth of Canada's acute care hospital beds are used for long-term care, and these costs are included in hospital sector expenditures.[162] This causes its hospital expenditures as a percentage of total expenditures to be even lower than those in the United States.

These comparisons clearly indicate that Canada spends fewer societal resources, as a percentage of GDP, for health care than does the United States. Canada spends less per capita for health care than the United States and it spends less of its aggregate health care expenditures in both hospital and physician services sectors.

Funding and Control In Canada, universal, comprehensive health insurance for hospital and physician services with private delivery of care is almost entirely publicly funded. Revenue sources include provincial taxes and federal transfer and cash payments to provinces. Alberta and British Columbia charge premiums, but since premiums are not based on risk they are, in effect, taxes,[163] with exemptions or subsidies for the aged, indigent, and unemployed.[164] Public funding eliminates financial access barriers to hospital and physician services and beneficiaries are not at financial risk.

Even the approximately 55 million United States Medicare and Medicaid beneficiaries may pay premiums, deductibles, or copayments.[165] This is similar to most of the private insurance plans that cover 188 million people or 77.5% of the population.[166] Thus, there is a range of financial risk and, correspondingly, financial access barriers to care, especially for the uninsured and the millions more who are underinsured.

The Hospital Sector A unique attribute of the Canadian system is that the provincial health ministries are the sole payor of care, and such centralized locus of control gives them monopsony—single-payor—power.[167] This payment method contrasts with that in the United States, where a patchwork of payors includes government, Blue Cross and Blue Shield, commercial insurers, and self-pay. The United States system is far less amenable to control.

Canadian provincial ministries of health prospectively set, either unilaterally or through negotiations, global budgets for each hospital. Within its budget, the hospital must provide all needed services.[168] This causes at least three results. First, the organizational stability contrasts with financial risk and instability in United States hospitals, where reimbursement is based on unit of service, per day, or per case (i.e., DRG). Second, Canadian hospitals are not volume driven as are United States hospitals. Third, the ministries control system capacity, new programs, technologies, and beds. Hospitals must obtain prior approval for expansion. If not approved, costs are not included in their global budget—a powerful form of centralized control. This control over system capacity results in indirect volume control and influences the behavior of hospitals. With global budgeting, "Canadian hospitals do not, at the margin, earn more by doing more."[169] They are not volume driven and are capacity bound.[170]

In the United States, reimbursement for hospital services is fragmented, involves multiple payors, is basically open ended and largely volume driven, and its complexity varies by type of payor. Other than to determine medical necessity, there are no direct volume controls, nor are there sector expenditure controls as in Canada. Reimbursement for Medicare beneficiaries is per case (admission) based on prospectively set DRGs. For other payors, reimbursement can be capitated (HMOs), negotiated payment based on federal DRGs, fee-for-service, percentage of charges, or actual charges, as for self-pay patients. Since all hospital reimbursement except HMOs is volume driven on a per-case or per-service basis, control of aggregate sector costs is difficult.

The United States system has built-in incentives for hospitals to have high admissions, high throughput, and high volume. In the United States health care environment, which is largely deregulated and is very competitive, there is little control over systemwide capacity and expansion.

The Physician Services Sector In Canada, private-practice physician services are reimbursed on a fee-for-service basis and are volume driven. Control is effected through two principal means. First, provincial governments negotiate fee schedules with provincial medical associations and prospectively set fees.[171] Second, five provinces with 80% of the population control aggregate physician expenditures by threshold-triggered discounting of fee schedules, recapturing by reducing future years' fee schedule increases, or, in Quebec, income capping provisions when aggregate sector expenditures exceed the prospectively set budget.[172] Thresholds limit provincial financial exposure by recouping distributions for increases in total physician volume of services by downward adjustments of future fee schedule increases, or by paying current fees at a discounted rate.[173] Thresholds do not set individual physician incomes, but they do affect total funds available and are a physician sector pseudo target income and indirect volume control mechanism.

Payment for physician services in the United States is fee for service and volume driven. A small but notable exception is some types of HMOs in which there is capitation or salaries. Reimbursement by most payors is based on usual, customary, and reasonable (UCR) charges.[174] Patients, however, are responsible for the difference between actual and UCR charges, except where physicians participating in publicly funded programs accept assignment.

In late 1989, the United States Congress enacted legislation requiring that physician fees be set for services to Medicare recipients, a change resulting from recommendations of the Physician Payment Review Commission[175] and the earlier work of Hsiao et al.[176] in developing resource-based relative values. As noted earlier, physician fees in Medicare Part B are based on a resource-based relative value scale (RBRVS) that was implemented in 1992. RBRVS is like DRGs and is derived from the product of the relative value scale times a conversion factor, with adjustments such as geographic cost considerations. RBRVS incorporates relative value units for three components: a work component, including physician time, a practice cost component, including office and staff expense, and a malpractice insurance premium component.[177] The act also requires the secretary of DHHS to establish Medicare volume performance standards to set rates of increase. Unlike some Canadian provinces, the Medicare volume performance standards do not establish expenditure targets but only affect the change in the Medicare fee schedule. Thus, it appears that this system will not control absolute volume through recapturing, as is done in most of Canada.

The United States federal policy to administratively set physician fee schedules for Medicare represents partial movement toward one element of the Canadian model—physician fee setting—and is significant for two reasons. First, it applies to services for 33 million Medicare beneficiaries, a group larger than the population of Canada. Second, other payors develop federal-like reimbursement methods, as happened following introduction of DRGs in the early 1980s. However, success of this policy may be limited without the monopsony attribute of the Canadian model and without prospective sector budgeting (i.e., expenditure targets).

Observations

The provincial- and territorial-based plans that provide universal, comprehensive health insurance for medically necessary hospital and physician services, with private delivery of care, public funding, and no financial access barriers to care, appear to work well in Canada. The system is not without its critics, however. Some argue that there is too much emphasis on acute versus preventive care and that resources are misallocated.[178] Delays for service are reported,[179] particularly for elective and high-technology procedures in hospitals. Hospitals may be capacity bound,[180] and introduction of advanced technology is less per capita than in the United States.[181] For example, Canada had only 12 magnetic resonance imaging units in 1989 (1 unit per 2,167,000 persons), whereas the United States had 900 units in 1987 (1 unit per 271,000 persons). Similarly, Canada had 32 open heart surgery units (1 unit per 813,000 persons) in 1989, whereas the United States had 793 units (1 unit per 307,000 persons) in 1987.[182]

Even its critics recognize that Canada's aggregate health care expenditures as a percentage of GDP and per capita are less than those of the United States. Health insurance in Canada is universal and comprehensive for hosptial and physician services and is publicly funded. Beneficiaries have access to care unimpeded by financial barriers. Canadian Medicare is one social program that achieves the objective of promoting the collective good for all Canadians.

While there are some in the United States who advocate adopting the second element of the Canadian model—prospective global budgeting for each hospital and the sector as a whole with single-source payors of care—this is unlikely to occur soon, if ever. There are inhibitors. First, such a radical change would provoke opposition from powerful special interests.[183] Second, health planning policy for hospital sector resource allocation and capacity control did not work in the 1970s and early 1980s. Third, consideration must be given to whether the inherent results of prospective global hospital budgeting—bound capacity, delays for some services, and restrictions on deployment of new technology[184]—are acceptable in the United States and whether Americans will give government power to be a sole-source, monopsony payor of care. In comparing the cultural differences between Canada and the United States, Kosterlitz observes that "the United States emphasis on individualism and mistrust of government contrasts sharply with Canadians' stress on collective good and government as its agent."[185] Fourth, the United States system is 10 times larger than Canada's. The logistics of implementation would be difficult at best, and perhaps unmanageable. Finally, the absence of widespread discontent of the population and less tolerance for higher taxes than in Canada seem to indicate that United States health policy will continue to be that of incremental change.[186] If so, and with public sentiment strongly favoring the use of private insurance, it is anticipated that policy initiatives to improve access to health care for the uninsured and underinsured will be based on private implementation with financial inducements by government.

SUMMARY

This chapter provides background information about the United States and Canadian health services systems. The discussion of United States health services includes a conceptual framework of its health care and health services system, a brief history of its early development, and data and commentary about various components. The result is to provide an understanding of the environment in which HSOs and their managers function. The system's enormity and complexity as well as the various elements are apparent. Users are urged to keep this chapter in mind and reference it when reading the following chapters. Continuous, comprehensive awareness of the environment and its effect is a crucial dimension of knowledge for successful managers. In that sense, one can never know too much; this reinforces the need for lifelong learning and the stimulation provided by organized continuing education efforts.

International health care expenditures for the 24 OECD countries give readers a perspective of the United States health care system relative to others in terms of aggregate health care expenditures as a percentage of GDP, per capita, and the portion that is publicly funded. Canada's universal, comprehensive health insurance system with private delivery of care is a model from which United States policymakers can learn. Attribute differences between the United States and Canada are emphasized.

The 1990s will be a decade in which the United States health services delivery system is likely to change in form and content to become very different from what it has been. Fewer services will be provided to inpatients in acute care hospitals, but those admitted will be more acutely ill. Higher intensity of illness will mean significantly higher costs in hospitals. Less need for inpatient care will result in hospitals closing or being converted to other uses. An increasingly common site of treatment will be the patient's home. Innovative relationships among various types of HSOs will deliver and finance health services in unique ways. The increase in the numbers and types of health services workers needed to support new technologies and services will raise salary costs. It is unlikely that health services costs will decrease, even though pressures to control them will probably result in moderation of increases. Physicians will be increasingly integrated into HSOs, which are likely to be part of comprehensive health care systems. These changes will require skillful and effective managers.

DISCUSSION QUESTIONS

1. What are the ramifications and implications for the health services system of the model developed by Blum? What are its strengths and weaknesses?
2. Describe and analyze the relationships among the various institutional and programmatic providers in the health services system.
3. Facilities and programs other than acute care hospitals are much more numerous and probably have a much greater effect on health status, yet the acute care hospital is the focal point of most attention directed at the health care system. What are the desirable and undesirable aspects of this attention from the standpoint of the acute care hospital provider and the consumer of health services?
4. Proliferation of types of health services personnel has continued unabated during the past several decades. What are the desirable and undesirable aspects of this fragmentation? If something should be done to slow or stop it, what should this be and how can it be achieved?
5. What changes in reimbursement to HSOs, especially acute care hospitals, have occurred since 1965? What forces in the macroenvironment were most important in causing these changes? Sketch and be prepared to defend a scenario that suggests the likely developments in reimbursement during the 1990s.
6. Federally supported state health planning has risen and fallen since passage of Medicare and Medicaid. Identify the advantages and disadvantages of statewide or areawide health planning from the standpoints of providers and consumers.
7. Describe how licensure, registration, and certification are different. What are the advantages and disadvantages of each from the standpoints of providers and consumers?
8. Resources consumed by the health services system, especially acute care hospitals, have soared uncontrollably since the late 1960s. What factors contributed, and in what proportions, to these increases? What new proposals to control costs are under consideration?
9. Review Tables 2.13, 2.14, and 2.15. What do you conclude about United States health care expenditures relative to those of other OECD countries?
10. Describe the major attribute differences between the United States and Canadian health care systems.

CASE STUDY 1:   GOURMAND AND FOOD—A FABLE[187]

The people of Gourmand loved good food. They ate in good restaurants, donated money for cooking research, and instructed their government to safeguard all matters having to do with food. Long ago, the food industry had been in total chaos. There were many restaurants, some very small. Anyone could call himself a chef or open a restaurant. In choosing a restaurant, one could never be sure that the meal would be good. A commission of distinguished chefs studied the situation and recommended that no one be allowed to touch food except for qualified chefs. "Food is too important to be left to amateurs," they said. Qualified chefs were licensed by the state with severe penalties for anyone else who engaged in cooking. Certain exceptions were made for food preparation in the home, but a person could serve only his own family. Furthermore, to become a qualified chef, a man had to complete at least 21 years of training (including four years of college, four years of cooking school, and one year apprenticeship). All cooking schools had to be first class.

These reforms did succeed in raising the quality of cooking. But a restaurant meal became substantially more expensive. A second commission observed that not everyone could afford to eat out. "No one," they said, "should be denied a good meal because of his income." Furthermore, they argued that chefs should work toward the goal of giving everyone "complete physical and psychological satisfaction." For those people who could not afford to eat out, the government declared that they should be allowed to do so as often as they liked and the government would pay. For others, it was recommended that they organize themselves in groups and pay part of their income into a pool that would undertake to pay the costs incurred by members in dining out. To ensure the greatest satisfaction, the groups were set up so that a member could eat out anywhere and as often as he liked, could have as elaborate a meal as he desired, and would have to pay nothing or only a small percentage of the cost. The cost of joining such prepaid dining clubs rose sharply.

Long ago, most restaurants would have one chef to prepare the food. A few restaurants were more elaborate, with chefs specializing in roasting, fish, salads, sauces, and many other things. People rarely went to these elaborate restaurants since they were so expensive. With the establishment of prepaid dining clubs, everyone wanted to eat at these fancy restaurants. At the same time, young chefs in school disdained going to cook in a small restaurant where they would have to cook everything. The pay was higher and it was much more prestigious to specialize and cook at a really fancy restaurant. Soon there were not enough chefs to keep the small restaurants open.

With prepaid clubs and free meals for the poor, many people started eating their three-course meals at the elaborate restaurants. Then they began to increase the number of courses, directing the chef to "serve the best with no thought for the bill." (Recently a 317-course meal was served.)

The costs of eating out rose faster and faster. A new government commission reported as follows: (1) Noting that licensed chefs were being used to peel potatoes and wash lettuce, the commission recommended that these tasks be handed over to licensed dishwashers (whose three years of dishwashing training included cooking courses) or to some new category of personnel. (2) Concluding that many licensed chefs were overworked, the commission recommended that cooking schools be expanded, that the length of training be shortened, and that applicants with lesser qualifications be admitted. (3) The commission also observed that chefs were unhappy because people seemed to be more concerned about the decor and service than about the food. (In a recent taste test, not only could one patron not tell the difference between a 1930 and a 1970 vintage but also could not distinguish between white and red wines. He explained that he always ordered the 1930 vintage because he knew that only a really good restaurant would stock such an expensive wine.)

The commission agreed that weighty problems faced the nation. They recommended that a national prepayment group be established which everyone must join. They recommended that chefs continue to be paid on the basis of the number of dishes they prepared. They recommended that every Gourmandese be given the right to eat anywhere he chose and as elaborately as he chose and pay nothing.

These recommendations were adopted. Large numbers of people spent all of their time ordering incredibly elaborate meals. Kitchens became marvels of new, expensive equipment. All those who were not consuming restaurant food were in the kitchen preparing it. Since no one in Gourmand did anything except prepare or eat meals, the country collapsed.

Question

1. Read and analyze the fable of Gourmand. How well does the analogy fit the United States health care system? How do health services managers assist the nation in avoiding the fate of the Gourmandese?

NOTES

1. *Healthy America: Practitioners for 2005*, 55. Durham, NC: Pew Health Professions Commission, October 1991.

2. Blum, Henrik L. *Expanding health care horizons: From a general systems concept of health to a national health policy*, 2d ed., 34. Oakland, CA: Third Party Publishing Company, 1983.

3. Blum, Henrik L. *Planning for health: Development and application of social change theory*, 96–100. New York: Human Sciences Press, 1974.

4. Data taken from the National Center for Health Statistics, 1987 and 1988; and from Thompson-Hoffman, Susan, and Inez Fitzgerald Storck. *Disability in the United States: A portrait from national data*, 37. New York: Springer Publishing Company, 1991.

5. Spencer, Gregory. *Projections of the population of the United States, by age, sex, and race: 1988–2080*, 8. Bureau of the Census, U.S. Department of Commerce, 1989.

6. National Center for Health Statistics, Public Health Service, U.S. Department of Health and Human Services. *Health United States 1990*, 185. Washington, D.C.: U.S. Government Printing Office, 1991.

7. Schieber, George J., and Jean-Pierre Poullier. International health care spending: Issues and trends. *Health Affairs* 10 (Spring 1991): 109.

8. Public Health Service, U.S. Department of Health and Human Services. *Directory of facilities obligated to provide uncompensated services, by state and city as of March 1, 1989*, i. Washington, D.C.: U.S. Government Printing Office, 1989.

9. U.S. Department of Health and Human Services, Public Health Services, National Institutes of Health. *Basic data relating to the National Institutes of Health*, 7. Washington, D.C.: U.S. Government Printing Office, 1990.

10. National Center for Health Statistics, *Health United States 1990*, 188.

11. National Center for Health Statistics, *Health United States 1990*, 189.

12. Pickett, George E., and John J. Hanlon. *Public health administration and practice*, 9th ed., 83. St. Louis: Times Mirror/Mosby College Publishing, 1990.

13. National Center for Health Statistics, *Health United States 1990*, 137.

14. Indian Health Service, Public Health Service, Department of Health and Human Services. *Trends in Indian health 1990*, 10. Washington, D.C.: U.S. Government Printing Office, 1990.

15. Department of Veterans Affairs. Total quality management. Washington, D.C., 1991.

16. Association of American Medical Colleges. *American medical education: Institutions, programs, issues*, 32. Washington, D.C., 1989.

17. Association of American Medical Colleges, *American medical education*, 11.

18. Sirrocco, Al. *Characteristics of facilities for the mentally retarded, 1986*, 8. Washington, D.C.: Division of Health Care Statistics, National Center for Health Statistics, Centers for Disease Control, Public Health Service, U.S. Department of Health and Human Services, 1989.

19. Sirrocco, *Characteristics*, 9.

20. Sirrocco, *Characteristics*, 15.

21. Norback, Judith. *The mental health yearbook/directory 1979–80*, 200. New York: Van Nostrand Reinhold Co., 1979.

22. National Center for Health Statistics, *Health United States 1990*, 158.

23. Association of American Medical Colleges. *Council of Teaching Hospitals: Selected activities report—May 1990*, 1. Washington, D.C., 1990.

24. Association of American Medical Colleges, *Council of Teaching Hospitals*, 1.

25. Association of American Medical Colleges, *Council of Teaching Hospitals*, 1.

26. Association of American Medical Colleges, *American medical education*, 11.

27. Association of American Medical Colleges, *American medical education*, 12–13.

28. National Center for Health Statistics, *Health United States 1990*, 160.

29. National Center for Health Statistics, *Health United States 1990*, 160.

30. Singer, Allen M. Projections of physician supply and demand: A summary of HRSA and AMA studies. *Academic Medicine* 64 (April 1989): 235.

31. Schwartz, William B., Frank A. Sloan, and Daniel N. Mendelson. Why there will be little or no physician surplus between now and the year 2000. *New England Journal of Medicine* 318 (April 7, 1988): 892–897; Schwartz, William B. and Daniel N. Mendelson. No evidence of an emerging physician surplus: An analysis of change in physicians' work load and income. *Journal of the American Medical Association* 263 (January 26, 1990): 557–560.

32. Association of University Programs in Health Administration. Staff report, 5. Arlington, VA, 1991.

33. Accrediting Commission on Education for Health Services Administration. *Self-study guide for graduate programs in health services administration*, 6. Arlington, VA, 1990.

34. Association of University Programs in Health Administration, personal communication, November 1991.

35. American Hospital Association. *Professional credentialing statutes*, 1. Chicago, November 1990.

36. Association of American Medical Colleges. *U.S. medical school finances: Part I and part II, 1989–1990*, 2. Washington, D.C., 1991.

37. National Center for Health Statistics, *Health United States 1990*, 169.

38. National Center for Health Statistics, *Health United States 1990*, 169.

39. National Center for Health Statistics, *Health United States 1990*, 165.

40. Association of Canadian Medical Colleges. *Canadian Medical Education Statistics*, Vol. 13, Tables 1, 26a. Ottawa, Ontario, Canada, 1991.

41. Peterson, Edward S., Anne E. Crowley, Joseph Rosenthal, and Robert Boerner. Medical Education in the U.S. 1979–1980. *Journal of the American Medical Association*. 244 (December 26, 1980): 2810–2823.

42. Association of American Medical Colleges, *U.S. medical school finances*, 5.

43. Johns Hopkins University. The flexible medical admissions program at The Johns Hopkins University School of Medicine. Baltimore, 1991.

44. American Board of Medical Specialties Research & Ed-

ucation Foundation. *Annual report & reference hand-book—1991*, 66. Evanston, IL, 1991.

45. Rich, Spencer. Report questions discipline by state medical units. *Washington Post* (June 3, 1990): A17.

46. American Dental Association. *Annual report: Dental education—1990–1991*, 4. Chicago, 1991.

47. American Dental Association, *Annual report*, 22.

48. American Dental Association, *Annual report*, 11.

49. Council on Dental Education, American Dental Association. *Dentistry: A changing profession*. Chicago, 1980.

50. American Dental Association. *State dental boards that license specialists*. Chicago, 1990.

51. American Podiatric Medical Association. Podiatric medicine. Bethesda, MD, 1991.

52. Bullough, Vern L., and Bonnie Bullough. *The care of the sick: The emergence of modern nursing*, 137–138. London: Croom Helm, 1979.

53. 1991 AJN Guide: State boards of nursing and RN licensure regulations. *American Journal of Nursing* 91 (April 1991): 20–27.

54. American Nurses Association. The nursing shortage: Situation & solutions, 7. Kansas City, MO, 1991.

55. American Nurses Association, The nursing shortage, 7, 8.

56. American Nurses Association, The nursing shortage, 3, 5.

57. Green, Jeffrey. Increased enrollment difficult for nursing schools to swallow. *AHA News* 27 (August 26, 1991): 1.

58. *Nursing Data Source 1991*, Vol. I, 36. New York: National League for Nursing, 1991.

59. ANCC certification (pamphlet). Kansas City, MO: American Nurses Credentialing Center, 1991.

60. *ANA certification catalogue*. American Nurses Association, Kansas City, MO, 1983.

61. ANCC certification, 1991.

62. The American Dietetic Association. *Laws that regulate nutritionists*. Chicago, 1990, updated 1991.

63. The American Society of Radiologic Technologists. Information Sheet. Albuquerque, NM, 1991.

64. Schafft, Gretchen Engle, and James F. Cawley. *The physician assistant in a changing health care environment*, 6. Rockville, MD: Aspen Publishers, Inc. 1987.

65. National Commission on Certification of Physician Assistants, Inc., personal communication, September 13, 1991.

66. Stuart, Sherri. 2001: A PA odyssey. *Journal of the American Academy of Physician Assistants* 4 (September 1991): 24a.

67. Cawley, James F. Hospital physicians' assistants: Past, present, and future. *Hospital Topics* 69 (Summer 1991): 15.

68. AHA tracks shortages in health care personnel. *AHA News* 25 (January 2, 1989): 1.

69. Business facts. *AHA News* 25 (March 1989): 7.

70. Division of Regulatory Affairs, Office of Health Planning. *Status report on state certificate of need programs*, 1. Washington, D.C.: U.S. Department of Health and Human Services, 1983.

71. O'Donnell, James W. The rise and fall of federal support. *Provider* (December 1987): 6.

72. Thomas, Constance. Certificate of need: Taking a new look at an old program. *State Health Notes* 114 (June 1991): 1.

73. Developments in state and local planning. *TODAY in Health Planning* (newsletter) 1 (June 1991): 9.

74. Thomas, Certificate, 1.

75. Cohen, Harold A. *Health Services Cost Review Commission*. Baltimore, 1983.

76. Kent, Christina. Twenty years of Maryland rate regulation. *Medicine & Health* (Perspectives insert) 45 (August 19, 1991).

77. Kent, Twenty years.

78. Kent, Twenty years.

79. This section is adapted from History of peer review. Washington, D.C.: Health Care Financing Administration, n.d. (Unpublished report received December 1991.)

80. Ready, Tinker. PROs under assault by government, consumers. *Healthweek* 4 (February 12, 1990): 6, 44–45.

81. Health Care Financing Administration. *DRGs definitions manual*, 7th rev., 809. Washington, D.C.: U.S. Government Printing Office, 1990.

82. Schneider, Don P., Brant E. Fries, William J. Foley, Marilyn Desmond, and William J. Gormley. Case mix for nursing home payment: Resource utilization groups, version II. *Health Care Financing Review* Annual Supplement (1988): 51.

83. Fries, Brant E., Gunnar Ljunggren, and Bengt Winblad. International comparison of long-term care: The need for resident-level classification. *Journal of the American Geriatrics Society* 39 (January 1991): 12–13.

84. Outpatient payment reform: The next budget-cutting target. *Hospitals* 64 (January 20, 1990): 42.

85. DRG-like system is front runner for OPD reform. *Health Care Competition Week* 8 (August 5, 1991): 3.

86. DRG-like system, 3–4.

87. News at deadline. *Hospitals* 64 (November 5, 1990): 8.

88. A discussion that provides extensive background on development of RBRVS and compares it with payment to Canadian physicians is found in Rakich, Jonathon S., and Edmund R. Becker. U.S. physician payment reform: Background and comparison to the Canadian model. *Health Care Management Review* 17 (Spring 1992): 9–19.

89. Grimaldi, Paul L. RBRVS: How new physician fee schedule will work. *Healthcare Financial Management* 45 (September 1991): 58, 60.

90. Grimaldi, RBRVS, 74.

91. Has HCFA "broken faith" with MD fee schedule? *Medical Staff Leader* 20 (August 1991): 8.

92. Has HCFA "broken faith," 1.

93. Grimaldi, RBRVS, 74.

94. Koska, Mary T. Hospitals: Begin strategic planning for RBRVS. *Hospitals* 65 (February 20, 1991): 28–30.

95. Joint Commission on Accreditation of Healthcare Organizations. *Committed to quality: An introduction to the Joint Commission on Accreditation of Healthcare Organizations*, 14. Oakbrook Terrace, IL, 1990.

96. Harris-Wehling, Jo, and Michael G.H. McGeary. Medicare: A strategy for quality assurance, IV: Medicare conditions of participation and quality assurance. *QRB* 17 (October 1991): 321.

97. Joint Commission, *Committed to quality*, 10.

98. Koska, Mary T. JCAHO: Pilot hospitals' input updates agenda for change. *Hospitals* 64 (January 5, 1990): 50.

99. American Medical Association, Chicago, personal communication, November 1991.

100. American Nurses Association. *This is the ANA*. Kansas City, MO, 1977.

101. American Hospital Association. *AHA Hospital Statistics*, 202. Chicago, 1991.

102. Federation of American Health Systems. *1991 annual report: The national health policy reform debate*, 10. Little Rock, AR, 1991.

103. American Osteopathic Hospital Association, personal communication, 1991.

104. American Osteopathic Association. *Background information on the osteopathic medical profession*. Chicago, 1991–1992.

105. American Health Care Association. *Profile: The American health care association*. Washington, D.C., 1991.

106. American Association of Homes for the Aging, personal communication, October 25, 1991.

107. Group Health Association of America. Information sheet. Washington, D.C., 1991.

108. Medical Group Management Association, personal communication, November 1991.

109. Accrediting Commission on Education for Health Services Administration. *1991–1992 ACEHSA Commissioners*. Arlington, VA, 1991.

110. Council on Education for Public Health. Council on Education for Public Health (pamphlet). Washington, D.C., 1991.

111. American Assembly of Collegiate Schools of Business. *Addendum to the AACSB Accreditation Council policy manual*, 21. St. Louis, 1990.

112. National League for Nursing. Fact sheet: The National League for Nursing. New York: 1991.

113. American Board of Medical Specialties Research & Education Foundation, *Annual report*, 62–63.

114. Koska, Mary T. Specialty board proliferation causes confusion. *Hospitals* 63 (August 5, 1989): 58.

115. Koska, Specialty board, 58.

116. John T. Dunlop on working with businesses and insurers. *Trustee* 41 (November 1988): 7.

117. Health benefits' costs surging despite employers' strategies. *AHA News* 27 (February 4, 1991): 3.

118. Blue Cross and Blue Shield Association. *Names of regular member plans*. Chicago, 1991.

119. Health Insurance Association of America, *Source book of health insurance data, 1982–83*, 7. Washington, D.C., 1982–83.

120. Department of Health and Human Services. *National medical expenditure survey: A profile of uninsured Americans, research findings 1*. Publication No. PHS 89-3443: 1. Washington, D.C.: U.S. Government Printing Office, 1989.

121. The material in this section is excerpted from Southby, Richard F., and Jonathon S. Rakich. International health care expenditures. *Hospital Topics* 69 (Spring 1991): 8–13.

122. Organization for Economic Cooperation and Development. *Financing and delivering health care: A comparative analysis of OECD countries*. OECD Social Policy Studies No. 4. Paris, 1987; Organization for Economic Cooperation and Development. *Health care systems in transition: The search for efficiency*. Paris, 1990.

123. Poullier, Jean-Pierre. Health care expenditure data: An international comparison from the OECD. In *Health care systems in transition: The search for efficiency*, 121. Paris: Organization for Economic Cooperation and Development, 1990; Schieber, George J., and Jean-Pierre Poullier. An overview of international comparisons of health care expenditures. *Health Care Financing Review* Annual Supplement (1989): 1; Schieber, George J., and Jean-Pierre Poullier. An overview of international comparisons of health care expenditures. In *Health care systems in transition: The search for efficiency*, 9. Paris: Organization for Economic Cooperation and Development, 1990.

124. Organization for Economic Cooperation and Development, *Financing and delivering*, 60.

125. Organization for Economic Cooperation and Development, *Financing and delivering*, 62; Schieber and Poullier, Overview of international, 9.

126. Poullier, Health care expenditure, 120.

127. Case, Karl E., and Ray C. Fair. *Principles of economics*, 61. Englewood Cliffs, NJ: Prentice Hall, 1989.

128. Schieber and Poullier, Overview of international, 12.

129. Blendon, Robert J., Robert Leitman, Ian Morrison, and Karen Donelan. Satisfaction with health systems in ten nations. *Health Affairs* 9 (Summer 1990): 185–192.

130. Blendon, Leitman, Morrison, and Donelan, Satisfaction with health, 186.

131. Blendon, Leitman, Morrison, and Donelan, Satisfaction with health, 188.

132. Blendon, Leitman, Morrison, and Donelan, Satisfaction with health, 189.

133. Gabel, Jon, Howard Cohen, and Steven Fink. Americans' views on health care: Foolish inconsistencies? *Health Affairs* 8 (Spring 1989): 105.

134. Jajich-Toth, Cindy, and Burns W. Roper. Americans' views on health care: A study in contradictions. *Health Affairs* 9 (Winter 1990): 149–151.

135. Jajich-Toth and Roper, Americans' views, 151.

136. Jajich-Toth and Roper, Americans' views, 149.

137. Jajich-Toth and Roper, Americans' views, 153–154.

138. Material in this section is excerpted with permission from Rakich, Jonathon S. Canada's universal-comprehensive health care system. *Hospital Topics* 69 (Spring 1991): 14–18; Rakich, Jonathon S. The Canadian and U.S. health care systems: Profiles and policies. *Hospital & Health Services Administration* 36 (Spring 1991): 25–42. (By permission. Copyright 1991, American College of Healthcare Executives).

139. Evans, Robert, and Gregory L. Stoddart. *Medicare at maturity*, xi. Calgary, Alberta, Canada: The University of Calgary Press, 1989.

140. Battistella, Roger M., and Thomas P. Weil. National health insurance reconsidered: Dilemmas and opportunities. *Hospital & Health Services Administration* 34 (Summer 1989): 139–155; Butler, Stuart M., and Edmund F. Haislmaier, eds. *Critical issues: A national health system for America*. Washington, D.C.: The Heritage Foundation, 1989; Enthoven, Alain C., and Richard Kronick. A consumer-choice health plan for the 1990s: A universal health insurance system designed to promote quality and economy—part I. *New England Journal of Medicine* 320 (January 5, 1989): 29–37; Enthoven, Alain C., and Richard Kronick. A consumer-choice health plan for the 1990s: A universal health insurance system designed to promote quality and economy—part II. *New England Journal of Medicine* 320 (January 12, 1989): 94–101; Haislmaier, Edmund, F. Perception vs. reality: Taking a second look at Canadian health care. *Backgrounder* (The Heritage

Foundation) 10 (January 31, 1991): 1–21; Himmelstein, David U., and Stephanie Woolhandler. A national
health program for the United States: A physicians' proposal. *New England Journal of Medicine* 320 (January
12, 1989): 102–108; Levey, Samuel, and James Hill.
National health insurance—the triumph of equivocation. *New England Journal of Medicine* 321 (December
21, 1989): 1750–1754; Marmor, Theodore R., and
Rudolf Klein. Costs vs. care: American's health care
dilemma wrongly considered. *Health Matrix* 4 (Spring
1986): 19–24; National Leadership Commission on
Health Care. *For the health of a nation, executive summary*, 1–10. Washington, D.C., 1989; Neuschler, Edward. *Canadian health care: The implications of public
health insurance*. Washington, D.C.: Health Insurance
Association of America, 1990.

141. Iglehart, John K. Canada's health care system (part 1).
      New England Journal of Medicine 315 (July, 17, 1986):
      202.

142. Crichton, Anne, David Hsu, and Stella Tsang. *Can-
      ada's health care system: Its funding and organization*,
      28. Ottawa, Ontario, Canada: Canadian Hospital Asso-
      ciation, 1990; Deber, Risa B., and Eugene Vayda. The
      environment of health policy implementation: The On-
      tario, Canada example. In *Oxford textbook of public
      health*, edited by W. Holland, vol. III, 442. Oxford, En-
      gland: Oxford University Press, 1985; Statistics Can-
      ada. *Canada year book 1990*, part 3, 9. Ottawa, On-
      tario Canada: Ministry of Supplies and Services, 1989.

143. Health and Welfare Canada. *Canada Health Act, an-
      nual report, 1986–87*, 7–8. Ottawa, Ontario, Canada:
      Department of National Health and Welfare, 1986/87.

144. Evans and Stoddart, *Medicare at maturity*, x; Statistics
      Canada, *Canada year book 1990*, part 3, 9.

145. Vayda, Eugene, and Risa B. Deber. The Canadian
      health care system: An overview. *Social Science and
      Medicine* 18 (1984): 191.

146. Health and Welfare Canada, *Canada Health Act*, 3.

147. Health and Welfare Canada, *Canada Health Act*, 11;
      Sutherland, Ralph W., and M. Jane Fulton. *Health care
      in Canada: A description and analysis of Canadian
      health care services*, 49–53. Ottawa, Ontario, Canada:
      The Health Group, 1988.

148. Taylor, Malcolm G. *Health insurance and Canadian
      public policy*, 2nd ed., 101. Montreal, Quebec, Can-
      ada: The Institute of Public Administration in Canada
      and McGill-Queens University Press, 1987; Taylor,
      Malcolm G. The Canadian health care system 1974–
      1984. In *Medicare at maturity*, edited by R.G. Evans
      and G.L. Stoddart, 4–5. Calgary, Alberta, Canada:
      The University of Calgary Press, 1989.

149. Crichton, Hsu, and Tsang, *Canada's health care*, 32–
      33; Taylor, Canadian health care, 7.

150. Statistics Canada, *Canada year book 1990*, part 2, 18.

151. U.S. Department of Commerce. *Statistical abstract of
      the United States, 1990*, 13. Washington, D.C.: U.S.
      Government Printing Office, 1990. Population data dif-
      fer from those on Table 2.6 because of different data
      sources.

152. Organization for Economic Cooperation and Develop-
      ment, *Health care systems*, 198.

153. Organization for Economic Cooperation and Develop-
      ment, *Health care systems*, 155.

154. Statistics Canada. *Hospital statistics preliminary an-
      nual report 1988–89*, 2. Health Reports, Supplement
      5, vol. 2, No. 2. Ottawa, Ontario, Canada: Canadian
      Centre for Health Information, 1990.

155. American Hospital Association. *Hospital statistics,
      1988–89*, 1. Chicago, 1989.

156. Health and Welfare Canada. Department of National
      Health and Welfare, Health Policy Division, Policy,
      Communications and Information Branch, personal
      communication, 1991.

157. Schieber, George J., and Jean-Pierre Poullier. Interna-
      tional health care spending: Issues and trends. *Health
      Affairs* 10 (Spring 1991): 113.

158. Schieber and Poullier, International health care expen-
      diture trends: 1987, 170–172.

159. Ontario Health Insurance Plan. *OHIP general guide*,
      24. Toronto, Ontario, Canada: Ontario Ministry of
      Health, 1987.

160. Crichton, Hsu, and Tsang, *Canada's health care*, 133–
      134; Ontario Health Insurance Plan, *OHIP general
      guide*, 18.

161. Health and Welfare Canada. *National health expendi-
      tures in Canada, 1975–1987*, 32. Ottawa, Ontario,
      Canada: Department of National Health and Welfare,
      Policy, Communications and Information Branch,
      1990; Health Care Financing Administration. National
      health expenditures, 1988. *Health Care Financing Re-
      view* 11 (Summer 1990): 25.

162. Health and Welfare Canada. *National health expendi-
      tures in Canada, 1975–1985*, 181. Ottawa, Ontario,
      Canada: Department of National Health and Welfare,
      Policy, Communications and Information Branch,
      1987.

163. Evans, Robert G., Jonathan Lomas, Morris L. Barer,
      Roberta J. Labelle, Catherine Fooks, Gregory L. Stod-
      dart, Geoffrey M. Anderson, David Feeny, Amiram
      Gafni, George W. Torrance, and William G. Tholl.
      Controlling health expenditures—the Canadian reality.
      New England Journal of Medicine 320 (March 2,
      1989): 573.

164. Iglehart, John K. Canada's health care system (part 2).
      New England Journal of Medicine 315 (September 18,
      1986): 780; Statistics Canada, *Canada year book 1990*,
      part 3, 10.

165. U.S. Department of Commerce, *Statistical abstract*,
      97.

166. U.S. Department of Commerce, *Statistical abstract*,
      100.

167. Kosterlitz, Julie. Taking care of Canada. *National Jour-
      nal* 21 (July 7, 1989): 1793; Himmelstein and Wool-
      handler, National health program, 105.

168. Barer, Morris L., Robert G. Evans, and Roberta J. La-
      belle. Fee controls as cost control: Tales from the frozen
      north. *The Milbank Quarterly* 66 (1988): 9; Deber and
      Vayda, Environment of health, 444; Evans, Robert G.
      Finding the levers, finding the courage: Lessons from
      cost containment in North America. *Journal of Health
      Politics, Policy and Law* 11 (Winter 1986): 595.

169. Evans, Finding the levers, 595.

170. Rakich, Canadian and U.S. health, 34.

171. Barer, Evans, and Labelle, Fee controls, 12; Lomas,
      Jonathan, Catherine Fooks, Thomas Rice, and Roberta
      J. Labelle. Paying physicians in Canada: Minding our
      Ps and Qs. *Health Affairs* 8 (Spring 1989): 83; Vayda
      and Deber, Canadian health care, 191.

172. Lomas, Fooks, Rice, and Labelle, Paying physicians, 83.
173. Lomas, Fooks, Rice, and Labelle, Paying physicians, 86.
174. Ginsburg, Paul B. Physician payment policy in the 101st Congress. *Health Affairs* 8 (Spring 1989): 7.
175. Physician Payment Review Commission. *Physician Payment Review Commission: Annual report to Congress, 1989.* Washington, D.C., 1989.
176. Hsiao, William C., Peter Braun, Daniel Dunn, and Edmund R. Becker. Results and policy implications of the resource-based relative-value study. *New England Journal of Medicine* 319 (September 29, 1988): 881–888; Hsiao, William C., Peter Braun, Daniel Dunn, and Edmund R. Becker. Resource-based relative-values. *Journal of the American Medical Association* 260 (October 28, 1988): 2347–2353.
177. United States Code Annotated. Title 42, The Public Health and Welfare, 1990 (supplementary pamphlet covering the years 1984–1989), 335–349. St. Paul, MN: West Publishing Co., 1990.
178. Rachlis, Michael, and Carol Kushner. *Second opinion: What's wrong with Canada's health-care system and how to fix it,* chpt. 1 and 2. Toronto, Ontario, Canada: Collins, 1989.
179. Walker, Michael. From Canada: A different viewpoint. *Health Management Quarterly* 11 (First Quarter 1989): 12.
180. Rakich, Canadian and U.S. health, 35.
181. Rublee, Dale A. Medical technology in Canada, Germany, and the U.S. *Health Affairs* 8 (Fall 1989): 180; 178–81. Walker, Michael. Why Canada's health care system is no cure for America's ills. *International Briefing* (The Heritage Foundation) 19 (November 13, 1989): 6.
182. Rublee, Medical technology, 180.
183. Enthoven and Kronick, Consumer-choice health plan—part II, 100.
184. Levey and Hill, National health insurance, 1752.
185. Kosterlitz, Julie. But not for us? *National Journal* 21 (July 22, 1989): 1871.
186. Levey and Hill, National health insurance, 1751.
187. From Lave, Judith R., and Lester B. Lave. Health care: Part I. *Law and Contemporary Problems* 35 (Spring 1970). Reprinted by permission. Copyright © 1970, 1971 by Duke University.

BIBLIOGRAPHY

American Board of Medical Specialties, Research and Education Foundation. *Annual report & reference handbook—1991.* Evanston, IL, 1991.

American Hospital Association. *AHA hospital statistics.* Chicago, 1991.

Association of American Medical Colleges. Council of Teaching Hospitals: Selected activities report—May 1990. Washington, D.C., 1990.

Association of American Medical Colleges. U.S. medical school finances: Part I and Part II, 1989–1990. Washington, D.C., 1991.

Barer, Morris L., Robert G. Evans, and Roberta J. Labelle. Fee controls as cost control: Tales from the frozen north. *The Milbank Quarterly* 66 (1988): 1–62.

Battistella, Roger M., and Thomas P. Weil. National health insurance reconsidered: Dilemmas and opportunities. *Hospital & Health Services Administration* 34 (Summer 1989): 139–155.

Blendon, Robert J., Robert Leitman, Ian Morrison, and Karen Donelan. Satisfaction with health systems in ten nations. *Health Affairs* 9 (Summer 1990): 185–192.

Blum, Henrik L. *Expanding health care horizons: From a general systems concept of health to a national health policy,* 2d ed. Oakland, CA: Third Party Publishing Company, 1983.

Blum, Henrik L. *Planning for health: Development and application of social change theory.* New York: Human Sciences Press, 1974.

Bullough, Vern L., and Bonnie Bullough. *The care of the sick: The emergence of modern nursing.* London: Croom Helm, 1979.

Butler, Stuart M., and Edmund F. Haislmaier, eds. *Critical issues: A national health system for America.* Washington, D.C.: The Heritage Foundation, 1989.

Crichton, Anne, David Hsu, and Stella Tsang. *Canada's health care system: Its funding and organization.* Ottawa, Ontario, Canada: Canadian Hospital Association, 1990.

Deber, Risa B., and Eugene Vayda. The environment of health policy implementation: The Ontario, Canada example. In *Oxford textbook of public health,* edited by W. Holland, vol. III, 441–461. Oxford, England: Oxford University Press, 1985.

Enthoven, Alain C., and Richard Kronick. A consumer-choice health plan for the 1990s: A universal health insurance system designed to promote quality and economy—Part I. *New England Journal of Medicine* 320 (January 5, 1989): 29–37.

Enthoven, Alain C., and Richard Kronick. A consumer-choice health plan for the 1990s: A universal health insurance system designed to promote quality and economy—Part II. *New England Journal of Medicine* 320 (January 12, 1989): 94–101.

Evans, Robert G. Finding the levers, finding the courage: Lessons from cost containment in North America. *Journal of Health Politics, Policy and Law* 11 (Winter 1986): 585–615.

Evans, Robert G. Split vision: Interpreting cross-border differences in health spending. *Health Affairs* 7 (Winter 1988): 17–24.

Evans, Robert G., Jonathan Lomas, Morris L. Barer, Roberta J. Labelle, Catherine Fooks, Gregory L. Stoddart, Geoffrey M. Anderson, David Feeny, Amiram Gafni, George W. Torrance, and William G. Tholl. Controlling health expenditures—the Canadian reality. *New England Journal of Medicine* 320 (March 2, 1989): 571–577.

Evans, Robert G., and Greogry L. Stoddart. *Medicare at Maturity.* Calgary, Alberta, Canada: The University of Calgary Press, 1989.

Fries, Brant E., Gunnar Ljunggren, and Bengt Winblad. International comparison of long-term care: The need for resident-level classification. *Journal of the American Geriatrics Society* 39 (January 1991): 10–16.

Gabel, Jon, Howard Cohen, and Steven Fink. Americans' views on health care: Foolish inconsistencies? *Health Affairs* 8 (Spring 1989): 103–118.

Ginsburg, Paul B. Physician payment policy in the 101st Congress. *Health Affairs* 8 (Spring 1989): 5–20.

Grimaldi, Paul L. RBRVS: How new physician fee schedule

will work. *Healthcare Financial Management* 45 (September 1991): 58, 60, 64, 66, 68, 70, 72, 74, 76.

Haislmaier, Edmund F. Perception vs. reality: Taking a second look at Canadian health care. *Backgrounder* (The Heritage Foundation) 10 (January 31, 1991): 1–21.

Harris-Wehling, Jo, and Michael G.H. McGeary. Medicare: A strategy for quality assurance, IV: Medicare conditions of participation and quality assurance. *QRB* 17 (October 1991): 320–323.

Health and Welfare Canada. *National health expenditures in Canada, 1975–1987.* Ottawa, Ontario, Canada: Department of National Health and Welfare, Policy, Communications and Information Branch, 1990.

Health Care Financing Administration. National health expenditures, 1986–2000. *Health Care Financing Review* 8 (Summer 1987): 1–36.

Health Care Financing Administration. National health expenditures, 1988. *Health Care Financing Review* 11 (Summer 1990): 1–54.

Himmelstein, David U., and Stephanie Woolhandler. A national health program for the United States: A physicians' proposal. *New England Journal of Medicine* 320 (January 12, 1989): 102–108.

Hsiao, William C., Peter Braun, Daniel Dunn, and Edmund R. Becker. Resource-based relative-values. *Journal of the American Medical Association* 260 (October 28, 1988): 2347–2353.

Hsiao, William C., Peter Braun, Daniel Dunn, and Edmund R. Becker. Results and policy implications of the resource-based relative-value study. *New England Journal of Medicine* 319 (September 29, 1988): 881–888.

Iglehart, John K. Canada's health care system (part 1). *New England Journal of Medicine* 315 (July 17, 1986): 202–208.

Iglehart, John K. Canada's health care system (part 2). *New England Journal of Medicine* 315 (September 18, 1986): 778–784.

Jajich-Toth, Cindy, and Burns W. Roper. Americans' views on health care: A study in contradictions. *Health Affairs* 9 (Winter 1990): 149–157.

Joint Commission on Accreditation of Healthcare Organizations. *Committed to quality: An introduction to the Joint Commission on Accreditation of Healthcare Organizations.* Oakbrook Terrace, IL, 1990.

Koff, Sondra Z. *Health systems agencies: A comprehensive examination of planning and process.* New York: Health Sciences Press, Inc., 1988.

Kosterlitz, Julie. But not for us? *National Journal* 21 (July 22, 1989): 1871–1875.

Kosterlitz, Julie. Taking care of Canada. *National Journal* 21 (July 7, 1989): 1792–1797.

Levey, Samuel, and James Hill. National health insurance—the triumph of equivocation. *New England Journal of Medicine* 321 (December 21, 1989): 1750–1754.

Levit, Katharine R., Helen C. Lazenby, Cathy A. Cowan, and Suzanne W. Letsch. National health expenditures, 1990. *Health Care Financing Review* 13 (Fall 1991): 29–54.

Lomas, Jonathan, Catherine Fooks, Thomas Rice, and Roberta J. Labelle. Paying physicians in Canada: Minding our Ps and Qs. *Health Affairs* 8 (Spring 1989): 80–102.

Marmor, Theodore R., and Rudolf Klein. Costs vs. care: American's health care dilemma wrongly considered. *Health Matrix* 4 (Spring 1986): 19–24.

Neuschler, Edward. *Canadian health care: The implications of public health insurance.* Washington, D.C.: Health Insurance Association of America, 1990.

1991 AJN Guide: State boards of nursing and RN licensure regulations. *American Journal of Nursing* 91 (April 1991): 20–27.

Organization for Economic Cooperation and Development. *Financing and delivering health care: A comparative analysis of OECD countries.* OECD Social Policy Studies No. 4. Paris, 1987.

Organization for Economic Cooperation and Development. *Health care systems in transition: The search for efficiency.* Paris, 1990.

Pickett, George E., and John J. Hanlon. *Public health administration and practice,* 9th ed. St. Louis: Times Mirror/Mosby College Publishing, 1990.

Poullier, Jean-Pierre. Health care expenditure data: An international comparison from the OECD. In *Health care systems in transition: The search for efficiency,* 119–126. Paris: Organization for Economic Cooperation and Development.

Rachlis, Michael, and Carol Kushner. *Second opinion: What's wrong with Canada's health-care system and how to fix it.* Toronto, Ontario, Canada: Collins, 1989.

Rakich, Jonathon S. Canada's universal-comprehensive health care system. *Hospital Topics* 69 (Spring 1991): 14–19.

Rakich, Jonathon S. The Canadian and U.S. health care systems: Profiles and policies. *Hospital & Health Services Administration* 36 (Spring 1991): 25–42.

Rublee, Dale A. Medical technology in Canada, Germany, and the U.S. *Health Affairs* 8 (Fall 1989): 178–181.

Schafft, Gretchen Engle, and James F. Cawley. *The physician assistant in a changing health care environment.* Rockville, MD: Aspen Publishers, Inc., 1987.

Schieber, George J., and Jean-Pierre Poullier. International health care expenditure trends: 1987. *Health Affairs* 8 (Fall 1989): 167–177.

Schieber, George J., and Jean-Pierre Poullier. International health spending: Issues and trends. *Health Affairs* 10 (Spring 1991): 106–116.

Schieber, George J. and Jean-Pierre Poullier. An overview of international comparisons of health care expenditures. *Health Care Financing Review* Annual Supplement (1989): 1–7.

Schieber, George J., and Jean-Pierre Poullier. An overview of international comparisons of health care expenditures. In *Health care systems in transition: The search for efficiency,* 9–15. Paris: Organization for Economic Cooperation and Development, 1990.

Schneider, Don P., Brant E. Fries, William J. Foley, Marilyn Desmond, and William J. Gormley. Case mix for nursing home payment: Resource utilization groups, version II. *Health Care Financing Review* Annual Supplement (1988): 39–52.

Schwartz, William B., and Daniel N. Mendelson. No evidence of an emerging physician surplus: An analysis of change in physicians' work load and income. *Journal of the American Medical Association* 263 (January 26, 1990): 557–560.

Schwartz, William B., Frank A. Sloan, and Daniel N. Mendelson. Why there will be little or no physician surplus between now and the year 2000. *New England Journal of Medicine* 318 (April 7, 1988): 892–897.

Singer, Allen M. Projections of physician supply and demand: A summary of HRSA and AMA studies. *Academic Medicine* 64 (April 1989): 235–240.

Southby, Richard F., and Jonathon S. Rakich. International health care expenditures. *Hospital Topics* 69 (Spring 1991): 8–13.

Spencer, Gregory. *Projections of the population of the United*

States, by age, sex, and race: 1988–2080. Washington, D.C.: Bureau of the Census, U.S. Department of Commerce, 1989.

Statistics Canada. *Canada year book 1990.* Ottawa, Ontario, Canada: Ministry of Supplies and Services, 1989.

Sutherland, Ralph W., and M. Jane Fulton. *Health care in Canada: A description and analysis of Canadian health care services.* Ottawa, Ontario, Canada: The Health Group, 1988.

Taylor, Malcolm G. The Canadian health care system 1974–1984. In *Medicare at maturity,* edited by R.G. Evans and G.L. Stoddart, 3–40. Calgary, Alberta, Canada: The University of Calgary Press, 1989.

Taylor, Malcolm G. *Health insurance and Canadian public policy,* 2nd ed. Montreal, Quebec, Canada: The Institute of Public Administration in Canada and McGill-Queens University Press, 1987.

Vayda, Eugene, and Risa B. Deber. The Canadian health care system: An overview. *Social Science and Medicine* 18 (1984): 191–197.

Walker, Michael. From Canada: A different viewpont. *Health Management Quarterly* 11 (First Quarter 1989): 11–14.

Walker, Michael. Why Canada's health care system is no cure for America's ills. *International Briefing* (The Heritage Foundation) 19 (November 13, 1989): 1–14.

3 / Ethical Considerations

A moral twilight zone has developed . . . in the past 10 years, as the power equilibrium has shifted from physicians to administrators. CEOs are ill prepared to make the decisions traditionally made by doctors and nurses about moral dilemmas.

Leonard Fleck, Center for Ethics and
Humanities in Life Sciences,
Michigan State University[1]

Ethical issues arise in all types of health services organizations (HSOs). The most significant occur in acute care hospitals, usually because the highest levels of technology are applied in them. It is a measure of the uniqueness and complexity of HSOs that when a matter raises ethical issues, there are often legal dimensions. Ethical and legal problems arise independently of one another, but one of them rarely occurs alone; many times managers find both.

This chapter discusses the ethical aspects of health services management. Because of the interaction of ethics and law, an introductory section describes sources of law, as well as the relationships between the law and ethics, and it thus serves as background for both this chapter and Chapter 4, "Legal Considerations."

SOURCES OF LAW

Ethics and law have a dynamic relationship, and it is useful to review briefly the development of the law. Every society has a code or system of laws that distinguishes acceptable and unacceptable behavior and penalizes those who behave unacceptably. *Law* is a system of principles and rules of human conduct prescribed or recognized by society and enforced by a public authority. This definition includes criminal and civil law. *Ethics* is the study of standards of conduct and moral judgment. When referring to a profession, it is the system, principles, or code of that group.

Criminal law has a moral underpinning in that it reflects society's sense of right and wrong—its moral code (ethics). This is true also for civil law, which governs relations among individuals, such as contracts and commercial transactions. Here, however, the underlying moral principles are more obscure. Some societies regarded the law as a gift from the gods; Plato's Greece is an example. Beyond the written law, which reflects the most significant concerns of society, however, are other considerations. The early Greeks recognized the importance of an unwritten form of law incorporating concepts of fairness that may have been too elusive or varied in their application to be readily incorporated into a codification. This tradition was continued by the courts of equity, established and known in England as chancery, which were transplanted to American legal practice. Plato considered the written law an oversimplification that could not take account of the nuances, conditions, and differences among persons and situations in a dispute. He believed the best method of resolving a dispute was one in which a philosopher applied an unwritten law. His own experiences proved this impossible in practice, however, and Plato later accepted a written form of law in which the authorities become servants of the law and administer it without regard to who is involved in the dispute.[2] This principle of "a rule of law, not of men" is reflected in the Anglo-American legal system.

There are times when orderliness and continuity must yield to requirements of justice in a particular case. This is known as *equity*. Equity seeks to do justice to the parties in a dispute that is unique and is unlikely to occur again. Aristotle recognized this problem:

> When therefore the law lays down a general rule, and thereafter a case arises which is an exception to the rule, it is then right, where the lawgiver's pronouncement because of its absoluteness is defective and erroneous, to rectify the defect by deciding as the lawgiver would himself decide if he were present on the occasion, and would have enacted if he had been cognizant of the case in question.[3]

Such a principle of law permits the right result to occur in a specific case in which blindly following the law would provide no remedy, or one that is unsatisfactory.

Bodenheimer, a scholar of jurisprudence, divides sources of law into two major categories, formal and nonformal.

> By formal sources, we mean sources which are available in an articulated textual formulation embodied in an authoritative legal document. The chief examples of such formal sources are constitutions and statutes . . . executive orders, administrative regulations, ordinances, charters and bylaws of autonomous or semiautonomous bodies . . . treaties and certain other agreements, and judicial precedents. By nonformal sources we mean legally significant materials and considerations which have not received an authoritative or at least articulated formulation and embodiment in a formalized legal document. Without necessarily claiming exhaustive completeness for this enumeration, we have subdivided the nonformal sources into standards of justice, principles of reason and consideration of the nature of things (*natura rerum*), individual equity, public policies, moral convictions, social trends, and customary law.[4]

Including charters and bylaws of autonomous or semiautonomous bodies as formal sources of law has special significance for health services managers because most HSOs have such documents. Courts look to these documents to determine the rights and obligations of those affected. Chapter 7, "How HSOs Are Organized," describes how states issue charters so that corporations and limited partnerships can be established. The importance of professional staff bylaws in the HSO is also discussed in Chapter 7.

Bodenheimer's definition of formal sources of law includes the codes of ethics that professional associations use to guide affiliates. The interpretations of such writings provide a basis for later guidance in application and decision making. Written provisions with interpretations have the virtues of consistency and predictability. Codes include what a profession considers to be minimally acceptable behavior. Codes also state the profession's goals and strivings—what is to be achieved—as well as philosophy and mission. Formal sources eliminate the need for nonformal sources, except when the former lack comprehensiveness or require interpretation.

RELATIONSHIP OF LAW TO ETHICS

Democratically derived laws generally reflect the views of justice and fairness held by a majority of the population. Nonetheless, many people may have contrary views and may consider the law unjust or immoral and be willing to risk punishment for breaking it. A classic example in American history is the Volstead Act, which amended the Constitution to prohibit the manufacture and distribution of alcoholic beverages. Violation of the law was rampant until its repeal in 1933. The abortion issue suggests the complexity of the relationship between ethics (morality) and law. Abortion is legal, but it is clear that many consider it unethical or immoral.

The link between law and ethics might be viewed as one to one—anything lawful is ethical and vice versa. This is not necessarily true. The law represents the minimum performance expected from members of society. Professions demand compliance with the law, but they add to it and hold members to a higher standard. Thus, even if the law does not require *any* member of society to perform a particular act, a professional code of ethics may require all members of that profession to do so. For that professional such an act (or failure to act) is thus legal, but not ethical.

Models showing the relationship of law and ethics were developed by Henderson.[5] Figure 3.1 suggests the succession of events that causes corporate decisions to come to public scrutiny and a determination as to whether they are legal or ethical, or both. This judgment is necessarily after the fact, despite management's efforts to predict the effects of actions. This model suggests the impossibility of knowing whether those who eventually judge the decision will consider it legal (law enforcement officials) or ethical (a profession or the general public). This adds uncertainty to HSO decision making. Predicting an action's legality is usually more accurate than judging whether it is ethical.

Figure 3.2 shows the combinations of legal, illegal, ethical, and unethical factors involved in corporate decision making. Decisions made in Quadrant I are both ethical and legal and are easily identified: managers who obey the law are acting legally and ethically. Quadrant II includes decisions that are ethical, but illegal. Codes such as that of the American College of Healthcare Executives require obeying the law as minimal ethical conduct. This blanket prohibition makes it virtually impossible that a health services manager could justify as ethical an act that is illegal. A possible exception occurs when an overriding moral reason compels one to disobey the law (e.g., it is more immoral to obey the law because of the harm caused than to disobey it).

Quadrant III includes decisions that are unethical but legal. This suggests the concept that ethical standards, especially in a profession, require a higher standard than does the law. Examples include failing to take all reasonable steps to protect patients from malpractice in an HSO, or managerial self-aggrandizement at the expense of patients.

Quadrant IV includes activities that are illegal and unethical. Examples are easy. Codes of ethics require that the law be obeyed; any decision that breaks the law is illegal and unethical. Embezzlement is in this quadrant, as is failing to meet fire safety regulations or filing a false Medicare report.

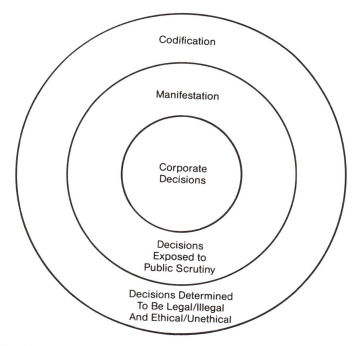

Figure 3.1. The relationship between law and ethics. (From Henderson, Verne E. The ethical side of enterprise. *Sloan Management Review* 23 [Spring 1982]: 37–47; reprinted by permission. Copyright © 1982 by the Sloan Management Review Association. All rights reserved.)

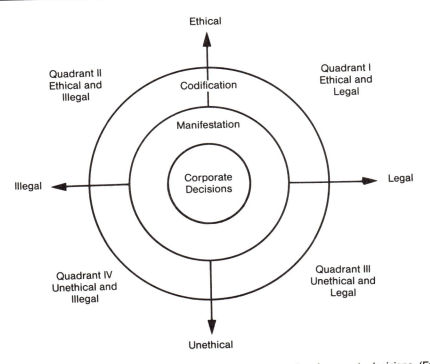

Figure 3.2.   A matrix of possible outcomes concerning the ethics and legality of corporate decisions. (From Henderson, Verne E. The ethical side of enterprise. *Sloan Management Review* 23 [Spring 1982]: 37–47; reprinted by permission. Copyright © 1982 by the Sloan Management Review Association. All rights reserved.)

MORAL PHILOSOPHIES

Three theories of moral philosophy are used extensively in western culture: teleology, deontology, and natural law. They provide a basis for the study of morals (ethics) and assist one in determining the moral rightness or wrongness of a decision.

Teleology

The word *teleology* comes from the Greek root *telos*, which means end. The most prominent modern theory of morality using this concept is called *utility theory;* the person who follows it is a *utilitarian.* The underlying premise is that the moral rightness or wrongness of an act or decision is judged by whether it brings into being more good (utility) or ungood (disutility) than alternative decisions. Classical utilitarianism's most prominent exponent was the English philosopher John Stuart Mill (1806–1873). Utilitarians have no independent right or wrong to guide them. They look at the consequences of an act—the "good" is independent of the "right." Utilitarians are sometimes called consequentialists because they judge actions by their consequences.

Utilitarianism is divided into act utility and rule utility. Act utility assesses each decision and determines its consequences when judging moral rightness or wrongness. Rule utility is more formal. It assesses various courses of action and measures their consequences. This allows a determination of which is the best course of action in general, and this is the action that should be taken, even though it may not produce the most good every time. The rule utilitarian has determined that on the whole a certain decision produces the most utility. Utility in a modified form is the basis for cost-benefit analysis. A summary statement that describes utilitarian theory is "the end justifies the means."

Deontology

Deontology is a theory about morality based on the presence of an independent right or wrong. It does not consider consequences as does utilitarianism. The word *deontology* is derived from the Greek *deon*, meaning duty. The best known proponent of the role of duty was the German philosopher Immanuel Kant (1724–1804). Briefly, his philosophy holds that the end is unimportant because human beings have duties to one another as moral agents, and these duties take precedence over consequences. For Kant, an act is moral if it arises from good will and if one consequently acts from a sense of duty. The Kantian test of morality is whether the action can meet the categorical imperative that requires that we act in accordance with what we wish to become a universal law. What is right or wrong for one person is right or wrong for everyone, in all places and at all times. According to Kant, an action is right only if it can be universalized without violating the equality of human beings. For example, Kantians see it as logically inconsistent to argue that a terminally ill person should be euthanized, because this amounts to saying that one can improve life by ending it. Deontology may be summarized as never treating humanity simply as a means, but rather always as an end.[6] Another summary is to practice the golden rule—do unto others as you would have them do unto you.

Natural Law

The third important moral philosophy is *natural law*. Mill defined the good in terms of the good produced; Kant rejected ethical theories based on desire or inclination and argued that there is an independent right. Natural law states that ethics (morality) must be grounded in a concern for human good. It is, therefore, teleological (consequential). It contends that the good cannot be defined only in terms of subjective inclinations; rather, there is a good for human beings that is objectively desirable, although not reducible to desire.[7] The natural law is based on Aristotelian thought as interpreted and synthesized with Christian dogma by St. Thomas Aquinas (1226–1274).[8] It assumes a natural order in relationships and a predisposition among rational persons to do, or refrain from doing, certain things. Because human beings are rational, we are able to discover what we should do, and in that attempt we are guided by a partial notion of the eternal law that is linked to our capacity for rational thought. Since natural law guides what rational persons do, it serves as the basis for the positive law, some of which is reflected in statutes. A summary statement of the basic precepts of natural law is that one should do good and avoid evil.

Natural law should be contrasted with legal positivism, which became prominent about 100 years ago, and which is based on an aversion to metaphysical speculations and to the search for ultimate principles that was reflected in the work of Aquinas. According to Bodenheimer, "The legal positivist holds that only positive law is law; and by positive law he means those judicial norms which have been established by the authority of the state."[9]

John Rawls and the Concept of Social Contract

The work of a contemporary American philosopher, John Rawls, is an extension of the deontological thinking of Immanuel Kant. In *A Theory of Justice*, Rawls develops the elements of a social contract between free, equal, and rational persons. To explain this social contract Rawls uses the hypothetical constructs of an original position and a veil of ignorance. The original position and veil of ignorance assume persons remain self-interested and rational, but know nothing of their individual talents, intelligence, social and economic situation, health, or the like. Rawls argues that such persons would agree to certain principles of justice: "First, each person is to have an equal right to the most extensive basic liberty compatible with similar liberty for others. Second, social and economic inequalities are to be arranged so that they are both (a) reasonably expected to be to everyone's advantage, and (b) attached to positions and offices open to all."[10] He reasons that rational, self-interested persons would reject utilitarianism and select instead the concepts of right and justice as precedent to the good. Rawls bases this conclusion on an assessment that rational self-interest dictates that one act to protect the least well off, since anyone could be part of that group.

PHILOSOPHICAL BASES FOR ETHICS[11]

Figure 3.3 shows that the ethical theories described above are the basis for principles, rules, and specific judgments and actions. Ethical theories do not necessarily conflict; diverse philosophies may reach the same conclusion about a particular action, albeit through different reasoning or by use of varying constructs.

Ethical theories and derivative principles guide development of the rules that produce specific judgments and actions. Four principles are important for health services managers: respect for persons, beneficence, nonmaleficence, and justice. Utility is included as an adjunct to beneficence. These principles should be reflected in the organization's philosophy, as well as the manager's personal ethic.

Respect for Persons

The principle of respect for persons has four elements. The first, *autonomy,* requires that one act toward others in a way that allows them to govern themselves—to choose and pursue a course of action. To do so, a person must be rational and uncoerced (unconstrained). Sometimes patients are or become nonautonomous (e.g., the physically or mentally incapacitated). They are owed respect, nonetheless, even though special means are needed for them to be autonomous. Autonomy underlies the need to obtain consent for treatment, as well as the general way an organization views and interacts with patients and staff.

Autonomy is in a state of dynamic tension with paternalism, a concept that suggests someone else knows what is best for the person. The Hippocratic oath is antecedent to paternalism in the patient–physician relationship. It urges physicians to act in the patient's best interests—as they judge those interests. Giving primacy to autonomy limits paternalism to very specific circumstances.

The second element of respect for persons is *truth telling.* In general parlance this requires managers to be honest in all activities. Depending on how absolute a position is taken, this also eliminates white lies, even if they are told because it is (correctly) believed that knowledge of the truth would cause harm to the individual learning it. The necessity of telling the truth to patients is

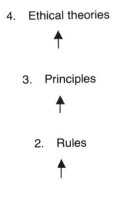

4. Ethical theories

3. Principles

2. Rules

1. Particular judgments and actions

Figure 3.3. Hierarchy of relationships. (From Beauchamp, T.L., and James F. Childress. *Principles of biomedical ethics,* 3d ed., 6. New York: Oxford University Press, 1989; reprinted by permission.)

less certain, however, depending on the circumstances. Some patients would suffer mentally and physically if told the truth about their illnesses. Should this happen, physicians would not meet their obligation of *primum non nocere* (first, do no harm). The modern expression of this concept is nonmaleficence, which is discussed below.

Confidentiality is the third element of respect for persons. It requires managers and clinicians to keep secret what they learn about patients. For managers, this duty applies as well to staff, organization, and community. The need to meet legal requirements causes major exceptions to confidentiality.

The fourth element of the principle of respect for persons is *fidelity*—doing one's duty, keeping one's word. This is sometimes called promise keeping. Like the other three elements, fidelity allows managers to meet the principle of respect for persons.

Beneficence

The second principle, beneficence, is rooted in the Hippocratic tradition and is defined as acting with charity and kindness. As applied in health services, however, it is a broader, more positive duty as compared with the principle of nonmaleficence. Nonmaleficence means refraining from actions that aggravate a problem or cause other negative results. Beneficence and nonmaleficence are endpoints on a continuum.

Beneficence may be divided into: 1) providing benefits and 2) balancing benefits and harms (utility). Conferring benefits is firmly established in medicine, and failing to provide them when one is able to do so violates the professional duties of clinician and manager. Balancing benefits and harms (utility) is the philosophical basis for cost-benefit analysis as well as other efforts to balance risks and benefits. It is like the principle of utility espoused by the utilitarians; however, here utility is only one of several considerations and, as noted below, has more limited application.

The positive duty suggested by the principle of beneficence requires the organization and its managers to do all they can to aid patients. There is a lesser duty to aid persons who are potential rather than actual patients. This distinction and its importance varies with the philosophy and mission of the organization and whether it serves a defined population. Thus, a hospital emergency department has no duty under the principle of beneficence to scour neighborhoods for persons needing its assistance. This duty changes, of course, when one of these individuals becomes a patient.

The second dimension of beneficence is balancing the benefits and harms of an action. This flows from a positive duty to act in the patient's best interests because one cannot act with kindness and charity if risks outweigh benefits. Regardless of its interpretation, utility cannot justify overriding the interests of patients and sacrificing them to the greater good.

Nonmaleficence

The third principle applicable to managing HSOs is nonmaleficence. Like beneficence, it has historical roots in medicine. Nonmaleficence is in effect *primum non nocere*—first, do no harm. This dictum to guide physicians' actions is equally applicable to health services managers. Nonmaleficence gives rise to specific moral rules, but neither the principle nor the derivative rules can be absolute because it is often appropriate (with the patient's consent) to inflict harm (e.g., take a blood sample) to avoid worse harm (e.g., performing a surgical procedure).

The principle of nonmaleficence most commonly applies to an HSO's relationships with patients. It also raises duties managers have to HSO staff, however, and there may be circumstances in which these two sets of duties conflict. Putting staff at extraordinary risk for their health and safety is inconsistent with the manager's duty to them, even when this results in meeting the principle of beneficence to patients. Balancing benefits and harms also suggests application of the concept of utility discussed above. The problem of acquired immunodeficiency syndrome (AIDS) raises these issues, and they are discussed later in this chapter.

Justice

The fourth principle, justice, is very important in certain types of managerial decision making (e.g., allocating the organization's resources). However, it applies as well to how patients and employees are treated in ways that have nothing to do with resource allocation (e.g., personnel policies). What is just, and how does one know when justice is achieved?

Philosophies treat this principle differently. Rawls defines justice as fairness. Partly, the definition requires that all persons get their just deserts or what they are due. But how are fairness and just deserts defined? Aristotle defines justice as equals treated equally, and unequals unequally. This concept of equity is common in public policy analysis. Equal treatment of equals is reflected in liberty rights such as freedom of speech for all. Unequal treatment of persons unequally situated is used to justify progressive income taxes and redistribution of wealth. This concept of justice is expressed in health services by expending greater resources on those more ill and more in need. These concepts of justice are helpful; however, they do not solve the problems of definition and opinion that are so troublesome for managers. Macro- and microallocation of resources have been extensively considered in the literature. Crucial to clinicians and managers who seek to act justly is that they consistently apply clear criteria in decision making.

Summary

Moral philosophies and derivative principles provide a framework for honing a personal ethic and using it to analyze and solve ethical problems. Like philosophers, managers are unlikely to agree fully with a moral philosophy. Most will be eclectic in developing or reconsidering a personal ethic. In general, however, the principles of respect for persons, beneficence, nonmaleficence, and justice are useful in defining the relationships among patients, managers, and organizations. They may carry different weights and take precedence over one another, depending on the issue being considered. Justice requires, however, that they be consistently ordered and weighted when similar problems are considered.

CODES OF ETHICS

A major problem with applied ethics is that many written and unwritten codes influence or guide human behavior. They arise from family background, religious orientation and training, professional affiliations and allegiances, and an often ill-defined personal code of moral conduct—an amalgam of intellect, reasoning, experience, education, and relationships. Codes are often vague or contradictory. Often, it seems there are few answers, only difficult questions and choices.

One attribute of professionalism is a strong element of service to society. This tends to minimize one's private life and maximize one's public life. Activities that violate a professional code may be subject to disciplinary action. Professions face a dilemma, however, in determining how much scrutiny to give nonprofessional activities. The relationship between private and public lives is especially problematic if, for example, a member's personal conduct scandalizes the profession. Few health services managers seem to have determined the boundary between private and professional lives. How far beyond the HSO and one's professional and public life may the profession go? Similarly, organizational culture and philosophy (discussed in Chapter 1) have an important interaction with a manager's personal ethic.

A well-developed organizational philosophy does not eliminate the need for a manager to have a personal ethic. A personal ethic is a framework for decision making and permits refinement of guidelines, judgments, and actions. It bears repeating that each of us is a moral agent whose actions (and nonactions) have moral consequences—consequences for which we are responsible. Conduct cannot be excused by claiming we are following orders, regardless of the source of those orders. Orders from lawfully constituted public authorities such as courts pose special problems. Moral agents who believe that such orders are unjust may engage in civil disobedience. In doing so, however, they must be prepared to bear societally imposed sanctions. Ethical (moral) implications of acts must be considered independent of the act itself.

Occasionally, conflicts arise between the HSO's ethic (expressed in its philosophy) and a manager's personal ethic. An HSO is bureaucratic and assumes a life of its own. The manager must think carefully about the implications of acquiescing in specific expressions of an HSO's philosophy. Again, this is the concept of moral agency. It may seem easier to go along in order to get along than to risk one's position and economic association by speaking out. Failing to speak out, however, violates our duty as moral agents. The dilemma of whether to be a whistleblower confronts few managers. This does not mean that HSOs have no problems that warrant speaking out. Managers cannot go about their daily tasks without considering the moral context of what they do. Likenesses, and differences, between organizational and personal ethics must not be forgotten.

HEALTH SERVICES CODES OF ETHICS

Institutions

Many of the associations noted in Chapter 2, "The Health Care Delivery System," have ethical guidelines. Among them is the American Hospital Association (AHA), the major trade association for hospitals. Its revised guidelines, adopted in 1987, include sections on community role, patient care, and organizational conduct. Members are urged to improve community health status and deliver high-quality, comprehensive services efficiently. There is emphasis on coordination with other HSOs. Specific provisions address the need for informed consent, confidentiality, and mechanisms to resolve conflicting values among patients and families, clinical staff, employees, the organization, and the community. Religious and social beliefs and customs of patients should be accommodated if possible, but the HSO's ethics are not subordinate to those of the patient. This suggests the importance of developing a philosophy *and* informing patients of it before treatment.

The American Health Care Association (AHCA) serves long-term care facilities (nursing facilities). It has no specific code of ethics, but members should follow the patients' bill of rights adopted by the AHCA. It discusses balancing rights and enumerates the rights of residents in long-term care facilities. These rights are concerned with fair treatment, information, communication, choice, and privacy. The focus is on minimizing the dehumanizing aspects of institutional care. Some states require nursing facilities receiving Medicaid monies to abide by a patient bill of rights based on that of the AHCA.

The Professions

One hallmark of a profession is that it has a code of ethics to define acceptable and unacceptable behavior; such codes are common in health services. Usually, language is general and performance standards are so vague that enforcement is difficult, if not impossible. Law is a notable exception, however, because lawyers are officers of the court and have a positive duty to report information that raises a substantial question as to another lawyer's honesty, trustworthiness, or fitness. Their ethics have judicial sanction because it is common for the highest court in the state or jurisdiction to adopt with few modifications the Code of Professional Responsibility of the American Bar Association (a private group) as its rules of professional conduct. Courts appoint a board of professional responsibility to enforce the rules and review and investigate complaints, which are heard by a special panel of judges. Adverse action by this panel can result in penalties ranging from probation and admonition to suspension or termination of the practice of law.

Even with vigorous enforcement, a code guides only those who want to do the right thing but who need help determining what that is. Someone who wants to get away with something is always at the fringe of a profession and will be dissuaded neither by principles of ethical conduct nor by legal requirements.

Managers

American College of Healthcare Executives   The American College of Healthcare Executives (ACHE) has had a Code of Ethics since 1939, 6 years after its founding. The code has evolved from a general and vague document to one that in the 1987 version specifically addresses the problems faced by affiliates. Examples include conflict of interest, using confidential information, honesty in advertising, working to assure access to health services, and maintaining professional competence. The 1987 code for the first time recognizes the concept of moral agency. It also identifies a positive duty for each affiliate to report violations. There continue to be many general statements to which it would be difficult to apply performance measures, but the code has become much more specific.

The ACHE Committee on Ethics investigates complaints about an affiliate's allegedly unethical actions. After investigation, the validity of the allegations is determined and a recommendation is made. Affiliates are entitled to due process, and the Code has a grievance (appeal) procedure. The maximum disciplinary action is expulsion. Affiliation is not linked to licensure, but if ACHE affiliation is considered to be important by employers and colleagues, expulsion will inhibit employment and career opportunities and is, therefore, a significant action. The deterrent effects of disciplinary action are speculative; nonetheless, applying the Code vigorously enhances its importance in the professional activities of affiliates.

Research prior to the 1987 iteration of the ACHE Code of Ethics showed that ACHE affiliates considered a code important. They believed the current code should be more comprehensive and specific in guiding decision making on ethical problems and that there should be more emphasis on enforcement and anonymous reporting to affiliates of the disposition of cases. Affiliates were also interested in learning more about ethical problems.[12] A vital, living code prepares affiliates to solve ethical issues. The Code, however, focuses almost exclusively on administrative ethics. Virtually no attention is paid to the vast array of biomedical ethical issues that may directly or indirectly confront the health services manager.

American College of Health Care Administrators   The Code of Ethics of the American College of Health Care Administrators (ACHCA), revised in 1989, guides managers of long-term care facilities (nursing homes), primarily the nursing facilities discussed in Chapter 2. Members must meet four "expectations," which are divided into prescriptions and proscriptions. The expectations state that the welfare of those receiving care is paramount; the manager must remain professionally competent; and other managers must be encouraged to meet their responsibilities to the public, the profession, and other colleagues. Issues receiving specific attention include quality of services; confidentiality of patient information; continuing education; conflicts of interest; fostering knowledge, supporting research, and sharing expertise; and providing information to the Standards and Ethics Committee of actual or potential code violations. No enforcement or appeals process is described.

Physicians

The American Medical Association (AMA) is the preeminent professional association for allopathic physicians, and its Principles of Medical Ethics are addressed exclusively here. The AMA's first code was adopted at its founding in 1847 and was based on the Code of Medical Ethics developed by the English physician and philosopher Sir Thomas Percival in 1803.[13] Several iterations have appeared since. Deleted from the 1957 version in 1980 was the prohibition that made it unethical for members to "voluntarily associate professionally with anyone" who did not practice a method of healing founded on a scientific basis—a prohibition aimed at chiropractors.

Also deleted was the prohibition on soliciting patients, which prevented physician advertising. Both changes resulted from lawsuits against the AMA. Allopathic medicine has limited association with chiropractors, but many physicians advertise.

The 1980 version of the Principles is less specific than the 1957 version. The code of ethics of organized medicine is moving in a direction opposite to that of the ACHE, whose code has become more specific. Like the ACHE Code, the AMA Principles include a positive duty for members to "strive to expose those physicians deficient in character or competence, or who engage in fraud or deception."[14] The AMA publishes the opinions of its judicial council. These interpretations of ethical issues aid physicians in understanding the Principles.

In analyzing the 1980 revisions of the AMA Principles, Veatch notes a significant change:

> The most dramatic feature of the . . . new AMA Principles is the opening to an ethics based on notions of rights and responsibilities rather than benefits and harms. It is the first document in the history of professional medical ethics in which a group of physicians is willing to use the language of responsibilities and rights.[15]

The new Principles (1980) address patient rights and confidentiality. The previous iteration allowed breaking patient confidentiality when it was in the interests of the patient or society, as well as when the law required it. Such interests were judged by the physician. The 1980 iteration requires physicians to "safeguard patient confidence within the constraints of the law." The paternalistic dimension is gone. The new Principles are a major change in the AMA's view of the physician–patient relationship.

Nurses

The Code for Nurses, developed by the American Nurses Association (ANA), was first adopted in 1950 and revised in 1985. The preamble states that clients are the primary decision makers in matters concerning their own health, treatment, and well being, and "the goal of nursing actions is to support the client's responsibility and self-determination to the greatest extent possible."[16] The absence of paternalism in this statement is notable.

The preamble includes a list of principles that govern interactions with clients that are similar to the ethical principles identified above. The introduction states that the code "serves to inform both the nurse and society of the profession's expectations and requirements in ethical matters."[17]

The code has 11 provisions, many of them specific. An interpretative statement follows each. One provision is like the AMA requirement that caregivers have a positive duty to expose unethical or incompetent practice. It states that "the nurse acts to safeguard the client and the public when health care and safety are affected by the incompetent, unethical, or illegal practice of any person."[18]

PATIENT BILLS OF RIGHTS

Further guidance about ethical relationships between health services consumers and the HSO and its employees comes from patient bills of rights. Titles vary, but bills of rights have been published by numerous organizations, including the AHA, the Joint Commission on Accreditation of Healthcare Organizations (Joint Commission), the Department of Veterans Affairs (DVA), and the American Civil Liberties Union (ACLU). As expected, the AHA is institution oriented, and the philosophy in its bill of rights is very different from that of the ACLU. The DVA "Code of Patient Concern" and the Joint Commission's "Patient Rights" lie between them.

All bills of rights reflect the law concerning issues such as confidentiality and consent. That of the ACLU, however, is much more demanding—almost strident—in its view of patients' rights than are the others, especially that of the AHA. Some AHA provisions are paternalistic, and recognize that there are times when it is in the best interests of patients not to be told about their medical condition. The ACLU mandates an advocate for each patient, that patients have full access to their medical records while hospitalized, and that they receive a copy at discharge. This rarely happens, however. The ACLU bill also details the information to be given to the patient when obtaining consent.

Although some provisions of these bills of patient rights reflect the law, none is legally binding. If adopted by an HSO, a bill of patient rights sets an ethical tone for its relationship with the patient. It may serve as a formal source of law. The effectiveness of a bill of patient rights is limited by the HSO's willingness to make its contents known to patients and to develop processes to encourage and monitor its use.

ETHICAL ISSUES AFFECTING GOVERNANCE AND MANAGEMENT

Fiduciary Duty

Fiduciary duty is an ethical (and legal) concept that arose from Roman jurisprudence and means that a relationship has certain obligations and duties. The most important is that the fiduciary (person in a position of trust) may not use the position for personal gain and must act only in the best interests of the person or organization. Governing body members of corporations organized both for profit *and* not for profit have a fiduciary duty, the breach of which can lead to personal liability.[19] However, the legal standard to judge breach of this fiduciary duty is different for the two types of governing bodies. Here, the concepts of trust and trustee have specific meanings.

Fiduciary duty applies when someone manages and controls assets (the trust) that are directed to a specific use by gift or bequest. Many trusts are established to benefit not-for-profit (charitable) corporations, although a trust may benefit individuals. Hospitals are common examples; others include schools of nursing and special funds for education of health services personnel.

Fiduciaries have primary duties of loyalty and responsibility:

> Loyalty means that the individuals must put the interest of the corporation above all self-interest, a principle based on the biblical doctrine that no man can serve two masters. Specifically no trustee is permitted to gain any secret profits personally, to accept bribes, or to compete with the corporation. . . .[20] The fiduciary duty of responsibility means that members of the governing board must exercise reasonable care, skill, and diligence proportionate to the circumstances in every activity of the board. In other words, the trustees can be held personally liable for negligence, which can be an affirmative act of commission or omission.[21]

"Trustee" is commonly used to describe governing body members of not-for-profit HSOs. Technically, the legally correct term for those who are not actually fiduciaries of a trust is "director" or "corporate director." Directors of not-for-profit organizations prefer the title trustee, probably because it distinguishes them from for-profit HSOs, where the title "director" is used.

The most significant court case involving "trustees"* of an HSO is *Stern et al. v. Lucy Webb Hayes National Training School of Deaconesses and Missionaries, et al.*[22] The suit was brought by David M. Stern on behalf of his minor son and other patients of Sibley Hospital as a class. The hospital is one of the activities controlled by the "trustees" of the Lucy Webb Hayes School. The plaintiffs alleged that patients at Sibley had paid too much for care because several "trustees" had engaged in mismanagement, nonmanagement, and self-dealing. It was alleged also that the problems resulted from a conspiracy between those "trustees" and various financial institutions. The court found no evidence of a conspiracy, but determined that:

> The charitable corporation is a relatively new legal entity which does not fit neatly into the established common law categories of corporation and trust . . . . [T]he modern trend is to apply corporate rather than trust principles in determining the liability of the directors of charitable corporations,

---

*The corporate board was called a board of trustees and its members were known as trustees even though no trust was involved and they functioned like corporate directors.

because their functions are virtually indistinguishable from those of their "pure" corporate counterparts.[23]

This determination meant that the Sibley "trustees" were held to a lesser standard of care than a true trustee.

The case is complex. It is sufficient to state that the named "trustees" were found to have violated their fiduciary duties, even when held to the lesser, corporate standard. Mismanagement occurred because the named "trustees" ignored the investment sections of yearly audits, they failed to get enough information to vote intelligently on opening new bank accounts, and in general they failed to exercise the most cursory supervision over hospital funds. Nonmanagement resulted from the same failure to exercise supervision, but was most starkly shown because the named "trustees" were repeatedly elected to the investment committee but did not object when it did not meet in over 10 years. Self-dealing was shown by the facts that thousands of dollars were kept in noninterest-bearing checking accounts, interest-bearing accounts paid less than market conditions would have permitted, and one "trustee" advised approval *and* voted to approve a contract for investment services with a corporation of which he was president. The court found, however, that no named "trustees" had gained personally, even though they were associated with organizations that benefited from the transactions. The absence of a conspiracy seemed important to the court in its ruling.

The court ordered the named "trustees" removed but found no personal liability. To prevent future problems, the court ordered the board to adopt a written investment policy, conduct a review to determine that all hospital assets conformed to the policy, and have a regular process for disclosing business affiliations. In the meantime, the board had adopted AHA-recommended guidelines on conflicts of interest. Although long after the fact, it was evidence of the board's good faith. The guidelines shown in Figure 3.4 are the 1990 iteration published by the AHA. They are identical to those adopted by the Sibley board in 1975 and reflect the corporate director rather than the true trustee standard.

Conflict of Interest

A potential major problem in any organization is conflict of interest. It occurs in HSOs in several ways. The examples of self-dealing in the Sibley Hospital case are one type. A conflict of interest also occurs when a person has multiple obligations that demand loyalty and the decisions based on these loyalties are different or in conflict. It is the problem of serving two masters that was noted earlier. The problems of conflict of interest for governing bodies, managers, and professional staff are discussed in Chapter 7. This section describes the elements of conflict of interest and how it might be avoided.

The ACHE Code of Ethics states that:

> A conflict of interest may be only a matter of degree, but exists when the healthcare executive:
> −is in a position to benefit directly or indirectly by using authority or inside information, or allows a friend, relative or associate to benefit from such authority or information. (or)
> −uses authority or information to make a decision to intentionally affect the organization in an adverse manner.[24]

This definition should guide managers in avoiding conflicts of interest. The phrase "a matter of degree" correctly suggests that limited behavior of some types is unlikely to cause, or is presumed not to raise, a question of conflict of interest, whereas exaggerated behavior of the same type does. Usually, an inexpensive lunch bought by an equipment salesman for a manager poses no problem. An all-expenses-paid 2-week vacation suggests a conflict of interest. Large gifts are presumed to encourage or reward certain behavior. The Code's guidance is that the executive shall "Accept no gifts or benefits offered with the expectation of influencing a management decision."[25] This is stringent, but appropriate.

An example of extravagant gifts and kickbacks occurred at the Cedars of Lebanon Hospital, where the chief executive officer (CEO) engaged in unethical and illegal activities.[26] These included self-dealing because the CEO was part-owner of a firm that contracted with his hospital for architectural consulting services that were never done. The CEO falsified board minutes to cover up the fraudulent contract. In another transaction the CEO received over 2,500 shares of stock (market value $75,000) in a computer company from which the hospital had purchased a $1.8 million diagnostic computer to be used for multiphasic screening. Underutilization caused a loss of over $2,000 per day. The CEO bribed public officials to get approval for construction permits and loans to build an unneeded addition. To ease a desperate cash flow problem the CEO broke the law by not paying federal withholding taxes on employees' salaries. The Cedars of Lebanon case has several examples of law breaking, which makes the activities unethical in themselves. The conflicts of interest are obvious. The important lesson is, however, that the problems occurred because the board was inattentive to what its CEO was doing. As a result the hospital was forced into receivership and the CEO went to prison.

There are more subtle examples of conflict of interest, however. Is it ethical for a manager to use a position of influence and power to gain personal aggrandizement of titles and position at the expense of patient care or other HSO activities? Is it ethical for a manager to be lax in developing and implementing an effective patient consent policy and process? Is it ethical for a manager to

---

Disclosure of certain interests of governing board members

Whereas, The proper governance of the nation's health care institutions depends on governing board members who give of their time for the benefit of their health communities, and,

Whereas, The giving of this service, because of the varied interests and backgrounds of the governing board members, may result in situations involving a dual interest that might be interpreted as conflict of interest, and,

Whereas, This service nevertheless carries with it a requirement of loyalty and fidelity to the institution served, it being the responsibility of the members of the board to govern the institution's affairs honestly and economically, exercising their best care, skill, and judgment for the benefit of the institution; and

Whereas, The matter of any duality of interest or possible conflict of interest can best be handled through full disclosure of any such interest, together with noninvolvement in any vote wherein the interest is involved;

Now, therefore, be it resolved: That the following policy of duality and conflict of interest is hereby adopted:

- Any duality of interest or possible conflict of interest on the part of any governing board member should be disclosed to the other members of the board and made a matter of record, either through an annual procedure or when the interest becomes a matter of board action.

- Any governing board member having a duality of interest or possible conflict of interest on any matter should not vote or use his personal influence on the matter, and he should not be counted in determining the quorum for the meeting, even where permitted by law. The minutes of the meeting should reflect that a disclosure was made, the abstention from voting, and the quorum situation.

- The foregoing requirements should not be construed as preventing the governing board member from briefly stating his position in the matter, nor from answering pertinent questions of other board members since his knowledge may be of great assistance.

Be it further resolved: That this policy be reviewed annually for the information and guidance of governing board members, and that any new member be advised of the policy upon entering on the duties of his office.

Figure 3.4.   Conflict of interest statement of the American Hospital Association. (From American Hospital Association. *Management advisory on functions of hospital executive management*, 2. Chicago, 1990; reprinted by permission of the American Hospital Association, copyright 1990.)

screen all reports and information given to the governing body and prepare them in the best light with regard to management's competence? Is it ethical for a manager who believes there are problems in a clinical department to fail to investigate? Is it ethical for managers who have concerns about their personal capacity to meet the demands of their position to remain in it? These examples raise ethical questions that are not easily answered.

Because conflicts of interest can be so subtle, only continued questioning and self-analysis will identify them. Intensified competition is likely to increase the frequency of conflicts of interest, but the ACHE Code and the AHA statement can help reduce or eliminate them. These guidelines focus on disclosing to the governing body actual or potential conflicts of interest and having managers avoid matters where conflicts might exist.

Confidential Information

HSOs are rife with confidential information about patients, staff, and the organization. Using this information properly is an ethical (and legal) obligation for managers. Problems occur if confidential information is used to benefit a manager or other persons with whom the manager is associated or related, or to harass or injure. Such problems can involve any manager, as well as governing body members. The ACHE code views this problem broadly and asks affiliates to "respect professional confidences" and "to assure the existence of procedures that will safeguard the confidentiality and privacy of patients, clients and others served."[27]

Misuse of confidential information includes leaks about governing body decision making so that advantageous sales or purchases can be made by the insider's associates, selling or giving patient medical information to the media or attorneys; and providing the HSO's marketing strategies to competitors. An example raising potential conflict of interest *and* confidential information problems occurs when a manager serves on the governing body of a potentially competing HSO or a planning agency. Fidelity to one's own HSO conflicts with the duty to objectively consider another HSO's certificate of need, for example. In addition, and more subtly, the manager becomes privy to information important to that manager's own HSO. One cannot ignore information learned in that role. A competitive marketplace makes it difficult to cooperate with other HSOs because of the potential for conflicts of interest and the antitrust implications.

Ethics and Marketing[28]

All HSOs market themselves, and they have always done so. Marketing occurs in the medical staff lounge, on community health day, in new employee orientation, and in press releases. Applying the four P's of marketing—product, place, promotion, and price—to health services is not difficult; health services marketers have adapted them with a new vocabulary—service, consideration, access, and promotion (SCAP). However, the new milieu of the competitive marketplace makes marketing problematic for many HSOs. Regardless, there seems to be general agreement that competition itself is desirable, and this seems to necessitate marketing.

Health services organizations are unique in historic purposes and context when compared with the typical business enterprise. They are different in purpose, type of activity, public service orientation, charitable motives, religious affiliations and history, profit status (many HSOs are not-for-profit organizations), close ties to several professions, the presence of large groups of professionals, labor intensity, and the emotional and psychological aspects of the service. Health service is a social enterprise with an economic dimension, not an economic enterprise with a social dimension.

The HSO can carry out its mission only if it remains solvent. "No money, no mission" has become a platitude, but it succinctly states the dilemma. HSOs must set limits on uncompensated care. Ethical issues arise in deciding whether to provide carriage trade and high-technology services or provide services benefiting the underserved or uninsured. Even a limited general duty of beneficence obliges the HSO to provide services that assist all groups and to be a community resource. Some HSOs offer services that generate surpluses that subsidize uncompensated care and fund programs for the underserved. Although laudable, these efforts raise other ethical questions.

Need Versus Demand   Discussion of HSO marketing often produces disagreement about whether demand is created or met. An element of this disagreement is which health services merit creation of demand and which do not. Little dispute is raised over screening for hypertension or colorectal cancer. Conversely, cosmetic surgery is often cited as an example of "unnecessary" demand. It is claimed that face lifts, tummy tucks, or liposuction waste health resources (whether or not they are self-paid) that should be available for other uses. This is a subjective definition of need. Reasonable persons could reach different conclusions, based on scientific fact, as to what patients "need" and whether the demands that arise from that need are appropriately put on the system. Perhaps services such as cosmetic surgery should not be defined as health services at all, but as consumer services, like haircutting and bodybuilding, that happen to use parts of the health system.

Epidemiological studies develop health data about populations. These studies include incidence and prevalence rates of disease, as well as psychological and physical problems, that are outside traditional definitions of illness. The problem of subjectivity arises when persons judging and evaluating these data apply their personal values to determine need for services. The process is not objective—either in determining what should be studied or in deciding what to do with results.

Debate about need is most heated when questions of marketing ethics are included, especially if marketing is to be used to determine potential demand or to encourage persons to seek elective procedures. Most troubling in this debate is the suggestion that meeting potential demand is unethical. Potential demand is a physical or psychological condition about which the individual either is unaware or is not convinced to take action, and conditions that are untreated because of financial barriers. Examples include dental care, hammer toes, hemorrhoids, cataracts, and psychiatric services.

If the World Health Organization definition of health ("Health is a state of complete physical, mental, and social well-being and not merely the absence of disease or infirmity."[29]) is applied, all efforts to improve health are beneficial. It is instructive to consider wellness activities. The possibilities seem limitless because all facets of life could be affected to improve health status and prevent medical problems. Beyond wellness activities are questions of how to treat demand from those who want to use disposable income as they wish, regardless of how foolish it might seem. Should they be denied elective procedures such as cosmetic surgery because some judge these procedures only a marginal improvement in the quality of life, or because the condition is not life threatening? This infringement on autonomy would be a major shift in freedom of choice.

The debate over appropriateness of coronary artery bypass surgery for patients with mild or moderate symptoms of heart disease is an example of an expensive therapy with mixed results. Cardiac surgeons note the procedure's usefulness for occluded coronary arteries and the relief of angina. Cardiologists and internists are inclined to treat these diagnoses medically, and they rely on data that show similar long-term results for patients in some categories when managed with a medical rather than a surgical regimen. Cost differences between the two are enormous.

It is not clear where or by whom the line should be drawn. Except for the occasional hypochondriac or the Munchausen syndrome* patient, it is rare that someone seeks treatment without reason. When demand for health care is viewed as a bell-shaped curve, it is most cost effective to

---

*Munchausen syndrome is "a condition characterized by habitual presentation for hospital treatment of an apparent acute illness, the patient giving a plausible and dramatic history, all of which is false."[30]

focus on the middle. When that group hears about new medical problems or diagnoses and treatment, they respond rationally. They are the worried well—persons not clinically ill but who are concerned about their health.

Responsible Marketing   How do HSOs market to patients and potential patients in a fashion consistent with an ethical obligation to avoid creating "unnecessary" demand, but at the same time fulfill their obligation to seek out and serve those who might be in need? This is the dilemma.

The AHA developed a statement on the purposes of hospital advertising—an important part of marketing. They are public education about available services, public education about health care, public accountability, public support, and employee recruitment. These efforts are undertaken in the contexts of truth, accuracy, and fairness. Comparisons with other providers, claims of prominence, and promotion of individual professionals are to be avoided.[31]

Responsible marketing is an elusive but important concept. If profits and return on investment are primary, HSOs will have a very different view of marketing and competition. Minimally, responsible marketing means tempering desires and potential demand with an effort to judge value and usefulness. This view of the patient has elements of paternalism, but it means that HSO decision makers have determined that certain expenditures and goals are more worthwhile than others, which is consistent with the purpose of the mission statement and their expertise as providers.

Future of Competition   There is a political science theory suggesting that, over time, enemies take on one another's attributes. This concern deeply troubles not-for-profit HSOs, which see themselves as historically incorporating a mindset and attitude different from for-profit HSOs. They fear that if they must aggressively compete for market share and position they will necessarily stress financial considerations and economic survival and lose sight of caring and humanitarian motives.

Significant in this regard are prospective payment systems, one permutation of which is diagnosis-related groups (DRGs)—the Medicare payment scheme. The effect of DRGs on the ethics of health services delivery is only now being identified. It has been suggested that the pressures of DRG payment will lead to an adversarial relationship between patients and HSOs (and perhaps physicians), and that patients' interests will be smothered in demands of efficiency and economic survival. Such results may occur under any payment system or type of ownership and will occur whenever caregivers and managers lose sight of their reason for being. Doing more with less and demands for efficiency need not be at variance with efforts to operationalize the principles of respect for persons, beneficence, nonmaleficence, and justice. It remains for all who are involved in organizing, planning, and delivering health services to keep these principles firmly in mind.

In retrospect, historical attitudes about competition, lack of profit motive, and not-for-profit status have been both a boon and a bane in health services. The absence of strong economic incentives, such as profit, contributed to HSOs' feeling good about themselves because they were doing good, rather than concentrating on doing it well *and* efficiently. An important contributing factor was that government programs, primarily Medicare, paid provider costs. This rewarded the inefficient and saved such HSOs from themselves.

Conflicts of Interest in Managed Care[32]

The potential for conflicts of interest is inherent in managed care because the goals, purposes, and objectives—the interests—of the management and staff of the managed care plan may be at variance with the interests of patients (members). The tension between plan and patients (and potential patients) occurs as early as the marketing stage, when benefits packages and market segments are identified. Although the *potential* for conflicts of interest is unavoidable, its presence and consequent negative effects can be minimized—if it is recognized and kept in mind by clinicians and managers. The potential for conflicts of interest is present when there are two allegiances (duties to a third party and to the patient) and one set of duties cannot be met without dereliction of the other.

Marketing and Operations   Can potential conflicts of interests lead to actual conflicts when no relationship has been established between a managed care plan and those at whom its marketing is directed? Arguably, no. Nonetheless, many plans have a self-image that is public service oriented and morally demanding. If marketing ignores or seeks to exclude high-risk groups ("cream skimming"), this causes a variance between historic and current mission and purpose. Furthermore, the plan may have to ignore high-risk groups because it has a greater duty to current than potential patients. It must be asked, however, whether any marketing strategy that focuses on healthy, low-risk groups is ethical.

Although not a conflict of interest, plan marketing must take into account the possible need to "keep one's light under a basket." If a managed care plan is, or is perceived to be, a leader in a certain technique or in treating a medical condition and this fact becomes known, it is likely there will be adverse selection—the plan may be inundated with new patients needing that treatment. Since higher quality may result in higher costs, the plan may also get into a vicious cycle as a good reputation for high quality (and good results) causes more high-risk persons (who may need expensive care) to join. As the plan finds itself straining against this adverse selection problem, quality may diminish for other patients, or the plan may have to restrict benefits or increase premiums. Thus, it is in the plan's interests to minimize the appearance of providing extraordinary quality care and, instead, to be seen as a place where medical services of good quality are delivered, but where nothing exceptional is available.

In addition to potential conflicts of interest that may be associated with marketing, there are other ways for the interests of a managed care plan and its patients to conflict. It is in the interests of both that the plan remain financially strong and well functioning to meet patient needs in a timely and effective fashion. Beyond this obvious congruence, however, there is ample opportunity for divergence.

As a bureaucracy, staff, clinicians, and managers have the goal of maximizing position, power, and income (and rewards) with the least disruption of homeostasis. Achieving these goals, especially maximizing income, may minimize service whether or not that is technically consistent with the contract. The bureaucratic response may even be at variance with the long-term survival of the plan. The patient has a primary interest in regaining or retaining health and paying the least to do so. Patients also want to maximize use of services consistent with their perceived need for them. If patients stay well with minimum costs and utilize existing services appropriately, goals of plan and patients are congruent. It is rarely that simple.

The major source of potential conflicts of interest is in utilizing services. In this regard, patients may be divided into those who are appropriate utilizers and those who overutilize, whether purposefully or not. The plan's interests and the interests of appropriate utilizers generally remain congruent; however, to be competitive, the plan must control overutilizers. Even appropriate utilizers are potential financial threats to a plan in a competitive environment, and it may seek to make them underutilizers in order to trim costs. In such situations, there is potential for conflicts of interest.

How do potential conflicts of interest, as shown by incongruent plan and patient goals, become true conflicts? Managed care plan marketing will describe the primary care and specialty services available. Limits are likely, however, and those on specialty or other expensive services will be downplayed. Beyond marketing, constraints may limit hours and services and accept queues, especially for self-limiting medical conditions. The public is usually unaware that queues have the economic value of reducing operating costs. Most plans have an escape valve for these pressures by providing walk-in emergency services or treating walk-in patients during office hours. A furor resulted when the CEO of a major east coast prepaid health plan admitted publicly there was a specific policy about the presence of queues and noted their value in reducing demand for certain services. In the long term these policies will have an anti-marketing effect and cause disenrollment. It is an effective short-term measure, nonetheless.

Physician Incentives and Other Constraints   For patients, subtle and potentially more serious constraints are directed at managed care plan physicians. Here, there is a potential conflict of interest not only between plan and patient but, in terms of professional ethics, between physician and patient. The Hippocratic oath requires physicians to act in the best interests of the patient—a paternalistic professional ethic. The AMA Principles of Medical Ethics suggest that patients' interests must be foremost as physicians choose the level and content of care.

In the final analysis this problem must be resolved by the physician, but the plan provides the context that facilitates or inhibits how this decision is made. Initially, there is a self-selection bias when physicians choose where to practice. Those who cannot accept the rules imposed by a plan will seek employment elsewhere. Once employed, however, a whole range of actions by the plan may modify behavior. Listed in order of increasing severity, they are economic disincentives and incentives, peer pressure, nonrenewal, and dismissal.

The following constraints are common in managed care plans: limits on referrals (especially outside the plan) and hospitalization, financial disincentives (and incentives), quotas on the number of patients who must be seen (used in staff-model health maintenance organizations [HMOs]), and peer review. Peer pressure plays an important role in most of these constraints, both positively and negatively. Constraints are positive when they encourage *judicious* but appropriate use of medical resources—this may account for the fact that managed care plans usually have much lower use of ancillary services and hospital days. When do constraints become excessive, however, thus depriving members of needed service? When do constraints infringe on the principles of nonmaleficence and beneficence? There is no simple or single answer because constraints are a function of the plan's willingness, prompted by the manager as a conscience and moral agent, to institute safeguards that balance competitiveness and financial viability on one side of the equation with protecting the patient on the other side.

Besides physician-oriented constraints that may result in conflicts of interest, other examples are found in the organizational and managerial functioning. Having a complicated decision-making process (e.g., significant committee involvement and several levels of review) may slow approval of new procedures, techniques, or equipment that deliver technically more competent care but raise plan costs. Such complexities may be more prevalent in not-for-profit plans than investor-owned plans. The presence of complex processes in not-for-profit plans may result from a greater degree of democracy, however, and not a deliberate attempt to diminish access. The effect may be the same, nonetheless. For-profit plans tend to have a narrower management pyramid and give the CEO more authority. A complex management structure in an investor-owned plan is less likely to diminish the organization's ability to conserve resources to the potential detriment of patients.

The plan may forego purchase of high-technology diagnostic and treatment equipment, or it may contract with physicians or for inpatient care of members at hospitals without such equipment. Such strategies lower cost. If lower costs enhance financial integrity and guarantee continued availability of services to patients the interests of plan and patients are congruent. For those who might have benefited from the technology, however, it is not an advantage—it is a conflict of interest.

Minimizing Conflicts of Interest   How do managed care plans and their managers prevent, or at least minimize, conflicts of interest? An indispensable first step is to acknowledge that potential conflicts of interest are inherent in the relationship between managed care plans and patients, as well as between physicians and the plan and physicians and patients. Awareness enables avoidance. Beyond that, checks and balances are needed. One solution is to have an ombudsman or consumer relations specialist. In addition, there are due process procedures for members who wish to have a matter reviewed. The success of such programs depends on enlightened management and on the personal characteristics of those involved. Plans may use the managing physician or gatekeeper concept to determine whether patients receive needed services. This role may conflict with financial and other incentives that constrain plan physicians. Federally qualified HMOs, for example, must have an effective grievance procedure for members. This requirement provides some protection, but to be useful the member must at least suspect the care was inadequate. This is a determination the patient may be incapable of making.

Independent audits of utilization review data and audits of data from similar plans are ways management determines that utilization is appropriate. Internal and external comparisons alert managers to problems that may result from conflicts of interests. Awareness of how conflicts of interest arise will help prevent them or minimize their effect. Such activities are essential if managers are to meet their ethical obligations to patients.

BIOMEDICAL ETHICAL ISSUES

Resource Allocation

The ethical implications of allocating resources are receiving increasing attention. Whether at the macro or micro level, resource allocation is an important application of the principle of justice and necessitates making decisions—who gets what, when, and how. This means that value-laden criteria such as worth, usefulness, merit, or need are often used. When government is involved, decisions sometimes are based on political motives. Like governments, HSO macroallocation decisions determine which equipment will be purchased and whether to begin a new program. Microallocation includes a physician's willingness to refer, a patient's geographic access to services and technologies, and economic considerations. Often, micro-level decision making is guided (in a sense, prejudged) by policies and procedures established by government and HSOs.

A solution commonly suggested is to apply the "greatest good" (utility) principle of utilitarianism to allocation decisions; this is often done by economists and policy analysts. It is at best a partial answer because applying only principles of utility may allow us to ignore considerations of human need, fairness, and justice.

Numerous macroallocation theories have been proposed. At one end of a continuum is egalitarianism, which requires that all technologies be available to all persons. This position is based on the concept that human beings are entitled to equal health services. Hyperegalitarianism is extreme egalitarianism and holds that, if a technology is not available to all, none may have it. At the other end of the continuum is a theory that health services are not a right that is to be guaranteed by society; rather, they are a privilege to be earned. This hyperindividualistic position holds that caregivers such as physicians have no obligation to render services to any who cannot afford them, unless they choose of their own free will and humanitarian instinct to provide them. Between these extremes is a view that society is obliged to encourage, develop, and perhaps even provide health services in limited situations. Charles Fried has suggested that *routine* services should be available to all—what he calls a "decent minimum"—but that high-technology services are limited in several ways and should be available on a different basis.[33]

Helpful theories of microallocation—allocation to individual patients—of exotic life-saving services have been developed by James Childress and Nicholas Rescher. They consider the problem of how (by what criteria) decisions about who gets what are to be made. Both start with medical criteria to determine need and appropriateness for treatment. Thereafter, they diverge.

Childress rejects subjective criteria (utilitarianism) because these comparisons demean persons and run counter to the inherent dignity of human beings. He argues that the only ethical system of allocation is one that views all persons needing a specific treatment as equals. To properly recognize human beings, treatment should be provided on a first-come, first-served basis or, alternatively, through random selection, as by a lottery.[34]

Rescher's approach has two tiers. The first consists of basic screening for factors such as constituency served (service area), progress of science (benefit of advancing science), and prospect of success by type of treatment or recipient (e.g., denying dialysis to the very young or very old). The second tier considers individual patients and judges biomedical factors (e.g., relative likelihood of success for that patient, life expectancy) and social aspects such as family role, potential future contributions, and past services rendered. If *all* factors are equal for two persons, Rescher uses random selection to make a final choice.[35] The social aspects are the most difficult because they result from value judgments. Rescher considers it irrational, however, to choose based on chance (after meeting medical criteria), as Childress advocates.

Each of these microallocation theories has advantages and disadvantages, and the resulting decisions are not likely to satisfy everyone. They guide users, however, in addressing the issues and problems in an organized fashion through decision-making frameworks. The choice of patients for the exotic life-saving treatment may be unpredictable, in the case of random allocations (Childress), or "rational" and almost totally predictable (Rescher). It may be a matter of primarily subjective criteria (Rescher) or left to chance and in that sense fair to all needing that treatment (Childress). Awareness of how choices are made allows the public to understand that the system is fair. Kantian principles of respect for persons and not using persons as means to ends are reflected in Childress's theory. Rescher's criteria are predominantly utilitarian. Few HSOs address the ethical dimensions of resource allocation issues in an organized, formal fashion.

Consent

The ethical and legal aspects of consent are similar, but ethical expectations are higher. The concept began in the law as protecting a person's right to be free from nonconsensual touching. This right at law *and* in ethics has expanded and includes autonomy (part of the principle of respect for persons) and self-determination, as well as a reflection of the special relationship of trust and confidence (fiduciary relationship) between physician and patient. This reflects Kant's concept of the equality of human beings. The law recognizes that failing to obtain adequate consent can lead to legal action for battery, an intentional tort. In addition, an action for negligence can be brought if physicians breach a duty to communicate information needed by the patient to make a decision.*

Both general codes of medical ethics, such as the AMA Principles (1980 version), and specialized codes, such as the 1975 Declaration of Helsinki (relating to biomedical research), recognize the importance of consent. Emphasizing patients' rights or sovereignty is an idealized view. It challenges a tradition of medical paternalism that makes the physician a dominant authoritarian figure who decides what is in the patient's best interest.[37]

Questions of consent arise initially when a patient seeks treatment. Consent is usually implied because the patient has sought treatment. Consent is also implied in life-threatening emergencies. Elective, routine treatment requires only *general* consent, as compared with *special* consent, which must be obtained for invasive, surgical, or unusual types of procedures or if the patient is part of an experiment. Consent of both types must be voluntary, competent, and informed.

Voluntary means that consent is given without duress having substantially influenced the

---

*Contrast this view with a case in Japan in which a physician told a patient she had gallstones, rather than frightening her by telling her she actually had gallbladder cancer. She delayed surgery. The cancer spread and she died. Her family brought suit. The court said the patient herself was to blame because she had not followed the physician's advice to have the surgery and that the physician had no obligation to inform her of the true condition.[36]

decision. Getting voluntary consent from prisoners who are to be part of an experiment is probably impossible because being incarcerated greatly diminishes their independence. Voluntariness is also reduced when inducements to participate are so great that one ignores prudence and caution. Similarly, circumstances may be such that even small inducements may be sufficient; for example, a starving person who is offered a small sum of money may agree to participate in a dangerous experiment.

Beyond these obvious problems, voluntariness is an elusive concept. Patients who correctly or incorrectly fear physician abandonment are under duress and are likely to follow the physician's suggestions. Patients are influenced by family and friends and may be pursuaded (perhaps coerced) by them. It is possible that consent is never really voluntary. It has been suggested that a patient's personal freedom to accept or reject medical treatment is so reduced that it exists only as the right to veto unwanted procedures.[38] Such arguments amplify the importance of understanding the complex relationships in medicine and preclude simple answers about obtaining voluntary consent.

Competent consent means that patients know the nature and consequences of what is contemplated or the decision being made. The law presumes that unemancipated minors are incompetent, as are mentally ill or mentally handicapped persons.

The third element of consent is that it be *informed*. Some discussions incorrectly refer to "informed consent" as if the need to be informed were the only criterion. This ignores the two elements discussed above. Historically, the courts adopted a *legal* standard for informed consent that required full disclosure of the nature of the condition for which treatment was proposed, as well as all significant facts about the condition, and an explanation of the likely consequences and difficulties. This standard is based on the amount of information a reasonable physician would give in the same or similar circumstances. By comparison, *ethical* criteria suggest more active patient participation. Criteria developed by the President's Commission state that patient sovereignty with complete participation in the process is preferred. It recognizes such participation as a goal, however, rather than an easily achievable relationship.[39] The President's Commission view has major implications for the majority legal standard.

More recently, a number of courts have adopted a standard based on what a typical (reasonable) patient would want to know. A legal criterion oriented to patient sovereignty is used in a few jurisdictions: what would that specific patient want to know? The latter legal standard is consistent with the position taken by the President's Commission and reflects the emerging ethical view that a covenant (contract) between patient and physician should guide their relationship.

HSOs have processes and procedures that address the legal aspects of informed consent; these are covered in Chapter 4. Notable here is that HSOs are likely to apply a legally oriented consent process, whose primary purpose is self-protection. It is typical for little emphasis to be placed on an ethical relationship that requires a higher standard of the HSO. This approach is utilitarian and is legally prudent. It ignores, however, a positive ethical obligation to the patient based on the principle of respect for persons.

Experimentation

Ethical issues of experimentation were raised in the early 19th century by an American physician, William Beaumont, and a French physiologist, Claude Bernard. Beaumont developed a personal code on experimentation in 1833 that was similar to those of today: 1) at times there is no alternative to experimenting on human beings, 2) a need exists for the experimenter to be conscientious and responsible, 3) random studies are unacceptable, 4) the experiment must be discontinued when it causes distress to the subject, and 5) the experiment must be abandoned at the subject's request.[40] Bernard wrote about using live animals in medical experiments (vivisection). He distinguished unacceptable from acceptable experimentation by asking whether the purpose is to mutilate or to learn; he argued that the purpose distinguishes the ethics.

There were no internationally recognized ethical codes on experimentation until after World War II. The Nuremberg Code of 1946 was primarily a reaction to Nazi "medical experiments." Concomitant with increasing human experimentation, several codes and sets of guidelines have been developed since. Some, such as the Declaration of Helsinki, are international. Others focus on American practice: the AMA's "Ethical Guidelines for Clinical Investigation" and the Department of Health and Human Services' (DHHS) "Regulations for the Protection of Human Subjects."

Of the four, DHHS regulations are the most specific, but they only apply to DHHS-funded research. The Food and Drug Administration (FDA), which regulates drugs and medical devices, approves them for general use only if its regulations on experimentation are followed. Only a few states require HSOs to follow requirements like those of the DHHS when they conduct non-federally funded research.[41] Surgical experimentation and new uses of drugs and devices (known as innovative treatment) are an almost totally unregulated gray area. Absent regulation, the patient-subject must rely on the voluntary, ethical conduct of the practitioner and the policies and guidelines of the HSO, if they exist.

If experimentation is defined as attempting new means, methods, and techniques, medicine has always experimented; without it there is no progress. Experimenting must continue, but protecting the subject is problematic. Issues raised include therapeutic versus nontherapeutic experimentation; competent, voluntary, and informed consent; and experimenting on incompetent subjects, such as those who are mentally ill or handicapped and children. The Nuremberg Code prohibits experimenting on children and by analogy other incompetent subjects. Other codes permit a legal guardian to provide consent.

Experimental treatment that might benefit the subject is therapeutic—the recipient is both patient and subject. Nontherapeutic experiments are those in which the subject is healthy, does not suffer from the problem for which the treatment is being tested, or cannot benefit from it in another way, such as diagnosis. More attention should be paid to the ethics of nontherapeutic experimentation because the patient does not benefit. Some assert that nontherapeutic, nondiagnostic experimentation must be based on fully informed consent and therefore it should not be performed on children and incompetent adults.[42]

A major emphasis for all codes is that the subject give voluntary, informed consent. Competence receives less attention. The Nuremberg Code has a provision that subjects may stop the experiment whenever they wish. This puts a heavy burden on subjects who may be incapacitated or intimidated by the experiment and probably lack the technical competence to know if their safety or well being is threatened. This weakness was corrected in the Declaration of Helsinki by requiring the use of an independent review committee to approve the experimental protocol. The declaration also increases the accountability for the medically qualified person in charge of the experiment.

No code excludes nontherapeutic experimentation; all recognize that volunteers for whom the experimental treatment offers no therapeutic benefit are needed for certain research. There is clear utilitarian language in all codes except that of the AMA, which is paternalistic. Utility balances the risk to the individual (for nontherapeutic research) with the benefit to society. In contrast, an emphasis on voluntary and informed consent is Kantian. DHHS regulations include this latter view, as well.

A major difficulty with codes other than DHHS regulations is that they do not clearly separate the physician's roles as healer and researcher. This puts a heavy burden on the physician because duality of interests can cause conflicts of interest for physician-researchers. What may be good for the subject as a patient is not necessarily the same as what is desirable for the experimental protocol or the researcher's interest in having a successful experiment. The problem is compounded in nontherapeutic research. AMA guidelines have a paternalistic view of the relationship between physician and patient-subject and expect the physician to exercise professional skill and judgment to act in the patient's best interests.

Numerous efforts to protect human subjects continue the philosophy first expressed in the Declaration of Helsinki. Most prominent is the *institutional review board* (IRB). IRBs protect human subjects, and their use is required by several federal agencies for federally funded or regulated research. Most important for the HSO are the IRB requirements of the DHHS and the FDA. Other agencies requiring the use of IRBs include the Environmental Protection Agency, the National Science Foundation, and the Consumer Product Safety Commission. Research involving human subjects that is funded wholly or partly by the DHHS (except certain educational practices and testing, interview procedures and observation, and collection of existing data) must be reviewed in a presided manner by an IRB. FDA requirements are similar and apply regardless of funding. Compliance is required because the goal is to obtain FDA approval to market drugs, biologicals, and medical devices.

DHHS requires an IRB that is competent to review research proposals for conformity with applicable law, standards of professional conduct and practice, and institutional commitment and regulation.[43] The IRB must have at least five members with varying backgrounds (at least one with nonscientific interests) who can review research proposals and activities like those commonly performed by the HSO. The IRB applies several requirements to proposed research; the experiment must minimize risk to subjects, determine that risks are reasonable compared to anticipated benefits, equitably select subjects, appropriately obtain and document consent from the subject or an authorized representative, monitor data to ensure safety, maintain confidentiality of information, and assure special protections when consent is obtained from subjects vulnerable to coercion or undue influence. In addition, special provisions identify what is needed for informed consent. The FDA uses similar elements of consent, but has provisions for emergencies and situations in which the subject cannot communicate or the legal representative is unavailable.

Death and Dying

Definitions   Historically, death has been defined as cessation of blood circulation and of circulation-dependent animal and vital functions such as respiration and pulsation. As technology developed, this definition proved inadequate. Table 3.1 summarizes various definitions of death.

In 1968, a Harvard Medical School committee developed criteria that defined irreversible coma. This development was important, but it raised other problems. The Harvard criteria were accompanied by a report stating that the patient's condition can be determined only by a physician and that, when the patient's condition is found to be hopeless, certain steps are recommended:

> Death is to be declared and *then* the respirator turned off. The decision to do this and the responsibility for it are to be taken by the physician-in-charge, in consultation with one or more physicians who have been directly involved in the case. It is unsound and undesirable to force the family to make the decision.[44]

This quotation is noteworthy because major changes in society's attitudes and perceptions have occurred since 1968. These include stress on patient autonomy as expressed through living wills and natural death act declarations, involving the family in decision making, and establishing institutional ethics committees. These changes diminish the centrality and primacy of the physician's role.

The Harvard criteria proved useful. Nonetheless, several criticisms have been raised. They are summarized by the President's Commission:

1. The phrase "irreversible coma" is misleading as applied to the cases at hand. "Coma" is a condition of a living person, and a body without any brain functions is dead and thus *beyond* any coma.
2. The writers of these [Harvard] criteria did not realize that the spinal cord reflexes actually persist or return quite commonly after the brain has completely and permanently ceased functioning.
3. "Unreceptivity" is not amenable to testing in an unresponsive body without consciousness.
4. The need adequately to test brainstem reflexes, especially apnea, and to exclude drug and metabolic intoxication as possible causes of the coma, are not made sufficiently explicit and precise.
5. Although all individuals that meet "Harvard criteria" are dead (irreversible cessation of all functions of the entire brain), there are many other individuals who are dead but do not maintain circulation long enough to have a 24-hour observation period.[45]

By mid-1990, 31 states and the District of Columbia had enacted the Uniform Determination of Death Act developed by the National Conference of Commissioners on Uniform State Laws. The Uniform Act includes alternate definitions of death. One uses brain death, defined as irreversible cessation of all functions of the entire brain, including the brainstem. The other uses irreversible cessation of circulatory and respiratory functions.[46] As suggested in Table 3.1, these criteria may be superseded by others that emphasize sociopsychological factors, the most prominent of which is the capacity for social interaction. Such a definition raises ethical issues about the

Table 3.1. Definition of death

Concept of death	Locus of death	Criteria of death
(philosophical or theological judgment of the essentially significant change at death)	(place to look to determine if a person has died)	(measurements physicians or other officials use to determine whether a person is dead—to be determined by scientific empirical study)
1. Irreversible loss of flow of vital fluids (i.e., the blood and breath)	Heart and lungs	Visual observation of respiration, perhaps with the use of a mirror Feeling of the pulse, possibly supported by electrocardiogram
2. Irreversible loss of the soul from the body	Pineal body(?) (according to Descartes) Respiratory tract?	Observation of breath (?)
3. Irreversible loss of the capacity for bodily integration	Brain	Unreceptivity and unresponsivity No movements or breathing No reflexes (except spinal reflexes) Flat electroencephalogram (to be used as confirmatory evidence) All tests to be repeated 24 hours later (excluded conditions: hypothermia and central nervous system drug depression)
4. Irreversible loss of consciousness or the capacity for social interaction	Probably the neocortex	Electroencephalogram

Adapted from Veatch, Robert M. *Death, Dying, and the Biological Revolution: Our Last Quest for Responsibility*, 53. New Haven, CT: Yale University Press, 1976. © Yale University Press. Used with permission. This table has been modified using material from the 1989 second edition.

Note: Death is defined as a complete change in the status of a living entity characterized by the irreversible loss of those characteristics that are essentially significant to it. The possible concepts, loci, and criteria of death are much more complex than the ones given here. These are meant to be simplified models of types of positions being taken in the current debate. It is obvious that those who believe that death means the irreversible loss of the capacity for bodily integration (3) or the irreversible loss of consciousness (4) have no reservations about pronouncing death when the heart and lungs have ceased to function. This is because they are willing to use loss of heart and lung activity as shortcut criteria for death, believing that once heart and lungs have stopped, the brain or neocortex will necessarily stop as well.

status of people with mental retardation, who may lack the capacity for social interaction. Similar definitions are not without precedent. One that includes the *potential* for social interaction has been applied to infants with Down syndrome who were allowed to die.

Life-Sustaining Treatment Among HSOs, hospitals and nursing facilities must solve ethical problems about discontinuing life-sustaining treatment. Historically, potential legal liability has made these facilities reluctant to discontinue life support without a judicial determination. The first such case receiving national attention, *In re Quinlan,*[47] occurred in 1976 when the New Jersey Supreme Court permitted the father of 21-year-old Karen Ann Quinlan to be appointed her guardian. It authorized him to discontinue all extraordinary procedures sustaining life if the family and physicians concurred that there was no reasonable possibility of her emerging from her persistent vegetative state and if there was consultation as to prognosis with the hospital ethics committee. This was one of the earliest enunciations of a role for ethics committees in hospitals. Quinlan was weaned from the respirator and transferred to a nursing facility, where she later died after being in a persistent vegetative state for 10 years.

The first case on life-sustaining treatment heard by the U.S. Supreme Court was *Cruzan v. Director, Missouri Department of Health*[48] in 1990. Nancy Cruzan had been in a persistent vegetative state since 1983, after being severely injured in an automobile accident. She was a patient in a Missouri state hospital, and a gastrostomy tube had been inserted to ease delivery of nutrition and hydration. Employees at the facility refused Cruzan's parents' request to have the gastrostomy tube removed and the parents filed suit. Ultimately, the Missouri State Supreme Court denied the parents' request and the U.S. Supreme Court agreed to hear an appeal. The Court affirmed the lower court decision by holding that the U.S. Constitution does not forbid the state of Missouri to require that the wishes of an incompetent person in a persistent vegetative state not to be kept alive by artificial means must be shown by "clear and convincing" evidence. The Court distinguished the rights of competent persons, who the Court assumed have a constitutionally protected right to refuse life-sustaining hydration and nutrition, from the rights of incompetent persons. The opinion noted that, while Missouri recognized there were circumstances when a surrogate may act for a patient in electing to withdraw hydration and nutrition and thus cause death, the state had established a procedural safeguard to ensure that the surrogate's action conforms with the wishes expressed by the patient while competent. The Court went on to grant broad latitude to the states to protect and preserve human life; it recognized their right to require a standard that "clear and convincing evidence" be presented as to the person's intentions regarding life continuation decisions. It also noted that the state is entitled to guard against potential abuses by surrogates who may not act to protect the interests of the patient and that the state may decline to include judgments about the quality of a patient's life. The Court did not, however, outline the limits of action a state could take.

In late 1990, Cruzan's parents were granted a second hearing in state court, which the state of Missouri did not oppose. New evidence convinced a judge that Nancy Cruzan would not have wanted to live in a persistent vegetative state and he ordered the feeding tube removed. "Anti-euthanasia" groups unsuccessfully sought to intervene. Cruzan died a few days later. In sum, in *Cruzan* the Court recognized broad state authority and responsibility to legislate processes for life continuation decisions.

Child Abuse The situation of "Baby Doe" seems similar to *Quinlan* and *Cruzan,* but has significant differences. "Baby Doe" is the name taken from a 1982 Indiana court case that was brought after parents declined to treat a newborn with Down syndrome who had tracheoesophageal atresia (no opening between stomach and intestine) and possible other anomalies. A court agreed that nontreatment was one medically recommended option. As expected, the untreated infant died. Baby Doe was unlike Karen Ann Quinlan or Nancy Cruzan in that he was not in a persistent vegetative state, nor was he terminally ill. A simple surgical procedure would have corrected the atresia, but not the underlying retardation.

That case and another in Illinois prompted DHHS to issue regulations prohibiting hospitals that received federal funds from denying needed care to infants with disabilities. DHHS claimed authority for the regulations under Section 504 of the Rehabilitation Act of 1973, which prohibits discrimination on the basis of disability. The regulations were legally challenged on procedural grounds because the period for public comment was too short. An attempt to promulgate a modified version of the regulations followed in 1983. Like the first, they proposed telephone hotlines to report alleged cases of withholding life-sustaining care from seriously ill newborns. An important change was the interpretation that the Rehabilitation Act did not require "impossible or futile acts or therapies that merely prolong the process of dying of an infant born terminally ill."

The original controversy had prompted Congress to address the issue of newborns with defects, and the Child Abuse Amendments of 1984 established treatment and reporting guidelines for severely disabled newborns. Withholding "medically indicated treatment" from disabled infants is illegal except when

> in the treating physician's(s') reasonable medical judgment, (i) the infant is chronically and irreversibly comatose; (ii) the provision of such treatment would merely prolong dying, not be effective in ameliorating or correcting all of the infant's life-threatening conditions, or otherwise be futile in terms of survival of the infant; or (iii) the provision of such treatment would be virtually futile in terms of the survival of the infant and the treatment itself under such circumstances would be inhumane.[49]

The law requires that all infants receive "appropriate nutrition, hydration, and medication," regardless of their condition or prognosis.

The law requires that health facilities designate persons to report suspected problems to state child protective services agencies. The agencies coordinate and consult with those persons and, after being notified of suspected medical neglect, may initiate legal action. The legal dispute on the second Baby Doe regulations reached the U.S. Supreme Court after the Child Abuse Amendments of 1984 were enacted. The Court held that the Rehabilitation Act of 1973 did not give the DHHS authority to issue regulations protecting newborns with defects. At that point, however, the issue had been made moot by the congressional action.

Advance Medical Directives (AMDs)

Living Will It is a paradox of modern medicine that patients retain a theoretical legal (and ethical) right to consent to treatment, but that the process can easily overwhelm their ability to control it. The living will was developed several decades ago to communicate one's wishes when one could not participate in decision making. "Living" and "will" seem contradictory because wills are the means by which a deceased's wishes are expressed. Here, however, the document has similar effect. It expresses an incapacitated person's wishes to those providing care; its primary purpose is to set limits. Absent state law, living wills have no legal status. A sample living will is shown in Figure 3.5.

Natural Death Act Statutes Public interest in living wills and highly publicized cases in which more treatment was provided than it seemed the patient wanted led to rapid state enactment of natural death acts, or death with dignity laws. In 1983 only 14 states had such statutes; by mid-1991 there were statutes in 43 states and the District of Columbia.[50] The natural death act declaration used in Virginia is shown in Figure 3.6. Properly executed natural death act declarations are legally binding on caregivers and can instruct them to withhold or withdraw life-sustaining treatment. Some statutes include penalties if these declarations are ignored. Such laws help solve the problem that the health services system encourages application of new technology but does

To My Family, My Physician, My Lawyer, And All Others Whom It May Concern

Death is as much a reality as birth, growth, and aging—it is the one certainty of life. In anticipation of decisions that may have to be made about my own dying and as an expression of my right to refuse treatment, I _____, being of sound mind, make this statement of
  (print name)
my wishes and instructions concerning treatment.

By means of this document, which I intend to be legally binding, I direct my physician and other care providers, my family, and any surrogate designated by me or appointed by a court, to carry out my wishes. If I become unable, by reason of physical or mental incapacity, to make decisions about my medical care, let this document provide the guidance and authority needed to make any and all such decisions.

If I am permanently unconscious or there is no reasonable expectation of my recovery from a seriously incapacitating or lethal illness or condition, I do not wish to be kept alive by artificial means. I request that I be given all care necessary to keep me comfortable and free of pain, even if pain-relieving medications may hasten my death, and I direct that no life-sustaining treatment be provided except as I or my surrogate specifically authorize.

This request may appear to place a heavy responsibility upon you, but by making this decision according to my strong convictions, I intend to ease that burden. I am acting after careful consideration and with understanding of the consequences of your carrying out my wishes. *List optional specific provisions in the space below.*

How to Use Your Living Will

The Living Will should clearly state your preferences about life-sustaining treatment. You may wish to add specific statements to the Living Will in the space provided for that purpose. Such statements might concern:

- Cardiopulmonary resuscitation
- Artificial or invasive measures for providing nutrition and hydration
- Kidney dialysis
- Mechanical or artificial respiration
- Blood transfusion
- Surgery (such as amputation)
- Antibiotics

You may also wish to indicate any preferences you may have about such matters as dying at home.

Important Points to Remember

- Sign and date your Living Will.
- Your two witnesses should not be blood relatives, your spouse, potential beneficiaries of your estate or your health care proxy.
- Discuss your Living Will with your doctors; and give them copies of your Living Will for inclusion in your medical file, so they will know whom to contact in the event something happens to you.
- Make photo copies of your Living Will and give them to anyone who may be making decisions for you if you are unable to make them yourself.
- Place the original in a safe, accessible place, so that it can be located if needed—not in a safe deposit box.
- Look over your Living Will periodically (at least every five years), initial and redate it so that it will be clear that your wishes have not changed.

Figure 3.5. A sample living will. (From Concern for Dying, 250 W. 57th Street, New York, NY; reprinted by permission.)

Written Natural Death Act Declaration

A declaration executed pursuant to this article may, but need not, be in one of the following forms, and may include other specific directions including, but not limited to, a designation of another person to make the treatment decision for the declarant should he be (i) diagnosed as suffering from a terminal condition and (ii) comatose, incompetent or otherwise mentally or physically incapable of communication. Should any other specific directions be held to be invalid, such invalidity shall not affect the declaration.

Declaration made this _____ day of _____ (month, year).
I, _____ ,
wilfully and voluntarily make known my desire and do hereby declare:

CHOOSE ONLY ONE OF THE NEXT TWO
PARAGRAPHS AND CROSS THROUGH THE OTHER

If at any time I should have a terminal condition and my attending physician has determined that there can be no recovery from such condition, my death is imminent, and I am comatose, incompetent or otherwise mentally or physically incapable of communication, I designate .... to make a decision on my behalf as to whether life prolonging procedures shall be withheld or withdrawn. In the event that my designee decides that such procedures should be withheld or withdrawn, I wish to be permitted to die naturally with only the administration of medication or the performance of any medical procedure deemed necessary to provide me with comfort care or to alleviate pain.

If at any time I should have a terminal condition and my attending physician has determined that there can be no recovery from such condition and my death is imminent, where the application of life-prolonging procedures would serve only to artificially prolong the dying process, I direct that such procedures be withheld or withdrawn, and that I be permitted to die naturally with only the administration of medication or the performance of any medical procedure deemed necessary to provide me with comfort care or to alleviate pain.

In the absence of my ability to give directions regarding the use of such life-prolonging procedures, it is my intention that this declaration shall be honored by my family and physician as the final expression of my legal right to refuse medical or surgical treatment and accept the consequences of such refusal.

I understand the full import of this declaration and I am emotionally and mentally competent to make this declaration.

_____
(Signed)
The declarant is known to me and I believe him or her to be of sound mind.

_____
Witness

_____
Witness

Figure 3.6. Suggested form of Written Natural Death Act Declaration adopted by the State of Virginia. (From *Code of Virginia* 1950, 1990 Cumulative Supplement, vol. 7A, Title 54.1, Article 8, Section 2984, 197–198.)

less well in discontinuing it. Use of living wills and natural death act statutes is limited to circumstances in which the person is terminally ill.

Durable Power of Attorney   It is increasingly common to find "durable powers of attorney for health care" used in surrogate decision making in life continuation decisions. Powers of attorney are a legal means by which persons delegate authority to someone who acts for them. A power of attorney is durable when the grant of authority continues beyond the time the person granting it is incapacitated. By mid-1990, 25 states and the District of Columbia had statutes extending durable powers of attorney to health care decisions, and 18 of these and the District of Columbia specifically allow agents to make decisions regarding withdrawing or withholding life support. A number of other states have court decisions, attorneys general opinions, or special attention to this issue in their natural death act statutes.[51]

A sample durable power of attorney form is shown in Figure 3.7. Like the living will form in Figure 3.5, it may not meet specific state requirements but may be useful where statutes do not address the issue.

Do-Not-Resuscitate Orders   Many patients neither have living wills nor have signed AMDs that meet the requirements of a natural death act. This makes it particularly important that the HSO have policies and procedures that address questions about resuscitating the terminally ill and patients for whom life continuation decisions must be made, such as those in a persistent vegetative state. Many HSOs have "do-not-resuscitate" (DNR) policies that affirm the right of patients or surrogates to direct their caregivers as to the aggressiveness of life-saving efforts. DNR policies should identify which chemical and mechanical technology(ies) are included. The DNR order that is written should specify which technologies are to be applied to a patient.

A study at three Houston teaching hospitals showed that DNR orders are applied inconsistently.[52] The hospitals did not have DNR policies, and the study found that some DNR patients continued to receive chemotherapy, surgery, and admission to the intensive care unit. At the other extreme, some DNR patients received inadequate hydration and nutrition. Staff are often confused about what care to give these patients, perhaps because they disagree with decisions to keep some patients alive. The study found that in 10% of cases no decision had been reached on whether to try to keep the patient alive. This indicates attempts to decide about resuscitation in advance of crises are failing in a number of cases. In most no-decision cases, the subject of DNR orders had not even been brought up with the patient or family. Other studies of DNR orders reported similar findings.[53]

Another dimension of DNR orders is whether they are written equitably for patients with different diseases but similar prognoses. A study reported in 1989 found that DNR orders are much more likely to be written for patients with AIDS or inoperable lung cancer than for patients with other diseases with equally poor prognoses, such as cirrhosis or heart failure. The researchers did not uncover reasons for the differences.[54] Veatch considers the more important problem to be that of failing to undertake treatment because the physician assumes it is not in a patient's interests, or that the patient would not want it.[55] Such actions do not consider patient autonomy—either in independent decision making or in involved participation. Findings like these suggest major ethical issues in DNR orders for terminally ill patients in hospitals.

HSO Role in AMDs   Even if HSOs increasingly assist patients with AMDs, patients necessarily rely on caregivers to accept and follow them. Research suggests that caregivers often override the patient's expressed interests when medical problems are clearly correctable, however.[56] There is also evidence that, in the past, most acute care hospitals put the burden of preparing AMDs on patients, and that few advised patients about their use.

Major impetus was added to AMDs when Congress passed the Patient Self-determination Act, which was part of the Omnibus Budget Reconciliation Act of 1990. It requires HSOs participating in Medicare and Medicaid to give all patients written information on policies regarding

Durable Power of Attorney
for Health Care Decisions

To effect my wishes, I designate _____,
residing at _____ (Phone #) _____,
(or if he or she shall for any reason fail to act, _____
(Phone #) _____, residing at _____)
as my health care surrogate—that is, my attorney-in-fact regarding any and all
health care decisions to be made for me, including the decision to refuse life-
sustaining treatment—if I am unable to make such decisions myself. This power
shall remain effective during and not be affected by my subsequent illness, disability or incapacity. My surrogate shall have authority to interpret my Living
Will, and shall make decisions about my health care as specified in my instructions or, when my wishes are not clear, as the surrogate believes to be in my best
interests. I release and agree to hold harmless my health care surrogate from any
and all claims whatsoever arising from decisions made in good faith in the exercise of this power.

I sign this document knowingly,
voluntarily, and after careful delibera-
tion, this _____ day of _____,
19_____.

_____
(signature)
Address _____
_____

Witness _____
Printed Name _____
Address _____
_____

Witness _____
Printed Name _____
Address _____
_____

I do hereby certify that the within document was executed and acknowledged before me by the principal this
_____ day of _____, 19_____.

Copies of this document have been
given to:

_____
Notary Public

The Durable Power of Attorney for Health Care

This optional feature permits you to name a surrogate decision maker (also
known as a proxy, health agent or attorney-in-fact), someone to make health care
decisions on your behalf if you lose that ability. As this person should act according to your preferences and in your best interests, you should select this person
with care and make certain that he or she knows what your wishes are and about
your Living Will.

You should not name someone who is a witness to your Living Will. You
may want to name an alternate agent in case the first person you select is unable or
unwilling to serve. If you do name a surrogate decision maker, the form must be
notarized. (It is a good idea to notarize the document in any case.)

Figure 3.7. A sample durable power of attorney for health care decisions. (From Concern for Dying, 250 W. 57th Street, New York, NY; reprinted by permission.)

self-determination and living wills, and to inquire and document in the medical record whether a patient has an AMD and, if so, to ensure compliance with state law. Patients must be advised of their right under state law to refuse or select treatment, and they must be told about the HSO's policies for implementing these laws. The organization must also provide staff and community education about use of AMDs.[57] Performing these legally required activities allows HSOs to meet their commitment to the principles of respect for persons, beneficence, and nonmaleficence.

"Good Death" Euthanasia comes from the Greek *eu* (good) and *thanatos* (death). It means that death occurs because medical technology is not applied or that which was applied is withdrawn, *and* that supportive care and pain control make death pain free. The word "euthanasia" is commonly used, however, to describe an action that is assisted suicide, such as a morphine overdose. Mixed use blurs important distinctions. The concepts of letting someone die and helping a person to commit suicide are different, and the terminology should reflect this.

Euthanasia is classified as active or passive and voluntary or involuntary. Active euthanasia occurs when a patient's death is purposely hastened; this is the criminal act of homicide. Passive euthanasia means that either no extraordinary (disproportionate) means are used to prolong life or that extraordinary (disproportionate) means of prolonging life are withdrawn. Extraordinary (disproportionate) means are those that are excessively painful, expensive, or inconvenient to the patient *and* offer no reasonable hope of benefit. Proportionate and disproportionate are concepts whose application is limited to critically, usually terminally, ill patients. Voluntary and involuntary have to do with the patient's wishes.

Summary Death and dying is an ethical issue that is only now being defined in the law. This contributes to the surrounding uncertainty. If the physician–patient relationship is viewed as stressing patient sovereignty, decisions about treatment come from the patient. Patients regularly lose control in a medical system dedicated to prolonging life and staving off death—perhaps at any cost. The problem is compounded by technologies that can continue life well into the dying process at high psychological and economic cost. Furthermore, the health services system has its own interests in preserving life and applying technology. It has been suggested that widespread use of AMDs might encourage systematic rationing of health care, especially to the elderly. If a right to die becomes a duty to die, the living will and its progeny, such as the natural death act declaration and the durable power of attorney, have created a Frankenstein monster.

Acquired Immunodeficiency Syndrome[58]

Background The virus that causes AIDS has proved to be an elusive foe. A great deal has been learned about the human immunodeficiency virus (HIV) since it was first identified in the early 1980s, but its spread continues. There have been a few scientific breakthroughs in understanding it, but there is neither a cure nor a vaccine. The major outbreak of AIDS in the general population that was predicted early in the epidemic has not occurred. The incidence rate of HIV among homosexuals has declined, but rapid spread has occurred among intravenous drug users and certain minority groups. In 1991, women were the fastest growing population of AIDS patients.[59] Meanwhile, prevention and education are receiving attention unprecedented in modern public health.

By 1991, over 100,000 deaths from AIDS had been reported in the United States since 1981.[60] AIDS has an average case fatality rate of 58%, which is among the highest of all diseases.[61] New drugs and improved treatment have increased life expectancy for persons with AIDS, but the near-term outlook is not bright. The Centers for Disease Control (CDC) estimates there will be 390,000–480,000 cases by 1993. Furthermore, it is estimated that 800,000–1.2 million Americans are already infected with HIV and will eventually require care.[62] A preliminary, but disputed, report in mid-1991 suggested that the AIDS epidemic may have peaked in 1990 and that the number of new cases had fallen significantly.[63]

Economic and social burdens of treating persons with AIDS are inequitably distributed because of the concentration of AIDS patients in major metropolitan areas and, within them, at a few inner city hospitals.[64] The geographic distribution of persons with AIDS may be changing, however. Their dispersion to nonurban, low-incidence areas will spread social and economic burdens and bring some relief to urban hospitals, but will probably do little to change the basic concentration of the cases.

One estimate of lifetime, median per case costs of treating persons with AIDS is about

$24,000. At $60,000 and $75,000, other estimates are considerably higher.[65] Estimates reported in 1991 showed average costs of $32,000 to treat a person with AIDS during any calendar year and an average of $85,333 between the time AIDS is diagnosed and the time the patient dies. It is estimated that the cumulative medical costs of treating all persons with AIDS in the United States from diagnosis to death will total $10.4 billion by 1994.[66]

Financing AIDS care is very difficult because much of what happens is outside the HSO's control. For example, a hospital must provide emergency treatment to all, and there is little choice if someone must be admitted. When the AIDS epidemic primarily affected middle-class whites, there was usually ample insurance. Even then, AIDS patients unable to work often lost their private insurance. As their assets were depleted these individuals might be covered by Medicaid, or Medicare, if they were classified as disabled. As the demographics of the epidemic changed, however, the number of uninsured patients increased dramatically. Funding treatment through public programs such as Medicare and Medicaid is equitable only if persons with AIDS have adequate access and if funding is sufficient to give HSOs the reimbursement they need. Increased effectiveness and use of nonhospital providers, including nursing facilities, hospice, and home health agencies, should reduce costs and deliver care in more apppropriate settings.

Some commentators attribute the decline in medical school applications to concerns about treating AIDs patients. Concentrations of such patients in metropolitan hospitals has implications for postgraduate medical education because residency program approval may be withdrawn if residents do not get experience with a wide range of illnesses. Large numbers of AIDS patients may cause problems for other staff, too.

Currently, HIV testing for HSO staff and patients is voluntary. This is likely to change, however, in large part because there is a strong move to classify AIDS as a sexually transmitted and communicable disease, which will put it into the mainstream of public health, where case finding, contact tracing, and testing are routine. Recently, the desirability of treating HIV differently from other communicable diseases has been questioned,[67] and the value of routine testing has been advocated.[68] A 1991 study of physicians and nurses found that 57% and 63%, respectively, favor mandatory testing of health care workers.[69] At its annual meeting in mid-1991, the AMA House of Delegates rejected mandatory HIV testing of health care workers and patients. Instead, the delegates voted to test physicians, medical students, and health care workers "when appropriate."[70]

Early in the AIDS epidemic, the CDC recommended use of universal precautions by health workers, which include handwashing, use of protective barriers (gloves, masks, and the like), and care in use and disposal of needles and other sharp instruments. Recent clinical developments allow HSOs to treat AIDS more effectively. Better prepared staff with specialized clinical skills and availability of new drugs have increased longevity for persons with AIDS. The result will be more episodes of hospitalization, as well as treatment at other types of HSOs, especially nursing facilities.

The AIDS epidemic raises significant ethical issues for the HSO and its managers. These include: 1) protecting staff providing care to HIV-positive patients, 2) protecting patients and staff from HIV-positive staff, and 3) maintaining the confidentiality of HIV-positive staff and patients. The legal dimensions of AIDS are discussed in Chapter 4.

Protecting Staff from Patients The major premise of all HSO relationships is that the HSO's primary duty is to staff. This duty is supported by fidelity, part of the principle of respect for persons, and by the principle of nonmaleficence: through its managers the organization must provide a safe work place. In addition, the duty is buttressed by the theory of utility: the greatest good for the greatest number—a result achievable only with an effective health services work force, which, in turn, is possible only if there are safe working conditions. Legal obligations support this duty to staff, too.

If protecting staff is an ethical priority, it is necessary to create and maintain an environment consistent with the obligation to provide health services to the community and treat persons with AIDS. HIV is present in all body substances of those who are HIV positive, but it seems to be spread only by sexual intercourse or intimate contact with body substances, particularly blood. The risk for health services workers is low, but a major concern nonetheless. The CDC and the Occupational Safety and Health Administration have developed guidelines for universal precautions that should be used in all HSOs.

Some physicians and staff are reluctant or unwilling to treat AIDS patients. There have been reports of surgeons who demand preoperative HIV testing of patients and who refuse to operate on those who are positive. In 1987, the AMA Council on Ethical and Judicial Affairs issued a statement that it is unethical for physicians to refuse to treat AIDS patients whose medical conditions are within their competence.[71] Nurses and staff have been disciplined for refusing to treat AIDS patients; some have been fired. Given the nature of the controversy, it is unlikely that statements or disciplinary action will convince some caregivers to treat persons with AIDS.

In mid-1987, the AHA issued recommendations reflecting the growing concern about clinical management of AIDS patients.[72] These recommendations were consistent with CDC guidelines that universal use of blood and body substance precautions is the best protection for caregivers. The guidelines suggest that *all* patients' blood and body substances be considered hazardous and that *all* patients be subject to the infection-control guidelines originally established for hepatitis and active AIDS patients. This means that isolation and biohazard precautions should be used for all patients (whether or not they are known to have AIDS) and that measures of protection from body substances and patient contact be taken accordingly. This approach was specifically recommended rather than conducting routine HIV testing of patients.

A few hospitals test all admissions for HIV. Patients who refuse will be admitted but treated with extra precautions, even though using extra precautions is at variance with the requirement for universal precautions. In late 1987, the AHA spoke out against routine testing of staff, and it continues to hold that position because, in its view, "adherence to universal precautions is the most effective means of reducing the risk of infection for hospital staff and patients."[73]

In late August 1987, the CDC confirmed that three hospital staff members exposed to AIDS-infected blood had acquired AIDS, and its revised recommendations allowed hospitals more latitude in conducting routine testing. Since then the CDC has documented 40 cases of health services workers who became infected with HIV through occupational exposure.[74] Some experts think that HIV among health services workers is significantly underreported and that there are many other cases.[75] Three large studies estimate the risk of contracting HIV after accidentally being stuck with a contaminated needle as about 1 in 250.[76] Surgeons are at higher risk. A study reported in 1991 found that they came into contact with patients' blood an average of 18.6 times per 100 procedures involving an incision; this compared with 2.7 times for nurses and technicians assisting in the operating room.[77]

The general risk of caregivers being infected by exposure to blood and body substances from HIV-positive patients is low and is far less than the risk of becoming infected with hepatitis. Nonetheless, it is troublesome that one study found high levels of noncompliance with universal precautions. A study conducted at the Johns Hopkins University Hospital Emergency Department found that physicians used universal precautions only 38% of the time. Other categories complied more often: residents 58% and nursing staff 44%. Housekeeping staff complied most often— 91% of the time. The staff blamed low compliance on time pressures (38%) and interference of precautions with procedural skills (33%).[78] These low levels of compliance occurred despite ready availability of gloves, gowns, and the like, and despite efforts to educate staff about risks. The study also revealed that the rate of infected emergency department patients at Johns Hopkins increased from 5.2% to 6.0% in one year. Encouraging compliance poses a special challenge to managers, and further research about how to achieve it must be undertaken. Enhanced education can be only a small part of the answer. Management must identify and correct structure and process inhibitors that reduce the staff's willingness or ability to use universal precautions.

HSOs that follow CDC and AHA guidelines—the ethical, clinically correct, and legally prudent course—treat all patients as if they are HIV positive. The August 1987 CDC guidelines suggested that hospitals judge whether their patients' characteristics were such that all admissions should be tested. In guidelines issued in September 1991, the CDC took a significant step toward patient testing by proposing that acute care hospitals "routinely offer and encourage" voluntary testing and counseling of patients for HIV. It is believed that such a policy will assist physicians in diagnosing medical conditions, aid in early management of HIV infection, and allow instruction of infected persons about proper behavior.[79] All HSOs should address the question of testing patients early and specifically.

Protecting Patients from Staff Some caregivers are HIV positive, but do not have active AIDS and wish to continue treating patients. Several highly publicized cases have involved physicians.

In 1991, the AMA stated

> that HIV infected physicians should either abstain from performing invasive procedures which pose an identifiable risk of transmission or disclose their sero-positive status prior to performing a procedure and proceed only if there is informed consent. As a corollary, physicians who are at risk of acquiring HIV infection, and who perform invasive procedures, should determine their HIV status.[80]

In 1991, the CDC reported three cases of possible HIV transmission from a dentist to his patients.[81] HIV-positive caregivers pose a risk of infection to patients and other staff from HIV *and* from the opportunistic diseases that afflict AIDS patients, including tuberculosis and *Pneumocystis carinii* pneumonia. Immunosuppressed patients are at great risk. Also significant, but subtle, is the fact that HIV affects the brain, sometimes long before other symptoms appear. This means use of HIV-positive staff is problematic.

In July 1991, the CDC issued new recommendations to prevent transmission of HIV to patients during exposure-prone procedures. These recommendations reemphasized universal precautions. Mandatory testing of health workers for HIV seropositivity was *not* recommended. Restrictions on the practice of health workers was not recommended for invasive procedures unless the procedures are exposure prone.[82] CDC expected that medical experts and medical specialty groups would develop lists of exposure-prone procedures. They refused to do so, however, arguing that there are no known cases of transmission of HIV from physicians to patients. Revised recommendations issued by CDC in late 1991 suggested that the emphasis should be on identifying those infected health care workers who do not meet standards of infection control or who may be unfit to practice.[83] As yet, no medical professional group has sought mandatory testing. There have been numerous calls for mandatory testing of health workers from the public sector, which have been echoed in Congress, however.

Currently, dedicated AIDS units are rare, primarily because most HSOs, including hospitals, have few AIDS patients. Hospitals with large numbers of AIDS patients typically admit them to general medical/surgical floors, even in acute phases of the disease. Managers reason that privacy is better protected; extra workload is spread among caregivers, especially nurses; and staffing and work assignment problems are eased.

Despite the uncertainty of statutory and case law, HSOs should identify HIV-positive staff (including physicians): it is ethically appropriate *and* legally prudent to prohibit HIV-positive staff from performing exposure-prone invasive procedures. In meeting their ethical duty of nonmaleficence—do no harm—staff themselves should want to know if they are a risk to patients. Because of the opportunistic diseases they contract, staff who have AIDS are a risk to patients, many of whom are immunosuppressed or physically weakened. HIV-positive staff also pose some risk to other staff and nonpatients. Such implications should cause managers to err in favor of caution in assignments, at least until legal parameters are established. Furthermore, as HIV-positive staff become increasingly immunosuppressed, infectious diseases common in HSOs are a risk to them. If the HSO is to discharge its ethical obligation to staff, such information must be considered in job assignments. Given that a great deal is unknown about HIV and its transmissibility, HIV-positive staff should be encouraged to accept nonpatient care jobs whether or not they perform invasive procedures. Protecting staff confidentiality is crucial to the success of this effort.

An equally compelling and more subtly evident reason for routine staff testing is suggested by preliminary evidence showing that HIV induces neuropsychiatric problems. Manifestations include impaired coordination and cognitive difficulties that may occur before physical symptoms are apparent. In normal clinical practice deficits in performance may be attributed to simple, random error rather than a medical condition. Serious problems may occur before a pattern is detected, and diminished competence may be apparent only in retrospect, most likely after some untoward event. The ethical (and legal) duty of employers to monitor staff and prevent harm to patients is well established.

Confidentiality   HSOs must be alert to special problems of confidentiality that surround AIDS. Within the constraints of state law, however, the first obligation must be to safeguard staff. Given preliminary evidence on compliance with universal precautions, at least in one hospital emergency department, identifying HIV-positive patients may be an additional stimulus to encourage staff compliance.

Some suggest that identifying patients as HIV positive will lead to two-class medicine. This charge is baseless. The potential for this problem has existed for the decade since HIV was first identified and patient charts and rooms were marked with biohazard notices, as well as other, less publicly obvious codes. Thus far, there is no evidence that patients with AIDS have received care different from other patients.

A dedicated AIDS unit similar to intensive care or cardiac care units has a certain appeal. Confidentiality problems are often cited when dedicated AIDS units are discussed. This risk is overstated because staff know (as they should) which patients have AIDS, and since AIDS has been so widely publicized it is likely that family or visitors are aware that it is a possibility, especially in the final stages. Second, concentrating AIDS patients allows special training and equipment to be brought to bear to protect staff and to enhance treatment. Third, only the staff wishing to work with AIDS patients would do so, perhaps stimulated by economic or other incentives. Finally, a dedicated unit minimizes any drift toward second-class care because the availability of staff and other resources would be readily apparent, whereas such lapses could be more easily overlooked or hidden on a general medical/surgical floor.

Summary   To date, few HSOs have been established exclusively to treat AIDS. Even though case loads may justify it, few dedicated AIDS units have been established. This may change as the public becomes more willing to accept persons with AIDS and as the financial effect becomes more acute. It is quite possible that public agencies will establish or staff AIDS hospitals, nursing facilities, hospices, outpatient facilities, and other special programs.

Hospitals must find ways to provide efficacious acute, episodic treatment and to assist HSOs, especially nursing facilities and hospices, that are alternative sources of care. Financing care will remain problematic for all providers. Caring for AIDS patients while protecting staff remains a major ethical challenge, and one in which managers will have the most significant role.

AIDS has ethical, managerial, and legal dimensions and nuances that make it as complex an issue as any that managers face. Within the constraints of law, however, the ethical and managerial priorities must be staff, patients, and community.

PREVENTING AND SOLVING ETHICAL PROBLEMS

Organizational Culture and Philosophy

The organizational culture and philosophy must be compatible. The organizational philosophy sets the tone and should be used to lead the culture to a higher plane. Optimally, organizational philosophy and culture are mutually reinforcing.

The most significant factor in preventing and solving ethical problems is that the HSO's organizational philosophy be well defined. The organizational philosophy must emphasize protecting patients and furthering their interests. This results from applying the ethical principles of respect for persons, beneficence, and nonmaleficence. Williams and Donnelly stress this relationship and argue that accountability to the patient exceeds any duty or relationship between a governing body and other persons or entities, including the professional staff.[84] They argue that this accountability is so important that if a patient is harmed through clinical malpractice, but is unaware of it, the HSO should inform the patient. Williams and Donnelly argue that doing so is consistent with the fiduciary duty and ethical role of the governing body and the organization. This may seem radical, but it is consistent with the degree of trust the public has (and should have) in HSOs and appropriately describes the HSO's reciprocal duty. It is crucial to the HSO's ethical survival that there be basic congruity between its philosophy and the personal ethic of all staff, but especially its managers. Moral agency requires that these ethical guidelines be reflected in the manager's actions.

Institutional Ethics Committees[85]

It is recommended that complex HSOs, especially acute care hospitals, have an ethics committee with at least two subcommittees, each of which addresses different types of ethical issues. An alternative is to have an ethics committee for administrative issues and an ethics committee for biomedical ethical issues. Specializing in this fashion is necessary because a committee able to grapple with biomedical ethics problems is unlikely to be well prepared to solve administrative ethics problems. Further specialization may be needed within the two broad categories of administrative and biomedical ethics. For example, there may be need for an infant care review committee. Care must be taken that committee proliferation does not cause inefficient overlap. Because of the need to solve general, organization-wide issues and specific, perhaps technical, problems, the committee with subcommittees model may be most effective. Before considering ethical problems within the HSO, institutional ethics committees (IECs) must develop a statement of their ethic. This is not a description of how to solve problems, but a statement of general principles to guide deliberations and decision making. The overall framework is provided by the organizational philosophy and mission. Only by successfully engaging in deliberations can IECs be effective. This exercise is also useful to identify and minimize differences in members' personal ethics.

As initially conceived by the court in the Karen Ann Quinlan case, IECs had a very limited scope. They were prognosis committees that assisted in answering questions about the terminally ill, especially about continuing life support. In some organizations IECs with this role are called "god squads" since they are instrumental in determining whether to withdraw life support. IECs should have and usually do have a broader role.

Some of the first information about the structure, procedures, activities, and effectiveness of IECs used to solve biomedical ethical problems resulted from a national survey done for the President's Commission, which was published in 1983.[86] No hospital with fewer than 200 beds had an IEC. Even in large hospitals IECs were not ubiquitous, but most hospitals, especially those with teaching programs, had an IEC. The study estimated there were fewer than 100 IECs in hospitals.

The Quinlan decision encouraged hospitals to establish IECs. IECs were most common in New Jersey; 71% had been formed because of that case.

Surveys in 1983 and 1985 by the National Society of Patient Representatives showed rapid growth of IECs. In 1983, 26% of hospitals responding to the survey had IECs. This figure rose to 59% in 1985. Many were a response to the Baby Doe case. Since then, IECs have broadened their roles, and undertaken tasks such as developing DNR orders and patient consent policies, advising on withholding or withdrawing life support, and educational programs.[87] Although the methodology used in the surveys caused disproportionate numbers of large hospitals to respond, the findings on rapid growth are consistent with research by the American Academy of Pediatrics reported below. Findings of a later telephone survey show little recent growth in the number of IECs, however.[88] It has been suggested that ethics committees have matured, and it is time to reconsider their roles and determine whether they should be involved in new ways and in other aspects of the organization's activities.[89]

Membership   Data from the President's Commission study suggest that biomedical IECs are interdisciplinary.[90] Physicians were the most common members and averaged 5.25 per committee. Committees averaged one member of the clergy. Others found on fewer than half the committees were attorneys, laypersons, social workers, and physicians in graduate education programs. Administrators were present far less frequently than physicians, and served on about half the committees. Underrepresentation of managers may reflect too little interest in clinical matters generally—a problem that must be remedied. The commission found no strong community link, something that governing body members and persons from the service area provide. They bring an important perspective.[91]

Administrative IECs will have fewer clinical personnel and more representatives from the governing body and management. Clinical personnel must be included, because it is reasonable to conclude that research results suggesting HSOs are most effective when they involve clinicians in management decision making also apply to solving problems of administrative ethics.

Purposes and Roles   IECs should have three roles. The first is to assist in developing the organizational philosophy and policies on ethical issues. The experience and perspectives of an IEC's interdisciplinary membership will produce better reasoned and more thorough results. Education is the second role. The IEC's composition and experience make it a reservoir of knowledge and expertise. These resources should be available to the governing body and staff. Such attributes add sophistication and will improve the quality of clinical and administrative decisions.

The third role is case consultation, wherein the committee or individual members assist in understanding and solving ethical issues raised by specific cases. Research by the President's Commission found that major benefits of biomedical IECs included facilitating decision making by clarifying important issues, shaping consistent hospital policies about life support, and providing opportunities for professionals to air disagreements. The committees were not found to be very effective at increasing the ability of patients' families to influence decisions or educating professionals about issues relevant to life support decisions. The commission found that committees provided counsel and support to physicians, developed policy about care of the critically ill, reviewed ethical issues of patient care decisions, provided counsel and support to other professionals and patients and families, determined medical prognoses, made final decisions about life support, and determined continuing education needs.[92]

The study also made two general observations:

1. Committees that do exist are not involved in large numbers of cases. Existing committees reviewed an average of only one case per year.
2. The composition and function of committees identified in the survey would not allay many of the concerns of patients' rights advocates about patient representation and control. Committees were clearly dominated by physicians and other health professionals. The majority of committees did

not allow patients to attend or request meetings, although family members were more often permitted to do so. Yet, chairmen generally regarded their committees as effective.[93]

The latter conclusion suggests that health services managers must be alert to patient autonomy—a matter affecting several aspects of the organization, but especially resource allocation and consent. Anecdotal evidence suggests that many President's Commission findings remain true.

Relationships   IEC relationships vary with the IEC's role, and activities can be general and specific. General activities are organization wide and can be divided into biomedical and administrative ethics. Examples include reconsidering the organizational philosophy, developing a conflict of interest policy, or guiding macroallocation decisions. Specific activities are individual cases in which ethical questions arise. Examples include determining whether something is consistent with the organizational philosophy or a conflict exists.

The IEC should be proactive in developing and revising the organizational philosophy and in considering ethical implications of macroallocation questions. Similarly, it should take the initiative to review and revise the consent process. It may, however, choose a passive role and wait to be consulted in specific instances of conflicts of interest and misuse of confidential information (in the case of an administrative IEC) or in specific clinical matters (in the case of a biomedical IEC).

There is evidence from the President's Commission study that IECs involved in biomedical ethics problem solving were most effective when they waited to be consulted rather than interposing themselves. Consultation means committees make recommendations, not final decisions.[94] IEC participation in biomedical and administrative decision making may be optional or mandatory. Following advice given by an IEC could also be made optional or mandatory. The combinations are shown in Table 3.2.

Physicians are unlikely to accept mandatory-mandatory involvement by a biomedical IEC. Furthermore, this may not be desirable in the majority of situations, when a competent physician is willing to develop alternatives and communicate them effectively to the patient and other concerned persons. Even when the physician is unwilling to share decision making with the members of an ethics committee, however, there are benefits to having advice available.

An important aspect of organizing an IEC is the question of where it should reside organizationally. This issue was not addressed by the President's Commission study. Options include making the IEC a standing committee of the governing body, the professional staff organization, or the administration. The fear that physicians will dominate the IEC led some experts to suggest that it be a governing body or administration committee. Similarly, no committee member should represent a specific interest or group.

Infant Care Review Committees

The Child Abuse Amendments of 1984 direct DHHS to encourage establishment of infant care review committees (ICRCs) in hospitals with tertiary-level neonatal care units. ICRCs are specialized IECs that focus on the biomedical ethical problems of infants with life-threatening conditions. In the DHHS guidelines, ICRCs are ethics committees that provide information and education, recommend institutional policies and guidelines, and offer counsel and review of issues

Table 3.2. Optional versus mandatory use of an IEC

Involvement of committee in decision making	Acceptance and use of advice given by IEC
Optional	
Optional	Optional
Mandatory	Mandatory
Mandatory	Optional
	Mandatory

related to infant care. DHHS considers it prudent to establish an ICRC, but the HSO makes the final decision.

DHHS recommends that membership of an ICRC include persons from varied disciplines and perspectives because a multidisciplinary approach provides expertise to supply and evaluate pertinent information. The committee should be large enough to present diverse viewpoints, but not so large that effectiveness is hindered. Recommended membership includes a practicing nurse, a hospital senior manager, a social worker, a representative of a disability group, a lay community member, and a member of the facility's medical staff, who serves as chair.[95] The recommendation that there be a representative of a disability group is counter to the principle that specific groups not have representatives.

DHHS recommends that ICRCs have staff support, including legal counsel; that it recommend procedures to ensure that hospital personnel and patient families know of its existence, functions, and 24-hour availability; that it be informed about pertinent legal requirements and procedures, including state law; and that it keep records of deliberations and summary descriptions of cases and their disposition.[96]

DHHS's recommended form and activities for ICRCs are similar to those reported in a 1984 study of 710 hospitals with special care pediatric units. The American Academy of Pediatrics (AAP) found that, of the 426 respondents, 56% had ICRCs or IECs and 75% of those without committees were considering establishing one. The remaining 25% handle ethical problems by other means. The committee activity mentioned most often was consulting on difficult ethical decisions; this was followed by advising parents, advising physicians (when consulted), and educating staff. Developing hospital policies was rated as the third most important function. Committee composition was similar to that found by the President's Commission study.[97]

The percentage of hospitals with ethics committees reported in the AAP study is much higher than that found in the President's Commission study. AAP findings are consistent with those of the National Society of Patient Representatives. The Commission's research was done several years before the AAP study, and differences in findings suggest a major change in the interim, at least regarding numbers of ICRCs. The AAP report even commented that evidence suggested many committees were new. The AAP found that more managers were serving on ICRCs than were found on IECs by the President's Commission. More involvement of managers in biomedical ethics is desirable.

Specialized Assistance

Ethics Consultation Services   One way HSOs can provide specialized personnel to advise and assist in solving biomedical ethics problems is to establish an ethics consultation service (ECS). Doing so is like establishing a clinical service. The ECS is staffed by ethicists with graduate degrees in philosophy, often at the doctoral level, and clinical personnel, such as physicians or other caregivers. The clinicians have a special interest and/or preparation in ethics, and provide a bridge between the ethicists and the clinical staff attending the patient. They serve, too, as a resource to the ethicists. In this model, an ethicist is on call and the clinical member of the ECS participates as needed. The ECS reports to the IEC, and the IEC develops and recommends policy to the governing body. The IEC also is a sounding board for problems that arise in ethics consultation. A variant of this model uses a primary consultant who is assisted by other ECS members. Both the primary consultants and those assisting have various backgrounds, but they all have specialized training in ethics and participate in case reviews, ethics instruction, and ECS staff meetings.[98]

Ethicists   A less formal approach is found in larger hospitals, but the concept should not be limited to them. These hospitals have full- or part-time ethicists on their staffs. As with ECSs, the ethicists are often philosophers with doctoral degrees who may be university or medical school faculty and who consult on biomedical ethical issues. Organizations seeking the assistance of an ethicist should consider anyone with specialized preparation in ethics and its application in the health field. Here, as with ECS, the ethicist is the clinically oriented, problem-solving extension of an IEC.

Dispute Resolution The American Arbitration Association has conducted seminars to train hospice professionals to resolve disputes over patient care more effectively. Resolving disputes is necessary because staff have different views about issues and cases. Improved dispute resolution should weld the multidisciplinary group into a cohesive and mutually supportive team that can resolve their differences and maintain the quality of patient care. Such preparation would assist IECs, ICRCs, and IRBs, as well. It is optimistic to assume that the act of establishing an IEC means success. Preparation in resolving disputes will improve effectiveness.

SUMMARY

This chapter identifies administrative and biomedical ethical issues and describes how HSOs and their administrative and clinical staffs work with them. The importance of the link between the organizational philosophy and the personal ethic of managers is stressed. The ethical dimensions of more recent problems such as marketing, competition, and AIDS are discussed.

After being identified first in the 1970s, ethics committees have become important in HSOs. By the 1990s they are commonplace, many are specialized, and they have broad and varied missions. Ethics committees are interdisciplinary to grapple better with problems that often have legal as well as bioethics considerations.

HSOs are becoming adept at solving ethical problems. The HSO, through its managers, has an ethical responsibility to protect patients and further their interests. This duty incorporates principles of respect for persons, beneficence, nonmaleficence, and justice, and is more demanding than the law. It stresses the independent relationship between managers and patients. The manager's duty to protect patients and further their interests transcends other obligations and is one HSOs must formalize and aggressively implement.

DISCUSSION QUESTIONS

1. Describe the relationship between law and ethics. Which is the more demanding standard? Why? Identify and be prepared to explain examples other than those described in the chapter.
2. Identify health services laws or regulations based on: 1) a utilitarian philosophy, 2) a deontological philosophy, and 3) elements of both. How compatible are these philosophies when included in the same law or regulation?
3. What does a professional code of ethics reflect? How can enforcement be made meaningful? Must a profession "police" its standards? Why or why not?
4. Describe uses *and* limitations of codes of ethics that apply to HSOs. Should they be communicated to patients who use the HSO? If so, how?
5. What is the HSO's role regarding patient rights? Are some duties or obligations surpassed by the HSO's duty to patients? Give examples of where this occurs.
6. Define "fiduciary." Give some examples in and out of health services. Are HSOs and their services unique in terms of this concept? If so, how?
7. Define conflict of interest. Give examples in HSOs. How can HSOs minimize them? What is the manager's role?
8. What should be the role of managers in allocating resources at the micro *and* macro levels? What can be done to reduce the likelihood that ethical problems will arise?
9. Identify examples of experimenting in HSOs. Distinguish surgical experimentation from that involving drugs and devices. How can patients be protected?

10. Distinguish living wills and natural death acts. What is their effect on HSOs? How do managers ensure that HSOs interact effectively with patients in terms of such directives?

CASE STUDY 1:   "WHAT'S A MANAGER TO DO?"[99]

S.L. Rine joined the managerial staff of a large health services provider after gaining several years of experience. Rine is an affiliate of the American College of Healthcare Executives (ACHE) and wants to build the best set of credentials in the shortest possible time. Rine wants to become a CEO.

Rine is responsible for several support departments as well as some clinical areas. Rine realized quickly that the HSO is very political. Much of what happens at the senior level is the result of personal relationships and obligations.

One of Rine's departments, maintenance, is responsible for all grounds. Rine found that grounds crews were being sent to homes of senior members of the board to maintain their lawns, shrubs, and trees. Rine asked the maintenance director to explain and was told that the practice had a long history and he suggested that things were better left as they were. When Rine asked the director for a cost estimate of the grounds work being done at the private homes, the director refused to give it and said he wasn't about to incur the wrath of the board members who were benefiting. Rine pondered what to do.

Shortly after talking to the maintenance director, Rine had lunch with the laboratory director. Without discussing specifics Rine described the problem in maintenance. The laboratory director exclaimed, "That's nothing!" and went on to describe how two board members were selling reagents, supplies, and equipment to the laboratory at what she believed were higher than market prices. Rine asked if she had done anything about it; she replied that her predecessor had tried to stop the practice and had had to look for a new job. Rine pondered what to do.

Questions

1. Identify the ethical problems that face the board members and the managers. Do similar problems face those not directly involved?
2. Are the grounds maintenance and the sale of reagents, supplies, and equipment to the laboratory ethically different? State your reasons. Are the two likely to be distinguished in the "real world?"
3. What steps should managers like Rine take if they have the moral courage to risk their jobs to try to solve the problems? Short of risking their jobs, what steps could they take?
4. What sources of assistance are there for Rine outside the organization? How should they be involved?

CASE STUDY 2:   BITS AND PIECES[100]

John Henry Williams was pleased with his new job in the radiology department of Affiliated Nursing Homes and Rehabilitation Center. He was appointed acting department head because his predecessor, Mary Beth Jacobson, was scheduled for 6 months maternity leave. John Henry would be responsible for the equivalent of two full-time and one half-time technicians, an appointments clerk, and $250,000 in equipment. He would have authority to purchase supplies, including certain types of film. The annual value of these purchases was about $90,000. Most were obtained from three vendors, companies from which the Center had bought for years.

During her orientation for John Henry, Mary Beth emphasized how much she liked the meetings with sales representatives from the three vendors. Over the years, one had become a personal friend. Most meetings were held at the nice restaurant near the Center. Some were held in her office and, if so, they always brought along a "little something." When John Henry asked what she meant, Mary Beth gave some examples: perfume, a bottle of French brandy, and a pen set in a leather case. John Henry remembered thinking that his wife would like the perfume, but he was more interested in the lunches. It would be a chance to get away from the dreary cafeteria, as well as his boring sack lunches. Mary Beth described the lunches as nothing fancy. She estimated the cost to the sales rep as the same as the small gifts—in the $40–$50 range.

John Henry asked Mary Beth whether there was a policy about accepting gifts from vendors. Mary Beth was put out by the question—it implied something might be wrong with what she was doing. She responded curtly that the Center trusted its managers and allowed them discretion in such matters.

John Henry asked if accepting gratuities might suggest to other staff that her decisions were influenced by the pecuniary relationship with the sales reps. Mary Beth's anger flashed. "I know you think that this doesn't look right. That isn't fair! I work long hours as a manager and get paid very little extra. It takes more effort and time to order and maintain proper inventory. If things go wrong, it's my head in a noose. These gifts make me feel better about my efforts. My work has been exemplary. I'd be happy to talk to anyone who thinks otherwise!!"

Questions

1. Develop arguments that support Mary Beth's position on the gratuities she is receiving. List them in rank order.
2. Describe the importance of business custom in the relationship Mary Beth has with the sales representatives. Should this influence the ethics of the situation?
3. Develop a policy regarding gratuities that Affiliated Nursing Homes and Rehabilitation Center could use. Identify the underlying ethical principles and be prepared to defend the policy.
4. Describe incidents from your own experience that are similar to those described in the case. What detrimental effects did they have on the organization? Were they resolved? If so, how?

CASE STUDY 3: DEMARKETING TO AVOID BANKRUPTCY[101]

Chris Hines had finally gotten far enough into the stack of papers on her desk to see last month's emergency department (ED) activity report. She had already digested the grim news about the continued financial hemorrhage at Community Hospital. The total deficit was $500,000 and it was only the fourth month of the fiscal year. Because Community Hospital served a largely inner city population, many of whom were uninsured or whose care was paid by a chronically under-funded Medicaid program, there seemed little hope that the financial situation would improve.

As CEO, Hines knew that over 40% of Community Hospital admissions came through the ED and that about one half of these arrived by taxi, private automobile, or on foot. The other half were brought in by the ambulance service run by the city government. A couple of years previously Hines had tried to implement a plan to increase the number of elective admissions (and thus improve the payor mix) by encouraging physicians to bring their private patients to Community Hospital. It failed, however, largely because the physicians had difficulty getting their patients admitted—ER admissions were taking too many beds. Next, Hines tried to work with city officials to implement a new ambulance routing system that would send more patients to other hospitals and give Community Hospital a chance to improve its financial condition. They were unsympathetic.

Hines knew that Community Hospital's endowment would carry the hospital for about three years, but if they were not breaking even by then the hospital would close. Since there was nothing that could be done through the city, the key to survival, she concluded, lay with reducing the number of uninsured and Medicaid admissions through the ER.

Hines spoke with several marketing consultants, one of whom offered to work *pro bono*. They seized upon the idea of demarketing the ED. They reasoned that it was the ED's fine reputation in the community that was responsible for the 50% of patients who came to the ED other than by city ambulance. They identified ways the ED could be made less desirable. The plan included: reducing ED staffing to a minimum; closing the parking lot near the ED; reducing housekeeping coverage so the physical plant would be dirty and unkempt; deferring non–safety-related mainte- nance; changing triage policies and procedures and staffing to increase waiting time for non- emergency patients; using staff who were most likely to be rude and inconsiderate; and encourag- ing rumors that the closure of the ED was imminent.

They knew there might be repercussions beyond the ED, but they were desperate and be- lieved there was no choice but to take extreme actions.

Questions

1. Identify the ethical issues in the case. Who bears major responsibility for their presence? Their solution?
2. Outline a strategy that would save Community Hospital without using the plan developed by Hines and the marketing consultant. How is it superior? Inferior?
3. Develop arguments that support the action planned by Hines from a utilitarian perspective and from a Kantian perspective.
4. Describe the likely effects of the action planned by Hines on patients, staff, physicians, and managers.

CASE STUDY 4:   CHOICES

Randy Glenn had just fallen asleep when the phone rang. It was the night supervisor at the com- prehensive care center and hospital of which Glenn was the CEO. The supervisor was very agi- tated and had trouble getting her words out. It took a few minutes for the message to become clear. One of Glenn's nightmares had come true. The four-bed intensive care unit (ICU) was full and there was an emergency case. The new patient had been injured in a car accident. She had been stabilized in the emergency department, but her injuries were such that transferring her to another facility would almost certainly cause death. She had to get into the ICU in 1–2 hours.

The night supervisor recovered somewhat and described the patients currently occupying ICU beds and the new patient:

Patient A: Sixty-year-old female, comatose, stroke victim who has been in the ICU for 27 days; prognosis uncertain; retired, no family.

Patient B: One-year-old premature male with Down syndrome; has been in ICU since birth; hospital repaired a duodenal atresia (no opening between stomach and small intestine), parents opposed the procedure; child's social future uncertain.

Patient C: Thirty-six-year-old male who had emergency appendectomy, developed se- vere wound infection and probable septicemia, source of infection unknown; previous anaphylactic shock in reaction to antibiotics necessitates ICU; bach- elor; aged mother in city.

Patient D: Twelve-year-old female undergoing chemotherapy for leukemia with experi- mental drug; has been in remission three times; close monitoring of protocol and potential reaction to drug requires ICU care; family in city.

New Patient: Twenty-four-year-old female; college honor student in physics, scholarship winner; pregnant; engaged; no family known.

The supervisor ended by asking, "What should I do? How do I treat five patients with only four beds?" Indeed, what to do? thought Glenn. I wish I had paid more attention in my ethics course. Glenn pondered alternatives to the question asked by the supervisor as the garage door opened and the 10-minute trip to the facility began.

Questions

1. What should Glenn do? Why is it ethically best?
2. Identify the steps to be taken in reaching a decision.
3. Describe ways to minimize these problems in the future and to deal with them when they occur. Adding additional ICU beds is not acceptable.
4. What sources of assistance might be available to Glenn at this point? Which should Glenn develop for the future?

CASE STUDY 5: BENEFITING THE ELDERLY BY INFECTING THEM WITH INFLUENZA

New Horizons is a state-owned institution for care of the indigent elderly. As in many nursing facilities, influenza is a major problem among the patients. Influenza is usually not fatal in younger populations, but it has a significant mortality for the elderly, often because of complications such as pneumonia. A major drug company has been doing animal studies on a vaccine to protect against influenza. The vaccine is ready for clinical trials.

The administrator of New Horizons, Gregg Greeley, was contacted by the drug company about the feasibility of establishing a research unit. The unit would have about twenty patients at a time. The presence of drug company employees, including physicians, nurses, and ancillary personnel, would provide better care for those in the unit than is usually available at New Horizons. In addition, there would be money for better meals and other amenities. However, once the vaccine had been administered the patients would be deliberately exposed to influenza to determine if the vaccine protected them.

Many patients at New Horizons have children or relatives who are their guardians. Greeley called some of the guardians and found they had no problem consenting to the experiment. Several noted that persons in the unit would receive better quality care and, if they contracted influenza, would receive the advantages of that care.

Questions

1. Which moral philosophy supports the action contemplated by Greeley? Which does not?
2. Should residents have a voice in the decision? If so, how can their wishes be known and implemented?
3. What interests are being balanced? How and by whom should the interests be weighed?
4. If the experiment proceeds, how should residents be protected? What is Greeley's role?

NOTES

1. Fleck, Leonard. Speech to the American Hospital Association. *Catholic Health World* 5 (October 15, 1989): 3.
2. Bodenheimer, Edgar. *Jurisprudence: The philosophy and method of the law*, 6. Cambridge, MA: Harvard University Press, 1974.
3. Bodenheimer, *Jurisprudence*, 6.
4. Bodenheimer, *Jurisprudence*, 325.
5. Henderson, Verne E. The ethical side of enterprise. *Sloan Management Review* 23 (Spring 1982): 41–42.
6. Kant, Immanuel. *Fundamental principles of the metaphysics of morals*. Translated by Thomas K. Abbott. In *Knowledge and value*, ed. by Elmer Sprague and Paul W. Taylor, 535–558. New York, Harcourt, Brace and Co., 1959.
7. Arras, John, and Nancy Rhoden. *Ethical issues in modern medicine* 3d ed. Mountain View, CA: Mayfield Publishing Company, 1989.
8. Bodenheimer, *Jurisprudence*, 23.
9. Bodenheimer, *Jurisprudence*, 94.
10. Rawls, John. *A theory of justice*, 60 Cambridge, MA: The Belknap Press, 1971.
11. This section is adapted from Darr, Kurt. Moral philosophies and principles. In *Ethics in health services management*, 2d ed., 15–27. Baltimore: Health Professions Press, 1991; used by permission.
12. Darr, Kurt. Administrative ethics and the health services manager. *Hospital & Health Services Administration* 29 (March–April 1984): 120–136.
13. American Medical Association. *Current opinions of the Judicial Council*, vii. Chicago, 1982.
14. American Medical Association. *Principles of medical ethics*. Chicago, 1980.
15. Veatch, Robert M. Professional ethics: New principles for physicians? *Hastings Center Report* (June 1980): 17.
16. American Nurses Association. *Code for nurses with in-*

terpretive statements, i. Kansas City, MO, 1985.

17. American Nurses Association, *Code for nurses,* iii.

18. American Nurses Association, *Code for nurses,* 1.

19. Southwick, Arthur F. *The law of hospital and health care administration,* 2d ed., 122–123. Ann Arbor, MI: Health Administration Press, 1988.

20. Southwick, *Law of hospital,* 123–124.

21. Southwick, *Law of hospital,* 126.

22. *Stern et al. v. Lucy Webb Hayes National Training School of Deaconesses and Missionaries, et al.,* 381 Federal Supplement 1003 (1974).

23. *Stern v. Hayes,* 381 Federal Supplement 1003 (1974).

24. American College of Healthcare Executives. *Code of ethics.* Chicago, 1987.

25. American College of Healthcare Executives, *Code.*

26. Devolites, Milton C. *The Cedars of Lebanon Hospital.* Unpublished case study, The George Washington University Department of Health Services Administration, 1974.

27. American College of Healthcare Executives, *Code.*

28. This section is adapted from Darr, Kurt. Marketing in a competitive environment. In *Ethics in health services management,* 2d ed., 221–226. Baltimore: Health Professions Press, 1991; used by permission.

29. Hanlon, John J., and George E. Pickett. *Public health: Administration and practice,* 5. St. Louis: Times Mirror/Mosby, 1984.

30. *Dorland's illustrated medical dictionary,* 27th ed., 1640. Philadelphia: W. B. Saunders Company, 1988.

31. American Hospital Association. New survey shows rapid growth in hospital ethics committees. Press release, September 1, 1985.

32. This section is adapted from Darr, Kurt. Conflicts of interest and fiduciary duty. In *Ethics in health services management,* 2d ed., 103–107. Baltimore: Health Professions Press, 1991; used by permission.

33. Harron, Frank, John Burnside, and Tom Beauchamp. *Health and human values: A guide to making your own decisions,* 148. New Haven, CT: Yale University Press, 1983.

34. Childress, James F. Who shall live when not all can live? *Soundings, An Interdisciplinary Journal* 53 (Winter 1970): 339–355.

35. Rescher, Nicholas. The allocation of exotic medical lifesaving therapy. *Ethics* 79 (April 1969): 173–186.

36. Hiatt, Fred. Japan court ruling backs doctors. *Washington Post* (May 30, 1989): A9.

37. President's Commission for the Study of Ethical Problems in Medicine and Biomedical and Behavioral Research. *Making health care decisions.* Vol. 1. Washington, D.C.: U.S. Government Printing Office, 1982.

38. Katz, Jay. Informed consent—a fairy tale. *University of Pittsburgh Law Review* 39 (Winter 1977): 137–174.

39. President's Commission, *Making health care decisions,* Vol. 1.

40. Wiggers, Carl J. Human experimentation as exemplified by the career of Dr. William Beaumont. *Alumni Bulletin* (Case Western Reserve University School of Medicine) (1950): 60–64.

41. Darr, Kurt. *Ethics in health services management,* 2d ed., 208. Baltimore: Health Professions Press, 1991.

42. Ramsey, Paul. *The patient as person,* 252. New Haven, CT: Yale University Press, 1970.

43. U.S. Department of Health and Human Services. Basic HHS policy for protection of human research subjects. 46 C.F.R. 98 *et seq* (1981, as modified).

44. Harvard Medical School. A definition of irreversible coma. *Journal of the American Medical Association* 205 (August 5, 1968): 337–338.

45. President's Commission for the Study of Ethical Problems in Medicine and Biomedical and Behavioral Research. *Defining death: Medical, legal, and ethical issues in the determination of death.* Washington, D.C.: U.S. Government Printing Office, 25, 1981.

46. Uniform Law Commissioners, Chicago, IL. Personal communication, July 26, 1990.

47. *In re Quinlan,* 70 N.J. 10 (1976).

48. *Cruzan v. Director, Missouri Department of Health,* 110 S. Ct. 2841, (1990).

49. *Child Abuse Act Amendments of 1984,* Public Law 98-457 (October 9, 1984).

50. Legislative roundup. *Concern for Dying Newsletter* (Summer 1991): 4.

51. Medical durable power of attorney. Newsletter, Society for the Right To Die, June 14, 1990.

52. Evans, Andrew L., and Baruch A. Brody. The do-not-resuscitate order in teaching hospitals. *Journal of the American Medical Association* 253 (April 19, 1985): 2236–2239.

53. Bedell, Susanna E., and Thomas L. Delbanco. Choices about cardiopulmonary resuscitation in the hospital: When do physicians talk with patients. *New England Journal of Medicine* 320 (April 26, 1984): 1089–1093.

54. Wachter, Robert M., John M. Luce, Norman Hearst, and Bernard Lo. Decisions about resuscitation: Inequities among patients with different diseases but similar prognoses. *Annals of Internal Medicine* 111 (September 15, 1989): 525–532.

55. Morse, Susan. Final requests: Preparing for death. *The Washington Post* (July 15, 1985): B5.

56. Danis, Marion, Leslie I. Southerland, Joanne M. Garrett, Janet L. Smith, Frank Hielema, C. Glenn Pickard, David M. Egner, and Donald L. Patrick. A prospective study of advance directives for life-sustaining care. *New England Journal of Medicine* 324 (March 28, 1991): 882–888.

57. Hudson, Terese. Hospitals work to provide advance directives information. *Hospitals* 65 (February 5, 1991): 26.

58. This section is adapted from Darr, Kurt. Dealing with AIDS. In *Ethics in health services management,* 2d ed., 233–243. Baltimore: Health Professions Press, 1991; used by permission.

59. Gladwell, Malcolm, and William Booth. CDC considers redefining AIDS. *The Washington Post* (June 8, 1991): A10.

60. Mortality attributable to HIV infection/AIDS—United States, 1981–1990. *Morbidity and Mortality Weekly Report* 40 (January 25, 1991): 42.

61. Freedman, Gail. Hospital growing AIDS care is bumping other services. *HealthWeek,* 3 (August 1989): 5.

62. Estimates of HIV prevalence and projected AIDS cases: Summary of a workshop, October 31–November 1, 1989. *Morbidity and Mortality Weekly Report* 39 (February 23, 1990): 110–112, 117–119.

63. Suplee, Curt. AIDS epidemic may have peaked, report says. *The Washington Post* (June 15, 1991) A3.

64. Boodman, Sandra G. Up against it: In Newark, a public hospital fights the twin plagues of AIDS and drugs. *Washington Post* Health Section (September 5, 1989); AIDS update: An executive report. *Hospitals* 64 (May 5, 1990): 26–34.

65. Hay, Joel W. Projecting the medical costs of HIV/AIDS: An update with focus on epidemiology. In *New perspectives on HIV-related illnesses: Progress in health services research*. Proceedings of a conference sponsored by the National Center for Health Services Research and Health Care Technology Assessment. DHHS Publication No. (PHS) 89-3449. Washington, D.C.: U.S. Government Printing Office. 1989.

66. Agency for Health Care Policy and Research, Public Health Service, U.S. Department of Health and Human Services. Cost of treating HIV may surpass $10 billion by 1994. *Research Activities* (Agency for Health Care Policy and Research) 146 (October 1991): 1.

67. Bayer, Ronald. Public health policy and the AIDS epidemic: An end to HIV exceptionalism? *New England Journal of Medicine* 324 (May 23, 1991): 1500–1504.

68. Angell, Marcia. A dual approach to the AIDS epidemic. *New England Journal of Medicine* 324 (May 23, 1991): 1498–1500.

69. Agency for Health Care Policy and Research, Public Health Service, U.S. Department of Health and Human Services. Physicians, nurses, and AIDS: Preliminary findings from a national study. *Research Activities* 142 (June 1991): 2.

70. AMA House of Delegates: No mandatory testing for HIV. *AHA News* 27 (July 1, 1991): 3.

71. American Medical Association. Ethical issues involved in the growing AIDS crisis. In Reports of the Council on Ethical and Judicial Affairs. Chicago, 1987. The report states that "A physician who knows that he or she has an infectious disease should not engage in any activity that creates a risk of transmission of the disease to others. . . . disclosure of that risk to patients is not enough; patients are entitled to expect that their physicians will not increase their exposure to the risk of contracting an infectious disease, even minimally."

72. American Hospital Association. *AIDS/HIV infection: Recommendations for health care practices and public policy, Report and recommendations of the Special Committee on AIDS/HIV Infection Policy, 1987–1988*. Chicago, 1988.

73. Sabatino, Frank. To test or not to test health professionals for HIV? It's debatable. *AHA News* 27 (April 15, 1991): 8.

74. Sabatino, To test or not to test, 8.

75. Okie, Susan. HIV-infected workers undercounted. *Washington Post* (January 16, 1990): A5.

76. Okie, HIV-infected workers undercounted, A5.

77. Sabatino, To test or not to test, 8.

78. Koska, Mary. AIDS precautions: Compliance difficult to enforce. *Hospitals* 63 (September 5, 1989): 58.

79. Green, Jeffrey, and Dona DeSanctis. CDC encourages HIV testing of hospital patients. *AHA News* 27 (September 23, 1991): 1.

80. AMA House of Delegates, 3.

81. Sabatino, To test or not to test, 8.

82. Centers for Disease Control. Recommendations for preventing transmission of human immunodeficiency virus and hepatitis B virus to patients during exposure-prone invasive procedures. *Morbidity and Mortality Weekly Report* 40 (July 12, 1991): 1–8.

83. CDC backs off listing 'exposure-prone' procedures. *AHA News* 27:48 (December 9, 1991), p. 3.

84. Williams, Kenneth J., and Paul R. Donnelly. *Medical Care Quality and the Public*. Chicago: Pluribus Press, 1982.

85. This section is adapted from Darr, Kurt. Organizational responses to ethical problems. In *Ethics in health service management*, 2d ed., 75–90. Baltimore: Health Professions Press, 1991; used by permission.

86. President's Commission for the Study of Ethical Problems in Medicine and Biomedical and Behavioral Research. *Deciding to forego life-sustaining treatment: Ethical, medical, and legal issues in treatment decisions*, 443–457. U.S. Government Printing Office, Washington, D.C.: 1983).

87. American Hospital Association, New survey (press release).

88. Right-to-die: An executive report. *Hospitals* 63 (November 20, 1989): 34.

89. Cohen, Cynthia B., ed. Ethics committees. *Hastings Center Report* 20 (March/April 1990): 29–34.

90. President's Commission, *Deciding to forego*, 450.

91. Mannisto, Marilyn M. Orchestrating an ethics committee: Who should be on it, where does it fit? *Trustee* 38 (April 1985): 18–19.

92. President's Commission, *Deciding to forego*, 451.

93. President's Commission, *Deciding to forego*, 448.

94. Freed, Benjamin. One philosopher's experience on an ethics committee. *Hastings Center Report* 11 (April 1981): 20–22.

95. Department of Health and Human Services, Office of Human Development Services. Services and treatment for disabled infants; Model guidelines for health care providers to establish infant care review committees. *Federal Register* 50 (April 15, 1985): 14893.

96. Department of Health and Human Services, Services and treatment for disabled infants, 14893.

97. Summary: Survey of Infant Care Review Committees. Paper delivered at the Annual Meeting of the American Academy of Pediatrics, Chicago, IL, September 18, 1984.

98. Fletcher, John C., Margo L. White, and Philip J. Foubert. Biomedical ethics and an ethics consultation service at the University of Virginia. *HEC Forum* 2 (1990): 89–99.

99. Adapted from Darr, Kurt. *Ethics in health services management*, 2d ed., 120–121. Baltimore: Health Professions Press, 1991; used by permission.

100. Adapted from Darr, Kurt. *Ethics in health services management*, 2d ed., 108. Baltimore: Health Professions Press, 1991; used by permission.

101. Adapted from Darr, Kurt. *Ethics in health services management*, 2d ed., 224–225. Baltimore: Health Professions Press, 1991; used by permission.

BIBLIOGRAPHY

American College of Health Care Administrators. *Code of ethics*. Alexandria, VA, 1989.

American College of Healthcare Executives. *Code of ethics*. Chicago, 1987.

American Medical Association. *Guidelines on clinical investigation*. In *Current opinions of the Council on Ethical and Judicial Affairs of the American Medical Association*. Chicago, 1989.

American Medical Association. *Principles of medical ethics.* Chicago, 1980.

American Nurses Association. *Code for nurses with interpretive statements.* Kansas City, MO, 1985.

Angell, Marcia. A dual approach to the AIDS epidemic. *The New England Journal of Medicine* 324 (May 23, 1991): 1498–1500.

Arras, John, and Nancy Rhoden. *Ethical issues in modern medicine,* 3d ed. Mountain View, CA: Mayfield Publishing Company, 1989.

Bayer, Ronald. Public health policy and the AIDS epidemic: An end to HIV exceptionalism? *New England Journal of Medicine* 324 (May 23, 1991): 1500–1504.

Beauchamp, Tom L., and James F. Childress. *Principles of biomedical ethics,* 3d ed. New York: Oxford University Press, 1989.

Bodenheimer, Edgar. *Jurisprudence: The philosophy and method of the law.* Cambridge: Harvard University Press, 1974.

Centers for Disease Control. Recommendations for preventing transmission of human immunodeficiency virus and hepatitis B virus to patients during exposure-prone invasive procedures. *Morbidity and Mortality Weekly Report* 40 (July 12, 1991): 1–8.

Childress, James F. Who shall live when not all can live? *Soundings, An Interdisciplinary Journal* 53 (Winter 1970): 339–355.

Cohen, Cynthia B., ed. Ethics committees. *Hastings Center Report* 18 (August/September 1988): 23–28.

Cohen, Cynthia B., ed. Ethics committees. *Hastings Center Report* 19 (January/February 1989): 19–24.

Cohen, Cynthia B., ed. Ethics committees. *Hastings Center Report* 19 (September/October 1989): 21–26.

Cohen, Cynthia B., ed. Ethics committees. *Hastings Center Report* 20 (March/April 1990): 29–34.

Cranford, Ronald E., and A. Edward Doudera, eds. *Institutional ethics committees and health care decision making.* Ann Arbor: Health Administration Press, 1984.

Danis, Marion, Leslie I. Southerland, Joanne M. Garrett, Janet L. Smith, Frank Hielema, C. Glenn Pickard, David M. Egner, and Donald L. Patrick. A prospective study of advance directives for life-sustaining care. *New England Journal of Medicine* 324 (March 28, 1991): 882–888.

Darr, Kurt. Administrative ethics and the health services manager. *Hospital & Health Services Administration* 29 (March/April 1984): 120–136.

Darr, Kurt. *Ethics for health services managers.* Case Studies in Health Administration, vol. 4. Chicago: Foundation of the American College of Hospital Administrators, 1985.

Darr, Kurt. *Ethics in health services management,* 2d ed. Baltimore: Health Professions Press, 1991.

Darr, Kurt, Beaufort B. Longest, Jr., and Jonathon S. Rakich. The ethical imperative in health services governance and management. *Hospital & Health Services Administration* 31 (March/April 1986): 53–66.

DeGeorge, Richard T. *Business ethics,* 3d ed. New York: Macmillan Publishing Company, 1990.

Department of Veterans Affairs, *Code of patient concern.* Washington, D.C.

Engelhardt, H. Tristam, Jr. *The foundations of bioethics.* New York: Oxford University Press, 1986.

Estimates of HIV prevalence and projected AIDS cases: Summary of a workshop, October 31–November 1, 1989. *Morbidity and Mortality Weekly Report* 29 (February 23, 1990).

Fletcher, John C., Norman Quist, and Albert R. Johnson. *Ethics consultation in health care.* Ann Arbor: Health Administration Press, 1989.

Fletcher, John C., Margo L. White, and Philip J. Foubert. Biomedical ethics and an ethics consultation service at the University of Virginia. *HEC Forum* 2 (1990): 89–99.

Frankena, William K. *Ethics,* 2d ed. Englewood Cliffs, NJ: Prentice Hall, 1973.

Harvard Medical School. A definition of irreversible coma. *Journal of the American Medical Association* 205 (1968): 337–338.

Hay, Joel W. Projecting the medical costs of HIV/AIDS. *Research Activities,* (Agency for Health Care Policy and Research) 126 (February 1990).

Henderson, Verne E. The ethical side of enterprise. *Sloan Management Review* 23 (Spring 1982): 37–47.

Joint Commission on Accreditation of Healthcare Organizations. Rights and responsibilities of patients. In *Accreditation Manual for Hospitals, 1992,* xi–xv. Chicago, 1991.

Kant, Immanuel. *Fundamental principles of the metaphysics of morals.* Translated by Thomas K. Abbott. In *Knowledge and value,* edited by Elmer Sprague and Paul W. Taylor, 535–558. New York, Harcourt, Brace and Co., 1959.

Katz, Jay. Informed consent—a fairy tale. *University of Pittsburgh Law Review* 39 (Winter 1977): 137–174.

Lynn, Joanne, and James F. Childress. Must patients always be given food and water? *Hastings Center Report* 13 (October 1983): 17–21.

Mortality attributable to HIV infection/AIDS—U.S., 1981–1990. *Morbidity and Mortality Weekly Report* 40 (January 25, 1991).

Office of Human Development Services, U.S. Department of Health and Human Services, *Child abuse and neglect prevention and treatment program* (final rule); and *Model guidelines for health care providers to establish infant care review committees* (notice). 45 C.F.R. Part 1340 (April 15, 1985).

Pellegrino, Edmund D., and David C. Thomasma. *For the patient's good: The restoration of beneficence in health care.* New York: Oxford University Press, 1988.

President's Commission for the Study of Ethical Problems in Medicine and Biomedical and Behavioral Research. *Summing up; Compensating for research injuries* (2 vols); *Deciding to forego life-sustaining treatment; Defining death; Implementing human research regulations; Making health care decisions* (2 vols); *Protecting human subjects; Screening and counseling for genetic conditions; Securing access to health care* (3 vols): *Splicing life; Whistleblowing in biomedical research* (various reports). Washington, D.C.: U.S. Government Printing Office, 1980–1983.

Ramsey, Paul. *The patient as person.* New Haven, CT: Yale University Press, 1970.

Rawls, John. *A theory of justice.* Cambridge, MA: The Belknap Press, 1971.

Rescher, Nicholas. The allocation of exotic medical lifesaving therapy. *Ethics* 79 (April 1969): 173–186.

Ross, Judith Wilson, and Deborah Pugh. Limited cardiopulmonary resuscitation: The ethics of partial codes. *Quality Review Bulletin* 14 (January 1988): 4–8.

Wachter, Robert M., John M. Luce, Norman Hearst, and Bernard Lo. Decisions about resuscitation: Inequities among patients with different diseases but similar prognoses. *Annals of Internal Medicine* 111 (September 15, 1989): 525–532.

Wiggers, Carl J. Human experimentation as exemplified by the career of Dr. William Beaumont. *Alumni Bulletin* (Case

Western Reserve University School of Medicine) (1950): 60–64.

Williams, Kenneth J., and Paul R. Donnelly. *Medical care quality and the public*. Chicago: Pluribus Press, 1982.

World Medical Assembly. *Declaration of Helsinki*. Recommendations guiding medical doctors in biomedical research involving human subjects, adopted by the 18th World Medical Assembly, Helsinki, Finland, 1964, and revised by the 29th World Medical Assembly, Tokyo, Japan, 1975.

4 / Legal Considerations

For law is order, and good law is good order.
Aristotle (384–322 BC), Politics[1]

Chapter 3, "Ethical Considerations," identified sources of ethics and law and discussed ethics in the context of health services management. Formal and nonformal sources of law were distinguished and ethics and law were contrasted. It was suggested that professional codes tend to be internalized, but whether or not they are internalized, codes must be consistent with the law. Codes of ethics are a formal source of law that usually establish a higher standard for professions than does the law.

Chief sources of formal law are constitutions, statutes, executive orders, administrative regulations, ordinances, charters, bylaws of autonomous or semiautonomous bodies, treaties and certain other agreements, and judicial precedents. All types, even treaties, may affect health services organizations (HSOs). Health services managers must have a basic understanding of formal law and its effect on the HSO.

PUBLIC PROCESSES THAT PRODUCE THE LAW

The Constitution is the basic law of the United States; most nations have similar documents that establish their governments. The federal system was established after the American Revolution when sovereign states relinquished specific authority. These enumerated powers are interpreted by the United States Supreme Court. Powers not delegated to the federal government are reserved to the states. This is important because of the police power of the state noted in Chapter 2, "The Health Care Delivery System." Each state's constitution establishes its form of government and identifies the rights of citizens.

The Legislative Process: Proposing and Enacting Laws

Statutes are enacted by state legislatures and the United States Congress. Comparable legislative activities are performed by local government when ordinances are passed. After enactment, these laws and ordinances are binding but may be challenged in court if they violate constitutionally protected rights or were improperly enacted because of procedural irregularity. The legislative branch relies on the executive branch to implement and enforce the laws.

Paradigmatic of these processes is that which occurs in the United States Senate and House of Representatives. Rather than describe the legislative process, this section describes how HSOs are properly involved in making laws that affect them.

Influence of HSOs It is noteworthy that after massive federal financing of health services began in 1965, the field of health care became highly politicized. The focus of this change has been in the nation's capital. Legislation proposed and enacted by Congress that has a direct effect on the health services field became increasingly subject to the influences of lobbyists, political action committees (PACs), and various other special interest groups, all of which seek to ensure that the laws proposed reflect their primary concerns. Thus, doing nothing will result in laws that are at variance with what is necessary and desirable from the standpoint of HSOs.

The management model shown in Figure 1.6 suggests that HSOs should and do affect their external environment (see the change loop [6]). One way this occurs is by presenting their views of current law and proposed legislation through a trade association or PAC. Another is by bringing a lawsuit (see The Judicial Process).

Trade Associations The offices of hundreds of trade associations are located in Washington, D.C., and its metropolitan area. Major health services associations have Washington offices so they can participate in developing federal laws and regulations that affect them. Prominent health services associations in Washington are the American Hospital Association (AHA), the American Medical Association (AMA), and the Federation of American Health Systems (FAHS). At their best, associations, through their lobbyists, provide legislators and staffs with information important in drafting legislation. Similarly, they provide information when regulations are drafted. Information from association experts may enhance the outcome of legislation, but it is certain that associations seek to further their special interests. It is arguable, however, that the quasi-public role of many health services associations means their interests have much in common with those of the public.

Associations make their positions known at several points. They might draft bills or specific language, either of which must be introduced by a representative or senator to enter the legislative process. Bills may be amended at various points in the process, including in committee or subcommittee, on the floor, or in conference between the two houses of Congress. During the legislative process, or to learn more about problems before drafting bills, committees or subcommittees may hold hearings at which persons from the health field give testimony. Hearings are held consistent with the committee chair's interests, however, and there is usually a political dimension.

The myriad of bills and subjects makes personal, in-depth knowledge by a member of the House or Senate almost impossible to achieve, and this makes staff very important. In addition to that occurring at hearings, a great deal of formal and informal interaction occurs between lobbyists and both committee staff and a congressional member's personal staff. This interaction occurs outside public scrutiny, but this should not suggest that something illegal or immoral is occurring. Staffers are aware that lobbyists present information in the way that is most advantageous for the special interest or association they represent. At the same time, the information may be crucial to understanding the bill or its ramifications, if enacted. A cardinal rule among lobbyists is that truthfulness is essential. If caught in a lie or purposely misleading the member or staff, the lobbyist's greatest asset—credibility—is gone, probably irretrievably. This description of lobbying and lobbyists does not state the obvious: There are dishonest legislators and special interest groups who seek to do more than express a viewpoint and make a convincing argument. These are the rare exception as measured by great numbers of such contacts, despite the bad publicity that sometimes occurs.

PACs In the past decade, most major HSO trade associations have organized PACs whose purpose is to make campaign contributions to incumbents or challengers. PACs permit aggregation and targeting of contributions and protect contributors that are often charitable organizations (as defined in the Internal Revenue Code) from losing their tax-exempt status. One of the first PACs was established by the AMA; the AHA soon followed.* Defenders of PACs argue that federal election laws prohibit gifts of a size that will significantly influence decisions of elected officials; the real purpose and value of contributions is to ensure access to lawmakers—a subtle but important distinction. This view is reflected by the fact that many PACs contribute to both opponents in a race.

The Regulatory Process: Administrative Law and Rule Making

Once enacted, laws must be implemented. This is done by the executive branch, which has numerous departments and agencies, in addition to independent regulatory bodies such as the

---

*Federal Election Commission data for 1989 and 1990 show contributions from PACs for the AMA to be $2,380,000 to 478 members of Congress; for the AHA, $503,000 to 304 members; and for the FAHS, $174,000 to 129 members.

Federal Trade Commission. All of these were established by Congress and all implement relevant laws and enforce their provisions. Because of their rule-making and regulatory activities, many departments and agencies in fact have legislative authority. This has only recently been the case, because as late as the 1930s the Supreme Court held that delegation of legislative authority by Congress was unconstitutional.[2]

Implementation of Law Through Regulations   To be implemented, laws must be made specific, and this is done through regulations that are issued by the executive department or agency with jurisdiction. The implementation process is governed by the Administrative Procedures Act of 1946, as amended. Requirements include notice of proposed rule making, proposed regulations, and final regulations. The steps preceding final regulations permit interested parties to comment on provisions and suggest their own versions. The department or agency may issue interim regulations that both test the effect of the proposed regulations and regulate until final regulations are prepared and put through the process.

During the period of public comment, affected HSOs are able to comment on and influence the content of final regulations. It is most cost effective to influence the process at this point. Primary targets are the bureaucrats who write the regulations. Sometimes, efforts are directed at the president, the Congress, or both to cause them to intervene in the issuance of regulations. HSOs and their professional associations have been successful on some occasions and unsuccessful on others. One example of failure occurred when, despite the efforts of hospitals and their trade associations, the National Labor Relations Board used its rule-making power to define administratively the bargaining units allowed in acute care hospitals (see Chapter 18, "Labor Relations").

Actions at the various steps in the implementation process appear in the *Federal Register,* which is published every working day. Final regulations are published there and compiled in the *Code of Federal Regulations.*

Multiple Functions of the Regulatory Process   The regulatory process is correctly seen as incorporating the functions and activities of the executive, legislative, and judicial branches. It is legislative in that regulations are issued pursuant to laws that have been enacted. The regulations must reflect the law and congressional intent, and have general (prospective) application, but in most cases there is significant latitude for interpretation in the rule-making process. Regulators have executive authority through their enforcement powers. They can require compliance by bringing complaints, by issuing directives such as cease and desist orders, and by levying fines. This may be done pending a decision in the agency's hearing and review process, or in an emergency can be done prior to a hearing. Finally, there is a judicial or quasi-judicial dimension in the regulatory process when a specific dispute regarding compliance has arisen. Hearings and reviews are held before hearing officers or administrative law judges who are part of that agency. They have a degree of independence because they are appointed for a specific term by the president and can only be removed for cause.

For the HSO, challenging a regulatory decision by engaging in the administrative hearing and review process is time consuming and expensive. Outside legal counsel expert in administrative law is needed to work with retainer or in-house corporate counsel. As a practical matter, individual HSOs have little choice but to comply with a regulation or, if the administrative ruling is adverse, to simply accept it without appeal to the courts. The costs and energy needed for a legal challenge are such that they can only be undertaken by a major HSO or an association. Recently enacted federal legislation that permits recovery of costs by successful challengers may change this.

An important development of the past several decades is the increasing complexity and significance of administrative law and the rule-making processes. Some political scientists argue that the bureaucracies have become a fourth branch of federal government. For example, although not typical, the discussion of the Baby Doe regulations in Chapter 3 shows that the federal courts can be brought into the rule-making process if required procedures are ignored. Generally, the parties must use the appeal and review process of the administrative agency or department. When this process has been exhausted, appeals are made to the federal courts.

The Judicial Process: Court Systems

HSOs are commonly involved in state and federal courts, both as plaintiffs (those bringing civil legal action) and defendants (those against whom civil legal action has been brought). In addition, associations often submit legal briefs as a friend of the court (*amicus curiae*) in both court systems. Such briefs bring to the court's attention legal precedents and other pertinent information from that group's special perspective in an effort to apprise the court of the likely effect of its decision on such interests.

Courts and Jurists   A full discussion of the various courts and their jurisdiction and authority is beyond the scope of this book. For our purposes, it is sufficient to state that there are two basic court systems—state and federal—that are generally similar. State and federal systems have trial courts (county and district courts, respectively), intermediate courts (appeals courts), and supreme courts. (Some states reverse the terms "supreme" and "appeals" and the appeals court is the highest court.) "Judge" is the title of jurists in courts other than the highest state and federal courts; "justice" is the title of members of state supreme courts and the Supreme Court of the United States. The nomination of state judges and justices by the governor is ratified by the legislature, typically the senate. Some states elect rather than appoint both judges and justices, although it is more common for judges than justices to be elected. If elected, terms of 10 or 15 years are common. Federal court judges and justices are nominated by the president with confirmation by the Senate; they serve for life.

Appointment insulates the judiciary from politics, and this results in more predictable and consistent court-made law. Of course, judges and justices appointed by a governor or president are likely to have compatible political philosophies. The need for legislative confirmation and the almost universal review of nominees by a committee of the bar, however, almost always results in appointment of competent and ethical individuals.

Stare Decisis and Res Judicata   The courts are a source of formal law through the mechanism of two central doctrines. *Stare decisis* is a Latin phrase meaning that courts will stand by precedent and will not disturb a settled point.[3] The doctrine rests on the principle that the law by which people are governed, to the extent possible, should be fixed, definite, and known. Courts and potential litigants can look to previously decided cases with similar facts to guide them. Predictability and consistency are important attributes of the law, and whimsical changes and uncertainty must be avoided not only with judge-made law but with legislative enactments. Nonetheless, precedents are occasionally overturned.

The second doctrine, *res judicata* (also a Latin phrase), means a matter has been judged, or a thing has been judicially acted upon or decided.[4] Therefore, it will not be heard again unless there has been a substantial problem in the original judgment because of factual error, misrepresentation, or fraud, or if there is significant new information not available earlier. This legal doctrine is important because, once appeals have been exhausted, the case is settled and usually will not be reopened. The doctrine of *res judicata* also adds stability and predictability to the law.

Executive Orders

Another source of formal law is the executive order. Some authority derives directly from the Constitution—the president's role as commander-in-chief of the armed forces, for example. In other cases authority is delegated by the Congress permitting the president to act in specific circumstances such as emergencies. A common domestic example occurs when the president declares a geographic location to be a disaster area, which qualifies it for federal assistance. This is one of the few examples in which executive orders might affect HSOs.

CONTRACTS

A contract is an agreement between two or more parties that identifies certain rights and obligations—they agree to do or not do certain things. There is reason for considering understandings between private persons or between private persons and government as another source of formal law. Bodenheimer notes:

> There would seem to be no reason, for example, why a collective bargaining agreement, constituting an accord which governs the hiring, discharge, wage rates, working hours, and disciplining of employee groups, should not be deemed a source of law just as much as a labor code enacted by a legislature which deals with exactly the same subjects. It must be kept in mind that a valid collective bargaining agreement may serve in court suits as well as arbitration proceedings as the sole legal foundation for the recognition and adjudication of substantial rights and the obligations on the part of employers and employees.[5]

The decision maker in disputes in which a contract is involved must first look to the generally applicable law and then interpret the private agreement in light of it. Thus, the contract's provisions become important.

Elements of a Contract

A valid contract has a number of elements. It is: 1) an agreement (which is reached after an offer and an acceptance), 2) for which there is a consideration (something of value), that is 3) reached by parties who have the legal capacity to contract, and 4) the objective of which is lawful. This is a straightforward statement, but applying such terms and concepts has built a vast body of statutory and case law.

HSOs make contracts with a wide variety of businesses and persons to provide goods and services. Examples include contracts buying supplies, equipment, and services; selling maintenance or laundry services; employing various personnel; and stipulating collective bargaining agreements. Many transactions are not and need not be in writing (e.g., a dietitian calls a greengrocer to bring vegetables with payment on delivery). However, states treat oral contracts differently than written contracts, and oral contracts may not be legally binding if they exceed a certain dollar amount or if their duration exceeds a certain length of time. Managerial control of contracts is maintained by using purchase orders that, when sent to the seller, constitute an offer to buy or, if sent in response to a previous offer to sell, constitute the acceptance. Increasingly, HSOs sell services. Hospitals sell laboratory services to physicians, or contract with health maintenance organizations (HMOs) to provide hospital care. Visiting nurse agencies sell therapists' services to nursing facilities. Such services are usually offered at predetermined prices, although cost-plus contracts may be used.

Breaches of Contract

Breaches of contract are rare when compared to the total number of contracts HSOs execute each year. Several defenses are available when a breach of contract occurs. They range from the fact that the contract is impossible to complete to mistakes by the parties about a material fact. Examples of impossibility are destruction or unavailability of the subject matter, death or illness, and legal prohibition. When these are not present, however, and the contract is simply breached, three types of remedies are available: rescission for a material breach, specific performance, and damages. Rescission means that the contract is null and void and the parties are put back into their original positions in relation to each other, insofar as possible. Specific performance requires the party who is in breach to do what was agreed in the contract. If neither rescission nor specific performance is the appropriate remedy, the aggrieved party may seek money damages.

Breaches of contract almost always involve lawyers and legal fees, and often a trial, even if one party is clearly right and the other is clearly wrong. Consequently, breaches should be avoided. One of the best ways to do this is to have competent legal counsel involved in drafting and negotiating all contracts. Binding arbitration is increasingly used to resolve disputes, and contracts should include a provision requiring it should the need arise. Arbitration is a low-cost, alternative means of dispute resolution and has become a standard provision in commercial contracts.

TORTS INVOLVING INDIVIDUAL PROVIDERS

Distinguishing Tort from Contract Liability

A principle of Anglo-American legal tradition is that persons are responsible for the harm they cause, whether they have acted intentionally or unintentionally (negligently). Such responsibility falls in the domains of both contract and tort obligations. The word "tort" is derived from the Latin *tortus,* or "twisted." Even when its common use in the English language faded, it remained in the law and acquired a technical meaning.[6]

A tort is a civil wrong other than a breach of contract, for which courts provide a remedy in the form of an action for damages.[7] For the action to be successful, certain elements must be present: there must be a duty, a breach of that duty, and resulting harm that is causally linked to the defendant. Intent is important because the defendant may be liable for punitive damages in addition to actual damages, depending on the intent and actual circumstances.

Contract liability is distinguished from tort liability primarily by the nature of what is protected:

> The distinction between tort and contract liability, as between parties to a contract, has become an increasingly difficult distinction to make. It would not be possible to reconcile the results of all cases. The availability of both kinds of liability for precisely the same kind of harm has brought about confusion and unnecessary complexity. . . . Tort obligations are in general obligations that are imposed by law—apart from and independent of promises made and therefore apart from the manifested intention of the parties—to avoid injury to others. By injury here is meant simply the interference with the individual's interest or an interest of some other legal entity that is deemed worthy of legal protection. . . . Contract obligations are created to enforce promises which are manifestations not only of a present intention to do or not to do something, but also a commitment to the future. They are, therefore, obligations based on the manifested intention of the parties to a bargaining transaction.[8]

The distinctions between a breach of contract and a tort seem straightforward, but, as the quote suggests, actual application can be confusing. This is especially true in the breach of an implied warranty, which is a hybrid of contract and tort. In general, there is an implied warranty that goods are fit (merchantable) for the usual and customarily intended purposes for which they are used. This concept has evolved into strict liability by which the seller warrants the quality and safe condition of the goods. Cases in the early 1970s began to apply this concept to some hospital activities such as blood transfusions as a result of which the patient became infected with serum hepatitis. In consequence, nearly all states "enacted statutes intended to reverse the result of these cases. Some of the statutes provide only that the furnishing of blood by a hospital or a blood bank is a service and not the sale of a product."[9] Distinguishing between a product and a service is important, because strict liability does not apply to a service. The concept of implied warranty has been extensively applied to various products and to medical devices, however.

Intentional Torts

Some torts arise from intentional rather than negligent conduct. The intent is not necessarily hostile nor based on a desire to do harm; rather, there is an intent to "bring about a result which will invade the interests of another in a way that the law will not sanction."[10] Types of intentional torts most likely to affect HSOs include battery, defamation, false imprisonment, invasion of privacy, wrongful discharge of an employee, and wrongful disclosure of confidential information. Assault is often linked to battery, but is distinguished in that assault must raise a reasonable apprehension of a harmful or offensive contact. A further distinction is that an assault can occur with no physical touching. It was noted in Chapter 3 that ethical consent must be informed, voluntary, and competent. Legal requirements for consent to treatment are similar and must be met to avoid a successful suit for battery.

Upon admission of any patient, an HSO should obtain general consent for routine treatment. A sample general consent form is shown in Figure 4.1. The HSO should also participate in obtaining specific (special) consent for nonroutine diagnostic procedures, as well as all surgical procedures. A sample special consent form is shown in Figure 4.2. Sometimes, getting specific consent is the physician's responsibility, and the HSO's role is only to determine that the medical record contains a signed statement. In such cases, the patient signs an authorization that allows HSO staff to participate in treatment rendered by the physician. Nonparticipation in the consent process by HSOs is a less prudent course of action and is inconsistent with the desirable ethical relationship between patient and HSO, as well as the increasingly broad legal liability of HSOs.

A major element of informed consent is how much to tell the patient, and a judgment must be made as to the extent of the patient's knowledge. One of three legal standards applies to the decision of how much information to give the patient: 1) the information that would be given by the reasonable physician, 2) the information that would be given to the reasonable patient, and 3) as a distinctly minority view, the information that this specific patient would want to have. A legal concept known as therapeutic privilege allows a physician to withhold information if, in the physician's judgment, the patient might be harmed by having it.

As suggested when the ethical aspects of consent were discussed in Chapter 3, it is often difficult for patients to give truly informed consent because of a myriad of factors that include education, intellect, emotional status, and general physical and psychological condition. Informed consent might be impossible despite diligent attempts by the HSO. Regardless, the effort must be made, and the HSO should provide an effective process in which it can occur. Some suggest that to give truly informed consent, the patient would have to be as well qualified as the physician who obtains it. Typically, however, patients put themselves in the physician's hands and accept recommendations for treatment.

Negligent Practice

Negligence can be defined as omitting to do something that a reasonable person (e.g., physician, nurse, manager) who was guided by reasonable considerations ordinarily regulating human affairs would do, or doing something a reasonable and prudent person would not do.[11] This seems straightforward enough, but volumes have been written to define and apply the concept of "reasonable person." What the reasonable person would do is called *the standard of care*. It is used to measure the performance of the act (actions) in question—the alleged negligence. If the plaintiff, the party with the burden of proof, convinces the finder of fact (either a jury or a judge hearing the case without a jury) by a preponderance of evidence that the act (actions) deviated from the standard of care, the finder of fact will find for the plaintiff—the person who has brought the suit. "Preponderance of evidence" refers to evidence that produces the stronger effect or impression, has a greater weight, and is more convincing as to its truth. Consequently, its effect is greater. If the party having the burden of proof does not meet that burden by a preponderance of the evidence, the finder of fact must find for the defendant.

The person who engages in tortious conduct is always liable to pay damages. Increasingly, however, the HSO is also named a defendant because of various legal theories to be discussed later. There are four elements needed for actionable negligence:

1. There must be a duty on the part of the caregiver (physician or other person) to provide care of a certain quality (standard of care).

The George Washington University/Medical Center

Authorization for Medical Care and Treatment
Authorization for Release of Medical Records to Third-Party Payers
Release of Responsibility for Personal Property/Valuables

1. I have come to George Washington University's Hospital for medical treatment. I ask the health care professionals at the Hospital to provide care and treatment for me that they feel is necessary. I consent to undergo routine tests and treatment as part of this care. I understand that I am free to ask a member of my health care team questions about any care, treatment or medicine I am to receive.

2. Because George Washington University's Hospital is a teaching hospital, I understand that my health care team will be made up of hospital personnel and medical students in addition to my attending physician and his/her assistants and designees. Hospital personnel include, but are not limited to, nurses, technicians, interns, residents, and fellows.

3. I understand that as part of my care and treatment, samples of my blood, urine, stool and tissues may be removed from me from time to time. I permit the University to use any leftover blood, urine, stool and tissues for research. (If I do not want the University to so use leftover portions, I may stop the University from doing so by writing "no" in the following block and writing my initials after it [   ].) If additional samples are needed for the research, I will be asked at that time.

4. I am aware that the practice of medicine is not an exact science and admit that no one has given me any promises or guarantees about the result of any care or treatment I am to receive or examinations I am to undergo.

5. I agree to the University's and/or my physician sending copies of my medical records (or information from my medical records) to my insurance provider(s) or other sources of payment, which may include my employer. I understand that this information will be sent when it is needed for payment of my medical bills. I release and forever discharge The George Washington University, its employees and agents and my attending physician from any liability resulting from the release of my medical records or information from them for payment purposes.

6. **Release of Responsibility for Personal Property/Valuables:** I understand that George Washington University is not responsible for any personal property or valuables that I keep with me while I am at the hospital, even if placed in a hospital provided locker. Personal property includes, but is not limited to, clothing, shoes and baggage. Valuables include, but are not limited to, money, credit cards, dentures, eyeglasses, hearing aids and jewelry. I understand, therefore, that I should send my valuables and as much of my property as possible home with my family/friends. I realize that I can request the University's Cashier's Office to store valuables I cannot send home.

7. I am currently a Tissue/Organ donor: ☐ YES   ☐ NO

EMERGENCY UNIT PATIENTS ONLY

8. I understand that it may be helpful for my personal physician to be involved in the care I receive while I am in The George Washington University Emergency Unit. I therefore allow an Emergency Unit physician to contact my personal physician, Dr. _____. (If I do not wish my physician to be contacted, I may stop the University from doing so by writing "no" in the following block and writing my initials after it [   ].)

9. I agree to the University's sending copies of my Emergency Unit record to my personal physician named above. (If I do not wish the University to send a copy to my physician, I may stop the University from doing so by writing "no" in the following block and writing my initials after it [   ].)

AFFIRMATION

I have read this form and understand it. All of my questions about what it says have been answered. I am signing it of my own free will. I understand that by signing it, I am agreeing to it.

_____   _____
Signature of patient (or parent, legal guardian or   Date/Time
next-of-kin. Please indicate which.)

_____   _____
Witness to affirmation and signature   Date/Time

Figure 4.1.   Sample general consent form. (Reprinted by permission of The George Washington University Medical Center.)

THE GEORGE WASHINGTON UNIVERSITY MEDICAL CENTER

PATIENT'S REQUEST FOR PROCEDURE OPERATION AND TREATMENT

(PATIENT IDENTIFICATION)

PATIENT

1. I, _____ ,(or

_____ as ☐ Parent ☐ Guardian ☐ Representative (Check One)

acting on his/her behalf), request the procedure/operation/treatment set out below.

2. I have requested that Dr(s). _____ perform

and supervise my procedure/operation/treatment which has been explained to me to be:

_____

My doctor's explanation informed me about my medical condition as well as the common foreseeable benefits and risks of the procedure/operation/treatment as well as of its reasonable alternatives, if any.

3. I know, too, that during my procedure/operation/treatment it may become apparent to my doctor that in his/her professional judgment further procedures, operations or treatments may be necessary. I therefore authorize modification or extension of this permit to include that which my doctor's professional judgment indicates to be necessary under the circumstances.

4. I understand that if a member of the Department of Anesthesiology is to participate in my care for general, regional or monitored anesthesia care, a separate consent will be obtained for these services.

5. If my doctor has indicated to me that I will require a local anesthetic as part of my procedure/operation/treatment, I authorize its administration. I acknowledge that my doctor has explained the benefits and risks of my receiving a local anesthetic as well as of the reasonable alternatives, if any. Further, I understand that during my procedure/operation/treatment, unforeseen circumstances may require alternative methods of anesthesia, such as general, and I therefore authorize modification of anesthesia administration which my doctor's professional judgment indicates to be necessary under the circumstances.

6. Should the need arise during my operation or immediate post-operative period, I also consent to the administration of blood and/or blood products. Further, I understand that despite careful testing and screening of blood and blood products by collecting agencies, I may still be subject to ill effects as a result of receiving blood transfusion and/or blood products. The following are some, but not all, of the potential risks that I am told can occur: fever and allergic reactions, hemolytic reactions, transmission of diseases such as hepatitis, AIDS, and cytomegalovirus (CMV), and fluid overload.

7. Knowing that The George Washington University Medical Center is a teaching institution, I understand that along with my doctor and his/her assistants and designees, other Medical Center personnel such as residents, trainees, nurses and technicians will be involved in my procedure/operation/treatment and care under his/her supervision.

8. I consent to appropriate routine tests and treatments as part of my medical care associated with this procedure/operation/treatment.

9. I agree to the appropriate disposal of any tissue or part removed from my body during the procedure/operation/treatment.

10. I understand the University's teaching mission and agree to the presence of appropriate observers during my procedure/operation/treatment for the advancement of medical education and care.

11. I also agree that photographs of my procedure/operation/treatment may be taken and utilized for research, teaching, or other scientific purposes as long as my identity is not disclosed.

PATIENT AFFIRMATION

By signing this request form, I am indicating that I understand the contents of this document, agree to its provisions, and request the procedure/operation/treatment as set forth in #2 be performed. I know that if I have concerns or would like more detailed information, I can ask more questions and get more information from my attending physician. I am also acknowledging that I know that the practice of anesthesiology, medicine and surgery is not an exact science and that no one has given me any promises or guarantees about the designated procedure/operation/treatment or its results.

I fully understand what I am now signing of my own free will.

WITNESS TO AFFIRMATION AND SIGNATURE	DATE	TIME	PATIENT SIGNATURE (or Parent, Guardian or Representative)		DATE

PHYSICIAN ATTESTATION

I, Dr. _____ , attest that this patient or the representative named above has been informed about the common foreseeable risks and benefits of undergoing the procedure/operation/treatment as well as its reasonable alternative(s), if any. Further, questions with regard to this procedure have been answered to his/her apparent satisfaction.

PHYSICIAN SIGNATURE	DATE

7540-76-519

2. There must have been a breach of that duty; that is, the care provided must not have met the established standard of the reasonable provider of that type of care.
3. The breach of duty must have been a substantial factor in the cause of the harm (proximate cause).
4. The patient must have been injured.

Absent any of these elements, the plaintiff patient cannot recover on a theory of negligence.

With few exceptions, state law in the United States places no positive legal duty on one person to aid another. This is also true for physicians and other caregivers, unless a contract establishes a duty. Once care is undertaken, however, the patient may not be abandoned, and care may be discontinued only if alternate provisions have been made and the patient is protected from harm. The tort of abandonment is a cause of action by a plaintiff.

Standard of Care   If providers have a duty to deliver services of a certain quality, how is that standard determined? Two basic standards are used to judge medical care. Historically, the most common was that of the locality where the provider practiced. Changes have occurred that include considering the practice in communities similar in size and medical resources. There have been other modifications to this standard of care, all in the direction of expanding the scope to that of the practice in adjacent areas and medical centers. Generally, providers are held to the standard of care that is appropriate under similar circumstances for practitioners of that type and that would be delivered with the same reasonable and ordinary care, skill, and diligence as those in good standing would ordinarily exercise in like cases. This is the "average standard of the profession test,"[12] and it is a national standard. Because there are different types of providers and various schools of medical theory about disease causation and cure (e.g., chiropractors and homeopaths, in addition to traditional [allopathic] medicine), the specific type of practitioner would be held to the standard for that particular type.

The breach of the standard of care must be proven by testimony from persons who are able to state what is normally expected of that type of practitioner delivering care with ordinary and reasonable care, skill, and diligence. This is done through expert witnesses. Historically, courts found a "conspiracy of silence" because physicians refused to testify as to the standard of care. Those who did were often discriminated against, disciplined, or ostracized by colleagues. This problem has lessened, but has not disappeared. Plaintiffs can use physicians who are regularly expert witnesses and who do not practice medicine, but they are easy targets for defense counsel seeking to discredit their testimony.

There are other ways to establish a breach of the standard of care: the treating physician's own statements; calling that physician as a hostile or adverse witness; using standard medical textbooks or similar sources; or invoking a doctrine known as *res ipsa loquitur* (the thing speaks for itself), which is a legal theory limited to specific circumstances. Sometimes, the negligence is a matter of common knowledge and expert testimony is not needed.

Proof of Negligence and Recovery of Damages   The final elements needed to prove negligence are causation and injury. There are several aspects of causation:

> In addition to proving that a physician was negligent, that is, failed to meet the standard of care, and that the patient was injured, a malpractice plaintiff must also prove that the injury resulted from the negligence. Although this element of proof is called "causation," the term has a different sense from that used in medical circles. The law considers an injury to be caused by a negligent act if the injury would not have occurred but for the defendant's act, or if the injury was a foreseeable result of the negligent conduct. The legal cause of an injury is often termed the proximate cause. Note that the plaintiff need not prove that the negligent act caused the result, but only the strong likelihood that it did. Also, the negligence need not be the sole cause, but only a significant factor in the injury. It must be remembered that the purpose of a malpractice trial is not to convict the defendants of malpractice, but to decide whether the loss caused by the injury should be allocated to the defendants. The standards of proof are thus lower than for a criminal trial, for example.[13]

To assist in solving problems of liability when two causes act together to bring about an event and either one of them alone would have brought the same result, some courts have adopted the concept of substantial factor. Was the defendant's conduct a substantial factor in bringing about the injury? An example of this concept is when two physicians are treating a patient essentially simultaneously in an emergency situation and both are negligent so that either could have brought about the plaintiff's injury. This concept was applied by the California Supreme Court in *Landeros v. Flood,* a medical malpractice case in which the defendant negligently failed to diagnose and report to the authorities a battered child syndrome and the plaintiff child was returned to the same environment, where the battering continued and further injuries were sustained. The court stated that

> an actor may be liable if his negligence is a substantial factor in causing injury, and he is not relieved of liability because of the intervening act of a third person if such act was reasonably foreseeable at the time of his negligent conduct.[14]

Damages awarded to the plaintiff can be actual, nominal, and/or punitive. Actual damages are awarded for past and future medical expenses, physical pain and mental suffering, and past and future loss of income. Nominal damages are paid when the plaintiff has proved the case but cannot prove the extent of damages. Punitive damages are awarded to the plaintiff when there is a desire to punish the defendant. These are also known as "exemplary damages" and can be likened to a fine levied against a defendant in a criminal case. They are appropriate when the conduct has been reckless, willful, malicious, or grossly negligent.

Malpractice "Crises"

In the late 1960s and early 1970s and again in the mid-1980s there were what have been called medical malpractice "crises" that resulted from unexpected and substantial increases in physician and hospital malpractice insurance premiums. Allegedly, these increases were prompted by adverse court decisions in cases of negligent practice and insurance carriers' fears that they had underestimated their potential liability. In both crises the premium increases caused physicians in some states to "go on strike" by declining to admit patients or provide certain types of care. Other physicians threatened similar action.

During the first of these malpractice crises, general concern prompted establishment of a Secretary's Commission on Medical Malpractice within the United States Department of Health, Education, and Welfare (DHEW) (now the Department of Health and Human Services [DHHS]) in 1971. Its 1973 report put the first crisis into perspective and found that: a claim was asserted for only one of every 226,000 patient visits to doctors; most doctors had never had a medical malpractice suit filed against them; and most hospitals, no matter how large, go through an entire year without having a single claim filed against them.[15] At that time, medical malpractice insurance premiums were less than 1% of total national health services expenditures. The Secretary's Commission also found, through analysis of claim files, that insurance carriers judged 46% of claims to be meritorious, a finding contradicting assertions that malpractice claims are generally baseless. The Commission's report suggested that medical malpractice is a problem.

The malpractice crisis in the 1980s was more regionalized, and the word "crisis" was heard less often. "The number of claims per physician rose nearly by half from 1980–86, and the average size of a claim more than doubled in real terms. Doctors saw premiums increase"—by 81% from 1982–1985—and again directed their anger at state legislatures, with some success.[16] Obstetricians were especially hard hit by malpractice insurance premium increases in some states. By the late 1980s there were signs the problem was diminishing: One major medical malpractice carrier reduced rates nationwide by 14.1%; and claims against physicians had declined from 10.2 to 6.7 per 100.[17] A 1991 report, however, showed that the number of physician malpractice claims increased for the first time since 1985.[18] This may be the prelude to a new round of increased medical malpractice claims and insurance premium increases.

Sources describing the second malpractice crisis are more diverse. A New York state study using mid-1980s data and reported in 1991 supports the Secretary's Commission finding from 1973 that malpractice is a real problem, not one imagined by lawyers and a fringe group of malcontent patients. It estimated that the fraction of medical negligence that leads to claims is probably under 2% and that "(p)erhaps half the claimants will eventually receive compensation."[19]

Reforms of the Malpractice System   After the crisis of the early 1970s, a number of states enacted tort reform. California's law, for example, now limits recovery by plaintiffs of non-economic damages (this primarily limits recovery for pain and suffering), caps plaintiff's legal fees, and allows juries to learn how much money the plaintiff has received from other sources. A 1991 assessment suggests that, by leaving the basic system in place, such reforms do not address the root of the malpractice problem. Caps on damages and attorneys' fees, for example, lower insurance premiums, but "patients with the most serious injuries are the ones who pay the price for the strategy."[20] A 3-year study of the Indiana Medical Malpractice Act found that, although premiums decreased, more people are getting more money than was paid out before the reform legislation was enacted in 1975. The study found that the average payment for claims of more than $100,000 was over $100,000 greater in Indiana than in Michigan and Ohio, two states without reforms. In addition, only about 33% of closed claims were settled without payment in Indiana, compared with 57% nationwide.[21]

In mid-1991, there was growing interest in some federal overhaul of the nation's malpractice system, even though malpractice traditionally has been an area of exclusive state control.[22] Any federal action is likely to be tied to other perceived problems such as excess testing, defensive medicine, and reimbursement. A seeming lack of aggressiveness by state licensing bodies in disciplining physicians is also likely to be an issue. Data from 1990 show that serious disciplinary actions (defined as license revocations, suspensions, and probations) declined by 4.8% from 1989. The 1,437 serious disciplinary actions by the 50 state licensing boards during 1990 reflected a decline from 2.64 per 1,000 to 2.52.[23] It was the second straight year of decline in the rate of disciplinary actions, and it meant that fewer than 0.5% of licensed physicians in the United States were disciplined by state licensing boards in 1990.[24]

Reforms such as a no-fault approach—wherein injured persons are compensated without a need to litigate—may dramatically increase rather than reduce costs. A study in Maine found that the time, financial costs, and, most significantly, contact with attorneys appears to discourage large numbers of people from seeking redress for medical malpractice injuries. The data suggested that very few people who believe they have experienced iatrogenic (physician-caused) illness or injury discuss these experiences with attorneys; those who do so appear to follow long and circuitous routes. Many more discuss the problem with health services professionals, including the professionals they hold responsible for the problems, and at a much earlier stage.[25]

Effects of Malpractice Suits   An important shift seems to have occurred in how the public perceives malpractice suits. A 1982 survey by the AMA found that nearly half of those queried thought that malpractice suits were justified. In early 1989, however, the same survey found that view was held by only 27%.[26] Business executives are taking a hard line about the effect of medical malpractice on health care costs. A poll found that 79% believed liability awards and malpractice insurance were the most important factors in driving up health insurance costs, a number far exceeding those who believed technology, inefficient hospitals, and unnecessary care were responsible.[27] The net result of these views may be that the number of claims and the level of awards by juries will decline, despite the apparently high levels of medical malpractice.

Analysis of the insurance industry suggests that market forces cause insurors to go through business cycles. When profits are good because of high premium income, new companies enter the market by writing medical malpractice insurance. As competition grows premiums are forced down; the resulting decline in profits forces some insurers out of the market. Those remaining can dramatically increase premiums. The problem is worsened by the fact that most carriers rely on nonpremium income from investments as a supplement. Adverse results of poor investment policies exacerbate the effects of increased competition.

There is little doubt that fear of malpractice lawsuits affects medical practice. Results include: distrust and antagonism between physicians and patients (physicans may see patients as potential lawsuits and screen them for attributes of litigiousness); increased insurance premiums as reflected in higher fees; and the practice by some physicians of defensive medicine, which is defined as altering medical practice because of a fear of potential lawsuits. Defensive medicine is seen as forestalling the possibility of lawsuits and providing a legal defense if lawsuits are instituted.[28] Defensive medicine is expensive in absolute terms, but this cost is not very significant compared to other expenditures. Data developed by the AMA show that, between 1982 and 1988, liability insurance premiums cost only 5.6% of a physician's total budget for professional expenses. Applying this percentage nationally means that premiums and damage payments totalled $5.7 billion of the $102.7 billion spent on physicians' services. The physicians surveyed estimated that costs of defensive medicine and the time they spent away from the office as a result of malpractice litigation cost $19.3 billion. Total professional liability costs of $25 billion were only 5% of total health services expenditures of almost $500 billion in 1987.[29] There is evidence that physicians' fears of iatrogenesis (medical problems caused by physician activity) because of too much testing are becoming a counterbalance to excessive use of ancillary services.

TORTS AND HSOs

Background

The previous discussion about torts focused on the role of the person who committed the civil wrong, whether intentionally or unintentionally (negligently). This section identifies and analyzes the legal theories used to find liability against the HSO where there is an employment relationship with physicians or others, or where the physician or other licensed independent practitioner is an independent contractor. HSO liability occurs through application of two theories: one is based on agency; the other is a general legal concept that the organization owes a duty to patients and others. It is these legal theories holding the HSO accountable that have been expanded most in the past several decades.

In the past, HSOs, notably hospitals, often avoided liability for the negligent acts of employees because of the legal theories of governmental immunity and charitable immunity. Governmental immunity still applies in some jurisdictions to government-owned HSOs. The theory was derived from the king's sovereign power to be free from civil actions. Only if this doctrine has been modified by statute, as in the case of the Federal Tort Claims Act, can an action be brought. Availability of this defense has been greatly reduced in the past several decades. Even more reduced is the doctrine of charitable immunity. It was based on the concept that the assets of HSOs serving in a charitable manner were unacceptably threatened if civil actions for medical malpractice could be brought against them. This protection has rapidly declined in the past several decades and is virtually unavailable as a defense.

Agency and Corporate Liability

There developed in English common law the legal concept that the master should be responsible for the servant's negligence. This is embodied in a Latin phrase, *respondeat superior*—let the master answer. Similarly, the principal is responsible for the acts of the agent. The negligence of servant or agent is imputed (vicarious liability) to the person best able to exercise control. An important pragmatic consideration underlying it, however, is that courts sometimes search for a "deep pocket," and the employer (principal) usually has one. This doctrine applies to HSO employees acting within the scope of their employment. It has limited applicability to caregivers who are independent contractors. Physicians are the most common type of independent contractor in HSOs. Because independent contractors exercise control over the means and methods of performing their tasks, the HSO is not liable for their negligent acts *by applying the theory of agency*. The issue is clouded when there is evidence of "apparent agency" and the patient has been led to believe that the HSO is an employer because the physician is held out as the employee.

The other legal theory by which HSOs are held liable is based on a general concept that an HSO owes a duty to patients (as well as others, such as visitors) to protect them from harm. This is known as corporate liability, an area of tort law that has rapidly expanded in the past several decades. Previously, this legal doctrine was used to permit recovery by visitors and patients who were injured because the HSO failed to keep buildings, grounds, and equipment in safe condition. In addition, the HSO is now seen to have a duty to take reasonable steps in selecting and retaining employees, as well as those who are there to provide care but are not employed (e.g., an independent contractor).

Southwick concludes that, although these two concepts of an organization's liability for medical malpractice remain somewhat separate, they have virtually merged into one:

> It should . . . be acknowledged that in the hospital setting there is no longer a viable distinction between the rules of *respondeat superior*, on one hand, and corporate or independent negligence, on the other. Essentially, the two theories have become one. . . . In the delivery of health care services in an institutional setting it is increasingly difficult to determine factually who is in control of whom. As allied health care professionals proliferate and are accorded a greater degree of independence from the direct supervision and control of the attending physician, the matter of the right to control another's actions becomes a very difficult question both as a matter of fact and of law. It therefore becomes necessary to place either sole or joint liability upon the institution which, in the final analysis, is ultimately responsible for arranging, providing, and coordinating the activities of a host of professional persons, all of whom must work together in the care of patients.[30]

This evolution in the law has major consequences for HSOs. They are not yet guarantors of the results of medical treatment, but the field is moving toward unequivocal accountability for all HSO activities that fall below the standard of care. HSOs use quality assessment, continuous quality improvement, and risk management to establish and maintain high levels of quality. These concepts are considered in Chapter 11, "Quality and Productivity Improvement," and Chapter 12, "Control, Risk Management, Quality Assessment/Improvement, and Resource Allocation."

DEVELOPING LEGAL AREAS

Acquired Immunodeficiency Syndrome–Related Litigation

By 1990, the number of acquired immunodeficiency syndrome (AIDS)-related lawsuits was already the largest number attributable to any one disease in United States legal history, and it was predicted that HSOs would become the most important focus of AIDS-related litigation in the next few years.[31] Chapter 3 provided a background on the AIDS epidemic. One of the areas of such litigation is the special risks present when staff members work with AIDS patients. The Occupational Safety and Health Act of 1974, administered by the Occupational Safety and Health Administration (OSHA), requires that employers provide employment and a place of employment that are free from recognized hazards that cause, or are likely to cause, death or serious physical harm. Universal blood and body substance precautions are required by OSHA. Such precautions are likely to be the focus of enforcement that uses a targeted basis as well as responding to employee complaints. OSHA is also expected to require employee educational programs about hazards and precautions, and to engage in its own educational activities.

In their efforts to protect staff, HSOs must be certain to avoid discriminating against the disabled—persons who have AIDS are defined as disabled. The rights of the disabled to have full and equal enjoyment of public accommodations were strengthened by passage of the Americans with Disabilities Act (ADA) in 1990, which combined protections for the disabled found in the Civil Rights Act of 1964, the Rehabilitation Act of 1973, and the Civil Rights Restoration Act of 1988.[32] The provisions of Title III are broad enough to protect the rights of patients and potential patients and reflect the fact that persons with AIDS, or who were thought to have AIDS, occasionally have been denied treatment.

> A health care provider may refer a person to another provider if the treatment or services required are outside the area of specialization. But an individual with a disability such as AIDS cannot be denied treatment because of that disability if the same services would be provided to a person without a disability.[33]

The second legal dimension concerns the risk to patients and staff from an employee infected with the human immunodeficiency virus (HIV). HSOs are subject to Section 504 of the federal Rehabilitation Act of 1973, which prohibits discrimination against otherwise qualified handicapped persons. The protections found in the Rehabilitation Act of 1973 for disabled but otherwise qualified applicants or employees were strengthened by the ADA. Title I addresses employment: "The act prohibits an employer from segregating or classifying an applicant or employee because of a disability; from contractual arrangements which will subject the employee with a disability to discrimination; or from using any standards which discriminate."[34] The ADA requires employers to make reasonable accommodations for disabled employees and, in addition, provides other protections. It is clear that the ADA will protect the application and employment of HIV-positive persons. It will be a question of fact as to whether or not an employee with frank AIDS is "otherwise qualified" in a health services setting, an issue that is addressed below.

In 1987, the United States Supreme Court considered a case analogous to that of an HIV-positive employee. In *Arline v. School Board of Nassau County, Florida*,[35] a teacher who had had three recurrences of tuberculosis was discharged because the school board considered her a health threat to students. Tuberculosis was found to be both handicapping and contagious, and the Court ruled that tuberculosis was a handicapping condition protected by the statute. The case was remanded for the trial court to determine whether Arline was otherwise qualified and whether she could have been accommodated in alternate employment.

In *Arline*, the Court stated in a footnote that it was not making a determination as to whether carriers of a contagious disease would be considered to have a physical impairment, or whether they would be considered handicapped under the act solely on the basis of contagiousness. Subsequent decisions by federal courts of appeal (courts lesser than the Supreme Court) have shown a willingness to assume that AIDS and HIV infections fall within the scope of section 504.[36] Additional federal protection for those persons who are HIV positive is found in the Civil Rights Restoration Action of 1987, which amended the Rehabilitation Act so that persons with a contagious disease or infection are protected if they do not "constitute a direct threat to health or safety" and are able to "perform the duties of the job."[37] Federal legislation is buttressed by handicap statutes in the 50 states and the District of Columbia.[38] The facts in *Arline* may be distinguished in several ways from those related to HSO staff with AIDS: chronic (tuberculosis) versus acute (the opportunistic diseases that eventually afflict persons who are HIV positive); type of setting; the risk to healthy students versus that to ill non-AIDS patients; and the well-established legal duties HSOs have to protect patients. When considering the facts of a case it is important to distinguish persons who are HIV positive from those with frank AIDS, who may be afflicted with a variety of diseases. Similarly, such considerations will affect applications of the ADA in HSOs.

Other legal aspects of AIDS focus on confidentiality, including reporting HIV infection and the duty to warn third parties. Legal protections against breaching medical confidentiality are well established in state law. With the AIDS epidemic, a majority of states have enacted new laws to safeguard the confidentiality and privacy of individuals infected or perceived to be infected with HIV.[39] The obligations of health services providers, including HSOs, to report certain communicable diseases are also well established. This was readily extended to AIDS. Efforts to extend reporting requirements to the results of the antibody test encountered difficulty, and only about one half of the states require it.[40]

Contact tracing is a historically important role of public health departments that is being applied to HIV infection. Duty to warn is more specific and defines the extent to which caregivers are legally obligated to protect third parties in immediate danger. In *Tarasoff v. Regents of the State of California*,[41] the Supreme Court of California held that if a psychotherapist reasonably believes a patient poses a direct threat to a third party, the psychotherapist must warn the endangered person. Most state supreme courts have adopted the reasoning in *Tarasoff,* but virtually all of them have limited their protective concern to identifiable third parties at risk of real and probable harm.[42] It seems likely that this legal doctrine will be applied to persons with HIV infection.

Antitrust Litigation

The federal government's interest in prohibiting private business activity that impedes competition in the marketplace dates from the Sherman Antitrust Act of 1890, passed "against a background of rampant cartelization and monopolization of the American economy."[43] In 1914, Congress passed additional antitrust legislation in the Federal Trade Commission Act and the Clayton Act. The Department of Justice and Federal Trade Commission (FTC) share responsibility for enforcement. States have laws patterned after the federal statutes.

Application of federal antitrust law in the health services field dates from the 1940s. In *AMA v. United States*,[44] the AMA and its Washington, D.C., affiliate society were convicted of a criminal violation of Section 3 of the Sherman Act because they had conspired to prevent Group Health Association (an HMO) from hiring and retaining physicians. A doctrine that the professions were immune from civil suit under antitrust developed in the law, and it was not until 1975 that the Supreme Court held that the learned professions, including physicians, were subject to it. Federal antitrust law is especially powerful, and terrifying for defendants, because successful plaintiffs are entitled to treble damages—that is, three times the damages that can be established. It is less well known that prevailing plaintiffs in a private antitrust action will have their attorneys' fees paid by a losing defendant.[45]

The first significant Supreme Court decision to apply antitrust principles in health services was *Hospital Building Co. v. Trustees of Rex Hospital* in 1976.[46] Space is too limited to describe more than the rudimentary aspects of the case, which involved two defendant hospitals that had cooperated with the local health planning council in developing a long-term plan for the community. Based on the plan, defendants opposed the plaintiff hospital's application for a certificate of need to expand its facility, arguing that it would duplicate facilities recommended by the planning council for defendant hospitals. After 14 years of litigation the case seems to have been concluded with application of a modified rule of reason.[47] Rule of reason means that if a challenged activity is not a per se violation of antitrust law (horizontal price fixing, allocation or division of a market, group boycotts and joint refusals to deal, and tie-in sales), courts compare the favorable and unfavorable effects of a restraint of trade on competition.[48]

Mergers have been of special interest to both the Department of Justice and the FTC because of the great potential they have for lessening competition. The case of *United States v. Rockford Memorial Corp.*[49] involved the merger of two not-for-profit hospitals. The merger was challenged in court by the federal government and was found to be prohibited under the Sherman Act. The court of appeals stated that Clayton Act restrictions on mergers apply to not-for-profit hospitals. (The government had failed to make this argument.) *Rockford* conflicts with the result in a similar case, *United States v. Carilion Health Systems, Community Hospital of Roanoke Valley,*[50] wherein the district court held that Clayton Act merger restrictions *did not* extend to not-for-profit hospitals. By refusing to hear the appeal of *Rockford,* the Supreme Court left considerable confusion as to application of federal antitrust law in mergers of not-for-profit hospitals. Such uncertainty is especially problematic when many hospitals and other types of HSOs face financial difficulties because of the inefficiencies of excess capacity and duplicative services. It has been argued, however, that *Rockford* does not prohibit hospital mergers. After listing several mergers, Higgins notes that:

> Of the five . . . mergers that were cleared to go forward, all were scrutinized by the FTC or Justice Department using the same standards that were applied in the *Rockford* case.
> It is difficult to deduce from that empirical evidence that the antitrust standards applied by the federal enforcement agencies—as is articulated in *Rockford*—compel a cessation of hospital merger activity.
> The(se) examples show that antitrust analysis is fact-specific. There are so many different combinations and fact patterns that only rarely do two transactions produce the same antitrust results. This phenomenon is particularly true in health care because of the wide variety of types of facilities and ownership, and because of the multiple legal structures used in mergers and affiliations.[51]

Peer review as part of quality assessment and improvement (QA/I) activities has resulted in antitrust actions against physicians and HSOs. Usually these cases arise in hospitals because the professional staff organization (PSO) formally reviews performance of its members. Staff members who lose privileges or are denied privileges because of peer review have challenged adverse decisions as anticompetitive actions based on economics, not QA/I. The case of *Patrick v. Burget*[52] in the early 1980s involved a physician who alleged federal antitrust violations by former colleagues at a clinic where he had practiced and by the hospital where his clinical privileges had been suspended following peer review.

The potential chilling effect such legal actions might have on peer review and other efforts to improve the quality of care stimulated Congress to enact the Health Care Quality Improvement Act of 1986 (HCQIA). The HCQIA provides immunity from private damage lawsuits under federal or state law (except civil rights laws) for any "professional review action" (which includes peer review) if that professional review action follows standards set out in the law. These standards include a reasonable belief that the action furthered the quality of health care and that the action was justified, there was a reasonable effort to obtain the facts, and the physician was given adequate notice and a fair hearing or such other procedures as were fair under the circumstances. (The HCQIA defines "physician" to include dentists.) Early court cases such as *Austin v. McNamara*[53] suggest that the immunities under HCQIA will be effective in encouraging peer review activities.

The HCQIA includes reporting requirements for several different types of entities regarding a variety of actions, and it establishes a national practitioner data bank to receive reports and provide information to authorized persons and organizations. For example, sanctions taken by boards of medical examiners (state licensing boards) must be reported. Health care entities are defined in the HCQIA as all hospitals and other health care entities that provide health care services and engage in professional review through a formal peer review process. They must report:

1. Professional review actions that adversely affect the clinical privileges of a physician for longer than 30 days.
2. Accepting surrender of clinical privileges of a physician
   a. while the physician is under investigation by the entity relating to possible incompetence or improper professional conduct, or
   b. in return for not conducting an investigation or proceeding.
3. If an entity that is a professional society takes a professional review action that adversely affects the membership of a physician in the society.

Reports are initially sent to the state board of medical examiners, which in turn must send them to the data bank. In addition, *any* entity (including an insurance company) that makes a payment under a policy of insurance, self-insurance, or otherwise to settle (or partially settle) or to satisfy a judgment in a medical malpractice action or claim must report certain information to the data bank. Here the statute is broader, and information about payments for the benefit of physicians *and* licensed independent practitioners must be reported. (Only here does the law include licensed independent practitioners other than physicians.) HSOs must make inquiries of the data bank when granting privileges to physicians *and* licensed independent practitioners and are presumed to know the information that is there.

The data bank became operational in the fall of 1990, and its full effects will not be realized for some years. It remains to be seen whether the HCQIA will actually encourage or discourage peer review. Some commentators argue that the need to report *any* payment discourages settlement—a straightforward business decision to settle a malpractice case might be interpreted as an admission of culpability by the physician. Indeed, a loophole in the law provides that, if an HSO agrees to pay the plaintiff if a physician is dropped from a lawsuit *before* settlement, the physician's name need not be reported to the data bank.[54] Such an action is within the letter, if not the spirit, of the law. It is likely, too, that disciplinary actions against physicians will be handled earlier and informally—for example, by the physician agreeing not to admit any more patients to a hospital and the hospital not renewing the physician's privileges at the next appointment cycle—rather than formally suspending the physician, which necessitates a report to the data bank.

Public statements by senior staff at the FTC make it clear that federal regulators will continue to focus on the health services field.[55] Particular interest in the early 1990s will be "sham IPAs"—independent practice associations that are nothing more than blatant price fixing arrangements.[56]

It is noteworthy that although most of the attention in antitrust litigation has been focused on federal activity—that of the Department of Justice and the FTC—a study in late 1990 found that, since 1985, state attorneys general have filed or investigated at least 70 antitrust cases in health services. Cases involved allegations of illegal group boycotts or concerted efforts by competitors against a third party, allegations of price fixing, anticompetitive mergers, and other suspected antitrust violations. The areas most frequently cited in the study for future attention by attorneys general were nursing homes, third-party payors, hospital mergers, mergers of large health maintenance organizations, and "sham" physician unions.[57]

Charitable Status of HSOs

As federal tax law developed, it recognized a special place for organizations that engage in charitable work. HSOs that are organized as not-for-profit corporations are eligible to apply for federal tax status as a tax-exempt organization. Such status gives numerous advantages, including exemption from federal income and excise taxes and the ability of donors to deduct their gifts to these organizations from federal income taxes. Most states accept the federal determination that an HSO is a charitable organization, and this provides the same tax advantages at the state level. In addition, tax-exempt HSOs usually pay no local property taxes.

Prior to 1969 the Internal Revenue Service (IRS) required that a tax-exempt hospital "must be operated to the extent of its financial ability for those not able to pay for the services rendered and not exclusively for those who are able and expected to pay."[58] In 1969, the IRS issued a new revenue ruling that removed the requirements of rendering service to those unable to pay and said that promotion of health was a sufficient charitable purpose that benefits the community as a whole. By operating an emergency room open to all and providing hospital care for all in the community able to pay the costs of it, a hospital was promoting the health of a class of persons broad enough to benefit the community. The IRS position was supported in the legal challenge that followed.[59] The net effect was that there could be less emphasis on treating those unable to pay without losing exempt status.

Recent developments, however, suggest that the issue is far from resolved either at the federal or state level. The stakes are high. The General Accounting Office estimates that the benefit of tax-exempt status to not-for-profit hospitals is worth $4.5 billion in saved income, use, sales, and property taxes, reduced costs through tax-exempt bond financing, and receipt of charitable donations.[60] The thrust in Congress seems to be to tie continued tax-exempt status for hospitals to minimum levels of charity care—probably to some percentage of the tax benefit of being tax exempt.

State officials in Texas and Utah have challenged hospitals' property tax exemption.[61] There have been numerous challenges of the tax-exempt status of hospitals by local governments in Pennsylvania. The rationale at both state and local levels has been that tax-exempt hospitals perform too little public service and charitable care to justify their special status. Some paid. Others fought and won, an example of which occurred in Burlington, Vermont.

A significant part of the problem, especially for hospitals, is that they are involved in activities such as joint ventures, diversification, and reorganizations, all of which have a distinct flavor of business, not charity. In addition, the media have been very attentive to the high levels of compensation earned by some HSO executives. These developments blur and diminish the perception of community benefits that so clearly distinguished not-for-profit HSOs in the past. If the public increasingly sees hospitals as businesses rather than charities, the efforts to eliminate or reduce the tax advantages of exempt organizations will grow.

Another problem ahead for the tax-exempt status of not-for-profit HSOs, especially hospitals, stems from the various collateral "businesses" that many undertake. Examples include filling prescriptions for persons who have not been hospitalized, sales to the general public of hearing aids through an audiology service, and selling or leasing durable medical equipment (DME). The test used by the IRS is whether the activity furthers the organization's exempt purpose. For example, revenue produced by a hospital cafeteria from serving patients and on-call staff is tax exempt because that activity furthers a hospital's exempt purpose; revenue derived from sales to the general public is not given the same treatment.[62] The problem has two dimensions: 1) whether unrelated business income jeopardizes tax-exempt status, and 2) the political implications of lobbying by for-profit businesses that believe they are experiencing unfair competition from tax-exempt HSOs whose tax status gives them an economic advantage and whose referrals allow them to channel patients to their own services. Congress has held hearings to investigate the extent of the problem of income unrelated to the exempt purpose.

A tax-exempt organization may participate in a limited amount of activity not related to its exempt purpose, provided that the activity is only an insubstantial part of its overall activities. "Insubstantial" is vague, but past experience provides some rules of thumb. Regardless, income from unrelated activities is taxed as unrelated business income—what the IRS calls unrelated business income tax.[63] The primary test used by the IRS to determine whether the unrelated business income tax applies to activities that do not constitute provision of health services is to distinguish between activities that benefit patients and those that benefit nonpatients. It is unlikely that a not-for-profit hospital, for example, will lose its federal tax-exempt status because of excessive unrelated activity.[64] Nonetheless, the consequences of losing tax exemption are so serious that caution is crucial.

In recent years, the IRS has looked closely at income earned through partnerships and joint ventures between exempt HSOs and taxable parties such as physicians.[65] Such arrangements raise questions of income unrelated to the exempt purpose as well as private inurement—a concept based on a requirement for exempt status that there may be no private benefit to individuals through the activities of an exempt organization. Arm's length arrangements such as reasonable salaries for services performed and lease of space at fair market value to a physician, for instance, are not considered inurement. The IRS has been especially vigilant as to arrangements that return substantial profits or capital gains to physicians who invest little in a joint venture with an exempt hospital. This focus is likely to continue.

THE LEGAL PROCESS

This discussion presumes a legal case involving a tort, not a breach of contract. A civil lawsuit begins when the plaintiff files a complaint with a court that has jurisdiction to hear the case. By reason of having been filed in a court, the complaint becomes an official document, and it is served on the defendant by a marshal or a sheriff's deputy. The defendant must respond to the complaint in a limited period of time. This response is known as an answer. The answer may deny in whole or in part the allegations stated in the complaint, or it may assert specific defenses, such as that the statute of limitations has expired and the suit may not be brought, the plaintiff assumed the risk, or the plaintiff was contributorily negligent. The defendant may also make certain motions before the court—for example, a motion to dismiss because the complaint fails to state a cause of action, or a motion to dismiss because the complaint was filed in a court that lacks jurisdiction.

Few cases are dismissed at this stage. The next phase is discovery. It is during this period that the parties to the suit attempt to learn about the opponent's case. The plaintiff seeks information to support the allegations and existence of tortious conduct; the defendant seeks to determine the strength of the plaintiff's case, and vice versa.

During discovery it is common for the plaintiff to make motions in court for production of documents needed to prepare its case. The defendant may sometimes ask the court to deny the motion for reasons such as a statutory privilege, relevance, and reasonableness of demands. In addition, information is obtained through written interrogatories and by taking sworn statements (depositions) of persons who have knowledge of the alleged injuries, or those who will testify as expert witnesses. There are limits to what documents must be produced. In all states, except in certain circumstances, the results of peer review are "privileged." This means they cannot be discovered. The discovery phase may take months or years, but statutes limit the length of time available. The procedural maneuvering to prevent opposing (usually plaintiff's) counsel from obtaining certain documents and information adds considerable time and expense to the proceedings.

Many cases are settled during the discovery process or when it is complete, primarily because the parties have learned enough about the accuracy of the allegations and the strength of the opposition's case to make an informed decision. States have developed various means to determine the merit of a claim of medical malpractice and to try to settle it. These are discussed below.

If the case has merit but there is no settlement, a trial date is set. The trial begins with opening statements by counsel in which they outline their cases and suggest what they will attempt to prove. The plaintiff's case is presented first, and counsel must prove "by a preponderance of the evidence" that the elements of a tort are present. This is done by introducing evidence consisting of documents and testimony by persons who may have observed the event or can offer other information, and by expert witnesses. Sometimes there is no direct evidence about the event but only a series of circumstances that lead to an inference of tortious conduct. The parties will object to introduction of evidence that damages their case. The judge rules on admissibility of the evidence and any motions made by counsel during the trial.

Witnesses are questioned in several steps. The party calling the witness asks questions first; this is called direct examination. After direct examination, opposing counsel asks questions to cross-examine the witness. Cross-examination permits counsel to "impeach" the witness by raising questions about the accuracy of the witness's memory, veracity, reputation, and the like. This tests the witness's testimony and allows the finder of fact (the jury or judge sitting without a jury) to weigh it. After cross-examination, there is redirect examination to allow counsel to "rehabilitate" the witness—to correct undesirable impressions that might have been left by cross-examination. The last round of questions is called re–cross-examination. A major theory of the law is that truth is most likely to emerge from this adversarial process, and the finder of fact thereby can determine the witnesses' credibility.

The defendant's case is presented following the plaintiff's and involves the same steps. When the evidence has been heard (and seen), the jury is "charged" by the judge. This means that the judge tells the jury in writing that if it determines that certain facts are present, the law requires it to find in certain ways. These instructions to the jury are crucial, and both sides submit proposed instructions from which the judge chooses. Of course, these instructions are cast by each of the parties in the light most favorable to its case. If there is no jury, the judge will retire to consider the evidence and render a decision. In some jurisdictions, the decision of finding for the plaintiff or defendant is reached separately from the determination of the amount of damages that should be awarded to the plaintiff if the finding is for the plaintiff.

At various times during the trial, the parties will make motions for the judge to consider and rule upon. For example, the defendant may move for a directed verdict after the plaintiff's case has been presented. If this motion is granted, which is rare, the trial ends because the judge has found for the defendant. Both parties may move for a directed verdict when all evidence has been presented. When the jury finds for one of the parties, the other may ask for a judgment notwithstanding the verdict or, alternatively, for a new trial. If the judge grants the former, which is rarely done, the jury verdict is overturned and judgment is entered for the other party. If the latter is granted, a new trial is set in the future. Each motion is supported by a brief that cites legal precedents and arguments as to why that motion should be granted.

If the defendant loses and the jury awards damages that the defendant believes are excessive as a matter of law, the defendant can petition the court for *remittitur*. If granted, the legal doctrine of *remittitur* allows the judge to decrease the award. Again, the defendant's motion is supported by a brief that cites the evidence presented and how it could not support the verdict. The plaintiff submits a brief in opposition. Similarly, the doctrine of *additur* allows a court to increase the amount of an inadequate award made by jury verdict.

The losing party may appeal the verdict. Appeals are based on alleged errors that were made by the trial court and that represent misapplication of the law by the judge. These appeals are entered in the appeals court (the intermediate level) or eventually in the supreme court. Typical of errors alleged by the losing party are permitting (or failing to allow) certain evidence, failing to grant a certain motion, the content of jury instructions, and the judge's decision to qualify or refuse to qualify an expert witness.

Trial and appeals court proceedings are very expensive. Discovery requires paying for reproduction of documents at a rate of several dollars per page, deposing the parties and witnesses, and paying expert witness fees. Such costs must be paid as they are incurred. There are major costs to defendants who must answer interrogatories, produce documents, and cope with the disruption and other aspects of defending the suit. Trial appearances by attorneys command much higher fees than those charged for other work. In addition, court costs must be paid. Appeals require that the stenographic record of the trial be transcribed. This record will be several thousand pages long for even a short trial and will cost thousands of dollars to prepare. High stakes, however, warrant such costs. Contingency fees for attorneys are suggested as a cause of the large number of medical malpractice suits. However, such financial arrangements permit patients who have been injured to seek redress even though they cannot pay the costs for an attorney to prepare and try the case.

SPECIAL CONSIDERATIONS FOR THE MANAGER

The preceding sections briefly summarized the law affecting HSOs. This section provides information about preventing medical malpractice and identifies special considerations once a complaint is served. The reader should see the HSO as having an independent ethical obligation to the patient and to the community separate from and more demanding than that arising from its legal duty.

Managers face a range of problems in effectively handling the legal and quasi-legal matters that regularly arise. These run the gamut from dealing with patients who have a grievance with the HSO and are potential litigants to providing instruction for staff members on proper maintenance of medical records.

Record Keeping

Anecdotal information suggests that HSOs lose many cases because they have inadequate records to support their contention that what was done met the standard of care. Without a written record, there are major problems proving what occurred. Legally, there is nothing magic about medical records and the information they can provide. In fact, courts prefer to have the person(s) who actually rendered the care present to testify. However, if a caregiver cannot show that a treatment was given or a drug administered through some written record, it must do so through oral testimony. This would be difficult a few weeks after the event; years later it is impossible. Personnel are highly mobile, memories fade, and the specific information needed simply cannot be provided. This makes complete and accurate medical records indispensable.

It is not uncommon that persons being sued or who fear suit alter the medical record. This is generally a criminal offense, and it certainly breaches a basic ethical duty. Pragmatically, however, it is likely the alterations will be discovered. When revealed, such conduct increases a jury's willingness to award damages, and the court may allow a claim for punitive damages. An effective risk management system requires that a responsible person obtain custody of the medical record at the first indication of a potentially compensible event in the HSO. This control should be exercised continuously until the dispute has been resolved, including any appeal.

A more common problem is that handwritten entries in the medical record are either difficult to read or illegible. Often, physicians have poor handwriting. The medical records committee or its equivalent must make special, continuous efforts to monitor and improve the legibility of all medical record entries. It must also be concerned that the record is properly organized, authenticated, completed properly and in a timely fashion, and readily available where it is needed.

Effective Use of House and Retainer Counsel

There are two basic ways HSOs obtain legal advice. Most common is that a retainer is paid to have an attorney available for consultation. The retainer guarantees access as needed. Considering the law's importance in managing HSOs and the need for ongoing advice and counsel, however, this is not the most desirable means. Increasingly, larger HSOs are hiring full-time attorneys as in-house counsel. In this arrangement, the attorney is a staff assistant to management and the governing body. One of these methods of having counsel available is essential. HSOs can no longer get by with free advice from a member of the governing body who is an attorney. The law as it affects HSOs is so specialized and frequently applied that a casual or informal relationship is insufficient.

Effective use of legal counsel poses problems no different from those of interacting with other technical staff. The specifics will vary, however, depending on whether counsel is in house or on retainer. Using in-house counsel encourages the attorney to be fully integrated into the various systems that alert management to legal problems or to prevent them from occurring. For example, an HSO could use an in-house attorney to direct the risk management program. Such involvement reduces dependence on management staff to recognize legal implications of problems. It is a paradox that, while frequent contact with in-house counsel enhances managers' knowledge in this regard, less intense involvement, which is usually the case with retainer counsel, requires managers to be more cognizant of potential legal problems and to involve counsel in a timely manner. Another advantage of in-house counsel is that the attorney is exclusively committed to that HSO and is not distracted by other clients. Furthermore, the attorney will become expert in the HSO's special problems and unique characteristics. The sum of these considerations is enhanced effectiveness.

Even with in-house counsel, certain areas of the law and activities such as trial work are often exclusively dealt with by attorneys specializing in them. If an insurance carrier is involved in a pending lawsuit, it will retain counsel to work on preparing and trying the case. Like medicine, the practice of law has become highly specialized. Having the appropriate skills will optimize the outcome.

Testifying

At some time during their professional careers, health services managers will probably testify in a legal proceeding. The most common testimony is that providing information as to how the HSO is organized or how it functioned in a particular circumstance. Less common is providing information about a problem that is personal knowledge of the manager (e.g., how the incident occurred).

Written interrogatories (questions) ask managers and staff to answer questions about organization, staffing, functions, and similar topics. These interrogatories are often the first step in the discovery process. They assist counsel to later request specific documents and information. Managers may also be deposed. This means that counsel for the opposing party asks questions of the manager while they are in each other's presence. When giving a deposition, the deponent (manager) is sworn to tell the truth. The attorney for the HSO is present, and a legal reporter makes a verbatim record. The HSO's counsel may object to the questions, but usually they are answered. If the testimony in the deposition is later introduced in court as evidence, the judge will be asked to rule on the objections counsel made during the deposition.

Health services managers may also testify as expert witnesses when the HSO with which they are, or were, affiliated is not a party to the lawsuit. Use of expert witnesses is widespread in legal proceedings involving HSOs, and this trend is likely to continue. Health services managers are qualified to testify as expert witnesses about management and organization of the types of HSOs about which they have specific knowledge. This knowledge is gained through experience and education. The expert, once accepted as qualified by the court, will be asked to render an opinion as to the appropriateness of the way in which the HSO in question organized and/or performed certain activities. Experts are used to establish the standard of care against which the HSO's performance is measured. Often, the response is elicited by means of a hypothetical question. This is less common than in the past, however, and questions are as likely to be formulated simply in terms of whether the performance of the HSO in question conformed with the standard of care.

Being an expert witness requires no special skills beyond a knowledge of one's field and a clear understanding of that practice as applied to the facts of the case. Since the finder of fact has the latitude of weighing the testimony of witnesses, it is incumbent upon the expert to testify in an honest and forthright manner. Anything short of this diminishes effectiveness.

Other Means of Dispute Resolution

Many lawsuits are settled between the time a complaint is served on the defendant and the start of trial. Some are settled even after trial begins. Settlement may occur at the initiative of the parties, who see the advantages of avoiding a costly trial and the uncertainty of the outcome (judges and juries are very unpredictable), controlling the result, and avoiding the negative publicity of a trial. Efforts at settlement are often prompted by the court because state law requires it or the judge believes the case could be settled.

Judicial means of resolving disputes are expensive and time consuming. Since the mid-1980s much attention has been given to alternative dispute resolution (ADR). ADR includes binding and nonbinding arbitration, mediation, mini-trials, and variations of these concepts. ADR techniques have special use in HSOs. Nonbinding arbitration and mediation have different purposes and processes and should be applied for specific types of disputes. Like binding arbitration, they are private, inexpensive, and efficient means of resolving disputes. The professional staff, especially, should be aware of the advantages of ADR, and their bylaws should reflect its use. Through its regional offices, the American Arbitration Association, a voluntary private organization, makes arbitrators and mediators available to resolve disputes of all types.

Many states use screening panels to determine whether medical malpractice claims have sufficient merit to proceed to trial. The panels were designed to identify nonmeritorious claims, reduce the burden on the courts, promote early disposition or settlement of meritorious claims, and reduce the cost of medical care by decreasing the volume of malpractice claims.[66] In 1980, some type of screening panel was used in 26 states.[67] By 1990, the number of states with screening panels was about the same; requirements and procedures vary considerably.[68] Typically, a screening panel is comprised of attorneys and physicians who render an opinion regarding the liability of a health care provider. Some states permit the panel to value damages if it finds at least one defendant liable. A screening panel's decision is nonbinding and, therefore, does not substitute for litigation.[69] Use of screening panels is mandatory in most states in which they are in use, but a number of states have voluntary systems.[70] Screening panel statutes have been struck down as unconstitutional in some states.

It is likely that in the future more hospitals will use voluntary binding arbitration to settle medical malpractice claims. "Voluntary" means that the parties may choose to engage in arbitration or not. If they do, however, the arbitrator's award is binding and judicial remedies may not be used. Such a program is used in Michigan.[71]

This discussion of ADR focused on medical malpractice. Many other types of legal problems occur in HSOs: disputes regarding sales agreements and employment and construction contracts; collection of debts; and matters such as zoning appeals. A provision that disputes are subject to binding arbitration is common in commercial and construction contracts and labor relations agreements. Arbitration and mediation could help solve the controversies regarding appointment and credentialing of licensed independent practitioner staff by HSOs, and such types of ADR are likely to be used more commonly in the future.

SUMMARY

This chapter provides a basic overview of the legal aspects of health services management and develops a general framework for managers to understand and analyze the legal aspects of problems. Greater understanding and appreciation of the law and its processes necessitate specialized course work and study of health services law. It should be clear, however, that the legal implications of HSO management have increased geometrically and are likely to continue to do so. This trend requires that managers have a basic understanding of the law as it affects the HSO and how to interact effectively with legal counsel. As with medicine, prevention is much more efficient than solving problems after they occur.

Managers know all too well that legal problems often have ethical dimensions, and vice versa. A basic aspect of this dynamic is that areas of the law are inadequately developed and there are instances in which law and ethics do not agree. This tension provides the manager with little guidance in decision making. The pragmatic reality, however, is that decisions must be made and actions taken. Regardless of the administrative and clinical aspects, the HSO, through its managers, has an ethical responsibility to protect patients and to act in their best interests. This standard is more demanding than that defined in the law.

DISCUSSION QUESTIONS

1. Identify formal sources of law in HSOs. How are they used? Is the emphasis on self-government and independence for groups such as the professional staff organization (PSO) consistent with external forces acting on HSOs, especially hospitals?

2. Describe processes that develop the law. What is the role of associations such as the American Association of Homes for the Aging, the American Hospital Association, and the Federation of American Health Systems? Is there a role for HSO managers?

3. How are standard of care and its breach determined? What are the roles of courts? Legislatures? Clinicians? Managers?

4. Is there compatibility between the HSO's role to act in the interests of patients (described in Chapter 3) and the need to defend itself against lawsuits for alleged malpractice?

5. State and federal regulatory processes are increasingly important to all HSOs. Identify examples of regulations affecting HSOs. Discuss the pros and cons from the standpoint of society and the HSO of the regulatory processes identified.

6. Contracts are necessary for HSOs to conduct business. Discuss examples of clinical and non-clinical contracts. What is the role of HSO managers in: 1) negotiating contracts, 2) monitoring compliance, and 3) resolving disputes?

7. The law distinguishes intentional torts and unintentional torts (negligence). What intentional torts affect HSOs? What should be the HSO manager's role in consent processes?

8. Meticulous record keeping is important to good medical treatment, and it is crucial to defending a malpractice action. Describe the manager's role in the process of record keeping.

9. Increasingly, attorneys are on the full-time staff of larger HSOs. What should managers seek in selecting an attorney? Identify the pitfalls of using in-house *and* retainer counsel.

10. Alternative dispute resolution (ADR) is advocated for all organizations. Describe this concept. Identify how various types of ADR could be used to settle disputes in HSOs.

CASE STUDY 1: REPORTING SUSPECTED CHILD ABUSE OR NEGLECT

Minnesota law requires physicians and other health services professionals to report suspected cases of child abuse or neglect to welfare authorities, the police, or both. Roosevelt Hospital is a large teaching institution in the state's only major metropolitan area. It has large emergency and outpatient departments. All attending physicians, house officers (residents), and clinical employees are told about the state law during new employee orientation, and this information is reiterated during hospital-sponsored continuing education programs. Roosevelt Hospital also has standard operating procedures that describe how to comply with the law. Forms to report suspected child abuse and neglect are provided.

You are the chief operating officer (COO) at Roosevelt. Your assistant told you last week that there has been a noticeable decline in the number of suspected child abuse and neglect cases being reported. This suggests to him that the staff may not be reporting cases as aggressively as last year. You are on your way to the American College of Healthcare Executives convocation, where you will be advanced to Fellow, so the matter must wait a week.

You get to the problem the following week. Most emergency and outpatient care is provided by house officers, so you ask the chief resident to meet with you. When she arrives she seems reluctant to discuss the matter. With some prompting, she confirms your assistant's interpretation of the data. She tells you that residents in pediatrics are the most unwilling to report suspected abuse and neglect when it appears not to be in the child's best interests. She tells you that most other residents and the attending staff agree about selective reporting.

To your horror, the chief resident recounts the details of two cases in which reports were made and the parents retained custody of the children. Both children suffered major trauma when the parents vented their frustration and anger about being reported. One child became paraplegic as the result of a spinal cord injury; the other had to have the fingers on one hand amputated because of burns sustained when his hand was held in a deep fryer.

The chief resident points out that the Oath of Hippocrates requires physicians to do what they believe to be in the best interests of the patient. She reminds you, rather sharply, that the child, not the parents, is the patient and the physician's moral duty lies with treating the child, not intimidating the parents. In addition, effective medical care is based on mutual trust. If parents see the hospital and physician as agents of the government informing on them, trust will disappear. Parents will avoid bringing children in for treatment if they are punished. She also notes that suspected abuse and neglect may not be substantiated on investigation. Being investigated by welfare authorities and police, however, stigmatizes the parents and violates the privacy of the family.

It is clear that the topic is both important and sensitive. You believe you are obliged to point out to the chief resident the opposing arguments from your perspective and that of the hospital.

Questions

1. What arguments can be made by the COO based on the law? Are the arguments based in morals or codes of ethics?
2. Should the COO use the significant formal managerial control that can be exercised over nursing and other employees to solve the problem? Why or why not?
3. Should the hospital take steps to modify state law by becoming involved in the political process? If so, what steps?
4. How much informal pressure should the COO put on the residents? What are the proper means of doing so?

CASE STUDY 2:   EFFECTIVE CONSENT

Alex Burkowski finished reading the incident report written by the supervisor of the cardiac catheterization lab and rescanned the letter from the former patient, Mr. Walter. This was the silly kind of thing that ate up his day, he thought. He wondered whether he or "Smokey the Bear" fought more fires.

As the director of risk management, Burkowski co-chaired the ad hoc interdisciplinary committee that had been established to review the consent policies at the large multispecialty group practice where he was employed. Now, he would have to try to get that committee moving again. At best, it would move only at glacial speed; at worst, it would be an exercise in futility.

He summarized the problem:

> Patient Walter admitted for catheterization. Patient alert during procedure; his cardiologist came to head of table to speak to him. Patient became alarmed about who was performing procedure (catheter visible to patient on television monitor). Cardiologist told him qualified cardiology resident was doing procedure. Procedure completed uneventfully. Patient very angry; told lab supervisor that no one told him someone other than "his doctor" would do the procedure—especially a "learner." Cardiologist can't remember if he informed patient about resident. No consent form in file.

Walter had threatened to sue, but Burkowski knew the law and understood that, absent an injury, it would be difficult for Walter to get damages. Burkowski started to write the memorandum to the committee, but he wasn't sure what to say.

Questions

1. What is the legal issue here? Whose concern is it? Do HSOs with medical education programs have a special legal obligation to patients in cases like this? If so, how is it met?
2. Outline the memorandum that Burkowski should write to the committee.

3. Burkowski seems to be as much a part of the problem as a potential part of the solution. If you were the CEO, what would you do? Why?

4. What is the ethical obligation here? What *should* the organization do regardless of the legal implications?

CASE STUDY 3: THE MISSING NEEDLE PROTECTOR

E.L. Straight is director of clinical services at Hopewell Hospital. As in most hospitals, there are a few physicians who deliver care that is acceptable but not of very high quality. They tend to make more mistakes than the others and have more patients who go "sour." After Straight took the position 2 years ago, new programs were developed and things seem to be getting better.

Dr. Cutrite has practiced at Hopewell longer than anyone can remember. He was once a brilliant general surgeon, but he has slipped physically and mentally, and Straight is considering ways to reduce his privileges. The process is incomplete, however, and Cutrite continues to do a full range of surgical procedures.

The operating room supervisor appeared at Straight's office one Monday afternoon. "We've got a problem," she said, somewhat nonchalantly, but with a hint of disgust. "I'm almost sure we left a plastic needle protector from a disposable syringe in a patient's belly—a Mrs. Jameson. You know, the protectors that are reddish-pink in color. They're impossible to see in a wound."

"Where did it come from?" asked Straight.

"I'm not sure," answered the supervisor. "All I know is that the syringe was in a used surgical pack when we did the count." She went on to describe the safeguards of counts and records. The discrepancy was noted when the records were reconciled at the end of the week. A surgical pack was shown as having a syringe that wasn't supposed to be there. When the scrub nurse working with Cutrite was questioned, she remembered that he had used the syringe, but when it was included in the count at the conclusion of surgery, she didn't think about the protective sheath, which must certainly have been on it.

"Let's get Mrs. Jameson back into surgery," said Straight. We'll tell her we have to check her incision and deep sutures. She'll never know we're really looking for the needle cover."

"Too late," responded the supervisor, "she went home the day before yesterday."

Damn, thought Straight. "Have you talked to Cutrite?"

The supervisor nodded affirmatively. "He won't consider telling Mrs. Jameson that there might be a problem and readmitting her," she said. "He warned us not to do anything, either," she added. "Cutrite claims it cannot possibly hurt her. Except for some discomfort, she'll never know it's there."

Straight called the chief of surgery and asked hypothetically about the consequences of leaving a small plastic cap in a patient's belly. The chief knew something was up, but didn't pursue it. He simply replied that it was likely there would be occasional discomfort, but probably no life-threatening consequences. "Although," he added, "one can never be sure."

Straight liked working at Hopewell Hospital and didn't relish crossing swords with Cutrite, who had declined professionally but was politically powerful. Straight had resisted fingernail biting for years, but that old habit was suddenly overwhelming.

Questions

1. What should Straight do? Why?
2. What sources of guidance can Straight use?
3. What steps should be taken to avoid similar problems in the future?
4. Is there anything disturbing about the attitudes of the operating room supervisor and chief of surgery? Explain.

CASE STUDY 4: IS THIS THE MOST EFFICIENT WAY?

Joan Vinson, the hospital COO, hated giving depositions. Plaintiffs' lawyers probed and pushed and leapt at any word that might give them an advantage. When the deposition was over she always felt wrung out, and there was a lingering feeling, a subtle implication, that somehow she was dishonest.

The case involved a claim that an emergency department (ED) triage nurse had misjudged the severity of a patient's arm injury. Delay in treatment allegedly exacerbated the injury and the plaintiff had a slight, permanent movement deficit. Usually this would not result in a lawsuit, but he was a semi-professional stock car driver and the complaint alleged the injury would make him less likely to win. The complaint demanded $50,000 in damages.

The hospital attorney told Vinson that proving damages would be very difficult and the case would probably settle for less than half the requested amount. He recommended, however, moving as slowly as possible. This would increase the plaintiff's attorney's expenses (it was a contingency case) and would make him more willing to settle.

Vinson had no doubt the triage nurse had erred. It had been a very busy night in the ED. The triage nurse was working a double shift because her replacement called in sick. When the plaintiff came to the ED the nurse had been working for 14 hours and was exhausted.

Vinson wanted to settle the suit, but she felt compelled to follow the attorney's advice. It just seemed to her that there had to be a better way to handle such problems, especially when liability wasn't really an issue.

Questions

1. What policy issue is present here? Describe the role of in-house or retainer counsel in a case such as this. Might either have a conflict of interest? Why?
2. Distinguish cases in which HSO staff are clearly negligent from those in which reasonable persons could disagree. What are the negative and positive aspects of contesting every case, regardless of merit?
3. What recommendations would you make to prevent the untoward event? Be prepared to support them.
4. Based on personal experience or facts known to you, describe an untoward event resulting from interacting with an HSO. What was the result? Did the HSO act honorably?

NOTES

1. Aristotle. *Politics,* translated by Benjamin Jowett, 287. New York: The Modern Library, 1943.
2. *United States v. Shreveport Grain and Elevator Company,* 287 U.S. 77 (1932).
3. *Black's law dictionary,* 5th ed., 1261. St. Paul, MN: West Publishing Co., 1979.
4. *Black's law dictionary,* 1174.
5. Bodenheimer, Edgar. *Jurisprudence: The philosophy and method of the law,* rev. ed., 340. Cambridge, MA: Harvard University Press, 1974.
6. Keeton, W. Page, ed. *Prosser and Keeton on the law of torts,* 5th ed., 2. St. Paul, MN: West Publishing Co., 1984.
7. Keeton, *Prosser and Keeton,* 2.
8. Keeton, *Prosser and Keeton,* 655–656.
9. Southwick, Arthur F. *The law of hospital and health care administration,* 352. Ann Arbor, MI: Health Administration Press, 1978.
10. Prosser, William L. *Handbook of the law of torts,* 4th ed., 31. St. Paul, MN: West Publishing Co., 1971.
11. *Black's law dictionary,* 930.
12. American jurisprudence, 2nd ed., Supplement, Section 218, Vol. 61, March 1989.
13. Southwick, Arthur F. *The law of hospital and health care administration,* 2d ed., 69. Ann Arbor, MI: Health Administration Press, 1988.
14. *Landeros v. Flood,* 17 Cal. 3d 399 (1976).
15. U.S. Department of Health, Education, and Welfare. *Report of the Secretary's Commission on Medical Malpractice,* 14. Washington, D.C.: U.S. Government Printing Office, 1973.
16. Kosterlitz, Julie. Malpractice morass. *National Journal* 23 (July 6, 1991): 1683.
17. Malpractice: Calm before the storm? *Medicine & Health Perspectives* 43 (September 18, 1989): 37.
18. Physician-malpractice claims show increase for first time in six years. *AHA News* 27 (May 13, 1991): 3.
19. Localio, A. Russell, Ann G. Lawthers, Troyen A. Brennan, Nan M. Laird, Liesi E. Hebert, Lynn M. Peterson, Joseph P. Newhouse, Paul C. Weiler, and Howard H. Hiatt. Relation between malpractice claims and adverse events due to negligence: Results of the Harvard Medical

Practice Study III. *New England Journal of Medicine* 325 (July 25, 1991): 249.

20. Grant, Ruth Ann. Tinkering on tort reform not enough to solve problem: Experts. *AHA News* 27 (March 18, 1991): 2.

21. Grant, Tinkering on tort reform, 5.

22. Kosterlitz, Malpractice morass, 1682–1686.

23. Disciplinary actions against physicians in 1990 declined 4.8%. *AHA News* 27 (May 27, 1991): 3.

24. Disciplinary acts against physicians. *Washington Post* Health Section (June 18, 1991).

25. Meyers, Allan R. 'Lumping it': The hidden denominator of the medical malpractice crisis. *American Journal of Public Health* 77 (December 1987): 1547.

26. Malpractice: Calm before the storm?

27. Smith, Lee. A cure for what ails medical care. *Fortune* (July 1, 1991): 59.

28. U.S. Department of Health, Education, and Welfare, *Report of the Secretary's Commission,* 14.

29. Hudson, Terese. Experts disagree over the cost of defensive medicine. *Hospitals* 64 (August 5, 1990): 74.

30. Southwick, *Law of hospital and health care administration,* 2d ed., 580.

31. AIDS-related lawsuits will continue to rise, report shows. *AHA News* 26 (April 16, 1990): 3.

32. Stein, Robert E. The Americans with Disabilities Act of 1990. *Arbitration Journal* 46 (June 1991): 6–7.

33. Stein, Americans with Disabilities, 13–14.

34. Stein, Americans with Disabilities, 6–7.

35. *Arline v. School Board of Nassau County, Florida* 107 S.Ct. 1123 (1987).

36. Tegtmeier, James W. Ethics and AIDS: A summary of the law and a critical analysis of the individual physician's ethical duty to treat. *American Journal of Law and Medicine* 16 (1990): 251–252.

37. Beyer, Ronald, and Larry Gostin. Legal and ethical issues relating to AIDS. *Bulletin of the Pan American Health Organization* 24 (1990): 456.

38. Beyer and Gostin, Legal and ethical, 456.

39. Beyer and Gostin, Legal and ethical, 457.

40. Beyer and Gostin, Legal and ethical, 458–459.

41. *Tarasoff v. Regents of the State of California,* 17 Cal. 3d 342 (1976).

42. Beyer and Gostin, Legal and ethical, 461–462.

43. Posner, Richard A. *Antitrust law: An economic perspective,* 23. Chicago: University of Chicago Press, 1976.

44. *AMA v. United States,* 130 F. 2d 233, (D.C. Cir. 1942); aff'd, 317 U.S. 519 (1943).

45. Bierig, Jack R. Antitrust for physicians. In *Physician's survival guide: Legal pitfalls and solutions* (compilation of articles), 63–84. Chicago: American Medical Association and National Health Lawyers Association, 1991.

46. *Hospital Building Co. v. Trustees of Rex Hospital,* 425 U.S. 738 (1976).

47. Southwick, *Law of hospital and health care administration,* 2d ed., 227–229.

48. Southwick, *Law of hospital and health care administration,* 2d ed., 250.

49. *United States v. Rockford Memorial Corp.,* 898 F. 2d 1278 (7th Cir. 1990); *cert. denied,* 111 S. Ct. 295 (1990).

50. *United States v. Carilion Health Systems, Community Hospital of Roanoke Valley,* 707 F. Supp. 840 (W.D. Va, 1989); *aff'd without opinion,* 892 F. 2d 1042 (4th Cir. 1989).

51. Higgins, Daniel B. *Rockford* will not end hospital mergers. *Hospitals* 65 (April 5, 1991): 76.

52. *Patrick v. Burget,* 800 F. 2d 1498 (9th Cir. 1986); *reversed,* 486 U.S. 94 (1988); *rehearing denied,* 487 U.S. 1243 (1988).

53. *Austin v. McNamara,* 731 F. Supp. 934 (C.D. Cal. 1990).

54. Rushford, Greg. Data bank has a deficit. *Legal Times* 13 (April 22, 1991): 1.

55. McGinn, Paul R. U.S. vows vigilance on health antitrust. *American Medical News* 33 (October 26, 1990): 1.

56. McGinn, Paul R. Next antitrust target—IPAs. *American Medical News* 33 (October 26, 1990): 30.

57. Burda, David. Study by state attorneys general finds at least 70 antitrust cases in healthcare since 1985. *Modern Healthcare* 20 (December 17, 1990): 41.

58. Havighurst, Clark C. *Health care law and policy: Readings, notes, and questions,* 204. Westbury, NY: The Foundation Press, Inc., 1988.

59. Havighurst, *Health care law,* 204–205.

60. Hudson, Terese. Not-for-profit hospitals fight tax-exempt challenges. *Hospitals* 64 (October 20, 1990): 36.

61. Hudson, Not-for-profit hospitals, 36.

62. Henry, Wayne. Tax-exempt challenges warrant hospitals' attention. *Healthcare Financial Management* 45 (January 1991): 32

63. Henry, Tax-exempt challenges, 30, 32.

64. Henry, Tax-exempt challenges, 32.

65. Henry, Tax-exempt challenges, 32.

66. Carlin, Peter E. Medical malpractice pre-trial screening panels: A review of the evidence. *Intergovernmental Health Policy Project* (newsletter) (October 30, 1980): 13.

67. Carlin, Medical malpractice pre-trial, 15.

68. Macchiaroli, Jean A. Proposed model legislation to cure judicial ills. *George Washington Law Review* 58 (January 1990): 186.

69. Macchiaroli, Proposed model legislation, 186.

70. Macchiaroli, Proposed model legislation, 188.

71. Macchiaroli, Proposed model legislation, 186.

BIBLIOGRAPHY

American Medical Association and National Health Lawyers Association, *Physician's survival guide: Legal pitfalls and solutions.* Chicago, 1991.

Beyer, Ronald, and Larry Gostin. Legal and ethical issues relating to AIDS. *Bulletin of the Pan American Health Organization* 24 (1990): 454–468.

Bodenheimer, Edgar. *Jurisprudence: The philosophy and method of the law,* rev. ed., Cambridge, MA: Harvard University Press, 1974.

Corbin, Arthur L. *Corbin on contracts.* St. Paul, MN: West Publishing Co., 1952.

Havighurst, Clark C. *Health care law and policy: Readings, notes, and questions.* Westbury, NY: The Foundation Press, Inc., 1988.

Henry, Wayne. Tax-exempt challenges warrant hospitals' attention. *Healthcare Financial Management* 45 (January 1991): 30, 32, 34–38.

HIV-infected physicians and the practice of seriously invasive procedures. *Hastings Center Report* 19 (January–February 1989): 32–39.

Keeton, W. Page, ed. *Prosser and Keeton on the law of torts,* 5th ed. St. Paul, MN: West Publishing Co., 1984.

Localio, A. Russell, Ann G. Lawthers, Troyen A. Brennan, Nan M. Laird, Liesi E. Hebert, Lynn M. Peterson, Joseph P. Newhouse, Paul C. Weiler, and Howard H. Hiatt. Relation between malpractice claims and adverse events due to negligence: Results of the Harvard Medical Practice Study III. *New England Journal of Medicine* 325 (July 25, 1991): 245–251.

Macchiaroli, Jean A. Proposed model legislation to cure judicial ills. *George Washington Law Review* 58 (January 1990): 181–260.

Meyers, Allan R. 'Lumping it': The hidden denominator of the medical malpractice crisis. *American Journal of Public Health* 77 (December 1987): 1544–1548.

Posner, Richard A. *Antitrust law: An economic perspective.* Chicago: University of Chicago Press, 1976.

Recommendations for preventing transmission of human immunodeficiency virus and hepatitis B virus to patients during exposure-prone invasive procedures. *Morbidity and Mortality Weekly Report* 40 (July 12, 1991): 1–8.

Southwick, Arthur F. *The law of hospital and health care administration,* 2d ed. Ann Arbor, MI: Health Administration Press, 1988.

Stein, Robert E. The Americans with Disabilities Act of 1990. *Arbitration Journal* 46 (June 1991): 6–15.

Tegtmeier, James W. Ethics and AIDS: A summary of the law and a critical analysis of the individual physician's ethical duty to treat. *American Journal of Law and Medicine* 16 (1990): 249–276.

U.S. Department of Health, Education, and Welfare. *Report of the Secretary's Commission on Medical Malpractice.* Washington, D.C., U.S. Government Printing Office, 1973.

5 / Health Services Technology

*Some technologies increase costs. Some
technologies decrease costs. And some technologies
do both. Some raise costs in the short run, but
save dollars over the full course of treatment;
others lower costs by moving care to nonhospital
settings, but increase costs overall because care is
more accessible and used more often.*

*How technology affects costs depends on the
technology, where it is used, and—above all—
on how the concepts of costs and benefits are
defined. Indeed, that is the challenge.*

Frank E. Samuel, Jr., President, Health
Industry Manufacturers Association[1]

The advancement and diffusion of technology are among the most controversial developments in the provision of health care. Technological innovations have given health services providers the means to diagnose and treat an increasing number of problems and illnesses. These same advances have been criticized, however, for their effect on the practice of medicine and on national health care expenditures, which increased from almost $27 billion in 1960 to more than $800 billion in the 1990s and which are expected to be more than $1.6 trillion by the end of the decade.

The dramatic rise in health care costs in the past 30 years is partly related to the proliferation of new technologies, the increased use of existing tests and procedures including attendant personnel, and financing of the innovations. That part of the rise in health care costs attributable to utilization of technology is uncertain. One estimate suggests that as much as 50% of the rise in total health care expenditures in recent years resulted from use of new technologies and overuse of existing ones.[2] Estimates as high as 70% have been made.[3] Health care economists have conceptualized the issues in several ways. One theory examines the impact of technology on hospital costs as measured by discrete units such as the labor and nonlabor inputs of using technology. A second theory analyzes costs associated with specific hospital-based technologies. A third examines the impact of technology on treatment of specific conditions and types of illnesses over time. A fourth measures the impact of technology on total health care expenditures. One conclusion of this body of research is that utilizing technology increased the intensity of resources used to treat individual cases, and this increased costs.[4] Some evidence suggests that increased intensity also has been due to introduction of new technologies used on new categories of patients, in addition to the use of existing technologies in new ways.[5] More recent analysis concludes that technological change (new procedures, capabilities, and products) is the primary explanation of the historical increase in expenditure and in the measured price indices.[6]

Medical technology is defined as "any discrete and identifiable regimen or modality used to diagnose and treat illness, prevent disease, maintain patient well-being, or facilitate the provision of health services."[7] By this definition medical technology ranges from biologicals and pharmaceuticals, computed tomography (CT) scanners, transplants, and intensive care units to coronary artery bypass procedures and patient billing computers and other systems used to operate and manage HSOs. Medical technology would also include managerial technologies such as how care is organized and provided (e.g., home care) or may include other types of providers (e.g., physician assistants or nurse-practitioners), but the influence of these developments on management of HSOs is not considered here.

A useful typology categorizes medical technologies by their characteristics. Table 5.1 shows these relationships. It is notable that, overwhelmingly, the technologies listed are delivered to persons who are hospital inpatients. Increasingly, however, such technologies can be delivered in nonhospital and outpatient settings. The cost implications are obvious.

Another way to describe medical technology is based on charge to the user. Technologies such as laboratory tests, radiographs, and other ancillary services typically costing from $2 to $100 are considered low in cost compared to CT scans and organ transplantation, which are high in cost, ranging from $200 to $30,000–$200,000+, respectively. Much of the controversy over increasing costs focuses on high-cost technologies, but inexpensive technologies raise similar concerns because they are used in high volume and may be labor intensive. Studies of data from the 1950s and 1960s showed that the primary cost-raising changes had been rapid increases in use of relatively low-cost ancillary services, such as laboratories and x-rays, which are commonly called "little ticket" technologies. Data from the 1970s and 1980s, however, showed that the use of "little ticket" technologies hardly changed, but that several new and expensive "big ticket" technologies came into common use and raised costs considerably.[8]

Despite differences in how technologies are described, there is no question that the trend is toward increased development and use of technology. It is important to examine the factors behind this trend, and their effect not only on the system as a whole but on management of individual HSOs.

Table 5.1. Types of medical technologies

Type	Examples
Diagnostic	CT scanner Fetal monitor Computerized electrocardiography Automated clinical labs MRI Ambulatory blood pressure monitor
Survival (life saving)	Intensive care unit Cardiopulmonary resuscitation Bone marrow transplant Liver transplant Autologous bone marrow transplant
Illness management	Renal dialysis Pacemaker PTCA (angioplasty) Stereotactic cingulotomy (psychosurgery)
Cure	Hip joint replacement Organ transplant Lithotripter
Prevention	Implantable automatic cardioverter-defibrillator Pediatric orthopedic repair Diet control for phenylketonuria Vaccines for immunization
System management	Medical information systems Telemedicine

Source: Rosenthal, Gerald. Anticipating the costs and benefits of new technology: A typology for policy. In *Medical technology: The culprit behind health care costs?* Pub. No. (PHS) 79-3216, 79. Washington, D.C.: U.S. Government Printing Office, 1979, as updated using *The Medicare Coverage Process* (National Advisory Council on Health Care Technology Assessment, Office of the Assistant Secretary for Health, Department of Health and Human Services, [September 14, 1988]: Appendix I).

HISTORY AND BACKGROUND

Historically, the technology of modern medicine can be traced to the end of the 19th century. The most significant developments in the diagnosis, treatment, and management of disease, however, date from the 1950s, concomitant with the increasing prominence of the National Institutes of Health (NIH). The growth of NIH was sparked by a renewed interest in curing disease, which was in turn prompted by new knowledge in the basic sciences. By the 1950s, immunizations to fight infectious diseases and drug therapies to treat noninfectious conditions such as pernicious anemia, diabetes, gout, and hyperthyroidism were readily available. It was hoped that new technologies could be developed to cure or prevent chronic and life-threatening diseases such as cancer, heart disease, and stroke.

TYPES OF TECHNOLOGIES

Definitive Technologies

Technologies are described as definitive when they yield a cure or prevention that is directed at the central disease agent or mechanism.[9] Vaccines that prevent diseases are the clearest example. Some progress has been made in the ability to prevent cardiovascular disease, for example, but research in cancer, heart disease, and stroke has yielded primarily diagnostic and management technologies (halfway or add-on technologies) as opposed to curative or definitive technologies. Figure 5.1 illustrates availability of management and definitive technologies for a range of health conditions.

Halfway Technologies

Overwhelmingly, technologies are "halfway" or "add-on" technologies. Unlike technological innovations in other fields that increase productivity or improve performance, often at lower cost, innovations in medical care generally add on or generate additional costs while accomplishing something not previously possible.[10] A recent example of a halfway technology is brain electrical activity mapping (BEAM). Although BEAM testing provides a means of imaging the brain similar to that provided by CT scanners, positron emission tomography, and magnetic resonance imaging (MRI) scans, the information received from BEAM testing will improve a clinician's ability to diagnose an abnormality; it is used in addition to, not in place of, other types of imaging.[11]

Hospitals are especially quick to add such technology. No hospitals reported having MRI machines in 1984; by 1988, 10.6% had them.[12] This speed of generalization of MRI technology is astounding when one considers that an MRI unit may cost $1.5 million to buy and $200,000 to install.[13] In early 1991, the ability to measure and map sources of electrical activity in the heart, the neuromuscular system, and especially the brain was substantially enhanced with the introduction of magnetic source imaging (MSI). CT and MRI are useful to diagnose and treat pathologies that leave structural lesions, but MSI provides important supplemental information. MSI units cost $2 million,[14] but hospitals will undoubtedly be eager to purchase them because of the new diagnostic information they can provide.

In a 1990 survey, ultrasound was the type of equipment most likely to be found in hospitals— 91.1% reported having it. The top categories of technology that hospitals did not own but planned to acquire included MRI, neodymium-yttrium-aluminum-garnet lasers, and cardiac catheterization laboratories.[15] However, recently published data support earlier findings that hospitals are slow to abandon old (established) diagnostic technology even when newer technology could replace it.[16]

Competing Technologies

Another dimension of the use of technology has to do with competing types that may be equally effective but have very different costs. A current example is the controversy between the throm-

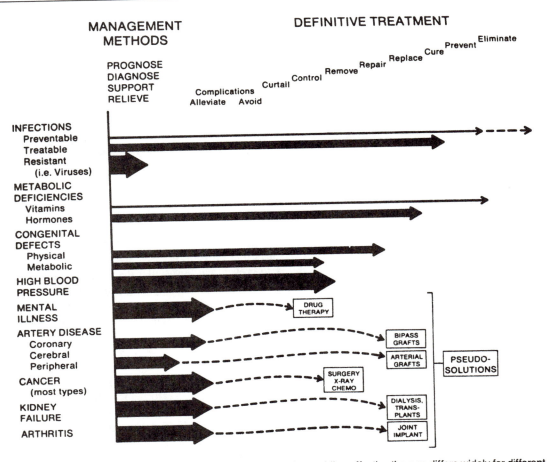

Figure 5.1. Advances in medical technology. Note: Progress in providing effective therapy differs widely for different conditions. For example, prevention, cure, and control have been attained for many infections. Many congenital malformations can be corrected by surgery, and high blood pressure can be effectively controlled. For conditions lacking definitive therapy, sophisticated technologies have been developed to replace or supplement the structure and function of affected organs. These technical triumphs should be regarded as pseudosolutions of value to current patients but not really directed toward the underlying causes and cures that must ultimately be developed for the benefit of future generations. (From Rushmer, Robert F. Technological resources for health. In *Introduction to health services,* edited by Stephen J. Williams and Paul R. Torrens, 2d ed., 298. New York: John Wiley & Sons, 1984; reprinted by permission. Delmar Publishers, Inc., Copyright 1984.)

bolytic agents, streptokinase and tissue-plasminogen activator (tPA), both of which are used to dissolve blood clots in persons with heart attacks. Streptokinase costs less than $200 per treatment, whereas tPA costs $2,200. Research shows that the two drugs produce similar results, but a large study found streptokinase to be safer because it poses a lower risk of stroke, the major potential side effect of treatment.[17] It has been suggested, however, that strong marketing efforts by the manufacturer of tPA will keep physicians convinced that it is superior.[18]

Cost-Saving Technologies

Few new technologies prevent disease either on an individual basis or for large groups of people (e.g., use of vaccines to protect future generations). Nonetheless, many reduce costs, especially when compared to old technologies used to treat the same disease. Examples include coronary angioplasty, arthroscopy, implantable infusion pumps, and lasers. These technologies may be used as halfway (add-on) therapies, but to the extent that they replace more costly treatment, the result will be lower costs to the patient and to the health services system. In this regard, costs and benefits are defined broadly and include aspects such as hospitalization and sick days avoided, early return to work, and quality of life, both short and long term. Any assessment of a technology must include these dimensions.[19]

EFFECT OF TECHNOLOGY ON HEALTH STATUS

Although halfway technologies improve diagnosis and management of many diseases (e.g., a CT scan might shorten a hospital stay and save other resources), their effect on health status is controversial. The modest increase in life expectancy from 1964 to 1985 of only 2.8 years for a 45-year-old male suggests that technological advances in medical care have had little effect on longevity. Alarming is the negative change in disability-free years, which are projected to *decline* by 7.3 years for a male born in 1964. It is argued that the decrease in disability-free years resulted from neglect of public health issues.[20] It also has been suggested that increased longevity may result from technological progress, but that it may not be reflected in standard health status statistics, such as life expectancy, until well into the future.[21] Notable, too, is that a cause of mortality may decline for no identifiable reason. For example, the death rate from coronary heart disease declined by about 40% from 1968 to 1987.[22]

Trying to credit technological advances with changes in health status indicators such as morbidity and disability raises other problems. It is paradoxical that saving a life through technological intervention may actually increase morbidity and disability. Technological advances may also improve the quality of life for persons with certain diseases. An example is a genetically engineered new drug for anemia that will be one of the most expensive drugs covered by Medicare. Epoetin will help 75,000 kidney dialysis patients at a cost of $500 million, and can be used to treat other causes of anemia.[23] Similarly, the acquired immunodeficiency syndrome (AIDS) epidemic has stimulated efforts to develop an artificial blood to substitute as a gas transporter carrying oxygen to the tissues and carbon dioxide back to the lungs. Such products are close to general availability, but the cost is expected to be about 50% higher than the cost of natural blood.[24] However, the advantages in protecting patients from AIDS, as well as other blood-borne diseases such as hepatitis, are obvious. Another example of a halfway technology is transplants. In 1989, 8,886 kidney, 2,160 liver, 1,673 heart, 412 pancreas, 89 lung, and 70 heart-lung transplants were performed.[25] Such halfway technologies improve the health status of patients but also increase health care costs considerably.

FORCES AFFECTING DEVELOPMENT AND DIFFUSION OF TECHNOLOGY

Medical Education and Practice

Among the most important factors that encouraged development and diffusion of technology after World War II were changes in medical training and the practice of medicine. Biomedical research programs funded through the NIH provided much of the impetus for medical schools to undertake research in the medical subspecialties, which led to growth of specialty departments within academic medical centers. Increasingly, medical school graduates went on to postgraduate training and then to practice in a medical specialty.

In 1949, 64% of physicians were general practitioners.[26] By 1965, 24% were general practitioners; by 1989 only 4% were.[27] Some physicians who are classified as specialists have many "generalist" functions and deliver significant amounts of primary care: internists (internal medicine), family practitioners, and pediatricians. Adding these three groups to the percentage who are general practitioners brings the total number of general care physicians to only 34.5%. This means that approximately two thirds of U.S. physicians are specialists.[28] Federal legislation in the 1970s sought to address this increasing imbalance in specialty distribution, but the technological focus of postgraduate medical training was unaffected. The almost exclusive specialty focus of residency training programs in acute care hospitals heightens the emphasis on technology.

Increased specialization in medical education meant physicians were trained to use technologic advances in their fields. Not surprisingly, they expected to use the same technologies in their practices. This desire to have state-of-the-art technology available and to use it as necessary, despite the cost, is called the technological imperative. Evidence of the technological imperative is most apparent in acute care hospitals and explains the proliferation of highly specialized technology in that setting. From the late 1960s to 1975, plant assets in community hospitals, as measured by the American Hospital Association (AHA), rose from an average of $20,000 per bed to an average of $33,440.[29] The average increased to $62,816 by 1977.[30] By 1989, the 50th percentile of net property, plant, and equipment was $95,826 per bed.[31] Contributing to this change has been the decline in the number of beds and the increase in acuity of illness of patients. The need to attract and retain physicians exaggerates the interest in having various technologies and increases the pressure to acquire, operate, maintain, and ensure their safe use.

The almost universal presence of technology does not suggest, however, that it is applied similarly nationwide. There are wide geographic variations in the treatments given to patients with the same diagnoses. These variations range from how often patients are admitted to an acute care hospital and how long they stay once there to whether, for example, they receive coronary artery bypass surgery when they have angina or are treated with a medical regimen of medication and modified diet. Another example of variation is the finding that physicians who have practiced longer than 15 years have a significantly greater number of inappropriate hospital admissions.[32] Finding wide variations in practice patterns raises doubts about medicine's scientific certainty and whether low-technology, less interventionist (as well as less expensive) treatments might not be equally effective as high-technology, more interventionist treatments. Understanding physician practice patterns and variation, as well as determining efficacy, will enable all HSOs to deliver medical services more efficiently and effectively.

Reimbursement

Third-Party Payment   Central to diffusion of technological advances into medical practice and the existence of the technological imperative was the availability of third-party reimbursement for medical services. In the traditional fee-for-service model of medical practice, the decision to utilize new technologies is usually made by individual physicians on the basis of findings that the technology yields benefit with a low probability of harm. Unlike other industries, innovations in medical technology have been judged not primarily on the basis of performing some function better or more efficiently, but rather on whether they will yield some benefit to individual patient care. Similarly, decisions to provide reimbursement for new technologies have been based on whether they are accepted and used by physicians. Manufacturers' prices for new technologies, particularly drugs and devices, tend to be high in order to recover research and development costs. Charges by HSOs at the point of delivery tend to be high to compensate for the skill and expertise involved in learning and offering a technology, as well as recovering the capital costs of acquiring it. Once established in the reimbursement system, these charges tended to remain high even after initial costs have been recovered.[33]

Assured payment for tests and procedures under cost-based reimbursement allowed HSOs to acquire technology knowing that the costs of capital investment and operation would be recovered. Consequently, in the past there were few incentives to evaluate the cost effectiveness of new technologies. Acquisition of technology is stimulated by the need for HSOs to attract both physicians and patients.

Diagnosis-Related Groups   In late 1983, the payment for Medicare patients in acute care hospitals was changed from cost-based reimbursement to a prospective payment system based on diagnosis-related groups (DRGs). The details of DRGs were discussed in Chapter 2, "The Health Care Delivery System." As noted, this program provides the incentive for acute care hospitals to do less, not more—the opposite of retrospective, cost-based reimbursement. Reimbursement is calculated using average cost per case. This should create an incentive to carefully evaluate acquisition of new technology, to use it more efficiently in treating individual patients as well as groups of similar cases, and to select cost-saving technologies whenever possible.

It was thought that hospitals providing a service infrequently would be unable to compete with those providing it frequently. In theory, the latter group would have lower average unit costs. It was also believed that since costs associated with using technology are not reimbursed separately, hospitals would have few incentives to adopt a new technology that increases cost per case by adding new operational costs. At this point, however, hospitals' acquisition and use of technology appears to be unchanged. It may be that only when Medicare payments are further reduced will the effect of DRGs on technology be felt.

Congress continues to try to reduce Medicare costs, primarily by reducing the DRG payment. It appears that those who feared the DRG system would stifle diffusion of new technology and adversely affect patient care were wrong; those who predicted that a hospital's need to be competitive and maintain admissions levels would necessitate acquiring technology were correct. Regardless, the long term influence of DRGs on hospitals and their use of technology remains to be seen. The real effect of DRGs may not match what was intended.[34]

Health Care Financing Administration In the late 1980s, the Health Care Financing Administration (HCFA) decided to apply more uniform and stringent standards by which to judge appropriateness of use of technology. In early 1989, HCFA issued proposed regulations to define for the first time the criteria "reasonable" and "necessary." Medicare uses these words to describe the new technology and procedures for which it will pay. The regulations state that, to be reasonable and necessary, the new technology and procedures must be "safe, effective, noninvestigational, and appropriate."[35] The regulations define these words in detail. New technologies and procedures meeting these criteria receive the significant financial endorsement of the federal government and are certain to be available in HSOs serving Medicare patients. The states chronically underfund Medicaid (state programs for the indigent that receive significant federal monies), and this makes it noteworthy that considerable resources are devoted to transplants. In 1988, only one state provided none of the seven types of transplant procedures covered (kidney, cornea, bone marrow, liver, heart, heart-lung, and pancreas); nine states provided all of them.[36]

The Public

A third force influencing diffusion of technology has been those benefiting from it—the public. Protected by third-party reimbursement from experiencing the direct costs of using state-of-the-art technology, patients, like physicians, believe themselves entitled to it. The practice of highly technical and specialty-oriented medicine, coupled with widely publicized advances in medical care, fostered patients' expectations that a technology is available to diagnose and treat every problem and that quality medical care necessarily involves extensive technology. A 1982 survey found that 51% of all respondents were unwilling "to limit the opportunities for people to use expensive modern technology"; an additional 14% were uncertain.[37] Thus, economically protected by third-party reimbursement, most patients have shared with physicians the expectation that all possible technologies should be available. Given this context, it is apparent that limiting use of technology will create unacceptable threats to the autonomy of patients and providers.

Competitive Environment

An increasingly important fourth force, especially in diffusion of technology, is competition. Pressures for acute care hospitals, as an example, to compete for physicians and patients push them to acquire and offer technology. This suggests that costs in competitive geographic areas will be higher than in noncompetitive areas. One study found that average costs per admission were 26% higher in the most competitive markets than in hospitals with no competitors within 16 miles.[38]

Discussion of a competitive environment in health services usually involves competition among HSOs. Increasingly, however, there are two additional important dimensions of competition: that between physicians and HSOs, and that among various physician specialties. Both are a function of technology.

Much new technology is portable. This allows physicians to bypass the acute care hospital, where such technology typically would have been located in the past. A common example is medical imaging. Physicians are unconstrained by regulations such as certificate-of-need requirements, and establishing an imaging center is a matter of raising capital and finding a location. Abuses have caused some states to regulate self-referrals, defined as physicians sending patients to facilities in which they have an ownership interest. Federal law prohibits physicians from referring Medicare and Medicaid patients to clinical laboratories in which they have an ownership interest. Legislation to expand the prohibition is being considered.

New technology, some of it less expensive to buy and less costly to operate, has blurred the traditional lines of various physician specialties and caused fierce competition among them. Ultrasound, lasers, laboratories, and mammography are examples. As evidence of this problem, a 1988 study by the American College of Radiology found that 60% of all imaging studies are done outside the hospital by nonradiologists.[39] This development has major implications for the specialties involved, as well as the potential to increase costs to the system.

FEDERAL GOVERNMENT
RESPONSES TO DIFFUSION OF TECHNOLOGY

As HSOs acquired increasing levels of technology, issues of cost, safety, and benefit emerged. It became clear that diffusion of new technology and its use had not been based on determining its cost–benefit ratio or cost effectiveness. Hospitals, especially, had not taken into account existing technological capabilities. In addition there had been no thorough examination of potential hazards associated with a technology. These concerns were the focus of federal legislation in the 1970s that sought to improve premarket evaluation of medical devices and influence utilization and acquisition of emerging technologies, particularly in acute care hospitals. The federal Medical Device Act, professional standards review organizations, certificates of need, and establishment of the congressional Office of Technology Assessment and the Department of Health and Human Services's (DHHS) National Center for Health Care Technology were the result.

Food and Drug Administration

Although the Food and Drug Administration (FDA) has been involved in premarket approval of drugs since 1962, evidence of the safety and efficacy of other medical technologies had not been required. The Medical Device Act Amendments of 1976 amended the Food, Drug, and Cosmetic Act to extend the FDA's premarket approval process to medical devices divided into three classes. The most stringent regulation (Class III) applies to devices that support life, prevent health impairment, or prevent an unreasonable risk of illness or injury. Manufacturers must obtain FDA approval before such devices may be marketed, a procedure that requires evidence of safety and efficacy.[40] FDA control of marketing new drugs and devices has been criticized as unnecessarily impeding introduction of technological innovations because of the time and money required to conduct clinical trials and obtain licensing. In the late 1980s, pressure on the FDA from those wanting rapid access to new drugs for treating the AIDS virus caused a reconsideration of FDA review processes, especially as they applied to drugs potentially beneficial in treating fatal illnesses.

Concomitant with greater regulation of medical devices has been the increased application of stricter product liability standards for medical devices. HSOs can be liable for defects in devices that are unknown to the manufacturer. HSOs may be responsible for going beyond the maintenance recommendations of the manufacturer, if necessary, and alerting the FDA about experience contrary to that reported by the manufacturer.[41] The potential for liability was enhanced when the Safe Medical Devices Act of 1990 (PL 101-629) codified the need for HSOs to report device-related problems to the manufacturers and/or the FDA. Reporting covers any incident in which any medical device may have caused or contributed to a patient's death, serious illness, or serious injury. Medical device is defined very broadly by the FDA and there are significant penalties for failing to report as required.[42]

Professional Standards Review Organizations and Professional Review Organizations

A more complete history of professional standards review organizations (PSROs) and how they were replaced by professional review organizations (PROs) beginning in 1984 is included in Chapter 2. In the context of medical technology, however, PSROs were established in 1972 as part of federal and state efforts to control health care costs by reducing use of technology and reviewing actual utilization and regulating acquisition of new technology. PSROs were to ensure that Medicare (and Medicaid) services were "medically necessary, met professional standards of care, and were provided in the most economical setting possible consistent with quality care."[43] Initially, the focus of review was appropriateness of acute care hospital admission and length of stay. Later, the services provided were also reviewed.

PSRO effectiveness was hampered by Medicare's interpretation of "reasonable and necessary." Usually this concept means that, if a procedure is no longer experimental and is accepted by the local community, it is deemed to be reasonable and necessary. Historically, actual indications for use were decided by the PSROs.[44]

PROs have a similar role regarding application of technology. They review the professional activities of physicians, other practitioners, and institutional and noninstitutional providers in rendering services to Medicare (and Medicaid, if states choose) beneficiaries. The review focuses on the necessity and reasonableness of care, quality of care, and appropriateness of the setting. Decisions of the PRO are ordinarily binding for purposes of determining whether benefits should be paid. Hospitals must have a contract with a PRO as a condition of receiving payment under Medicare.[45]

One example of a controversial procedure is coronary artery bypass graft (CABG). In the early 1980s, costs for CABG ranged from $15,000 to $40,000 per procedure, including a surgical fee of $2,500–$5,000. A 1983 NIH study found that CABG was a common and overutilized procedure; it was estimated that 25,000 of the 200,000 CABG procedures performed annually could be eliminated without jeopardizing patient care.[46] A more recent assessment concluded that "surgical therapy improves prognosis in high-risk patients, but the advantage over medical therapy declines with longer followup."[47]

In early 1991, the DHHS contracted with four hospitals to provide CABG to Medicare patients on a fixed-fee basis that included physician and hospital costs. Rates paid to the hospitals range from $21,000 to $35,000 and are a savings of 5%–30%, depending on the hospital. Current rates for CABG range as high as $42,000.[48] Contracts designating hospitals to provide specific services to Medicare patients will increase as HCFA makes further efforts to reduce costs. Other payors will likely do the same.

Certificate of Need

Enactment of certificate of need (CON) and Section 1122 legislation by the states in conjunction with the National Health Planning and Resources Development Act of 1974 regulated acute care hospitals' acquisition of new technology (and construction) by mandating approval of capital expenditures. CON legislation varied by state, but required acute care hospitals to justify their need for technologies costing more than $100,000–$150,000. Legislation enacted in 1981 and federal regulations implemented in 1984 increased the limits to $400,000 for major medical equipment and $250,000 for purchase of new institutional services, although actual state levels could be lower. During the 1980s, however, a philosophical shift at the federal level toward increased competition substantially reduced the support for regulatory efforts such as CON. As federal support declined, so did the interest of the states. As noted in Chapter 2, by 1991 only 39 states continued to have some type of CON program.

Assumptions underlying CON and health planning legislation were that availability of technology invites use and potential abuse and that the cost of technology is paid by all users. The CT scanner is an early example of a technology that became controversial because it was widely available and allegedly overused. Newer technology such as MRI, and alleged overuse of cesarean sections, have taken the spotlight more recently. These examples illustrate the problem inherent in the first assumption underlying CON legislation—providing quality health care does not require extensive use of technology. This assumption conflicted with societal expectations that all available technology should be used.

CON legislation was criticized for several reasons. One criticism was the emphasis on high-cost technologies with no attention to low-cost technologies. High-volume use of low-cost technologies could have a significant effect on health care costs. Electronic fetal monitoring was an example of a widely used, low-cost technology whose capital cost excluded it from CON review.[49]

A second shortcoming of CON regulation was its failure to consider operating costs associated with installing and using a technology. In 1977, for example, it was estimated that technical and professional operating costs associated with a CT scanner were a minimum of $300,000 annually.[50] Third, CON was criticized for decreasing competition among institutions in a particular market. Regulation of acute care hospital services and types of equipment eliminated a major incentive to compete. Finally, CON covered and continues to cover only hospital purchases of technology. As technology became increasingly portable, free-standing HSOs such as imaging centers have become ubiquitous. Physicians are a major force in such efforts, which compete directly with hospitals. For example, New Jersey has almost four times as many MRI scanners outside hospitals (primarily owned by physicians) as in them.[51]

Regulation such as that in the CON program was important in decisions made by acute care hospitals to acquire new technology. Given the myriad of new devices and equipment being developed, however, HSOs generally, and acute care hospitals especially, have had little help in conducting extensive reviews, nor have they had access to information and data on the cost effectiveness of technology. In addition, CON failed to consider the role of the acute care hospital's medical staff in acquiring and utilizing technology, as well as the hospital's need to attract and retain physicians. In the short term, regulating hospitals' acquisition of new technology did little to change physicians' behavior or generate useful information on which to base decisions.

Technology Assessment

A fourth type of government action, this one nonregulatory, established federal activities to evaluate technology. Technology assessment is defined as evaluating medical technology for evidence of safety, efficacy, cost, cost effectiveness, and ethical and legal implications, both in absolute terms and by comparison with other competing technologies.[52] The Institute of Medicine of the National Academy of Sciences estimated that, in 1983, only 2.9% of national health expenditures by all sources were spent on technology assessment.[53] Expenditures for technology assessment are declining. It is estimated that in 1988 the budgets of the most prominent technology assessment programs, added to related activities of industry, and exclusive of clinical trials, totaled approximately $50 million.[54]

The congressional Office of Technology Assessment, authorized in 1972 and fully operational since 1974, includes a Health Program as one of its nine programs. The purpose of this program is to help Congress understand and plan for the consequences of applying technology. The studies undertaken are varied and include implications of medical technology, efficaciousness of specific medical procedures, uses of health education, and quality of medical care. A major focus is the policy implications of medical technology.[55]

Concern about proliferation of medical technology and its benefits, costs, and risks caused Congress to enact the Health Services Research, Health Statistics, and Health Care Technology Act of 1978. The National Center for Health Care Technology (NCHCT) was established in the Public Health Service of DHHS as a clearinghouse for information on medical technology and a source of information on the safety and efficacy of new technologies. The act specified that cost effectiveness be taken into account in certain research and assessment activities. NCHCT was to make recommendations to HCFA as to cost effectiveness, appropriateness, and medical validity of various technologies that might be reimbursed by Medicare and Medicaid.[56] NCHCT was defunded in 1981, however, and its role as advisor to HCFA was transferred to the Office of Health Technology Assessment of the National Center for Health Services Research.[57] This Center was reauthorized in 1987 as the National Center for Health Services Research and Health Care Technology Assessment.[58]

In 1989, new legislation established the Agency for Health Care Policy and Research (AHCPR) in the Public Health Service to replace the National Center for Health Services Research and Health Care Technology Assessment. AHCPR's mission is to enhance the quality of patient care services through improved knowledge that can be used in meeting health care needs. Its activities are to:

Develop a broad base of scientific research, methods, and data.
Demonstrate and evaluate new ways to organize, finance, and direct health care services to improve delivery, access, and outcomes.
Assess technologies being considered for reimbursement by federally funded programs.
Facilitate development of practice guidelines and standardized measures of quality care.
Promote utilization of health services research findings through information dissemination.[59]

The role of AHCPR in technology assessment is muted. The congressional Office of Technology Assessment is likely to remain the major governmental source of information about technology, but its activities are limited to advising Congress. It is noteworthy that, although both agencies focus on a rather narrow federal interest, their recommendations are commonly followed by other third-party payors—thus broadening their potential impact considerably.

The lack of comprehensive federal activities has led to the conclusion that

There currently is no broad mechanism or system to sponsor and support research pertinent to assessment of health care technologies as applied to the delivery of health care; or to link the stages that a technology traverses beginning with basic research and ending with application, diffusion, or ultimately, discontinuation; or to take the lead in appropriately linking quality assessment and technology assessment.[60]

There are several private-sector efforts to actually assess technology or to aid potential users and purchasers in decision making. These include programs of the American College of Physicians, the American Medical Association, National Blue Cross/Blue Shield Association, the Health Industry Manufacturers Association, and the American Hospital Association. In addition, several programs are located in academic centers and teaching hospitals.[61]

Figure 5.2 shows technology assessment methods using an input-process-outcome sequence. Within these general methods are randomized clinical trials, evaluating diagnostic technologies, series of consecutive cases, case studies, registers and data bases, sample surveys, epidemiolog-

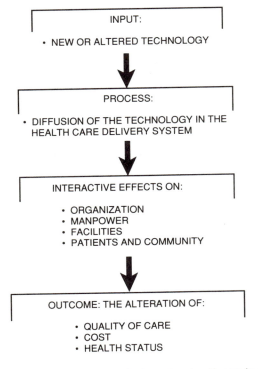

Figure 5.2. Technology assessment methods measure the impact on health care in an input-process-outcome sequence. (From Glasser, Jay H., and Richard S. Chrzanowski. Medical technology assessment: Adequate questions, appropriate methods, valuable answers. *Health Policy* 9 [1988]:269; reprinted by permission.)

ical methods, surveillance, quantitative synthesis methods (meta-analysis), group judgment methods,[62] cost-effectiveness and cost–benefit analyses, and mathematical modeling. Often forgotten, but important nonetheless, are the social and ethical issues of technology assessment.[63]

In summary, it is clear that assessing health care technology is not a high priority for either government or the private sector. This is difficult to understand given that hundreds of billions of dollars are spent in a health services system that is driven to a large extent by technology. The modest efforts being undertaken cannot develop the full range of information to comprehensively assist HSOs in using technology efficiently and effectively. HSO managers should be aware, however, that there are an estimated 50 technology assessment programs administered by government, industry, and professional societies.[64] This suggests that assessment, or at least some information about a technology, is probably available, but it may take some effort to find it.

HSO TECHNOLOGY DECISION MAKING

Assessment of technology at the HSO operating level is very different from that done by national public or private groups. Among the most important differences is that, when machine- and chemical-based technologies become generally available to HSOs, questions of safety and efficacy have been answered by the FDA. The efficacy and safety of new surgical techniques or innovative uses of already-approved machine- and chemical-based technologies, however, have few, if any, controls, except those applied by the HSO. Assessment of technology by the HSO includes: appropriateness for the patient population; financial feasibility, cost effectiveness, useful life, and operating costs; availability of trained technical personnel, expert physicians, and support services; availability of back-up technologies (e.g., open heart surgery if a coronary angioplasty fails); and limitations on reimbursement.[65]

Historically and presently, acute care hospitals have the most capital-intensive physical plants, and their physicians have been generally given great deference in decision making about equipment. This situation continues.[66] Physicians are believed to be technically trained to make decisions about acquiring technology, and a high level of technology is thought to be essential to attracting and retaining them. This has resulted in a situation in which hospitals sought to have everything.

Review and Planning

Partly in response to cost containment pressures and increased legal liability and partly because of competition, HSOs, especially acute care hospitals, are altering how they make decisions to acquire and use new technology and procedures and to ensure safe operation and maintenance. One approach has established annual review and financial planning processes for medical technologies separate from other capital expenditure decision making. This is crucial for financial planning because many major technologies become obsolete sooner than the useful life estimated for depreciation purposes. As a result, depreciation and replacement allowances rarely meet costs of replacement with more sophisticated equipment. If the rate of technological innovation and diffusion increases, this problem will become even more pressing. An example is the CT scanner, which sold for approximately $300,000 in 1973 with an estimated life of 5 years. Improved scanners costing more than $700,000 were available only 4 years later.[67] In 1990, prices for CT scanners ranged from $195,000 to $1.6 million.[68] Similarly, the cost of fluoroscopes with image intensifiers rose from $40,000 in 1965 to $200,000 in 1977.[69] By 1990, fluoroscopic units for cardiac catheterization cost as much as $600,000.[70]

The suggestion that hospitals develop a strategic technology plan is advice applicable to other HSOs. The purpose of such a plan is to guide technology acquisition, clinical staff development, and market strategies. The plan assesses emerging medical technology in a 5- and 10-year time frame and identifies the technology niches in which the HSO should focus its professional staff development and market strategies.[71]

Technology Evaluation and Acquisition Methods

An approach to decision making about technology was developed by the AHA and the Center for Health Services Research at the University of California, Los Angeles. The Technology Evaluation and Acquisition Methods (TEAM) assessment provided a way of organizing a review process, determining participation, and developing the criteria to be used. The process addressed what investigators identified as the four common problems acute care hospitals faced in evaluating and acquiring technology: treating requests for medical technology similar to requests for other capital expenditures; absence of multidisciplinary staff participation in hospital planning and evaluation of medical equipment requests; sporadic and unorganized physician participation in acquisition decisions; and reliance on the same staff members who request equipment to provide assessment of need and feasibility.[72]

The central objective of TEAM was that mini-assessments were conducted for each proposed technology as to: need and utilization; impact on staffing, space, and supply; impact on patient care; vendor and product evaluation; and financial impact. TEAM used elements of technology assessment (i.e., multidisciplinary review and impact assessment), but it was an alternative to technology assessment for making acquisition decisions efficiently and in a timely manner.[73]

TEAM was designed for acute care hospitals, but the model is applicable to other HSOs. TEAM used a standing committee, whose only purpose was to coordinate the evaluation of requests for technology and make recommendations to the capital budgeting committee. Committee members are from the governing body, professional staff organization (PSO), and employees, and should be drawn from several areas and specialties. The committee's major responsibility is to identify persons able to conduct comprehensive assessments for proposed acquisitions in each of the five areas noted in the previous paragraph. Those conducting the assessments need not be committee members. If no physicians are on the committee their input should be sought, especially in the assessment of the potential effect on patient care.

Review Committee   The request review committee should operate within the purview of the HSO's long-range strategic planning activities. The first step should determine whether acquiring new equipment or technology is consistent with the mission and long-range plan. One way to ensure this integration is to use the long-range plan as a guide to prioritize requests. As the HSO's policymaker, the governing body might also have input in assigning priorities. Based on this ranking, the committee should delegate the various assessment tasks that will form the basis for its final recommendations to the capital budgeting committee. Information gathered in the assessment phase will also prove useful in justifying expenditures for medical technology to regulatory agencies.

A second responsibility of the committee should be to follow up and evaluate technologies put into operation and the impact of services offered as a result. Such a process is useful in identifying the effect of accepted projects and is also useful to evaluate and modify the committee's assessment process.

The success of this endeavor depends largely on clear delineation of responsibilities for the request and assessment process among key groups in the HSO. The governing body's role is to work with the chief executive officer (CEO) to develop a policy that guides formation, implementation, and ongoing operation of a program such as TEAM and gives responsibility for it to the CEO. This policy should also outline a mechanism that ensures compatability of requests for technology with the HSO's mission statement and long-range plan. Finally, the governing body should play a key role in identifying the resources needed to acquire medical technology and in allocating them among the request review committee's recommendations.

CEO and PSO   As is true for implementation of all policy, primary responsibility for ongoing functioning of any technology request and assessment program lies with the CEO. As the presiding officer of the request review committee, the CEO should rank requests submitted and assign assessment tasks to committee members, hospital and PSO, or other specialists. In addition, the CEO should act as the committee's liaison with the governing body, departments, members of the PSO interested in initiating requests for medical technology, and regulators who review capital expenditures.

The PSO is a third party that is crucial in assessing and acquiring medical technology. Its most obvious role is to initiate requests to individual departments or clinical services, or directly through the CEO or administrative staff. Perhaps more important is participation in assessing the technology's impact on services offered by the HSO.

Current Methods of Technology Assessment

The AHA did not develop TEAM further, but more recent approaches are similar: 1) monitor and analyze new and emerging technologies; 2) assess the impact of new technologies on the HSO; 3) consider how specific technologies will affect staffing, delivery of care, and facility design; 4) evaluate economic considerations such as reimbursement, life-cycle costs, and cost and revenue shifting within the HSO; 5) analyze risks associated with new and replacement technologies; and 6) consider the impact of third-party payors on technology.[74]

Despite a paucity of assistance, acute care hospitals and other HSOs have grappled with the problem of technology assessment in ways not unlike those recommended in TEAM. There are private services available to HSO managers to provide information about technology and its effect on the HSO. The evidence suggests that hospital systems, which have significantly greater resources, have gone farthest in developing technology assessment methods. Criteria used by one hospital system are like those recommended for free-standing HSOs and include the technology's value to patients, to the system, and to third-party payors; overall cost effectiveness; fit with technologies already present; and influence on finances during the next decade. Such analyses are expensive—that hospital system spends $1 million annually on technology assessment.[75]

A decision to adopt any new technology necessitates answering questions about the cost of acquisition, maintenance, and replacement. Financing may be done out of current revenue, by borrowing, from reserves, through joint venture funds, or from donations resulting from charitable giving. Other strategies have been suggested: 1) merge interests with physicians and other HSOs and develop complementary plans to minimize duplication of expensive technology; 2) obtain manufacturer support for development, training, and maintenance of technology; 3) become a demonstration site for manufacturers; and 4) become a service center for other providers.[76] Survey data suggest that acute care hospitals primarily finance equipment acquisitions with internal funds and gifts, "because the vast majority of equipment purchases are relatively small."[77] In 1991, the average acute care hospital of less than 300 beds had a capital equipment budget of only $1.8 million; an average hospital of more than 500 beds spent $7.9 million.[78] In an era of diminished funding, successful managers must be creative to meet costs of technology.

Lack of a central clearinghouse for information about technology and the absence of assistance in understanding and assessing technology must be decried. Developing a generic prototype for technology assessment by communities and HSOs should be a national priority.

MANAGING MEDICAL TECHNOLOGY EQUIPMENT

The staggering increase in the amount and complexity of equipment directly and indirectly involved in patient care (Table 5.2), coupled with the enlarged legal liability for defects and equipment malfunction, necessitates use of specially trained staff to manage medical technology. Increasingly, clinical engineers are employed in HSOs; this is especially true in acute care hospitals. They manage biomedical equipment by monitoring safety, and by maintaining and repairing equipment. In these activities they are assisted by bioelectronic equipment technicians.

Related areas of activity in acute care hospitals that may not be the responsibility of clinical engineering exist in departments such as central supply, which inspects and has repaired under contract those devices widely used throughout the hospital, including intravenous pumps and suction equipment. Usually, acute care hospitals have critical care technicians who set up and check out equipment needed by specific patients. These technicians may or may not be part of the clinical engineering staff. In addition, larger HSOs may have computer technicians who repair and program the increasing numbers of personal and mini-computers used by staff.

Clinical engineers, bioelectronic equipment technicians, and critical care technicians must be distinguished from the engineers, technicians, and skilled personnel in plant operations (usu-

Table 5.2. Types of biomedical equipment

Diagnostic	Therapeutic	Monitoring	Housekeeping
Body potentials	Radiant energy	Body parameters	Patient
Blood	Resuscitation	Environment	Records and statistics
Radiant energy	Prosthetic & orthotic		Teaching
Laboratory	Special treatment		
	Surgical support		

From Shaffer, Michael J. Managing hospital biomedical equipment. In *Hospital organization and management,* edited by Kurt Darr and Jonathon S. Rakich, 4th ed., 273. Baltimore: Health Professions Press, 1990; reprinted by permission.

ally called engineering) who are responsible for proper functioning of electrical and mechanical equipment such as patient beds, lights, and air conditioning.

Shaffer suggests that three levels of effort should be directed at managing medical technology equipment:

Level 1: Corrective maintenance to repair broken equipment
Level 2: Preventive maintenance to ensure reliability
Level 3: Management to assure cost effectiveness[79]

These efforts reflect good management practice and satisfy requirements such as those of the Joint Commission on Accreditation of Healthcare Organizations (Joint Commission).

Joint Commission

Recognizing the need to establish formal programs to manage technology, the Joint Commission's *Accreditation Manual for Hospitals* specifies that:

There is an equipment management program designed to assess and control the clinical and physical risks of fixed and portable equipment used for the diagnosis, treatment, monitoring, and care of patients and of other fixed and portable electrically powered equipment.[80]

This standard has required characteristics:

Written criteria, which include characteristics of equipment function, clinical application, maintenance requirements, and equipment incident history, are used to identify equipment to be included in the program.

A current, accurate, unique inventory is kept of all equipment included in the program, regardless of the equipment's ownership or purpose.

The equipment management program is used to identify and document equipment problems, failures, and user errors that have or may have an adverse effect on patient safety and/or quality of care.[81]

Current Joint Commission standards for biomedical equipment are much more focused and demanding than previous standards.

Clinical Engineering

Based partly on the Joint Commission standards, a clinical engineering program should have five elements: 1) input to prepurchase evaluation (vendor evaluation), 2) careful inspection of newly acquired equipment with respect to safety and performance, 3) training personnel in the appropriate operation of equipment, 4) periodic inspection and preventive maintenance, and 5) record keeping on the maintenance and status of all equipment.[82] These activities are especially important because the HSO may be liable for negligence related to the equipment's use and to the education of users. Negligence related to use arises from a failure to inspect and properly install, operate, and maintain equipment. Negligence through failure to educate includes not providing warnings and instruction to appropriate personnel and/or not having adequate procedure manuals. In addition, the HSO must ensure that all equipment functions safely and effectively and that it can be used properly by the staff.[83]

Historically, the technicians who operated and maintained biomedical equipment had only rudimentary knowledge of its functioning and little ability to anticipate problems or safety hazards. Although the skills of technicians are still needed, new technology requires much more extensive training. As changes occur, decisions about the skills needed to manage technology and who is adequately trained are more difficult. In the past several decades the field of clinical engineering has trained engineers to work specifically with complex technology and to implement programs to ensure performance and safety of biomedical equipment in HSOs. Certification for clinical engineers was developed in the mid-1970s.[84] In 1990, however, only 400 clinical engineers were certified in the United States.[85]

Biomedical engineering is the broad term often used to encompass both clinical engineers and bioengineers. The functions of hospital clinical engineers emphasize administrative skills (Table 5.3); bioengineers are more research oriented. The needs and availability of in-house talent are important factors in making decisions on the types of engineering and technical personnel to employ. Boxerman and Arthur offer two guidelines:

> (1) technicians must be supervised by engineers, because despite their skills at performing a wide range of technical tasks, they require the guidance and direction of engineers; (2) clinical engineers rather than hospital engineers should provide technical supervision for the activities of those technicians involved with patient related or high-technology equipment. Included in this category is computer equipment, which will likely become an area of increasing concern for the clinical engineer."[86]

The concept of having a formal department of clinical engineering within acute care hospitals specifically, but HSOs generally, continues to evolve. Optimal organizational placement for

Table 5.3.   Clinical engineering functions

1.   DEVELOPMENT AND INTEGRATION OF NEW SYSTEMS
    Planning
        System concept and design
        Facility, equipment, and interface diagrams
        Manufacturing and test specifications
        Cost estimates
        Operational and maintenance procedures
    Purchasing
        Sales literature files
        Sales quotations
        Buying decisions
    New installation
        Contractor liaison
        On-site installation and checkout support
    Training
        Scheduled nurse/technician training courses
        Educational seminars
    Evaluation
        System performance
        Statistics
        Cost effectiveness

2.   OPERATION, MAINTENANCE, AND CALIBRATION
    Alignment and calibration
    Pre-operation preparation and checkout
    Routine performance/safety checks
    Equipment operation
    Failure repairs
    Incoming quality control inspection and test
    Spare parts inventories
    Schematic, instruction book, and reference library
    Operational improvements

3.   MEDICAL RESEARCH AND DEVELOPMENT SUPPORT
    Proposal development
    New equipment design and construction
    Model shop operation
    Evaluation testing

From Shaffer, Michael J., Joseph J. Carr, and Marian Gordon. Clinical engineering—an enigma in health care facilities. *Hospital & Health Services Administration* 24 (Summer 1979):81; reprinted by permission. © 1979, Foundation of the American College of Healthcare Executives.

this unit is undetermined. Traditionally, clinical engineering reported to an assistant administrator or a vice president and it served all biomedical equipment users. Although the relationship is typical of other services that support patient care, this approach has been criticized because the department is administratively distant from users and communication is problematic. To address this concern some hospitals have established departments of clinical engineering, which report to the medical director. A variation has clinical engineering as a division reporting to a major biomedical departmental user such as the clinical departments of anesthesiology or surgery. Critics believe these latter approaches expose clinical engineering to interdepartmental pressures and politics. A third possibility uses a matrix in which a centralized clinical engineering department is subdivided into teams that interact directly with user departments.[87] Figure 5.3 shows the primary relationships among engineers, technicians, and users.

Figure 5.4 shows a means of organizing biomedical equipment activities within an acute care hospital. This approach recognizes the importance of effective interactions between the providers and users of the service. There is more than one way to organize and offer biomedical equipment services. It is incumbent upon managers, however, to ensure that the functions outlined above are effectively performed in the HSO.

SUMMARY

This chapter examines the effect of technology on the health services system and its HSOs, especially acute care hospitals. The technological imperative is a prominent reality at macro and micro levels. A variety of initiatives, usually federally stimulated, have sought to control costs and guide HSOs in effective and efficient use of high technology. Often forgotten, however, is the aggregate financial effect of wholesale use of individually inexpensive technology. The prospective payment system (DRGs) for acute care hospitals is the latest effort to control Medicare costs and, thus, to affect technology, if only indirectly. Third-party payors are following the federal government in adopting variations of prospective payment. Vital for HSOs is that they effectively manage the technology necessary to retaining physicians and offering high-quality care.

Effective managers are boundary scanners. Medical technology is a critical aspect of this activity. Numerous not-for-profit and for-profit organizations offer their services to assist man-

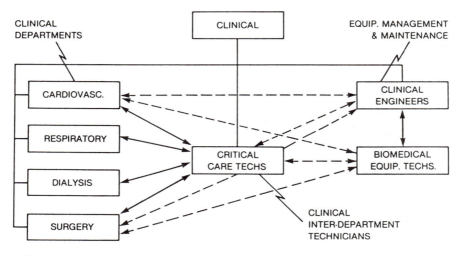

Figure 5.3. Engineer-technician-user interactions. (From Shaffer, Michael J. Managing hospital biomedical equipment. In *Hospital organization and management,* edited by Kurt Darr and Jonathon S. Rakich, 4th ed., 282. Baltimore: Health Professions Press, 1989; reprinted by permission.)

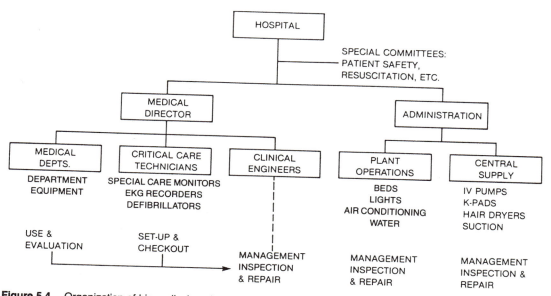

Figure 5.4. Organization of biomedical equipment. (From Shaffer, Michael J. Managing hospital biomedical equipment. In *Hospital organization and management*, edited by Kurt Darr and Jonathon S. Rakich, 4th ed., 283. Baltimore: Health Professions Press, 1989, reprinted by permission.)

agers in learning about new developments and providing new information about existing technology. There is no substitute, however, for the manager personally having a working knowledge of technology of all types.

The general framework of this chapter should be considered in combination with Chapter 3, "Ethical Considerations," and Chapter 4, "Legal Considerations." Solving problems encountered by HSO managers necessitates understanding and analyzing ethical and legal, as well as technological, components. These seemingly disparate elements are often present in complex combinations—their dynamics and interactions add significantly to the impact on the manager. A basic aspect of this dynamic is that major areas of the law are inadequately developed to deal with new technology, and in many instances ethics and the law do not agree on the correct course of action. This results in a tension and provides the manager with contradictory guidance in decision making. Nonetheless, the pragmatic reality remains that decisions must be made and actions taken.

DISCUSSION QUESTIONS

1. Describe the impact of medical technology on HSOs and the costs of health services. Link the theories of distribution of scarce life-saving technology described in Chapter 3 and problems HSOs have in dealing with medical technology.
2. What is the likely long-term effect of DRGs on introduction of new medical technology? What is the likely effect on use? What are the implications for patient care?
3. Technology is increasingly portable and available outside traditional HSOs. Portability is especially problematic for acute care hospitals. Identify the advantages and disadvantages from the standpoint of the HSO *and* the patient.
4. Trends suggest significant consumer interest in alternatives to traditional medicine. These include low- or no-technology treatment as found in holistic medicine, wellness care, and disease prevention. Suggest the implications for HSOs.

5. The control of development and generalization of medical technology is fragmented. Identify control points and suggest ways to improve them. Distinguish the private and public sector.

6. Equipment and other medical technology are present in HSOs because physicians ask for them and patients expect them. Describe changes in the external environment that affect availability and application of technology. What is management's role in resolving differences between expectations and realities?

7. Policy and financing debate focuses on high-cost technology such as transplantation. The chapter suggests that high-volume use of low-cost technology affects total costs. How can effects of low technology be assessed at the HSO level? At the societal level?

8. The internal management of biomedical equipment poses several problems for managers. How do managers involve clinical staff to solve these problems? Identify types of equipment that managers can purchase without involving clinical staff.

9. Competition is a major force in health services, and marketing may be crucial to HSO success. What are the relationships between marketing and acquisition and application of medical technology? Give examples from your experience or the literature.

10. Little attention is usually paid to nonclinical technology such as financial data systems, but such technology can dramatically affect HSO costs and effectiveness. Identify types of nonclinical equipment and their effects on managing HSOs. What links are there between clinical and nonclinical technology?

CASE STUDY 1: THE FEASIBILITY OF BEAM

Brain electrical activity mapping (BEAM) is a recently developed technology for imaging the brain. It significantly improves the physician's ability to localize an abnormality. In response to increased demands for this procedure from staff radiologists and local neurologists and reports in the literature of the usefulness of BEAM testing, Metropolitan Hospital has decided to investigate the possibility of acquiring access to BEAM testing. The options include contracting for use of a BEAM machine as well as actual purchase. A third option is to approach neighboring County Hospital about the possibility of sharing its recently acquired BEAM machine.

A major consideration regarding this decision is uncertainty about the future of reimbursement. It is likely that Medicare payments under DRGs will be reduced even further. In addition, other third-party payors are already requiring more stringent review of new technologies.

Because of this concern and the fact that all the options involve a major expenditure of capital funds, the chair of the governing body asked the CEO to form a committee and evaluate each of the options, including that of foregoing access to BEAM testing. They will use this assessment to make a final decision between the BEAM project and a proposed addition to the intensive care unit, a project that has the strong support of the surgical staff and has already been delayed twice.

Although the governing body would prefer to delay this decision until developments regarding reimbursement are better understood, several attending physicians think the use of BEAM testing is critical to their practices and have stated that, although they prefer the nursing staff at Metropolitan, they will be forced to admit certain patients to County in order to use BEAM. A rumor has just surfaced in the professional staff organization that several prominent members are considering developing a consortium to purchase and operate BEAM and other diagnostic equipment in a professional office complex under construction.

Questions

1. Propose the membership of a committee that will be assigned to assess the need for BEAM testing and the option to be selected.

2. What types of information should be presented to the governing body in the committee's final report?

3. What political and economic complications are present in the decision-making process?

4. How should these complications be addressed? Be specific in identifying the sequence of steps to be taken.

CASE STUDY 2:   "STAY OUT OF MY BACKYARD!"

Andrea Bevans, chief operating officer of Holy Name Hospital, knew it was a matter of when, not if. The memo she had just read was the first salvo in what promised to be another turf war within the professional staff organization (PSO). In the memo, the hospital's vascular surgeons demanded that radiologists not be allowed to perform invasive procedures using lasers. Bevans had heard about cold laser technology and wondered when it would cause repercussions on the PSO. She knew that certain lasers can be used safely within blood vessels because they generate little or no heat. These lasers dissolve unwanted tissue, leaving wanted tissue unharmed. To support their position, the vascular surgeons cited their concern for the quality of patient care. Bevans suspected there just might be an economic reason, too.

The memo stated that vascular surgeons had the background, training, expertise, and proven outcomes using surgical skills, and they could best learn and apply the new techniques, if those techniques were appropriate at all. To allow radiologists to work inside the vascular system by threading catheters into various blood vessels would violate previously tried and tested relationships and would cause other, unspecified, disruptions. The memo ended with a thinly veiled threat: "Should the hospital allow radiologists to perform invasive procedures using lasers, it may not be possible for members of the surgical staff to be available to treat untoward events, should they occur."

Bevans reread the memo and mused about the path of modern medicine. It had reached the point where many conditions were treatable without a scalpel. She thought briefly about "Bones," the physician on "Star Trek," who had only to pass a device over a patient's body to make a diagnosis. Is that where we're headed, she thought?

"But, enough of science fiction," she said to herself. "How do I solve yet another turf battle without too many casualties, not the least of whom could be me?"

Questions

1. Identify the quality of care issues. How are they similar to, but different from, the economic issues?

2. What information should Bevans have to understand the facts and issues? To whom should Bevans turn for advice?

3. Develop three options that Bevans could use. Identify and justify your choice of the best.

4. Identify three other quality/economic controversies that occur among institutional or personal health services providers.

CASE STUDY 3:   "LET'S 'DO' A JOINT VENTURE"

In 1985, a consortium of churches established Arcadia Lifecare Community (ALC) as a not-for-profit, tax-exempt corporation. It was located in the tidewater region of eastern Virginia near a major naval base. It had 200 independent living apartments and a 20-bed nursing facility. ALC featured indoor and outdoor recreational activities and emphasized maximum independence for residents.

By 1990, poor management had brought ALC to the brink of bankruptcy. It was rescued by a large loan from the consortium and put under professional management. ALC was soon on firm financial footing, and the board of directors determined that its services should be diversified. ALC developed a respite care program to provide weekend and day care for dependent persons and give relief to family members. It established a home hospice program.

The board hired a consultant to assist in strategic planning. Based on market analyses and community assessments, the consultant suggested several new programs. First on the list was a rehabilitation center. The consultant noted that there were no outpatient rehabilitation services in the area, that rehab tied in naturally with existing services (including the respite care and residential services), and that reimbursement was currently generous. Startup costs, including leasing space and equipping and staffing a rehabilitation center, were estimated at $500,000. The board was enthusiastic, but had less than $100,000 for a new venture. ALC was leveraged (mortgaged) to the maximum and there was no ready source of new capital.

As the board grappled with this question, the consultant suggested a joint venture with a group of physiatrists located about 35 miles away. The consultant proposed that they pool their capital and establish a for-profit subsidiary to offer rehabilitation services. A telephone call to the physiatry group showed it to be interested.

Questions

1. Critique what ALC is doing in terms of the technology that it has considered and is considering. Include both positive and negative aspects.
2. Identify additional compatible activities that ALC could undertake. Be specific as to how they fit.
3. Identify the benefits and risks of forming a joint venture with the physiatry group.
4. What is the role of ALC's managers, especially the CEO, in these activities?

CASE STUDY 4: "WHY CAN'T YOU KEEP MY LAB RUNNING?!"

Brent Jackson's secretary, Mark, had just buzzed and told him Dr. Farrington was calling. Jackson tensed as he picked up the telephone. This wasn't going to be pleasant, he thought. Farrington directed the pulmonary function laboratory and always seemed to be on the telephone complaining about one piece of equipment or another. The technician from Gateway Hi-Tech had not come as promised, and now Farrington had to cancel a procedure scheduled for the next morning. This time Farrington didn't threaten to have Jackson fired—which he had done before. It was clear, however, that his patience had run out. Something had to be done about equipment repair and maintenance.

Five years ago Jackson had joined Medical Associates, Inc., a large multispecialty group practice, as a strategic planner and marketer. Two years later he was promoted to a job with line management responsibility. His work was exemplary and he was asked to manage several other areas and departments.

When Jackson became responsible for biomedical equipment management there were two staff: a clinical engineer and a technician. The engineer left a few months later and recruiting for the past 18 months had been unsuccessful. The technician was well trained and worked hard, but there was too much to do. Jackson estimated there were about 300 pieces of diagnostic and therapeutic equipment, representing at least 200 different types. Some, such as the piece of equipment in Farrington's laboratory, were serviced under contract. Jackson had found, however, that such contracts were expensive and often unreliable. In addition, Jackson knew that there were many activities, such as evaluation of new equipment, training of staff, and preventive maintenance, that were getting little attention.

Farrington's complaints seemed to be only the tip of the iceberg. Jackson wasn't really sure where to start, but he knew something had to be done.

Questions

1. Develop a statement of the problem facing Jackson.
2. What alternative solutions are available to Jackson? Which would you choose? Why?
3. List the advantages and disadvantages of using contract equipment maintenance and repair companies.
4. Identify the steps Jackson should take if he chooses to develop a comprehensive in-house medical equipment management program.

CASE STUDY 5:   "ISN'T THERE A BETTER WAY?"

Alice Smith hated saying no to requests for new technology, but as vice president for clinical services at Community Hospital it was an unfortunate fact of her professional life. Smith had just shown Dr. Madeline Jones to the door of her office and she knew Jones was not happy. Jones, the acting chief of anesthesiology, had asked Smith to authorize $2,500 to modify an anesthesia machine. Although well educated and articulate, Jones was not able to explain how the modification would: 1) save money as the hospital struggled to survive under DRGs, and/or 2) measurably enhance patient care (the quality of surgical outcomes). Smith usually asked these questions, and she thought everyone on the clinical staff and in the hospital knew that.

As Smith sat down she mused about how her response to Jones would be viewed by the clinical staff, many of whom would hear the latest news about the "ogre" in administration by day's end. Smith knew she already had a reputation for being a hard nose. She didn't mind that. She feared, however, that hostility was building in the clinical staff and it would spill over into other relationships. The outcomes of Smith's discussions with various physician managers were very different. Some did their homework and could answer her questions; their equipment requests were usually granted. Smith knew this was seen as favoritism, but that simply wasn't true.

The intercom buzzer broke Smith's reverie. She knew there had to be a better way to make equipment-related decisions.

Questions

1. Develop a statement of the problem facing Smith.
2. Identify the positive and negative aspects of the situation that Smith has allowed and encouraged to develop.
3. Assume that Smith wants to enhance the ability of physicians to articulate their equipment requests. What steps should she take? With whom should she work most closely?
4. What are the positive and negative aspects of enhancing the clinical staff's ability to articulate their equipment requests? What other group(s) would benefit from the same assistance?

NOTES

1. Samuel, Frank E., Jr. Technology and costs: Complex relationship. *Hospitals* 62 (December 5, 1988):72.
2. Institute of Medicine, Committee for Evaluating Medical Technologies in Clinical Use. *Assessing medical technologies*, 9. Washington, D.C.: National Academy Press, 1985.
3. Stevens, William K. High medical costs under attack as drain on the nation's economy. *New York Times* (March 28, 1982):50.
4. An excellent review article of economic studies done to examine the economic impact of technology, including types of approaches taken, findings, and conclusions in Cotterill, Philip G. The impact of technology on health

care costs. In *Profile of medical practice 1980,* 107–121. edited by Gerald L. Glandona and Roberta J. Shapiro, Chicago: American Medical Association, 1980.
5. Showstack, Jonathan A., Steven A. Schroeder, and Michael Matsumoto. Changes in the use of medical technologies, 1972–1977: A study of 10 inpatient diagnoses. *New England Journal of Medicine* 306 (December 1982): 706–712.
6. Newhouse, Joseph P. Has erosion of the medical marketplace ended? In *Competition in the health care sector: Ten years later,* edited by Warren Greenberg, 53, 55. Durham, NC: Duke University Press, 1988.

7. Perry, Seymour, and M. Eliastam. The National Center for Health Care Technology. *Journal of the American Medical Association* 245 (June 26, 1981):2510–2511.
8. Scitovsky, Anne A. Changes in the costs of treatment of selected illnesses, 1971–1981. *Medical Care* 23 (December 1985): 1345–1357. Showstack, Jonathan A., Mary Hughes Stone, and Steven A. Schroeder. The role of changing clinical practices in the rising costs of hospital care. *New England Journal of Medicine* 313 (November 7, 1985):1201–1207.
9. Bennett, Ivan L., Jr., Technology as a shaping force. In *Doing Better, Feeling Worse,* edited by John H. Knowles, New York: W. W. Norton & Co., Inc., 1977. 128–129.
10. Bennett, Technology as a shaping force, 126.
11. Schriber, Jon. Brain Storms. *Forbes* 131 (June 6, 1983): 116–117, 121; American Hospital Association, Division of Management and Technology, *Executive briefing* (AHA Hospital Technology Series), 4. Chicago, 1982.
12. Souhrada, Laura. Biotechnology, cost concerns dominate in 1989. *Hospitals* 63 (December 20, 1989):32.
13. Russell, Louise B., and Jane E. Sisk. Medical technology in the United States: The last decade. *International Journal of Technology Assessment in Health Care* 4 (1988):275.
14. Moran, Elizabeth J. New technique opens windows to heart and brain. *Hospitals* 65 (February 5, 1991):60, 62.
15. Anderson, Howard J. Survey identifies trends in equipment acquisitions. *Hospitals* 64 (September 20, 1990):3.
16. Eisenberg, John M., J. Sanford Schwartz, F. Catherine McCaslin, Rachel Kaufman, Henry Glick, and Eugene Kroch. Substituting diagnostic services: New tests only partly replace older ones. *Journal of the American Medical Association* 262 (September 1, 1989):1196–1200.
17. Okie, Susan. Lowest-cost heart drug safer, researchers say. *Washington Post* (March 3, 1991):A4.
18. Streptokinase study will not dim tPA's popularity: Experts. *AHA News* 26 (March 19, 1990):3.
19. A useful discussion of the technology assessment process is found in Glasser, Jay H., and Richard S. Chrzanowski. Medical technology assessment: Adequate questions, appropriate methods, valuable answers. *Health Policy* 9 (1988):267–276.
20. Massaro, Thomas A. Impact of new technologies on health-care costs and on the nation's "Health." *Clinical Chemistry* 36 (B) (1990):1613.
21. Zeman, Robert K. Medicine: I'll take high tech. *Washington Post* (August 16, 1983):A17.
22. McKinlay, John B., Sonja M. McKinlay, and Robert Beaglehole. A review of the evidence concerning the impact of medical measures on recent mortality and morbidity in the United States. *International Journal of Health Services* 19 (1989):186.
23. Souhrada, Biotechnology, 32.
24. Martinsons, Jane. Limits on the use of artificial blood. *Medical Staff Leader* 18 (June 1989):3.
25. Business facts: Transplants performed in the United States in 1989. *AHA News* 26 (July 9, 1990):7.
26. Rogers, David E. The challenge of primary care. In *Doing better, feeling worse,* edited by John H. Knowles. New York: W. W. Norton & Co., Inc., 1977.
27. Roback, Gene, Lillian Randolph, and Bradley Seidman. *Physician characteristics and distribution in the U.S.,* 21. Chicago: American Medical Association, 1990.
28. Roback, Randolph, and Seidman, *Physician characteristics,* 21.
29. Phillips, Donald F. Technology: The honeymoon is over. *Hospitals* 52 (April 1, 1978):159.
30. Iglehart, John K. Looking ahead at technology. *Hospitals* 53 (June 1, 1979):88.
31. The comparative performance of U.S. hospitals. In *Health care investment analyst,* 84. Baltimore: Deloitte and Touche, 1990.
32. Agency for Health Care Policy and Research, Public Health Service, U.S. Department of Health and Human Services, Longer-practicing physicians may hospitalize more patients unnecessarily. *Research Activities* 136 (December 1990):3
33. Bunker, John P., Jinnet Fowles, and Ralph Schaffarzick. Evaluation of medical-technology strategies: Effects of coverage and reimbursement. *New England Journal of Medicine* 306 (March 11, 1982):622–623.
34. Russell and Sisk, Medical technology in the United States, 280–282.
35. Medicare program: Criteria and procedures for making medical services coverage decisions that relate to health care technology. Proposed Rule. 42 C.F.R. Parts 400 and 405. *Federal Register* 54 (January 30, 1989):4302–4318.
36. Intergovernmental Health Policy Project, The George Washington University, Washington, D.C. Medicaid coverage of organ transplants: Survey results. *State Health Notes* 87 (November 1988):6–7.
37. Reinhold, Robert. Majority in survey on health care are open to changes to cut costs. *New York Times* (March 29, 1982): Although the majority of respondents in the survey were unwilling to limit the opportunities for people to use expensive modern technology, they were willing to consider changes in the health care system that might reduce costs, such as having routine illnesses treated by a nurse or a doctor's assistant rather than by a doctor, and going to a clinic at which they would be assigned any available doctor instead of seeing their own private doctor.
38. Robinson, James C., and Harold S. Luft. Competition and the cost of hospital care, 1972 to 1982. *Journal of the American Medical Association* 257 (June 19, 1987): 3241–3245.
39. Robinson, Michele L. Turf battle rocks radiology. *Hospitals* 63 (November 5, 1989):47.
40. Russell and Sisk, Medical technology, 271.
41. Burroughs, John T., and Carl R. Edenhofer. Product liability actions in medical negligence: The barrier is breaking. *Journal of Legal Medicine* 4 (June 1983):218–229.
42. Alder, Henry C. Safe Medical Devices Act: What you need to know now to comply with the new law. *Health Facilities Management* 4 (November 1991): 14, 16, 18, 20, 22.
43. Lashof, Joyce C. Government approaches to the management of medical technology. *Bulletin of the New York Academy of Medicine* 57 (January–February 1981):40–41.
44. Lashof, Government approaches, 41.
45. Committee on Ways and Means, U.S. House of Representatives. *1990 green book: Overview of entitlement programs.* Washington, D.C.: U.S. Government Printing Office, 1990.
46. Cohn, Victor. Study says some coronary bypasses are unneeded. *Washington Post* (October 27, 1983):A5.
47. Killip, Thomas. Twenty years of coronary bypass surgery. *New England Journal of Medicine* 319 (August 11, 1988):368.
48. Medicare CABG centers chosen. *Health Policy Week* 20 (February 4, 1991):1–2.

49. Cohen, Alan B., and Donald R. Cohodes. Certificate of need and low capital-cost medical technology. *Milbank Memorial Fund Quarterly* 60 (Spring 1982):307–328.

50. Fineberg, Harvey V., Gerald S. Parker, and Laurie A. Pearlman. CT scanners, distribution and planning status in the United States. *New England Journal of Medicine* 297 (October 6, 1977):217.

51. Gaul, Gilbert M. One city's love affair with technology. *Washington Post* Health Section (November 6, 1990):14.

52. Perry, Seymour. Technology assessment in health care: The U.S. perspective. *Health Policy* 9 (1988):318.

53. Institute of Medicine. *Assessing medical technologies,* 37.

54. Perry, Seymour, and Barbara Pillar. A national policy for health care technology assessment. *Medical Care Review* 47 (Winter 1990):408.

55. Office of Technology Assessment, United States Congress. *The OTA health program.* Washington, D.C.: U.S. Government Printing Office, 1989.

56. Perry, Technology assessment, 320.

57. Iglehart, John K. Health policy report: Another chance for technology assessment. *New England Journal of Medicine* 309 (August 25, 1983):510.

58. National Center for Health Services Research and Health Care Technology Assessment, Public Health Service, U.S. Department of Health and Human Services. *Program profile: Office of Health Technology Assessment,* 2. Washington, D.C.: U.S. Government Printing Office, 1988.

59. Agency for Health Care Policy and Research, Public Health Service, U.S. Department of Health and Human Services. *AHCPR Program Note,* 1. Washington, D.C., 1990.

60. Perry and Pillar, National policy, 405.

61. Perry, Technology assessment, 322.

62. A concise discussion of consensus development conferences is found in Jacoby, Itzhak. Update on assessment activities: United States perspective. *International Journal of Technology Assessment in Health Care* 4 (1988):100–101.

63. Institute of Medicine, *Assessing medical technologies,* 70–175.

64. Jacoby, Itzhak, Ph.D., Professor and Director, Division of Health Services Administration, Uniformed Services University of the Health Sciences, F. Edward Hèbert School of Medicine, Bethesda, Maryland, personal communication, October 28, 1990.

65. Perry, Technology assessment, 323.

66. Souhrada, Laura. System execs overcome barriers to tech assessment. *Hospitals* 63 (August 5, 1989):38.

67. Sanders, Charles A. Taming the technological tiger. *Trustee* 31 (March 1978):24.

68. *Health devices sourcebook—the hospital purchasing guide,* B 457. Plymouth Meeting, PA: ECRI, 1990.

69. Sanders, Taming the technological tiger, 24.

70. *Health devices sourcebook,* B 407.

71. Coile, Russell C., Jr. The 'Racer's edge' in hospital competition: Strategic technology plan. *Healthcare Executive* 5 (January/February 1990):22.

72. McKee, Michael, and L. Rita Fritz. Team up for technology assessment. *Hospitals* 53 (June 1, 1979):119–122.

73. American Hospital Association. Trustee development program: The board's role in the planning and acquisition of clinical technology. *Trustee* 32 (June 1979):47–55.

74. Berkowitz, David A. Strategic technology management. *Healthcare Forum Journal* 32 (September/October 1989): 16–18; Sprague, Gary R. Managing technology assessment and acquisition. *Healthcare Executive* 3 (November/December 1988):26–29.

75. Souhrada, System execs, 39.

76. Miccio, Joseph A. The migration of medical technology. *Healthcare Forum Journal* (September/October 1989):24.

77. Anderson, Howard J. Survey identifies technology trends. *Medical Staff Leader* (October 1990):30.

78. Anderson, Survey identifies, 33.

79. Shaffer, Michael J. Managing hospital biomedical equipment. In *Hospital organization and management,* edited by Kurt Darr and Jonathon S. Rakich, 4th ed., 273. Baltimore: Health Professions Press, 1990.

80. Joint Commission on Accreditation of Healthcare Organizations, Standard PL 3: Plant, technology, and safety management. In *Accreditation manual for hospitals, 1992,* 131. Oakbrook Terrace, Illinois, 1991.

81. Joint Commission, *Accreditation manual,* 131.

82. Nobel, Joel J. Small hospitals manage clinical equipment. *Hospitals* 53 (June 1, 1979):132.

83. Shaffer, Michael J., and Marian R. Gordon. Clinical engineering standards, obligations and accountability. In *Management and clinical engineering,* edited by C. A. Caceres, 346–347. Dedham, MA: Artech House, 1980.

84. Boxerman, Stuart B. and R. Martin Arthur. Matching technical jobs with needs. *Hospitals* 54 (June 16, 1980):106.

85. Shaffer, Managing hospital, 281.

86. Boxerman and Arthur, Matching technical jobs, 112.

87. Shaffer, Michael J., Joseph J. Carr, and Marian Gordon. Clinical engineering—an enigma in health care facilities. *Hospital & Health Services Administration,* 24 (Summer 1979):92–93.

BIBLIOGRAPHY

Alder, Henry C. Safe Medical Devices Act: What you need to know now to comply with the new law. *Health Facilities Management* 4 (November 1991): 14, 16, 18, 20, 22.

Berkowitz, David A. Strategic technology management. *Healthcare Forum Journal* 32 (September/October 1989): 14–20.

Eisenberg, John M., J. Sanford Schwartz, F. Catherine McCaslin, Rachel Kaufman, Henry Glick, and Eugene Kroch. Substituting diagnostic services: New tests only partly replace older ones. *Journal of the American Medical Association* 262 (September 1, 1989):1196–1200.

Institute of Medicine, Committee for Evaluating Medical Technologies in Clinical Use. *Assessing medical technologies.* Washington, D.C.: National Academy Press, 1985.

Killip, Thomas, Twenty years of coronary bypass surgery. *New England Journal of Medicine* 319 (August 11, 1988): 366–368.

Massaro, Thomas A. Impact of new technologies on healthcare costs and on the nation's health. *Clinical Chemistry* 36 (1990):1612–1616.

McKinlay, John B., Sonja M. McKinlay, and Robert Beaglehole. A review of the evidence concerning the impact of medical measures on recent mortality and morbidity in the United States. *International Journal of Health Services* 19 (1989):181–208.

Medicare program: Criteria and procedures for making medical services coverage decisions that relate to health care technology. Proposed Rule. 42 C.F.R. Parts 400 and 405 *Federal Register* 54 (January 30, 1989):4302–4318.

Newhouse, Joseph P. Has erosion of the medical marketplace ended? In *Competition in the health care sector: Ten years later,* edited by Warren Greenberg, 41–56. Durham, NC: Duke University Press, 1988.

Office of Technology Assessment, United States Congress. *The OTA health program.* Washington, D.C.: U.S. Government Printing Office, 1989.

Perry, Seymour. Technology assessment in health care: The U.S. Perspective. *Health Policy* 9 (1988):317–324.

Perry, Seymour, and Barbara Pillar. A national policy for health care technology assessment. *Medical Care Review* 47 (Winter 1990):401–417.

Roback, Gene, Lillian Randolph, and Bradley Seidman. *Physician characteristics and distribution in the U.S.* Chicago: American Medical Association, 1990.

Russell, Louise B., and Jane E. Sisk. Medical technology in the United States: The last decade. *International Journal of Technology Assessment in Health Care* 4 (1988):280–282.

Scitovsky, Anne A. Changes in the costs of treatment of selected illnesses, 1971–1981. *Medical Care* 23 (December 1985): 1345–1357.

Shaffer, Michael J. Managing hospital biomedical equipment. In *Hospital organization and management,* edited by Kurt Darr and Jonathon S. Rakich, 4th ed., 272–286. Baltimore, MD: Health Professions Press, 1990.

Showstack, Jonathan A., Mary Hughes Stone, and Steven A. Schroeder. The role of changing clinical practices in the rising costs of hospital care. *New England Journal of Medicine* 313 (November 7, 1985):1201–1207.

III / Structuring Health Services Organizations

6

Concepts of
Organization Design

Hospitals are not inevitable institutions. They are constantly negotiated and renegotiated in response to immediate crisis and the practicalities of change.

Rosemary A. Stevens, "The Hospital as a
Social Institution . . ."[1]

Chapter 1 defined management as the process, composed of interrelated social and technical functions and activities (including roles), occurring within a formal organizational setting for the purpose of accomplishing predetermined objectives through the utilization of human and other resources. An important element of this definition is that management occurs in a *formal organizational setting,* which makes organizing a crucial function of managers. This chapter focuses on the key concepts of organizing and organization design as they influence organizational structures. Chapter 7, "How HSOs Are Organized," presents several types of health services organizations (HSOs).

Managers at all levels of HSOs are involved in the organizing function. Figure 6.1 shows that organization design begins by designating individual positions and progresses to large, fully integrated systems. Mintzberg[2] points out that the design of organizations begins with individual positions. Individual positions are building blocks for work groups, clusters of work groups, entire organizations, and integrated systems of organizations. Senior managers are concerned more with broad aspects of organizing, such as authority and responsibility relationships, departmentation, coordinating components, and perhaps formation of systems of organizations. In essence, they are concerned with how effectively the HSO is structured to meet its objectives. Middle-level managers are more concerned with organizing work groups and clusters of work groups. First-line managers are more directly concerned with organizing individual positions; their tasks include job design, work process flow, and work methods and procedures.

In the organizing function managers build the *formal organization,* the structure conceptualized and sanctioned by the HSO's senior managers and governing body. Coexisting with the formal organization, however, is the *informal organization.* It exists because people working together invariably establish relationships and interactions outside the formal structure. Thus, every HSO has a formal structure developed by management and an informal structure that reflects the wishes and preferences of the staff. Both formal and informal organization design concepts are considered in this chapter.

It may be useful to review the comprehensive model of management for HSOs in Figure 1.6 (Chapter 1), which shows that conversion of inputs to outputs takes place in a formal organizational setting with structure, tasks/technology, and people elements. "Structure" includes formally designed arrangements such as authority–responsibility relationships; grouping work activities into departments; and coordination, communication, information, and control mechanisms. "Tasks/technology" is work specialization: job design, work processes, methods and procedures, and logistical, material, and work flows. It also represents technological characteristics of the organizational setting, including equipment, people–machine relationships, and, to some degree,

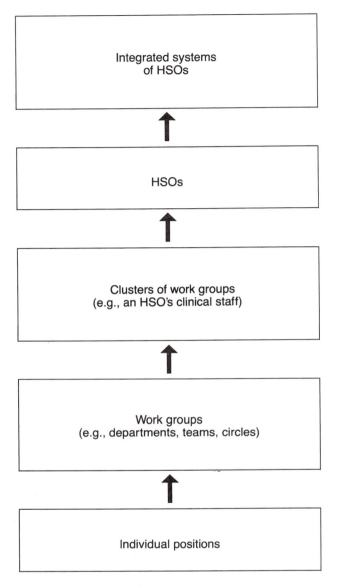

Figure 6.1. Levels of organizational design in HSOs.

information/knowledge used by management and other personnel in performing their duties and tasks. "People" are the human part of HSOs. People accomplish work, and it is only through them that work occurs. Managers accomplish work activity through people by integrating structure, tasks/technology, and people. In doing so, however, they must contend with the dynamics of formal and informal and individual behavior—positive and negative—including roles, perceptions, expectations, and values.

Essentially, the importance of organizing grows from the need for cooperation. When one considers the complexity of work done in HSOs and the diversity of the professional, technical, and support people who perform it, the need for cooperation is evident—a need that may be more important in HSOs than any other type of organization. Even within a single unit such as diagnostic radiology, a wide range of work is performed at many skill levels, and organizing this work is vital to overall effectiveness and efficiency, both of which concern the manager. An organization design is effective if it facilitates attaining the HSO's objectives; it is efficient if objectives are attained using minimum resources.

Managers in dynamic HSOs engage in organizing almost continuously. Some people erroneously assume that organization design is something managers do once, when a new organization is created, and then turn their attention elsewhere. Actually, organizing is ongoing and involves not only initial design, but routine redesign. The opening quote to this chapter states that HSOs are "constantly negotiated and renegotiated," and it is redesign that makes organization design an ongoing challenge. Leatt, Shortell, and Kimberly list circumstances in which HSO managers are likely to find design changes necessary:

1. *When the organization is experiencing severe problems.* Indicators of inadequate performance may be presented to the manager from external reviews such as accreditation processes, or from internal reviews such as financial statements and clinical audits. These problems may be identified at varying levels within the organization, for example, for a particular position, a workgroup, a department, or a total organization.
2. *When there is a change in the environment which directly influences internal policies.* In some circumstances there may be major changes in the environment, such as prospective payment for hospital services or capitation payment for all health services received by a given population. These changes may require a redesign and refocusing of key organizational groups.
3. *When new programs or product lines are targeted by the mission statement.* When an organization recognizes as high priority certain markets or product lines, an organization design change may be necessary to infuse resources into the new area. Conversely, when old programs are to be dropped, new structural arrangements may be necessary.
4. *When there is a change in leadership.* New leadership may provide considerable opportunity to rethink the way in which the organization has been designed. New leadership tends to view the organization from a different perspective and may bring innovative ideas to the reorganization.[3]

CLASSICAL ORGANIZATION DESIGN CONCEPTS

Although they have been modified over the years, the key organization design concepts that guide the formal structure of most HSOs were developed by a group of general administrative theorists who worked early in the twentieth century. Most important among these theorists were Henri Fayol, a French industrialist, and Max Weber, a German sociologist. The writings of Fayol[4] and Weber[5] and their colleagues represent what have come to be called the *classical concepts of organization design.*

Some people are surprised to learn that many basic design characteristics of modern HSOs are rooted in conceptualizations that are nearly a century old. This reflects the wisdom that went into the development of the classical concepts and says something about their durability. Williams and Huber note about these concepts:

> Most organizations are strongly influenced by classical theory. Some of its assumptions are questionable and many of its principles are deficient; its assertions are too sweeping, and its application has often led to undesirable results. It is, nevertheless, a brilliant expression of organization theory and a standard of reference which cannot be ignored or considered insignificant by theorist or practicing manager.[6]

Weber (1864–1920) is most often associated with the organizational form he termed "bureaucracy." His work is a logical beginning point in analysis of organizations because Weber thought that bureaucracy, in its pure form, represented an ideal or completely rational form of organization. The term "bureaucracy," usually associated with governmental organizations, raises a negative image for many. It has come to represent the undesirable characteristics of "red tape" found in many large organizations. These include duplication, delay, and general frustration. In Weber's conceptualization, however, the term meant something very different. He used it to describe a structure based on the sociological concept of rationalization of collective activities.[7]

Weber abstracted the concept of "ideal" organization from observing many actual organizations and combining them into his ideal bureaucracy model. This model was a basis for theorizing how work should be done in large organizations. The key features[8] Weber believed were necessary if an organization were to achieve the maximum benefits of ideal bureaucracy include:

1. *A clear division of labor* so that each task performed by employees is systematically established and legitimized by formal recognition as an official duty.
2. *Positions arranged in a hierarchy* so that each lower position is controlled and supervised by a higher one. The effect of this is a chain of command.
3. *Formal rules and regulations* to uniformly guide actions of employees. In Weber's view a system of rules ensures a rational approach to organization and a degree of uniformity and coordination that could not otherwise exist. The basic rationale for rules in Weber's model is that the manager uses them to eliminate uncertainty in performance of tasks resulting from differences among individuals. Beyond this, he believed that rules and regulations provide continuity and stability to an organization.
4. *Impersonal relationships* and avoidance by managers of involvement with employees' personalities and personal preferences. Weber believed this practice ensured that the bureaucrat did not permit emotional attachments or personalities to interfere with rational decisions.
5. *Employment based entirely on technical competence* and protection against arbitrary dismissal. Employees in the ideal bureaucracy are selected using rigid criteria that apply uniformly and impersonally to each candidate. Criteria are based on objective standards for the job established by the officials of the organization. Promotions in the ideal bureaucracy are awarded on the basis of seniority and achievement.

Originally published in 1916, the characteristics of Weber's ideal bureaucracy became "the design prototype for almost all of today's large organizations."[9]

Fayol's contributions to organization design were primarily based on his identification of a set of "principles" of management. Table 6.1 is an abbreviated version of Fayol's fourteen principles of management. Just as Weber's conceptualization of the ideal bureaucracy has significance in the design of today's organizations, many of Fayol's observations remain relevant. As Higgins notes,

> Virtually all organizations are still arranged according to the division of work using highly specialized labor, whether they are making . . . microchips or providing health care services. All organizations use the principle of authority; virtually all employ the unity of command concept; and all use some degree of centralization versus decentralization, and the scalar chain.[10]

The work of Fayol, Weber, and other early general administration theorists, such as Luther Gulick and Lyndall Urwick[11] and James Mooney and Alan Reiley,[12] is relevant to the design of modern organizations, including HSOs. However, each classical concept must be updated to reflect new information about how organizations are best structured to meet present and future needs of society as well as the needs of workers in them. To assist in that effort, the following sections present the most important and relevant classical concepts of organization design, along with a contemporary perspective on the concept. The key classical concepts that affect the principal concerns of managers as they design organizations are: 1) division of work, 2) authority and responsibility relationships, 3) departmentation, 4) span of control, and 5) coordination.

Division of Work

The Classical View The classical theorists—and before them the economist Adam Smith, author of *The Wealth of Nations,* published in 1776[13]—recognized the potential benefits of division of work. It was noted by Fayol as the first of 14 principles of management (see Table 6.1). Division of work or specialization of work permits employees to be more efficient. In the view of classical theorists, division of work provided significant economic benefits (efficiency). Importantly, it also enhances *proficiency* in performing work. For example, a transplant team reflects

Table 6.1. Fayol's 14 principles of management

1. *Division of Work.* This principle is the same as Adam Smith's "division of labor." Specialization increases output by making employees more efficient.
2. *Authority.* Managers must be able to give orders. Authority gives them this right. Along with authority, however, goes responsibility. Wherever authority is exercised, responsibility arises.
3. *Discipline.* Employees must obey and respect the rules that govern the organization. Good discipline is the result of effective leadership, a clear understanding between management and workers regarding the organization's rules, and the judicious use of penalties for infractions of the rules.
4. *Unity of Command.* Every employee should receive orders from only *one* superior.
5. *Unity of Direction.* Each group of organizational activities that has the same objective should be directed by one manager using one plan.
6. *Subordination of Individual Interests to the General Interests.* The interests of any one employee or group of employees should not take precedence over the interests of the organization as a whole.
7. *Remuneration.* Workers must be paid a fair wage for their services.
8. *Centralization.* Centralization refers to the degree to which subordinates are involved in decision making. Whether decision making is centralized (to management) or decentralized (to subordinates) is a question of proper proportion. The problem is to find the optimum degree of centralization for each situation.
9. *Scalar Chain.* The line of authority from top management to the lowest ranks represents the scalar chain. Communications should follow this chain. However, if following the chain creates delays, cross-communications can be allowed if agreed to by all parties and superiors are kept informed.
10. *Order.* People and materials should be in the right place at the right time.
11. *Equity.* Managers should be kind and fair to their subordinates.
12. *Stability of Tenure of Personnel.* High employee turnover is inefficient. Management should provide orderly personnel planning and ensure that replacements are available to fill vacancies.
13. *Initiative.* Employees who are allowed to originate and carry out plans will exert high levels of effort.
14. *Esprit de Corps.* Promoting team spirit will build harmony and unity within the organization.

From Robbins, Stephen P. *Management*, 3d ed., 38. Englewood Cliffs, NJ: Prentice Hall, 1991; reprinted by permission.

a careful division of work among a group of people. Each member performs specialized work and becomes proficient in it. The team is excellent because individual members make superior work contributions.

Technically, division of work means dividing work of the organization into "specific jobs having specified activities."[14] The content of a job is determined by what the person doing it is to accomplish. For example, the job of pharmacist in an HSO is defined by the activities a person in this position is expected to accomplish. These activities are different from those expected of someone with the job of nurse, vice president for professional affairs, or computer programmer.

Much of the world's work—and certainly that performed in HSOs—is performed by people who specialize in particular work through education and experience. Personnel specialization is a common way to divide work in HSOs because licensure and accreditation rules and policies require HSOs to employ people who have specific attributes. The work of physicians, nurses, technologists, and therapists, for example, is largely defined by licensure and certification. Personnel specialization implies expertise based on education and experience in the activities of a job. Concomitantly, HSOs, more so than most organizations, are structured to accommodate the specialties of people who work there.

Organizations, through the division of work, also encourage job or work specialization. Much specialization has a functional basis.[15] *Functionalization* is dividing the HSO's work based on functions to be performed. Division of work causes HSOs to be organized into numerous departments or units within which work is functionally similar but among which work is functionally dissimilar. For example, work in the dietary department is dissimilar from that in admitting. Within these departments, however, the work is functionally similar. Specializing has several advantages, including enhancing the HSO's ability to select, train, and equip people to do work by matching their activities with functions. In functionally specialized work people often learn the job more quickly than if work is not specialized. This allows managers to achieve greater levels of control because they can more easily standardize functionally specialized work.[16]

The Contemporary View The classical theorists who developed the concept of the division of work saw it as an untapped source of increased productivity. Examples of the potential economic benefits of work division and specialization abounded at the beginning of the 20th century. However, increased division of work had a negative side—people who perform specialized work may find it repetitive, monotonous, and unfulfilling. In response, *job enlargement* (combining tasks to create a new job with broader activities) and *job enrichment* (expanding responsibilities so work becomes more challenging and satisfying) programs are increasingly important in all types of organizations, including HSOs. Holt reports the use of job enrichment techniques in HSOs:

> In most hospitals, doctors, nurses, and technical specialists differentiate their jobs carefully. A patient being treated in an emergency room may be diagnosed by one doctor, have lab work evaluated by another, be treated by yet another, and be shifted among several specialists in the process. The doctors, laboratory specialists, and nurses all perform their specialized work with little concern for what the others are doing. In contrast, with integrated medical teams formed through job enrichment efforts, each team member is involved in team decisions and total care of the patient. In cardiac rehabilitation, for example, heart attack patients have been diagnosed, clinically treated, rehabilitated, and provided with extended care by a team of physicians, nurses, and counselors who stay with them from the initial incident to satisfactory recovery.[17]

The contemporary view is that, while the efficiency and proficiency benefits of the division or specialization of work are real, they must be balanced against negative consequences. Taken too far, division of work can become dysfunctional and should be countered with job enlargement or enrichment programs, but such programs need to be applied with care and thought. Mintzberg argues that:

> [T]he results of job enlargement clearly depend on the job in question. To take two extreme examples, the enlargement of the job of a secretary who must type the same letter all day every day cannot help but improve things; in contrast, to enlarge the job of the general practitioner (one wonders how . . . perhaps by including nursing or pharmacological tasks) could only frustrate the doctor and harm the patient. In other words, jobs can be too large as well as too narrow. So the success of any job redesign clearly depends on the particular job in question and how specialized it is in the first place.[18]

The contemporary view is that the benefits of work division and specialization for HSOs, as well as for their staff (especially those whose economic success depends on holding highly specialized professional and technical jobs), must be balanced against the dysfunctional effects of such specialization. This balancing takes the form of job enlargement and enrichment programs and is consistent with the widely popular *quality of work life* (QWL) movement. Organizations initiate quality of work life programs "to make the work environment more compatible with their employees' physical, social, and psychological needs."[19] The central purpose of such programs is to make work meaningful for people and to create an environment in which they can be motivated to perform and satisfied by the results of their work.[20]

Authority and Responsibility Relationships

The Classical View   Another important classical organization design concept relevant for organizations is establishment of authority and responsibility relationships over performance of work. Growing directly out of the division of work in organizations is the need to assign the responsibility for and authority over the performance of the work. *Authority* is the power derived from a person's position in an organization. It is sometimes called legitimate power and "is the ability to influence others to carry out orders or to do something they would not have done otherwise."[21] *Responsibility* is the obligation to perform certain functions or achieve certain objectives and, like authority, is derived from position in the organization.

Authority is *delegated* downward in organizations from higher levels of management to lower levels. This *scalar process*[22] results in a scaling or grading of levels of authority and responsibility in HSOs. The authority and responsibility of an HSO president are different from those of vice presidents, department heads, and individual employees. Vertical layers in an organization are the clearest evidence of the scalar process. Higgins notes:

> The scalar chain simply defines the relationships of authority from one level of the organization to another. In the scalar chain, individuals higher up on the chain have more authority than those below them. This is true of all succeeding levels of management from top management to the first-line employee. The scalar chain helps define authority and responsibility and, thus, accountability.[23]

Classical theorists distinguished two forms of authority relationships: *line authority* and *staff authority.* As organizational concepts, "line" and "staff" are best understood as a matter of relationships. A line relationship is one in which a superior exercises direct authority over a subordinate. This is *command* authority and is represented by the *chain of command* in an organization. The chain of command in an HSO is illustrated by the relationships among nurses on a unit to the head nurse of the unit, to the nursing supervisor, to the vice president for nursing, and finally to the president of the HSO. Each person in this chain has the authority, by virtue of organizational position, to issue directives to, and expect compliance from, persons lower in the chain.

Staff authority, in contrast, is *advisory* authority. "It is the authority that comes in the form of counsel, advice, and recommendation."[24] An HSO's in-house legal counsel has a staff position and cannot dictate the terms of a contract between the HSO and its unionized employees. However, the lawyer can advise the HSO's line managers (chief executive officer and vice president for human resources in this instance) about language and terms.

The Contemporary View   Classical theorists were obsessed with the concept of authority in organizations. In their view authority was "the glue that held the organization together."[25] Furthermore, they believed that the rights attached to one's position were the only important sources of power or influence in the organization. The classical theorists "believed that managers were all-powerful."[26] This might have been true 100 years ago, but no longer. Now, authority is seen as just one element in the larger concept of power in organizations.[27]

Power   There are numerous sources of power and influence in HSOs (this is discussed more fully in Chapter 14, "Leadership," in relationship to the power of leaders). The authority that derives from one's formal position is only one source. French and Raven[28] conceptualize interpersonal power with five distinct bases in organizations: legitimate, reward, coercive, expert, and referent. Only the first three bases derive from the manager's formal position.

Power derived from position in an organization is *legitimate power*. This formal authority resides in managers and exists because organizations find it advantageous to assign power to individuals so they can do their jobs effectively. All managers have some legitimate power or authority based on position. Managers also have *reward power,* which is based on their ability to reward desirable behavior and stems from the legitimate power granted to managers. Because of their position, managers control rewards such as pay increases, promotions, and work schedules, and this buttresses legitimate power. Managers also have *coercive power* because of their position. It is the opposite of reward power and is based on the ability to punish or prevent someone from obtaining desired rewards.

These sources of power in organizations are restricted to managers by definition; others are not. These other sources are quite important in HSOs and often mean that power and influence are spread beyond that reserved for managers.

Expert power derives from having knowledge valued by the organization. Expert power is personal to the individual who has the expertise. Thus, it is different from legitimate, reward, and coercive power, which are prescribed by the organization, even though persons may be granted these types of power because they possess expert power. For example, persons with expert power often rise to management positions in their areas of expertise. It is also noteworthy that, in organizations in which work is highly technical or professional, such as HSOs, expert power alone makes people powerful. For example, the power of physicians and other licensed independent practitioners is based on clinical knowledge and skills. Physicians with scarce expertise, such as transplant surgeons, have more expert power than physicians whose expertise is more readily replacable.

Referent power results when someone engenders admiration, loyalty, and emulation to the extent that the person gains the power to influence others. This is sometimes called charismatic power and is certainly not limited to managers. In organizations charismatic individuals wield considerable influence. As with expert power, referent power cannot be given by the organization as can legitimate, reward, and coercive power.

The contemporary view of authority and responsibility in HSOs is that they are still key concepts, heavily influencing the organization design. However, the classical views on the sources of authority have been expanded to include authority as only one of several sources of power. In this larger context power is not limited to managers.

Delegation   Another important contemporary development in the concept of authority and responsibility pertains to delegation. Almost without exception classicists thought decisions should be made at the lowest possible level in the organization and that this was compatible with good decisions. This means top management should not make decisions on routine matters that could be handled at a lower level. Mooney and Reiley stated that

> One of the tragedies of business experience is the frequency with which men [business in 1939 was an almost exclusively male domain], always efficient in anything they personally can do, will finally be crushed and fail under the weight of accumulated duties that they do not know and cannot learn how to delegate.[29]

The theory of delegation was first expounded by the classicists. It is now considered an integral part of the question of how centralized or decentralized decision making in organizations should be. Decentralization is closely related to delegation, but it is more. It is also a philosophy of organization and management. Decentralization requires more than handing authority or responsibility to subordinates. Organizations discover that decentralizing requires carefully selecting which decisions to push down and which to hold at or near the top.

Delegating authority decentralizes an organization and vice versa. Dale[30] developed criteria to determine the extent of decentralization in an organization:

1. The greater the number of decisions made lower down the management hierarchy, the greater the degree of decentralization.
2. The more important the decisions made lower down the management hierarchy, the greater the degree of decentralization. For example, a manager's ability to commit to capital expenditures indicates the degree to which authority has been delegated.
3. The more functions that are affected by decisions made at lower levels, the greater the degree of decentralization. For example, HSOs that permit all department managers to make marketing or personnel decisions in their areas of responsibility have greater decentralization than those that restrict these decisions to the functional departments of marketing or personnel/human resources.
4. The less checking required on decisions at lower levels of the organization, the greater the degree of decentralization. Decentralization is greatest when no check at all is made; less when superiors must be informed of the decision after it has been made; and still less if superiors must be consulted before the decision is made. The fewer people to be consulted, and the lower they are on the management hierarchy, the greater the degree of decentralization.

Departmentation

The Classical View   Every organized human activity—from a sand lot baseball game to the human genome project—has two fundamental and opposing requirements: *division* of work to be performed and *coordination* of the divided work.[31] Classical theorists recognized the relationship between dividing work and the need to then coordinate divided work to achieve satisfactory results. They developed the concept of *departmentation* (sometimes called *departmentalization*) as an organization design concept that partially addresses these dual concerns. Departmentation still heavily influences design of modern organizations and is "the grouping of jobs under the authority of (usually) a single manager, according to some common, rational basis."[32]

The classical view of departmentation is that it is a natural consequence of division and specialization of work. Since it is rational to specialize work, it is also rational to group similar workers into work groups. In turn, they are grouped into clusters of work groups until the organization has a superstructure (see Figure 6.1). Gulick and Urwick[33] noted four reasons for departmentation: purpose, process, persons and things, and place. Bases for departmentation have increased since, but the basic concept is largely unchanged. Mintzberg,[34] for example, suggests six bases for grouping workers into units and units into larger units:

> *Knowledge and skills:* workers are grouped by specialized knowledge and skills. Hospitals group surgeons in one department, pediatricians in another.
>
> *Work process and function:* workers are grouped by processes or functions performed. Departments of marketing or finance in HSOs are examples.
>
> *Time:* workers are grouped by when work is done. Hospitals and other HSOs are 24-hour-a-day operations. Some workers are grouped into day, evening, and night shifts.
>
> *Output:* workers are grouped by outputs, whether services or products. Many HSOs group workers by whether they produce inpatient or outpatient services.
>
> *Client:* workers are grouped by patient(s) served. It is common for some HSOs to establish work groups based on age or sex of patients. Geriatric and women's health programs are examples.
>
> *Place:* workers are grouped by physical location. A hospital system might operate ambulatory clinics downtown and in suburban locations.

A single HSO may use all these bases for grouping workers to design an effective organization.

No matter which basis is used, the act of grouping workers helps establish the means by which their work can be coordinated within the groups and with other work groups. Mintzberg[35] suggests that grouping (or departmentation) has at least four important implications for workers and their organizations:

1. Grouping sets up a system of common supervision. Once workers are grouped, a manager can be appointed to coordinate and control the work of the group.
2. Grouping facilitates sharing resources. People in work groups share a common budget, facilities, and equipment.
3. Grouping typically leads to common measures of performance. Shared resources on the input side and group-level objectives on the output side permit group members to be evaluated by common performance criteria. Common performance measures encourage group members to coordinate work.
4. Grouping encourages communication. Shared input resources and output objectives and close physical proximity encourage communication. This facilitates coordinating work of group members.

The Contemporary View   HSOs use all six of the bases of departmentation discussed above, including departmentation by function, the basis most favored by the classical theorists. This basis, reinforced by the specialized knowledge and skills of many workers, is clearly visible in HSOs. Nurses are in nursing service, pharmacists in the pharmacy, and so on. Even within departments, the departmentation concept is evident. For example, a large clinical laboratory (a result of functional departmentation) is comprised of even more functionally specialized work groups, such as blood bank, chemistry, and hematology.[36]

However, a contemporary change in HSOs is the increased focus on patients as the basis for departmentation or grouping. This probably results from increased competition for patients among HSOs. A direct outgrowth of this phenomenon is a significant increase in grouping workers on the basis of patients. Geriatric and women's health programs abound, as do comprehensive cardiac care programs marketed specifically to corporate executives.

One of the most important recent changes regarding HSO organization design is recognizing that rigidly departmented organizational structures, no matter what the basis for departmentation, face significant problems of coordination across departments and other divisions of workers. The bureaucratic form—what Burns and Stalker[37] call the *mechanistic* form, which stresses departmentation and hierarchy—works well in some circumstances but not others. The mechanistic form is effective in stable circumstances, but it is at a distinct disadvantage when flexibility to changing circumstances is more important. Organization designs that are more *organic*[38] work better in dynamic circumstances. As Gibson, Ivancevich, and Donnelly point out,

> The organic organization is flexible and adaptable to changing environmental demands because its design encourages greater utilization of the human potential. Managers are encouraged to adopt practices that tap the full range of human motivations through job design that stresses personal growth and responsibility. Decision making, control, and goal-setting processes are decentralized and shared at all levels of the organization. Communications flow throughout the organization, not only down the chain of command.[39]

Another significant contemporary organization design development in HSOs responds to difficulties encountered in managing large-scale projects that require the skills of people in different departments or encourages use of multidisciplinary approaches to patient care. *Project teams* use groups of workers drawn from different departments. Project teams do not replace the departmental structure. They are organic complements to the more mechanistic functional departmental structure and eliminate some of its rigidity in certain circumstances.

A situation in which a project team could be used is a decision to organize services into a comprehensive home health care program for the chronically ill. This effort would benefit from a team organized around the focus of the program—home services for the chronically ill. Team members are drawn from nursing, social services, respiratory therapy, occupational therapy, pharmacy, and physicians specializing in chronic disease. To market the program and to handle finance and reimbursement issues, expertise would be provided by team members drawn from the HSO's administration. A project manager would be named.

Project organization permits flexibility, enhances worker skill development, and enriches jobs for team participants. It has a negative side, however. Project organization can cause ambiguity for workers who participate in a project with its own manager while holding a position in their home department, which has a different manager. Project organization is time consuming because it relies on extensive communication, often in face-to-face team meetings. Furthermore, good project managers are scarce. They must be knowledgeable in the area of the project's focus *and* have good interpersonal skills. Managers accustomed to working in a departmented structure must adopt a new approach to the job to successfully manage projects. Management of project teams differs from managing departments along the dimensions illustrated in Table 6.2.

HSOs can easily use the project organization design by superimposing it on the existing functionally departmented design. This can be done in a few areas, such as the home care program noted earlier, or for the whole organization. Figure 6.2 is a *matrix design* for a psychiatric hospital in which functional managers head departments and program or product line managers

Table 6.2.   Differences in department and project management

Function	Department management	Project management
Planning	Repetitive with annual, monthly, weekly and daily issues that are similar from cycle to cycle	Single cycle of planning, broken into discrete phases
Communication	Clearly defined channels which emphasize chain of command and adherence to procedure	Must be more rapid, relies on both formal and informal channels; meetings are more frequent
Leadership	Generally hierarchical, multiple layers of administration	More streamlined; requires advocacy rather than administration for leadership
Roles and responsibilities	Clearly defined, supported by position descriptions, formal policy, and procedure documentation; social pecking order determined by job	Must be defined at the start of project and redefined as project progresses

From Stevens, George H. *The Strategic Health Care Manager,* 125. San Francisco, Jossey-Bass Publishers, 1991; reprinted by permission.

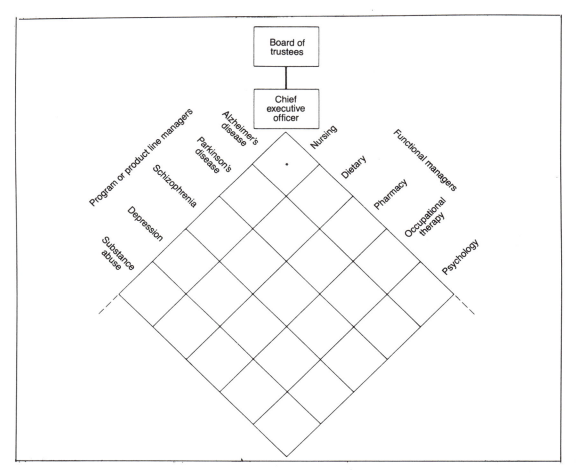

Figure 6.2.   A matrix design for a psychiatric hospital. (From Leatt, Peggy, Stephen M. Shortell, and John R. Kimberly. *Health Care Management: A Text in Organization Theory and Behavior,* 2nd ed. by Stephen M. Shortell and Arnold D. Kaluzny, 324. Delmar Publishers Inc., Albany, NY; Copyright 1988. Reprinted by permission)

head major clinical programs or product lines. Notice that the individual worker depicted is a member of nursing *and* the Alzheimer program.

Span of Control

The Classical View   An organization design question of fundamental concern to classical theorists was how large to make groupings of workers. How many should be grouped in a department, and on what basis was the decision made? In considering these questions, classical theorists developed the *span of control* concept. It was and remains an important organization design concept. Span of control is defined as the number of subordinates reporting directly to a superior.

Classical theorists generally agreed that managers should have limited numbers of subordinates reporting directly to them. Their conclusion was pragmatic and based on the ability of managers to exercise *control* over those who reported directly to them. Some theorists even specified numbers for the optimum span. Urwick[40] specified six as the maximum span if the manager was to maintain close control. Davis[41] distinguishes two types of span of control: executive and operative. Executive span refers to senior and middle-level management positions, operative to first-line management positions. Davis judged that an effective executive span of control could vary from three to nine, while the operative span could have as many as 30 reporting directly to a first-line manager.

How an organization answers the span of control question significantly affects its design. As seen in Figure 6.3, smaller spans of control produce "tall" organizations and larger spans produce "flat" organizations. The tall and flat structures in Figure 6.3 have equal numbers of positions, but the tall structure has five levels while the flat one has three. Complex HSOs usually have a tall pattern. This results from extreme differentiation and specialization of numerous and varied departments (e.g., laundry and nursing) and the consequent need for limited spans of control. Less complex HSOs, such as clinics or small nursing facilities, have flat structures.

The Contemporary View   The most important change in the span of control concept has been the recognition that several factors must be considered in determining the appropriate spans of control in an organization's design. In contemporary theory the factors that determine an appropriate span of control include:[42]

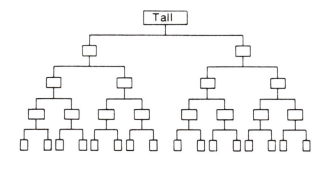

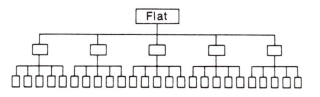

Figure 6.3.   Contrasting spans of control.

Level of professionalism and training of subordinates Professionalized and highly trained workers (characteristics prevalent in HSOs) require less close supervision, which permits wider spans of control.

Level of uncertainty in the work being done Complex and varied work requires close supervision, compared to simple and repetitive work. Close supervision requires narrow spans of control.

Degree of standardization of work Standardized and routinized work, whether professional, such as in a pharmacy or laboratory, or work such as food preparation, requires less direct supervision. Spans of control for standardized work can be wider than for less standardized work.

Degree of interaction required between managers and workers Work situations in which more interaction is needed between managers and workers require narrower spans of control. Effective interaction takes time. Increasing the number of people interacting increases demands for interaction. Interactions can be computed. The number of subordinates increases arithmetically, but the number of possible interactions between managers and subordinates increases exponentially because managers can interact with individuals and with combinations of individuals. The number of possible interactions between a manager and two subordinates, individually or in combination, is six. If the number of subordinates is five, potential interactions increase to 100; six subordinates mean 222 possible interactions between manager and subordinates.

Degree of task integration required If work being done in a group is integrated or interdependent, a narrower span of control may be needed. Integrating the work of a few people whose work is interconnected is easier than doing so for a large number of people.

The contemporary view is that the classical concept of span of control is highly relevant to HSO design. However, several contingencies must be recognized when applying it. A president with five or six vice presidents may be an appropriate span of control. At levels where work is standardized and routinized the spans can be much wider. Another factor is the nature of the work. It is easier to supervise 10 file clerks than 5 head nurses. Abilities and availability of managers must be taken into account. The training and personal qualities of some managers enable them to manage more subordinates than others, thus having a broader span of control. Similarly, better training and higher potential for self-direction of subordinates reduces the need for relationships with management and increases the number of subordinates a manager can supervise.

Coordination[43]

The Classical View The classical theorists, especially Fayol, thought the organization design concept of coordination was very important. Chester Barnard, another influential classical theorist, went so far as to say that, in most circumstances, "the quality of coordination is the crucial factor in the survival of the organization."[44] Fayol's conceptualization was representative of how classicists viewed coordination. He defined it as "pulling together all activities of the enterprise to make possible both its working and success."[45] He believed that a well-coordinated organization had distinct characteristics: each department works in harmony with other departments; each department knows the share of common tasks it must assume; and work schedules of all departments are integrated.

Fayol observed that organizations are poorly coordinated for several reasons: people in each department may know little about what happens in other departments; by focusing too much on their departments, managers have difficulty thinking of the organization's general interest; and managers create barriers between their departments and other departments. Fayol called this last point creating "water-tight compartments," a concept now called "protecting turf." Fayol noted that failing to consider the organization's general interest, which he judged disastrous for an organization, "is not the result of preconcerted intention but the culmination of nonexistent or inadequate coordination."[46]

Classical theorists saw coordination as a way to link various parts of an organization and considered it a vital concept for managers. The early theorists defined coordination in ways that remain valid. They saw it as consciously assembling and synchronizing different work efforts so they function harmoniously in attaining organization objectives.[47] Some authors now use *integration* to express this concept. Lawrence and Lorsch define integration as "the process of achieving unity of effort among the various subsystems in the accomplishment of the organization's tasks."[48] The two terms have very similar meanings.

The Contemporary View   The definition of coordination and recognition of its importance in organization design can be attributed to classical theorists, but a rich menu of *mechanisms of coordination,* the activities managers use to achieve coordination,* has been developed since. Experience with these mechanisms yields different levels of success depending on the situation. This led to a *contingency* view of coordination; no coordinating mechanism is always best. The extensive menu of coordinating mechanisms and the wisdom to see them in a contingency framework are contemporary developments.

It is more appropriate to use a contingency approach to coordination in HSOs than in many other types of organizations because of the large number of professionals working in HSOs. Scott[49] points out that, because activities of health professionals are complex, uncertain, and of great social importance, distinctive structural arrangements have evolved to support health professionals' autonomy. He identifies three types of structural arrangements. The *autonomous arrangement* is that in which an organization delegates to a professional group goal setting, implementation, and evaluation of performance. Management controls only the support staff. Historically, HSOs have had this arrangement with their professional staff organizations (PSOs). The *heteronomous arrangement* is that in which professionals are subordinated to management, with responsibilities delegated to professional groups. Nursing and social work typically have this relationship with HSOs. A third relationship between professionals and HSOs is the *conjoint arrangement,* in which professionals and management have equal power. Conjoint arrangements are an abstraction, but occasionally, in certain HSOs, the balance of power between PSO and management may be conjoint or something akin to it. The structural arrangement an HSO has with professional staff affects the choice of mechanisms used to coordinate their work with that of others.

Typologies of Coordination Mechanisms   The mechanisms that managers use to achieve coordination in HSOs may be categorized in several different ways. Litterer[50] suggests a typology of three categories: coordination through the hierarchy, the administrative system, and voluntary activities. *Hierarchical coordination* links various activities by placing them under a central authority. In a simple HSO this form of coordination is often sufficient. Complex HSOs have several levels and specialized departments and hierarchical coordination is more difficult. The chief executive officer is a focal point of authority, but it is impossible for one person to solve all coordinating problems in the hierarchy. Therefore, coordination through the hierarchical structure must be supplemented.

The *administrative system* is a second mechanism to coordinate activities in Litterer's typology. He notes that "A great deal of coordinative effort in organizations is concerned with a horizontal flow of work of a routine nature. Administrative systems are formal procedures designed to carry out much of this routine coordinative work automatically."[51] Work procedures such as mem-

---

*It should be noted that coordination is best discussed in conjunction with control. Because control is an extensive topic and involves much more than its relationship to coordination, however, it is treated separately in Chapter 12, "Control, Risk Management and Quality Assessment/Improvement, and Resource Allocation." It is noted here that coordination mechanisms unsupported by control mechanisms rapidly lose effectiveness. Control provides the muscle that allows coordination to be effective.

oranda with routing slips help coordinate operating units. To the extent these procedures can be programmed or routinized, it is not necessary to establish other specific means for coordination. For nonroutine and nonprogrammable events, administrative systems or actions such as coordinating committees may be required to provide integration.

A third type of coordination, according to Litterer, is through *voluntary action* when individuals or groups see a need for coordination, develop a method, and implement it. Much of this type of coordination depends on the willingness and ability of individuals or groups to voluntarily find ways to integrate their activities with other organizational participants. Achieving voluntary coordination is one of the most important yet difficult problems for the manager. Voluntary coordination requires that individuals have sufficient knowledge of organizational objectives, information about specific problems of coordination, and the motivation to do something about the problems. Fortunately, voluntary coordination in HSOs is facilitated by the professionalism of many of the staff. While their example is the hospital, the point applies to all HSOs when Georgopoulos and Mann observe that

> The hospital is dependent very greatly upon the motivations and voluntary, informal adjustments of its members for the attainment and maintenance of good coordination. Formal organizational plans, rules, regulations, and controls may ensure some minimum coordination, but of themselves are incapable of producing adequate coordination, for only a fraction of all the coordinative activities required in this organization can be programmed in advance.[52]

A primary force ensuring voluntary coordination is the value system focused on patient welfare, which is partly developed through the training and professionalism of HSO staff.

Mintzberg[53] categorizes the mechanisms of coordination available to managers as mutual adjustment, direct supervision, standardization of work processes, standardization of work outputs, and standardization of worker skills. Figure 6.4 illustrates these coordinating mechanisms, which can be summarized as:

Mutual adjustment—provides coordination by informal communications among those whose work must be coordinated. Like Litterer's voluntary actions noted above, work is coordinated by those performing it (see Figure 6.4a).

Direct supervision—like Litterer's hierarchical coordination, is a way of coordinating work that occurs when someone takes responsibility for the work of others, including issuing them instructions and monitoring their actions (see Figure 6.4b).

Standardization of work processes—is an alternative coordinating mechanism that programs or specifies the contents of work. HSOs standardize work processes when possible, such as standard admission and discharge procedures or standard methods of performing laboratory tests (see Figure 6.4c, Work processes).

Standardization of outputs—specifies the product or expected performance, with the process of how to perform the work left to the worker (see Figure 6.4c, Outputs).

Standardization of worker skills—occurs when neither work processes nor output can be standardized. If standardization is to occur in such situations, it must be through worker training (see Figure 6.4c, Input skills). This form is most frequently found in HSOs, where complexity of much of the work does not allow standardization of work processes or outputs. Standardization of worker skills and knowledge is an excellent coordinating mechanism. For example, "When an anesthesiologist and a surgeon meet in the operating room to remove an appendix, they need hardly communicate; by virtue of their respective training, they know exactly what to expect of each other. Their standardized skills take care of most of the coordination."[54]

Hage[55] provides another typology of coordination mechanisms. He includes four types: programming, planning, customs, and feedback. In using *programming,* organizations develop ex-

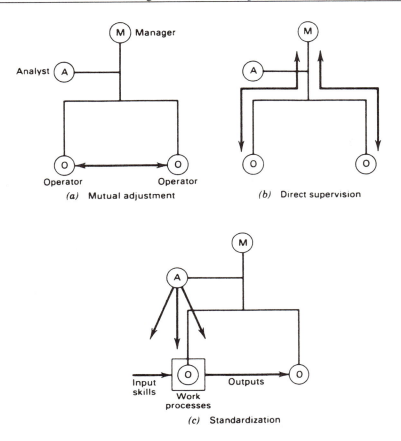

Figure 6.4. Mintzberg's five coordinating mechanisms. (From Mintzberg, Henry. *Structure in Fives: Defining Effective Organizations,* 5. Englewood Cliffs, NJ: Prentice Hall, Inc., 1983; reprinted by permission.)

plicit rules and prescriptions (called programs) that define jobs and the sequence of activities for all jobs in a department and, beyond that, for the organization as a whole. Programming allows staff to learn and do their jobs and reduces the need for communication except for questions about interpreting a rule. Programming an organization yields a result quite similar to Litterer's administrative system and is accomplished with rules, manuals, job descriptions, personnel procedures, promotion policies, and the like. HSOs rely heavily, but not exclusively, on programming as a means of coordination.

Planning differs from programming. A plan delineates objectives that the organization hopes to achieve and the means to achieve them. Planning and programming can, of course, be combined. Programs are specific means to achieve the HSO's planned objectives. Planning as a coordinative mechanism is exemplified by the need of planning in one unit to be made part of the whole. For example, overall expansion plans must be considered in the human resources planning that occurs in nursing service. In fact, all departmental plans should contribute to the objectives contained in the organization's plans. Senior managers are responsible for ensuring that all managers understand organizational objectives. It is the joint duty of all managers to determine whether their plans are compatible with all other plans. To the extent this is done, coordination is facilitated.

Customs are a coordination mechanism. Programming is a rational attempt to prescribe norms of behavior in organizations. Customs are norms developed over time that specify behavior of participants in an organization's social system. In this sense, customs may be more rational than programming rules because customs based on a history of trial and error are a distillation of good practice, whereas programming can result from a manager's ideal sense rather than lessons learned from reality. Customs are an important coordinating mechanism, but in complex HSOs they are not, in and of themselves, sufficient to achieve effective coordination.

Feedback, the fourth in Hage's typology of coordination mechanisms, occurs in verbal and nonverbal forms. Indeed, machines are often designed with feedback mechanisms to improve performance. In coordination, communication feedback indicates when the organization is not functioning well or when problems of conflict or inefficiency arise. Not all forms of communication represent feedback, but some, particularly those involving committees and horizontal communication, are likely to represent management's attempts to coordinate through feedback. Communication, including the role of feedback, is detailed in Chapter 15, "Communication." Committees usually include persons from several departments or functional areas and are concerned with problems requiring coordination. Such use of committees is well established in HSOs.

Other Coordinating Mechanisms   Other coordinating mechanisms are used in contemporary HSOs. Sometimes the "mechanism" is one person. For example, Lawrence and Lorsch[56] found that well-coordinated organizations often rely upon individuals, whom they term "integrators," to achieve coordination. Successfully playing an integrator role depends more on having professional competence than occupying a particular formal position. People are successful integrators because of specialized knowledge and because they represent a central source of information. Examples of effective integrators are found among all health professionals. In most HSOs individual nurses, regardless of formal position, often function as integrators linking physicians to the HSO's formal administrative structure. These same integrators often provide significant coordination among various departments and subunits, particularly as they relate to patient care. The integrator role is also played by people chosen to be program or product line managers in matrix structures (review Figure 6.2).

Another contemporary mechanism that can improve coordination is the *quality circle.* Quality circles are discussed in Chapter 10, "Managerial Problem Solving and Decision Making," as a problem-solving and quality improvement technique and in Chapter 16, "Organizational Change," as a way to involve people in organizational change. Originally developed in the United States but brought to a high art in Japan, this mechanism is gaining acceptance as a means of coordinating, especially at the operational level. It features small-group, problem-oriented meetings in which employees focus on changes needed to improve morale, productivity, or quality. Techniques used include nominal group process, multicriteria decision making, and critical incident examination. Quality circles improve communication and inspire more effective teamwork in HSOs, both of which contribute directly to enhanced coordination.

The contemporary view of coordination as an organization design concept is that it is vital to effective HSO performance and that managers can select from a long menu of coordinating mechanisms: administrative system; committees; customs; direct supervision; feedback; hierarchy; integrators; matrix designs; mutual adjustment; planning; programming; project management through task forces or teams; standardization of work processes, outputs, or worker skills; quality circles; and voluntary action. Managers in HSOs use various combinations of these mechanisms to achieve coordination; usually several are used concurrently.

Summary of the Classical Organization Design Concepts

The relationship of classical design concepts to the actual organizational structure of an HSO is readily seen in the schematic representation known as an *organization chart.* For example, the hospital organization chart in Figure 6.5 shows the basic nature of the *division of work.* Each unit in the chart represents a subdividing of work and suggests that staff in each unit specialize. The

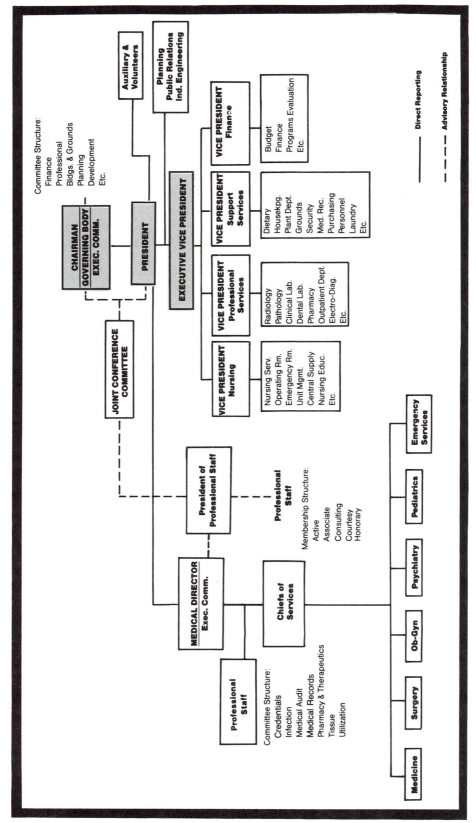

Figure 6.5. Organization chart of a general acute care hospital.

chart also illustrates *authority and responsibility relationships*. The vertical dimension generally shows who has authority over and responsibility for whom. Those higher in the chart generally have authority over those lower in it. People on the same level generally have equal amounts of authority and responsibility. The chart also depicts groupings of people into units in the *departmentation* process. The chart permits easy assessment of a *span of control* simply by counting the people with a direct reporting relationship to a manager. Finally, the chart suggests who is responsible for *coordinating* parts of the HSO, although the coordinating mechanisms they might use are not apparent in the chart.

Of course, organizational structures built upon the classical design concepts such as the one shown in Figure 6.5 do not show the entire organizational structure. Coexisting with this formal organization is an informal organization that is not visible in the organization chart.

THE INFORMAL ORGANIZATION

Existing within the formal pattern of authority–responsibility relationships is another important pattern—the *informal organization*. The formal organization is planned and prescribed, representing a deliberate effort to establish patterned relationships. A great deal of management time and effort is spent establishing and maintaining the formal organization. The results of this effort include development of an organizational structure such as that depicted in Figure 6.5, and related job descriptions, formal rules, operating policies, work procedures, control procedures, coordinating mechanisms, compensation arrangements, and other ways to guide employee behavior. However, many interactions among members of an organization are not prescribed by the formal structure. Relationships and interactions that arise spontaneously from activities and interactions of members, but are not set forth in the formal structure, make up the informal organization.

Formal and informal organizations coexist and are, in fact, inseparable. Blau and Scott point out that they are totally intermeshed:

> It is impossible to understand the nature of a formal organization without investigating the networks of informal relations and the unofficial norms as well as the formal hierarchy of authority and the official body of rules, since the formally instituted and the informally emerging patterns are inextricably intertwined. The distinction between the formal and the informal aspects of organization life is only an analytical one and should not be reified; there is only one actual organization.[57]

The formal and the informal organizations *together* constitute the organizational setting in which work is performed in HSOs. The formal organization is characterized by prescribed authority-responsibility relationships, division of work and departmentation, and the hierarchical structure. The formal organization is the *planned* interrelationships of people, things, and activities. By contrast, the informal organization is characterized by dynamic behavior and activity patterns that occur within the formal organization structure as a result of people working with other people—their interaction and fraternization across formal structural lines. Managers must pay careful attention to both formal and informal aspects of organization design.

The Nature of Informal Organizations

Keen awareness of and interest in informal organization design concepts stem from the famous Hawthorne studies of the 1930s.[58] These studies showed that informal organization is integral to the work setting. The informal organization arises from *social* interactions of persons in an organization. Much of what managers know about the informal organization is based on the work of sociologists and social psychologists, who study groups and the behavior of people in groups.

A *group* is "two or more persons, who come into contact for a purpose and who consider the contact meaningful."[59] As Wexley and Yukl[60] show, group members also depend on one another to achieve their objectives. Thus, groups have a purpose, although it may be implicit rather than stated, and there is interdependence among members. Groups in organizations can be classified as formal or informal groups. A *formal group* is one that "is intentionally created by managers and has specific tasks aimed at achieving organizational objectives. It is part of the [formal] organization structure."[61] Examples of formal groups include committees, quality circles, task forces, and project teams. In contrast, *informal groups*

> are not created by authority but rather evolve from spontaneous attractions among individuals who seek social reinforcement. They seldom have stated goals and lack the assumption of permanence. They can, however, be extremely influential, as when co-workers "network" communications or develop cohesive behavior.[62]

Three important facts emerge from these definitions and descriptions of the informal organization:

1. *The informal organization is inevitable.* Management can change or eliminate any aspect of the formal organization because management created it. The informal organization is not created by management and thus is less subject to management's preferences. As long as people are involved in formal organizations, there will be informal organizations.
2. *Small groups are the central component of the informal organization.* Group membership strongly influences overall behavior and performance of members. Many sociologists now believe that the small group, not the individual, is the basic component of organizations.
3. *Informal organization has both positive and negative consequences for the organization.* To capitalize on the advantages and minimize the disadvantages of the informal organization, the manager must understand the informal organization and, therefore, must understand groups in the organization.

Why People Form Informal Groups

When one considers why a human being does anything, the starting point is motivation. As discussed in Chapter 13, "Motivation," motivation theory begins with the premise that people are motivated by things that satisfy *their* needs. If the formal organization satisfied all the needs of participants, there would be no informal organization. Informal groups come into being because members' needs are not fully met by the formal organization.

What *needs* does the informal organization satisfy? Interpersonal contacts within the small group provide relief from the boredom, monotony, and pressures of the formal organization. Persons in groups are usually surrounded by others with similar values, and this reinforces their value system. Another reason people join informal groups is that groups accord informal status, which may be nothing more than belonging to a distinct little unit that is more or less exclusive. Informal group membership also provides a degree of personal security; the group member feels acceptance by peers as an equal and feels secure in their company. Group membership permits the individual to express views before sympathetic listeners. The group helps satisfy an individual's recognition, participation, and communication needs. The group member may even find an outlet for leadership drives. These important forms of satisfaction are available in the group—usually to a greater degree than in the formal organization. Another important reason for group membership is to secure information. The grapevine—the flow of informal information detailed in Chapter 15—is a phenomenon known to all who participate in organizations. Suffice it to say here that informal group membership gives members access to informal communication. The common denominator in all these reasons for group membership is that they meet specific needs of members that are not fully met by the formal organization. Informal groups arise and persist in the organization because they perform desired functions for their members.

Key Parameters of Informal Groups

Mondy and colleagues suggest that an informal group possesses identifiable characteristics:

> First, its members are joined together to satisfy needs. However, these needs may be completely different; one worker may want to make friends, another may be seeking advancement. Second, the

informal organization [group] is continuously changing. Relationships that exist one day may be gone the next. Third, members of various organizational levels may be involved. The informal organization does not adhere to the boundaries established by the formal one. A manager in one area may have close ties to a worker in another. Fourth, the informal organization is affected by relationships outside the [HSO]. A top-level manager and a supervisor may associate with each other because they are members of the same golf club. Finally, the informal organization has a pecking order: certain people are assigned greater importance than others.[63]

Beyond these characteristics, there are other key parameters of how informal groups form and operate that managers must know.

Leadership in Informal Groups   A key parameter of how informal groups function is leadership, even if it is unofficial. Leaders of informal groups have been studied extensively:[64]

1.   They possess attributes that group members perceive to be critical to satisfy *their* needs.
2.   They embody values of the groups from which they come. Leaders perceive these values, organize them into a philosophy, and verbalize them to members and nonmembers.
3.   They receive communications relevant to the group and communicate the new information to their group. Leaders are information centers for informal groups.

Informal group leaders serve several functions. The leader not only initiates action and provides direction, but resolves differences of opinion on group-related matters. Furthermore, the leader communicates group values and feelings to nonmembers, such as representatives of the formal organization. Leadership is retained only as long as the role is performed well.

Stages of Group Development   Another parameter of groups is how they are formed. Groups in work places, whether they are part of the formal organization (e.g., committees or quality circles) or are informal groups, generally develop in stages: forming, storming, norming, performing, and adjourning.[65]

In *forming*, the group is established by management or develops informally. This is a time when members become acquainted and learn about the tasks they are to perform or the benefits they might obtain from membership. *Storming* is characterized by conflict and potential conflict in the group. This has to be sorted out before progress can be made by the group, and sometimes the sorting out process is quite "stormy." In the *norming* stage members begin to function cooperatively as a group. Members establish the rules of conduct or "norms" for group members. As the name suggests, the *performing* stage is reached when the group is fully functional.

> Members are well organized, concerned about the group and its results, and are able to deal with task accomplishment and conflict in rational and creative ways. The primary concerns of the group at this stage are continuing to achieve results and adapting over time to changing conditions.[66]

The group dissolves in the final stage, *adjourning*, which is sometimes called dissolution. All groups eventually dissolve, either because the reasons for which they were formed are no longer relevant or because the group no longer serves the needs of its members.

Managers should know which stage of development a group is in because their reaction to a forming group will be different than their reaction to a performing group. The most appropriate reaction to an adjourning group might be to ignore it unless the manager considers it to be a positive force in the organization.

The Structure of Informal Groups   Another important variable in informal group formation and operation is the tendency of such groups to develop a complex structure of relationships. The structure of informal groups is determined by different *status* positions of members: group leader, primary group member, fringe group member, and out status. For example, Figure 6.6 shows the informal structure of a group of nine people working in one section of a clinical laboratory. The solid square in the center represents the *group leader*. Clustered around the leader are the other four members of the *primary group*. This close association is characterized by intense interaction and communication. The three people at the *fringe* are likely to be newcomers who are, in

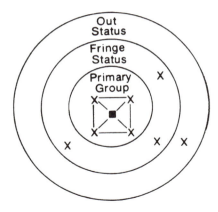

Figure 6.6.   Informal group sociometry.

effect, being evaluated by the primary group and who may become full members. If not accepted they move to *out status*. One person is already in out status. This has profound behavioral effects if the person in out status wants to belong to the primary group. Belonging to the formal group of employees in the laboratory section is no substitute for full membership in the informal group.

The informal organization is not limited to group membership. It also exists as people in the formal organization interact to accomplish work within the context of the formal organization. Figure 6.7 indicates the actual contacts between people in an organization. Not all contacts go through formal channels; in some, levels of the organization are bypassed, and in others, there is cross-contact from one chain of command to another. Contact charts do not show the reasons for informal relationships; they do, however, illustrate the complexity of the informal organization.

Positive Aspects of the Informal Organization

The informal organization serves useful purposes in an HSO, even though management does not create it and managers often see it as a problem. Indeed, the informal organization can be a problem for the manager. The formal organization reflects how managers prefer that people behave; the informal organization is reality. Problems with the informal organization arise when individuals

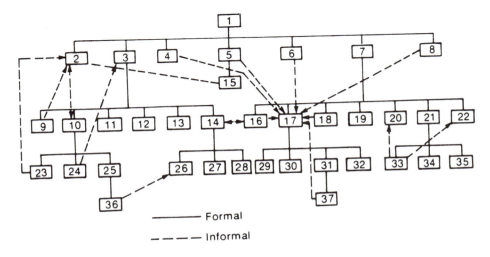

Figure 6.7.   A contact chart.

and groups that comprise it work at cross-purposes with objectives of the formal organization. A fact of organization life is that what is good for the employee is not always good for the employer and vice versa. An employee may want to meet objectives of both the informal group and the HSO, but these may conflict. The result is known as *role conflict*.

The situation of a typical head nurse in an HSO provides an example of role conflict. On the one hand, management expects head nurses to participate in managing the HSO and to plan, organize, and control activities in their units. On the other hand, head nurses are first-line supervisors who have close ties with staff nurses in their units. Often, they are former peers. Head nurses may still belong to informal groups formed by these people. The informal groups may have expectations of their head nurse members that do not coincide with those coming from management. In such circumstances nurses are role conflicted.

Even with such potential problems, however, managers should recognize that informal organizations can, and often do, make positive contributions to HSOs. Some of the more positive ones are listed below.

Informal Complements Formal   The primary benefit of the informal organization is that it blends with the formal organization to form a system that accomplishes work. Formal plans and policies can be too inflexible to meet the needs of a dynamic situation. Thus, the more flexible and spontaneous characteristics of informal organization are a great advantage if they permit, or encourage, deviations in the interest of contributing to organizational goals. Durbin was among the first to recognize the complementarity of the two: "Informal relations in the organization serve to preserve the organization from the self-destruction that would result from literal obedience to the formal policies, rules, regulations, and procedures."[67]

Informal Organizations Provide Social Values and Stability   Turnover may be caused by poor matching of person and job or may be due to pragmatic reasons such as offers of better jobs or family-related moves. However, many resignations occur because new employees cannot become primary members of one or more informal groups. Group membership is a means by which employees achieve a sense of belonging and security. If an organization is cold and impersonal and informal interpersonal contacts are not encouraged or, in some cases, even permitted, new employees may seek employment elsewhere. Of course, informal group membership can be carried to such an extreme that the workplace becomes a social circle, to the detriment of the organization's effectiveness and efficiency. Good management avoids this extreme, however, and provides an atmosphere in which workers, through informal relationships, can meet their human needs of acceptance and gregariousness.[68]

Informal Organizations Can Simplify the Manager's Job   The informal organization can make things easier for the manager in concrete ways *if* the manager maintains control of the situation. When informal group support is available to the manager, supervision in a much more general way is possible than when support is not available. Managers can delegate and decentralize more easily when informal groups are cooperative. The converse is true, as well. The manager must understand the informal organization and use it to advantage. As Mondy and colleagues note:

> Awareness of the nature and impact of informal organization often leads to better management decisions. The acceptance of the fact that formal relationships will not enable full accomplishment of organizational tasks should stimulate management to seek other means of motivation. Managers should seek to improve their knowledge of the nature of people in general and subordinates in particular. They should realize that organizational performance can be affected by the workers' willingness to grant cooperation and enthusiasm. Means other than formal authority must be sought to develop attitudes that support effective performance.[69]

Informal Organizations Are Communication Channels   A well-known benefit of the informal organization is that it provides another channel of communication; the *grapevine* can enhance managers' effectiveness if they study and use it. Chapter 15 has an in-depth discussion of informal communication in HSOs. The grapevine relays certain information to employees and can be used to determine their feelings and attitudes on issues. However, the grapevine can cause problems; the free flow of unfounded rumors can be quite destructive, for example. Neither formal nor information organizations can be effectively used if managers do not understand them.

Living with the Informal Organization

Existence of the informal organization within the formal structure is a fact of organizational life in HSOs. The formal and informal aspects of the organization must be balanced if optimal performance and goal attainment for individuals and the organization are to be achieved. If management tries to suppress the informal organization, it may create a destructive and dysfunctional situation. To protect members and make the work situation acceptable, the informal organization resists what it perceives as autocratic management. These opposing forces clash; the result is reduced effectiveness. This can cause undesirable outcomes such as work restriction, insubordination, disloyalty, and other manifestations of an antiorganization attitude.

The optimum situation occurs when the formal organization is strong enough to maintain a unified thrust toward attaining objectives, but simultaneously permits a well-developed informal organization to help maintain group cohesiveness and stimulate teamwork. In other words, it is ideal when the informal organization is strong enough to be a positive force but not so strong as to dominate the formal organization. Such a relationship is difficult to achieve, but managers can do two things to move the HSO toward this balance. First, they can seek to understand the informal organization and act to convince employees of their understanding and acceptance of it. Particularly important in conveying acceptance is that managers minimize the effect of their actions on the informal organization. Second, they can integrate the interests of the formal and informal organizations to the maximum extent. In doing this, managers should prevent actions through the formal organization that unnecessarily threaten informal relationships.

The informal relationships in HSOs are important to those who work in them and to the organizations. The informal organization deserves the attention of managers because it can complement the effectiveness of the formal stucture, thereby enhancing the organization's ability to fulfill its objectives. Furthermore, understanding "the informal organization reflects the manager's recognition that people in organizations are not mechanistic—they are instead changing, complex, and social beings."[70]

AN INTEGRATED VIEW OF ORGANIZATION DESIGN

Organizations, from the simplest enterprise to large, complex academic medical centers, have five interrelated parts. Mintzberg[71] labels them the strategic apex, the operating core, the middle line, the technostructure, and the support staff. *The strategic apex* are those people who set the strategic direction of an organization. In HSOs this includes the governing body, the president, and perhaps the vice presidents. *The operating core* are those who do the basic work of the organization. They take inputs and convert them to outputs—the products and services of the organization. In HSOs this includes the physicians, nurses, technologists, therapists, and others who provide health services.

The middle line are managers located between the executives in the strategic apex and people in the operating core. They are the middle of the organization's chain of command. Included are department heads and heads of other units and subdivisions. Examples include head nurses and nursing supervisors and directors of pharmacy, laboratory, and dietary services.

The technostructure consists of staff members who help plan and control the basic work of the organization. The people in the technostructure affect the work of others. The role of people in the technostructure is to *standardize* work. They are removed from direct operations—from the operating work flow—but "they may design it, plan it, change it, or train the people who do it."[72] The technostructure in HSOs includes industrial engineers, risk managers, and those who support efforts for continuous quality improvement, because they help standardize and improve work processes; strategic planners, budget analysts, and accountants, because they help standardize outputs; and people who recruit and train workers, because they help standardize the skills in the organization's workforce.

Support staff provide indirect services. In Mintzberg's conceptualization, they provide support to the organization's basic work, but do not do the basic work. In HSOs, support staff support provision of health services, but do not directly provide health services. Examples include fundraising and development, legal counsel, marketing, public relations, finance, and human resources management. Support staff differ from people in the technostructure primarily in that support staff do not focus on work standardization. Support staff provide services to the organization that permit it to do its basic work.

Mintzberg diagrams the five parts of organizations as shown in Figure 6.8. He points out that the structure depicted there

> shows a small strategic apex connected by a flaring middle line to a large, flat operating core. These three parts of the organization are shown in one uninterrupted sequence to indicate that they are typically connected through a single line of formal authority. The technostructure and the support staff are shown off to either side to indicate that they are separate from this main line of authority, and influence the operating core only indirectly.[73]

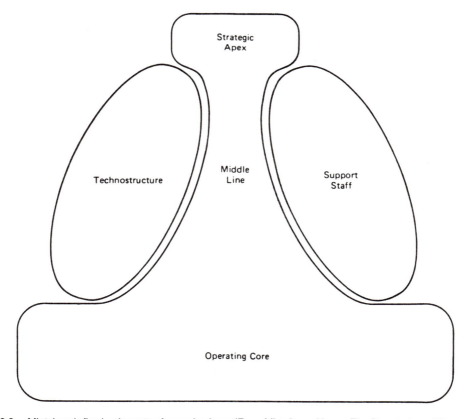

Figure 6.8. Mintzberg's five basic parts of organizations. (From Mintzberg, Henry. *The Structuring of Organizations,* 20. Englewood Cliffs, NJ: Prentice Hall, Inc., 1979; reprinted by permission.)

Mintzberg's conceptualization of the organization is like that resulting from the classical design concepts discussed earlier. The organization depicted in Figure 6.8, like those in Figures 6.3 and 6.5, has the classic pyramid shape. It, too, is built around authority relationships. In Mintzberg's view, the structures of almost all organizations can be included in one of five basic designs based on various configurations of the strategic apex, operating core, middle line, technostructure, and support staff. He labels these design alternatives as the simple structure, the machine bureaucracy, the professional bureaucracy, the divisionalized form, and the adhocracy.[74]

The simple structure, as the name implies, represents the simplest organization design (see Figure 6.9). It has a strategic apex that may be one person, such as the owner of a small enterprise, a physician in private practice, or the director of a small ambulatory care center. In addition, it has an operating core consisting of a group of workers. The middle line, technostructure, and support staff components are small or missing.

The machine bureaucracy resembles the mechanistic design described by Burns and Stalker[75] and the classical bureaucracy described by Weber.[76] This design (see Figure 6.9) is

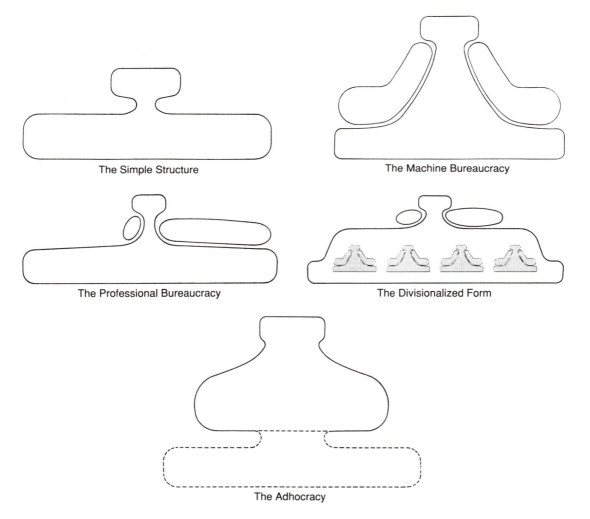

The Simple Structure   The Machine Bureaucracy

The Professional Bureaucracy   The Divisionalized Form

The Adhocracy

Figure 6.9. Mintzberg's five organizational configurations. (From Mintzberg, Henry. *The Structuring of Organizations,* 307, 325, 355, 393, 443. Englewood Cliffs, NJ: Prentice Hall, Inc., 1979; reprinted by permission.)

characterized by a large, well-developed technostructure and support staff because there is great emphasis on work standardization and a focus on marketing and financial and operational control systems. Major decisions are made in the strategic apex, which features rigid patterns of authority. Spans of control are narrow, decision making is centralized, and the organization is functionally departmented. This design typifies manufacturing organizations, although some hospitals, especially those owned by government,[77] also exhibit this design because so much of their work is routine and repetitive and their external environment tends to be stable.

The professional bureaucracy is characterized by an operating core composed primarily of professionals. This design is common in hospitals, universities, and other professionally dominated organizations, such as public accounting firms. The operating core is the heart of the organization, and decision making is decentralized to it. The technostructure is underdeveloped because work is largely done by professionals who do not need—indeed, do not permit—others to do their work. In larger professional bureaucracies, such as hospitals, support staff (see Figure 6.9) may be highly developed and diverse. This staff is needed to support the professionalized operating core.

The divisionalized form has independent units joined by a shared administrative overlay. In contrast to other designs this form is characterized by a large, well-developed middle line because division managers are responsible for their divisions and may be given considerable decision-making latitude (see Figure 6.9). Examples of divisionalized forms include corporations such as General Motors, federal and large state governments, and large, multiorganizational HSO systems. Systems of HSOs have become prevalent through corporate restructuring (creating several corporate entities to perform medical and nonmedical functions previously done by one corporation) and through active programs of merger and consolidation within the health services industry.

The divisionalized form has the advantage of decentralizing decision making to units within the larger organization. This same process, however, makes it more necessary and more difficult to coordinate activities of the divisions. Longest and Klingensmith, adapting Porter's[78] approach to achieving effective linkages among business units of a diversified corporation, suggest several ways of managing coordination among the units of a system:

- *Horizontal structure.* Organizational devices that cut across unit lines, such as partial centralization and interunit task forces or committees that facilitate communication.
- *Horizontal systems.* Management systems with a cross-unit dimension in areas such as planning, control, incentives, capital budgeting, and management information systems.
- *Horizontal human resource practices.* Human resource practices that facilitate unit cooperation, such as cross-unit job rotation, management forums and training.
- *Horizontal conflict resolution processes.* Management processes that resolve conflicts among units. Such processes can be usefully distinguished from horizontal structure and systems, and relate more to the style of managing an organization. The key is for senior management to install and operate a system that is fair in settling disputes among units.[79]

The adhocracy, the fifth of Mintzberg's organization designs, is akin to Burns and Stalker's[80] organic design. As Mintzberg describes it,

> Adhocracy is the most difficult of the five configurations [see Figure 6.9] to describe because it is both complex and nonstandardized. Indeed, adhocracy contradicts much of what we accept on faith in organizations—consistency in output, control by administrators, unity of command, strategy emanating from the top. It is a tremendously fluid structure in which power is constantly shifting and coordination and control are by mutual adjustment through the informal communication and interaction of competent experts.[81]

Describing the adhocracy is complicated by the existence of two forms of this configuration: the *operating* adhocracy and the *administrative* adhocracy.

In the operating adhocracy, "the operating and administrative work blend into a single effort. That is, the organization cannot easily separate the planning and design of the operating work—in other words, the project—from its actual execution."[82] As shown in the solid line adhocracy diagram in Figure 6.9, "the organization emerges as an organic mass in which line managers, staff, and operating experts all work together on project teams in ever-shifting relationships."[83] By contrast, administrative work in an adminstrative adhocracy is sharply separated from operating work. This is shown by the dashed line operating core in the adhocracy diagram in Figure 6.9.

The adhocracy often takes the form of a matrix structure or project teams with emphasis on activities in both the operating core and technostructure. Power in adhocracies shifts between professionals and technical experts. This design can be a free-form structure with frequently changing job descriptions and a flexible concept of authority. HSOs might use adhocracy in multi-disciplinary programs for the elderly, chronically ill, or women, or in the research-oriented departments (e.g., oncology or genetics) in academic medical centers. Mintzberg describes the adhocracy configuration as "one that is able to fuse experts drawn from different disciplines into smoothly functioning ad hoc project teams."[84]

Choosing an Organization Design

There is no magic formula by which managers choose one organization design over another. Furthermore, complex organizations have many different designs embedded in them as various parts try to match structure to strategy, management philosophy, and environmental pressures. In a large and complex HSO such as a teaching hospital, for example, the dental clinic may have a simple structure, the clinical laboratory may be structured as a machine bureaucracy, and the medical and surgical nursing units may be professional bureaucracies. The hospital might be one of several hospitals that are divisions of a multiorganizational system, with the system using the divisionalized form. Simultaneously, the hospital could have a project team of administrative experts in strategic management, marketing, finance, and information systems that, parallel to their regular staff positions and structured as an adhocracy, operates as a "consulting firm" selling expertise to clients such as smaller hospitals and physician groups. Table 6.3 summarizes key structural elements and situations in which these design options might fit.

A leading management theorist, Peter Drucker, gives good advice to managers who must select from among organization design options. He suggests that they evaluate the options against the following criteria:

- Clarity, as opposed to simplicity. The Gothic cathedral is not a simple design, but your position inside it is clear; you know where to stand and where to go. A modern office building is exceedingly simple in design, but it is very easy to get lost in one; it is not clear.
- Economy of effort to maintain control and minimize friction.
- Direction of vision toward the product rather than the process, the result rather than the effort.
- Understanding by each individual of his or her own task, as well as that of the organization as a whole.
- Decision making that focuses on the right issues, is action oriented, and is carried out at the lowest possible level of management.
- Stability, as opposed to rigidity, to survive turmoil, and adaptability to learn from it.
- Perpetuation and self-renewal, which requires that an organization be able to produce tomorrow's leaders from within, helping each person develop continuously; the structure must also be open to new ideas.[85]

SUMMARY

In carrying out the organizing function, managers build a formal organization structure. Coexisting with the formal structure is the informal organization, which is that set of interrelationships and interactions that occur among people in an organization but that lie outside the formally planned and sanctioned structure.

Formal organization structures are built on a set of organization design concepts whose roots can be traced back to general administrative theorists who lived early in the 20th century. Among them, Fayol and Weber made particularly important contributions to understanding the design of

Table 6.3. Key dimensions of Mintzberg's five organizational configurations

	Simple structure	Machine bureaucracy	Professional bureaucracy	Divisionalized form	Adhocracy
Key means of coordination	Direct supervision	Standardization of work	Standardization of skills	Standardization of outputs	Mutual adjustment
Key part of organization	Strategic apex	Technostructure	Operating core	Middle line	Support staff (with operating core in operating adhocracy)
Structural elements					
Specialization of jobs	Little specialization	Much horizontal and vertical specialization	Much horizontal specialization	Some horizontal and vertical specialization (between divisions and headquarters)	Much horizontal specialization
Training and indoctrination	Little training and indoctrination	Little training and indoctrination	Much training and indoctrination	Some training and indoctrination (of division managers)	Much training
Formalization of behavior—bureaucratic/organic	Little formalization—organic	Much formalization—bureaucratic	Little formalization—bureaucratic	Much formalization (within divisions)—bureaucratic	Little formalization—organic
Grouping	Usually functional	Usually functional	Functional and market	Market	Functional and market
Unit size	Wide	Wide at bottom, narrow elsewhere	Wide at bottom, narrow elsewhere	Wide at top	Narrow throughout
Planning and control systems	Little planning and control	Action planning	Little planning and control	Much performance control	Limited action planning (especially in administrative adhocracy)

(continued)

Table 6.3. *(continued)*

	Simple structure	Machine bureaucracy	Professional bureaucracy	Divisionalized form	Adhocracy
Liaison devices	Few liaison devices	Few liaison devices	Liaison devices in administration	Few liaison devices	Many liaison devices throughout
Decentralization	Centralization	Limited horizontal decentralization	Horizontal and vertical decentralization	Limited vertical decentralization	Selective decentralization
Situational elements					
Age and size	Typically young and small	Typically old and large	Varies	Typically old and very large	Typically young (operating adhocracy)
Technical system	Simple, not regulating	Regulating but not automated, not very complex	Not regulating or complex	Divisible, otherwise like machine bureaucracy	Very complex, often automated (in administrative adhocracy), not regulating or complex (in operating adhocracy)
Environment	Simple and dynamic; sometimes hostile	Simple and stable	Complex and stable	Relatively simple and stable; diversified markets (especially products and services)	Complex and dynamic; sometimes disparate (in administrative adhocracy)
Power	Chief executive control; often owner managed; not fashionable	Technocratic and external control; not fashionable	Professional operator control; fashionable	Middle-line control; fashionable (especially in industry)	Expert control; very fashionable

From Mintzberg, Henry. Organization design: Fashion or fit? *Harvard Business Review* 59 (January/February 1981): 107. Reprinted by permission of *Harvard Business Review*. Copyright © 1981 by the President and Fellows of Harvard College; all rights reserved.

organizations. Their work and that of several of their contemporaries form what are called the *classical concepts of organization design*. Five of these concepts are examined: division of work and specialization, authority and responsibility relationships, departmentation, span of control, and coordination.

The *division of work* refers to dividing the work of an organization into specific jobs having specified activities. For example, the job of pharmacist is defined by the activities a person in this position is expected to accomplish. The corollary of division of work is the specialization of workers. As a result of the boredom and monotony that can accompany divided and specialized work, it is sometimes necessary to implement job enrichment programs to offset these negative consequences of specialization.

Growing directly out of the division of work is a need to assign *responsibility* for and *authority* over performance of work. This assignment occurs through the technical process of delegation. This results in scaling or grading the levels of authority and responsibility in the HSO. Also inherent in the authority structure of organizations is the distinction between line and staff authority. Line authority is command authority and follows the chain of command. Staff authority is advisory authority.

A natural consequence of division and specialization of work is *departmentation*—grouping of jobs under the authority of one manager. Six bases for grouping workers are examined: knowledge and skills, work process and function, time, output, client, and place. The *span of control* concept is examined, with emphasis on the influence of span on the shape (tall or flat) of the organization. A number of contingency factors that help determine the proper span of control are discussed.

This chapter notes that rigidly applying the concepts of division of work, hierarchical authority, departmentation, and span of control results in mechanistic organization structures. While these are appropriate structures in some circumstances, they are inappropriate in others. Therefore, such organic organizational structures as project teams and matrix designs are considered as ways to reduce the rigidity of mechanistic designs.

The organization design concept of *coordination* is important in HSOs in which there is a high degree of division and specialization of work and functional departmentation coupled with a need to closely integrate the work. Several coordinating mechanisms are examined: the administrative system, committees, customs, direct supervision, feedback, hierarchy, integrators, matrix designs, mutual adjustment, plans, programming, project management through task forces or teams, standardization (of work processes, outputs, or worker skills), quality circles, and voluntary action.

The informal organization consists of relationships that occur spontaneously from the activites and interactions of staff in the organization, but that are not set forth in the formal structure. To a large extent, the nature of small groups explains the informal organization. If the manager is to fully realize the positive benefits of an informal organization and simultaneously minimize its negative impact, two things must be done: 1) the manager must understand the informal organization and accept it as a fact of organizational life; and 2) to the extent possible, the manager must integrate interests of the informal organization with those of the formal organization.

Mintzberg's five organizational designs are used to integrate the discussion. They are variations of organizations' strategic apex, middle line, operating core, technostructure, and support staff. The five configurations are simple structure, machine bureaucracy, professional bureaucracy, divisionalized form, and adhocracy. Situations in which each form fits are considered.

DISCUSSION QUESTIONS

1. What are the major characteristics of Weber's ideal bureaucracy as an organization form?
2. Discuss the concept of departmentation and apply it to a hospital, a nursing facility, and a small freestanding ambulatory center.

3. Why is coordination so important for HSOs and what are the mechanisms of coordination?
4. Discuss the relationships among span of control, delegation, and centralization-decentralization.
5. Discuss the characteristics of a matrix organization and how it differs from the "classical" functionally departmented organization.
6. Discuss the differences between a tall and a flat organization. Is one form better than the other? Why or why not?
7. Is decentralization better than centralization of authority and decision making?
8. Discuss why informal groups form. Identify their major characteristics.
9. Why is the function of organizing so important in HSOs?
10. Compare and contrast Mintzberg's five basic organizational configurations.

CASE STUDY 1:   A NEW APPROACH ON THE NURSING UNITS

A number of problems existed at Horizon Hospital, a large psychiatric facility. Turnover among nursing personnel was much higher than is typical for psychiatric hospitals, and relationships between the nursing service and members of the professional staff organization (PSO) were unusually poor. Psychiatrists and clinical psychologists often complained that their patients received inadequate attention from nurses and that their orders were not fully and promptly followed.

The hospital president asked the vice president for nursing to recommend a course of action to resolve the problems. He developed a plan to restructure the nursing units using a matrix design (as in Figure 6.2). The vice president's plan included a new structure, reporting relationships, authority and responsibility relationships, and a timetable for implementing the matrix design.

The president was impressed with the plan and believed it might improve the situation. However, when she showed the plan to the chief of staff and several members of the PSO, she was told in no uncertain terms that they would oppose it and would do nothing to implement the change.

Puzzled by their reaction, the president called the vice president into her office to discuss the next step.

Questions

1. Why do you think the PSO members reacted as they did?
2. Is there anything inherently wrong with the matrix design? Is it inappropriate for psychiatric hospitals?
3. What should the president and vice president for nursing do now?

CASE STUDY 2:   THE NEW ADMINISTRATIVE RESIDENT[86]

Jackie Johnson, the new and ambitious administrative resident at Goodhelp Rehabilitation Center, was eager to get things done and constantly looked for departments to streamline. One day she found a gold mine in the switchboard. She rolled up her sleeves when she found out that, although turnover was very low, there was a great deal of dissatisfaction among the switchboard operators. The eight operators were very close in age (mid-40s), socialized with one another after working hours, and frequently discussed personal matters. Johnson regarded Ms. Kelly, the chief operator, as very personable. She got along well with the public but constantly complained that the employees were overworked and underpaid.

Johnson checked with other hospitals in the area and found that, among switchboard operators, Goodhelp had one of the lowest rates of pay in town. When she approached the chief operating officer (COO) on the matter of higher pay, she was told it would be impossible to increase the pay for the operators at the present time.

Johnson set about to do what she could to help the operators. She found that they were working split shifts, and since in her opinion this obviously was not practical, she changed their working schedule. To her surprise, the chief operator reacted very unfavorably to the change in schedule. She then rearranged the work activities by hiring a receptionist so that the operators would be able to concentrate on running the switchboard. The receptionist was not given any cooperation by the switchboard operators, and the first two new employees in the position re-signed. Johnson felt that the chief operator was responsible for the operators' not accepting the new receptionists. She requested that the COO terminate the chief operator. The COO refused to do so. Johnson suddenly found herself in the position of having the switchboard in worse shape than when she started "reforming" it.

Questions

1. What do you think about Johnson's behavior?
2. Why did the telephone operators react as they did?
3. Why did the operators not help the receptionists?
4. If you were the COO, what would you do?

CASE STUDY 3: "I CANNOT DO IT ALL!"

When Arnold Brice was named president of Health Care, Inc., a health maintenance organization (HMO), he inherited a staff composed of vice presidents for marketing, finance, and professional services, and a medical director. Each member was capable in many ways, and Health Care, Inc., was on a solid financial footing with bright prospects. It was located in an expanding community; a 15%–20% annual growth rate was projected for the next 5 years.

Within a few weeks of joining Health Care, Inc., Brice perceived a serious flaw with his staff: none of them would make a decision, not even on rather routine matters such as personnel questions, choice of marketing media, or changing suppliers. This troubled him. Before long the situation seriously impeded his efforts to give thought to strategic plans for the HMO. To make matters worse, he found that the vice presidents routinely discussed their own problems among themselves—to the extent that a great deal of time was consumed in doing so. Yet even with all of this activity, the vice presidents frequently presented him with issues in their areas of responsibility and requested that he make the decision.

At a regular staff meeting, when every member of his staff had an issue requiring a decision, Brice finally blew up. Waving his arms in exasperation, he shouted (very uncharacteristically for him), "I cannot do it all! You are going to have to make these decisions yourselves."

The meeting broke up with the staff looking very puzzled, and Brice realizing that he had to do something besides shout at his staff.

Questions

1. Is this an organization problem? What factors might be contributory?
2. In terms of the organizing function, what can Brice do?

CASE STUDY 4: THE SECRETARIES[87]

There are three secretaries in the business office of Pleasant Valley Nursing Center. The secre-tarial output proved to be a bottleneck in the smooth flow of work in the office. The secretaries had been assigned to various sections of the business office, and the office manager discovered that when one secretary was overloaded with reports and other work, one or both of the other secre-taries often had time on their hands. The peaks and valleys of the secretaries' work loads were usually in contraposition as follows:

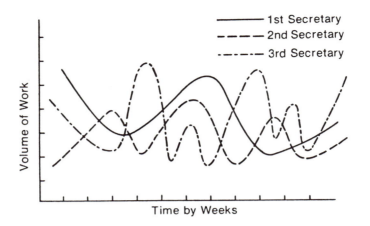

The business office manager decided to pool the work of the secretaries instead of assigning them to one section of the office. On Friday afternoon he called the three secretaries into his office and explained the new idea. They made little comment. Over the weekend, however, one of the secretaries called the business office manager and told him she was resigning effective the following Friday.

On Monday, the other two secretaries spoke to the business office manager and told him they did not like the new plan. They thought their job status would be lowered by the pooling arrangement. The business office manager pointed out they would be performing exactly the same work as before, at the same rate of pay, with the same titles. The secretaries said that they had been aware of the overload situation but had not done anything about it because they had thought they were doing things the way the business office manager wanted. The two secretaries then asked if they could work out a plan on their own.

Realizing that the pressure of his regular duties required his full attention, the business office manager shrugged his shoulders and told the secretaries to make their own arrangements. A replacement for the departing secretary arrived toward the end of that week.

Within a few weeks the three secretaries had devised a plan for synchronizing and interchanging work during rush periods. While the plan looked very much like a pooled arrangement of work, the secretaries were satisfied with the arrangement. The business office manager was also satisfied because the work flow had been smoothed and efficiency increased.

Questions

1. Why did the secretaries react as they did?
2. Using informal organization theory concepts, how could the business office manager have improved the process by which this change was initiated?

CASE STUDY 5: SOMEBODY HAS TO BE LET GO[88]

Ken was a senior vice president of one of the nation's leading quality consulting firms. In 4 years the makeup of the company had expanded from the founder, a secretary, 2 full-time trainers, and 4 part-time trainers to 125 full-time employees. Fifteen of these were full-time "account executives," trainers with limited sales and customer service responsibility. About 70% of the company's revenues came from offering training courses on continuous quality improvement to clients. Revenues and profits had grown by leaps and bounds, but early in the 4th year revenues dropped drastically as the economy hit a mild recession and expected sales from the company's biggest client, a national hospital chain, failed to materialize.

Ken was assigned the task of determining what to do structurally. Losses were projected for this quarter, and the president and chairman of the board—the founder—had decreed that members of the work force who were not productive had to be let go. A target number of 25 people had been set. Ken had been placed in charge of a three-person task force, and given one week to develop a plan, including the names of those to be released and the timing of their releases. All releases had to be completed within 3 weeks.

The company had grown so rapidly that it had not had time to complete job descriptions for any of the jobs in the company. It was common knowledge that a lot of people, including some account executives, were sitting around doing nothing a lot of the day. There had never been any evaluations of employees, other than those of the training staff.

At the end of the briefing session in which Ken was assigned this task, the president commented: "Good luck! You are going to need it."

Questions

1. If you were Ken, where would you start? How would you proceed?
2. How can you rationally make these choices?
3. What kind of design does this organization need?

NOTES

1. Stevens, Rosemary A. The hospital as a social institution, new-fashioned for the 1990s. *Hospital & Health Services Administration* 36 (Summer 1991): 165.
2. Mintzberg, Henry. *The structuring of organizations.* Englewood Cliffs, NJ: Prentice Hall, 1979; Mintzberg, Henry. *Structure in fives: Designing effective organizations.* Englewood Cliffs, NJ: Prentice Hall, 1983.
3. Leatt, Peggy, Stephen M. Shortell, and John R. Kimberly. Organization design. In *Health care management: A text in organization theory and behavior,* edited by Stephen M. Shortell and Arnold D. Kaluzny, 2d ed., 316. New York: John Wiley & Sons, 1988.
4. Fayol, Henri. *General and industrial management,* translated by Constance Storrs. London: Sir Isaac Pitman and Sons, Ltd., 1949.
5. Weber, Max. *The theory of social and economic organization,* translated by A.M. Henderson and Talcott Parsons. New York: The Free Press, 1947.
6. Williams, James C., and George P. Huber. *Human behavior in organizations,* 3d ed., 270. Cincinnati, OH: South-Western Publishing Company, 1986.
7. Weber, *Theory of social and economic organization.*
8. Weber, *Theory of social and economic organization.*
9. Robbins, Stephen P. *Management,* 3d ed., 39. Englewood Cliffs, NJ: Prentice Hall, 1991.
10. Higgins, James M. *The management challenge: An introduction to management,* 42. New York: Macmillan Publishing Company, 1991.
11. Gulick, Luther, and Lyndall Urwick, eds. *Papers on the science of administration.* New York: Institute of Public Administration, 1937.
12. Mooney, James D., and Alan C. Reiley. *Onward industry: The principles of organization and their significance to modern industry.* New York: Harper and Brothers, 1931.
13. Smith, Adam. *The wealth of nations.* London: Dent, 1910.
14. Gibson, James L., John M. Ivancevich, and James H.

Donnelly, Jr. *Organizations: Behavior, structure, processes,* 7th ed., 444. Homewood, IL: Richard D. Irwin, Inc., 1991.
15. Davis, Keith, and John W. Newstrom. *Human behavior at work: Organizational behavior,* 8th ed., 335. New York: McGraw-Hill Book Company, 1989.
16. Aldag, Ramon J., and Timothy M. Stearns. *Management,* 2d ed. Cincinnati, OH: South-Western Publishing Company, 1991; Holt, David H. *Management: Principles and practices,* 2d ed. Englewood Cliffs, NJ: Prentice Hall, 1990.
17. Holt, *Management,* 253.
18. Mintzberg, *Structuring of organizations,* 76–77.
19. Dunham, Randall B., and Jon L. Pierce. *Management,* 655. Glenview, IL: Scott, Foresman and Company, 1989.
20. Mintzberg, *Structure in fives,* 30.
21. Higgins, *Management challenge,* 253.
22. Davis and Newstrom, *Human behavior,* 335.
23. Higgins, *Management challenge,* 253–254.
24. Dunham and Pierce, *Management,* 372.
25. Robbins, *Management,* 289.
26. Robbins, *Management,* 290.
27. Pfeffer, Jeffrey. *Power in organizations.* Marshfield, MA: Pitman Publishing, 1981.
28. French, John R.P., and Bertram H. Raven. The basis of social power. In *Studies of social power,* edited by Dorwin Cartwright, 150–167. Ann Arbor, MI: Institute for Social Research, 1959.
29. Mooney and Reiley, *Onward industry,* 39.
30. Dale, Ernest. *Planning and developing the company organization structure,* 107. Research Report No. 20. New York: American Management Association, 1952.
31. Mintzberg, *Structuring of organizations;* Mintzberg, *Structure in fives.*
32. Higgins, *Management challenge,* 258.
33. Gulick and Urwick, *Papers on the science,* 15.
34. Mintzberg, *Structuring of organizations,* 108–111.
35. Mintzberg, *Structuring of organizations,* 106.

36. Longest, Beaufort B., Jr. *Management practices for the health professional,* 4th ed. Norwalk, CT: Appleton & Lange, 1990.
37. Burns, Tom, and George M. Stalker. *The management of innovation.* London: Tavistock Publications, 1961.
38. Burns and Stalker, *Management of innovation.*
39. Gibson, Ivancevich, and Donnelly, *Organizations,* 507.
40. Urwick, Lyndall. *The elements of administration.* New York: Harper & Row, 1944.
41. Davis, Ralph C. *Fundamentals of top management.* New York: Harper & Row, 1951.
42. Barkdull, Charles W. Span of control—a method of evaluation. *Michigan Business Review* 15 (May 1963): 27–29; Steiglitz, Harry. *Organizational planning.* New York: National Industrial Conference Board, 1966; Aldag and Stearns, *Management.* The number of relationships (R) with subordinates (n) is known as the Graicunas theory and is determined as follows: R = n (2^{n-1} + n − 1). See Higgins, *Management challenge,* 265–266.
43. This section draws heavily from Longest, Beaufort B., Jr., and James M. Klingensmith. Coordination and communication. In *Health care management: A text in organization theory and behavior,* edited by Stephen M. Shortell and Arnold D. Kaluzny, 2d ed., 234–264. New York: John Wiley & Sons, 1988.
44. Barnard, Chester I. *The functions of the executive,* 256. Cambridge, MA: Harvard University Press, 1938.
45. Fayol, *General and industrial,* 104.
46. Fayol, *General and industrial,* 104.
47. Haimann, Theo, and William G. Scott. *Management in modern organizations,* 2d ed., 126. Boston: Houghton Mifflin Company, 1974.
48. Lawrence, Paul R., and Jay W. Lorsch. Differentiation and integration in complex organizations. *Administrative Science Quarterly* 11 (June 1967): 1–47.
49. Scott, W. Richard. Managing professional work: Three models of control for health organizations. *Health Services Research* 17 (Fall 1982): 213–240.
50. Litterer, Joseph A. *The analysis of organizations,* 223–232. New York: John Wiley & Sons, 1965.
51. Litterer, *Analysis of organizations,* 227.
52. Georgopoulos, Basil S., and Floyd C. Mann. The hospital as an organization. *Hospital Administration* 7 (Fall 1962): 57–58.
53. Mintzberg, *Structuring of organizations;* Mintzberg, *Structure in fives.*
54. Mintzberg, *Structuring of organizations,* 6–7.
55. Hage, Jerold. *Theories of organizations: Forms, processes, and transformations.* New York: Wiley-Interscience, 1980.
56. Lawrence and Lorsch, Differentiation and integration.
57. Blau, Peter M., and W. Richard Scott. *Formal organizations,* 6. San Francisco: Chandler Publishing Co., 1962.
58. Roethlisberger, Fritz J., and William J. Dickson. *Management and the worker.* Cambridge, MA: Harvard University Press, 1939.
59. Mills, T.M. *The sociology of small groups,* 2. Englewood Cliffs, NJ: Prentice Hall, 1967.
60. Wexley, Kenneth N., and Gary A. Yukl. *Organizational behavior and personnel psychology,* 3d ed. Homewood, IL: Richard D. Irwin, Inc., 1977.
61. Higgins, *Management challenge,* 464.
62. Holt, *Management,* 366.
63. Mondy, R. Wayne, Judith R. Gordon, Arthur Sharplin, and Shane R. Premeaux. *Management and organizational behavior,* 222–223. Boston: Allyn and Bacon, 1990.
64. Scott, William G., and Terence R. Mitchell. *Organization theory,* 175–182. Homewood, IL: Richard D. Irwin, Inc., 1976.
65. Tuckman, Bruce W., and Mary Ann C. Jensen. Stages of small-group development revisited. *Group and Organizational Studies* 2 (Summer 1977): 419–427; Gersick, Connie J.G. Time and transition in work teams: Toward a new model of group development. *Academy of Management Journal* 31 (March 1988): 9–41.
66. Higgins, *Management challenge,* 468.
67. Durbin, Robert. *Human relations in administration,* 68. Englewood Cliffs, NJ: Prentice Hall, 1951.
68. Longest, *Management practices.*
69. Mondy, Gordon, Sharplin, and Premeaux, *Management and organizational,* 226.
70. Longest, *Management practices,* 118.
71. Mintzberg, Henry. Organization design: Fashion or fit? *Harvard Business Review* 59 (January/February 1981): 103–116; Mintzberg, *Structuring of organizations;* Mintzberg, *Structure in fives.*
72. Mintzberg, *Structuring of organizations,* 29.
73. Mintzberg, *Structuring of organizations,* 20.
74. Mintzberg, *Structuring of organizations;* Mintzberg, Organization design; Mintzberg, *Structure in fives.*
75. Burns and Stalker, *Management of innovation.*
76. Weber, *Theory of social and economic organization.*
77. Leatt, Shortell, and Kimberly, Organization design, 318.
78. Porter, Michael E. *Competitive advantage: Creating and sustaining superior performance.* New York: The Free Press, 1985.
79. Longest and Klingensmith, Coordination and communication, 260.
80. Burns and Stalker, *Management of innovation.*
81. Mintzberg, Organization design, 111.
82. Mintzberg, Organization design, 112.
83. Mintzberg, Organization design, 112.
84. Mintzberg, *Structuring of organizations,* 432.
85. Drucker, Peter F. New templates for today's organizations. *Harvard Business Review* 52 (January/February 1974): 51.
86. Adapted from Hamilton, James A. *Decision-Making in Hospital Administration,* 278–280. Minneapolis: University of Minnesota Press, 1960; used by permission.
87. From Longest, Beaufort B., Jr. *Business Management of Health Care Providers.* Chicago: Hospital Financial Management Association, 1975; reprinted by permission.
88. Adapted from Higgins, James M. *The Management Challenge: An Introduction to Management,* 311. New York: Macmillan Publishing Company, 1991; used by permission.

BIBLIOGRAPHY

Aldag, Ramon J., and Timothy M. Stearns. *Management,* 2d ed. Cincinnati: South-Western Publishing Company, 1991.

Barkdull, Charles W. Span of control—a method of evaluation. *Michigan Business Review* 15 (May 1963): 27–29.

Barnard, Chester I. *The functions of the executive.* Cambridge, MA: Harvard University Press, 1938.

Blau, Peter M., and W. Richard Scott. *Formal organizations.* San Francisco: Chandler Publishing Co., 1962.

Burns, Tom, and George M. Stalker. *The management of innovation*. London: Travistock Publications, 1961.

Dale, Ernest. *Planning and developing the company organization structure*. Research Report No. 20. New York: American Management Association, 1952.

Davis, Keith, and John W. Newstrom. *Human behavior at work: Organizational behavior*, 8th ed. New York: McGraw-Hill Book Company, 1989.

Davis, Ralph C. *Fundamentals of top management*. New York: Harper & Row, 1951.

Drucker, Peter F. New templates for today's organizations. *Harvard Business Review* 52 (January/February 1974): 45–53.

Dunham, Randall B., and Jon L. Pierce. *Management*. Glenview, IL: Scott, Foresman and Company, 1989.

Durbin, Robert. *Human relations in administration*. Englewood Cliffs, NJ: Prentice Hall, 1951.

Fayol, Henri. *General and industrial management*, translated by Constance Storrs. London: Sir Isaac Pitman and Sons, Ltd., 1949.

French, John R. P., and Bertram H. Raven. The basis of social power. In *Studies of social power*, edited by D. Cartwright, 150–167. Ann Arbor, MI: Institute for Social Research, 1959.

Georgopoulos, Basil S., and Floyd C. Mann. The hospital as an organization. *Hospital Administration* (Fall 1962): 50–64.

Gersick, Connie J. G. Time and transition in work teams: Toward a new model of group development. *Academy of Management Journal* 31 (March 1988): 9–41.

Gibson, James L., John M. Ivancevich, and James H. Donnelly, Jr. *Organizations: Behavior, structure, process*, 7th ed. Homewood, IL: Richard D. Irwin, Inc., 1991.

Gulick, Luther, and Lyndall Urwick, eds. *Papers on the science of administration*. New York: Institute of Public Administration, 1937.

Hage, Jerold. *Theories of organizations: Forms, processes, and transformations*. New York: Wiley-Interscience, 1980.

Haimann, Theo, and William G. Scott. *Management in modern organizations*, 2d ed. Boston: Houghton Mifflin Company, 1974.

Higgins, James M. *The management challenge: An introduction to management*. New York: Macmillan Publishing Company, 1991.

Holt, David H. *Management: Principles and practices*, 2d ed. Englewood Cliffs, NJ: Prentice Hall, 1990.

Lawrence, Paul R., and Jay W. Lorsch. Differentiation and integration in complex organizations. *Administrative Science Quarterly* 11 (June 1967): 1–47.

Leatt, Peggy, Stephen M. Shortell, and John R. Kimberly. Organization design. In *Health care management: A text in organization theory and behavior*, edited by Stephen M. Shortell and Arnold D. Kaluzny, 2d ed., 307–343. New York: John Wiley and Sons, 1988.

Litterer, Joseph A. *The analysis of organizations*. New York: John Wiley & Sons, 1965.

Longest, Beaufort B., Jr., *Management practices for the health professional*, 4th ed. Norwalk, CT: Appleton & Lange, 1990.

Longest, Beaufort B., Jr., and James M. Klingensmith. Coordination and communication. In *Health care management: A text in organization theory and behavior*, edited by Stephen M. Shortell and Arnold D. Kaluzny, 2d ed., 234–264. New York: John Wiley & Sons, 1988.

Mills, T. M. *The sociology of small groups*. Englewood Cliffs, NJ: Prentice Hall, 1967.

Mintzberg, Henry. Organization design: Fashion or fit? *Harvard Business Review* 59 (January/February 1981): 103–116.

Mintzberg, Henry. *Structure in fives: Designing effective organizations*. Englewood Cliffs, NJ: Prentice Hall, 1983.

Mintzberg, Henry. *The structuring of organizations*. Englewood Cliffs, NJ: Prentice Hall, 1979.

Mondy, R. Wayne, Judith R. Gordon, Arthur Sharplin, and Shane R. Premeaux. *Management and organizational behavior*. Boston: Allyn and Bacon, 1990.

Mooney, James D., and Alan C. Reiley. *Onward Industry: The principles of organization and their significance to modern industry*. New York: Harper and Brothers, 1931.

Pfeffer, Jeffrey. *Power in organizations*. Marshfield, MA: Pitman Publishing, 1981.

Porter, Michael E. *Competitive advantage: Creating and sustaining superior performance*. New York: The Free Press, 1985.

Robbins, Stephen P. *Management*, 3d ed. Englewood Cliffs, NJ: Prentice Hall, 1991.

Roethlisberger, Fritz J., and William J. Dickson. *Management and the worker*. Cambridge, MA: Harvard University Press, 1939.

Scott, W. Richard. Managing professional work: Three models of control for health organizations. *Health Services Research* 17 (Fall 1982): 213–240.

Scott, William G., and Terence R. Mitchell. *Organization theory*. Homewood, IL: Richard D. Irwin, Inc., 1976.

Smith, Adam. *The wealth of nations*. London: Dent, 1910.

Steiglitz, Harry. *Organizational planning*. New York: National Industrial Conference Board, 1966.

Stevens, George H. *The strategic health care manager*. San Francisco: Jossey-Bass Publishers, 1991.

Stevens, Rosemary A. The hospital as a social institution, new-fashioned for the 1990s. *Hospital & Health Services Administration* 36 (Summer 1991): 163–173.

Tuckman, Bruce W., and Mary Ann C. Jensen. Stages of small-group development revisited. *Group and Organizational Studies* 2 (1977): 419–427.

Urwick, Lyndall. *The elements of administration*. New York: Harper & Row, 1944.

Weber, Max. *The theory of social and economic organization*, translated by A. M. Henderson and Talcott Parsons. New York: The Free Press, 1947.

Wexley, Kenneth N., and Gary A. Yukl. *Organizational behavior and personnel phychology*, 3d ed. Homewood, IL: Richard D. Irwin, Inc., 1977.

Williams, James C., and George P. Huber. *Human behavior in organizations*, 3d ed. Cincinnati: South-Western Publishing Company, 1986.

7

How HSOs Are Organized

"It is a pretty good zoo," said young Gerald
McGrew, "and the fellow who runs it seems
proud of it, too."
Dr. Seuss, *If I Ran The Zoo*[1]

This chapter describes several common types of health services organizations (HSOs). A brief history of each genre is sketched, and information about functions, organizational structure, governance, management, professional staff organization (PSO), caregiver and support staff, and licensure and accreditation is provided. Included are acute care hospitals, hospices, managed care organizations, nursing facilities, ambulatory care organizations, birth centers, and home health agencies. The discussion is not exhaustive of the variety or complexity of the tens of thousands of HSOs, but the examples are paradigmatic. The chapter begins with a generic background about HSOs and how they are organized, including legal status; governing body role and functions, composition, and committees, and the relationship of the governing body to the chief executive officer; management functions, qualifications, and relationships; and PSO credentialing, membership, privileges, discipline, and integration, as well as the handling of impaired clinicians by the PSO.

BACKGROUND

Regardless of ownership, role, activity, or any other characteristic, all HSOs have a governing body (GB). These range from a GB as simple as one individual in a sole-proprietorship nursing facility, to the Central Office found in the Department of Veterans Affairs, to the complex arrangement found in an academic medical center hospital. The GB is the ultimate authority and decision maker for the HSO. It determines the HSO's direction and evaluates progress toward implicit and explicit goals. One of the GB's most important jobs is to select and evaluate the performance of the chief executive officer (CEO).

Each HSO has a CEO, although titles vary. As HSOs take on many of the accoutrements of business enterprise, they more frequently use corporate titles such as president and executive vice president. The GB delegates authority to the CEO. This includes managing the HSO's day-to-day operations consistent with policies approved by the GB. For many reasons, including HSOs' legal relationships and the financial demands on them, GBs are being held to a higher level of public accountability, and this necessitates a closer and more effective working relationship between the CEO and the GB. As with titles, this relationship is extraordinarily varied and may range from one in which the CEO is given great latitude in management decision making to one in which the CEO has little independence. The CEO evaluates performance of other managers in the HSO, and senior managers may be evaluated in cooperation with the GB.

By definition, an HSO has a clinical staff who deliver health and health-related services. The specific makeup of the clinical staff and its organization vary markedly among HSOs, even within the same type. In its broadest sense, clinical staff includes anyone who cares for patients. In this text, however, clinical staff is used to refer to the various types of licensed independent practitioners (LIPs),* the most common and clinically the most important of whom are physicians.

---

*The Joint Commission on Accreditation of Healthcare Organizations defines a licensed independent practitioner as "any individual who is permitted by law and by the hospital to provide patient care services without direction or supervision, within the scope of the individual's license and in accordance with individually granted clinical privileges."[2]

Increasingly, the clinical staff includes other types of LIPs who have significant independence in their interactions with patients. Examples are dentists, clinical psychologists, podiatrists, nurse midwives, and chiropractors. In acute care hospitals and some other types of HSOs, this clinical staff is a separate, unincorporated association with its own bylaws.

The association of clinical staff is commonly known as the medical staff organization because in the past it was composed almost exclusively of physicians. Increasingly, it will be called the *professional staff organization*, a title suggesting the broad range of preparation and activities of clinicians in it. That title and the acronym PSO are used here. Nonhospital HSOs are likely to already use PSO to designate their clinical staff. Regardless of title, the PSO is largely self-governing. Members of the PSO provide services personally and order other HSO staff to provide clinical or support services. Relationships among members of the PSO depend on the setting and the work being done. In some HSOs, such as a medical group practice, the numbers of physician and nonphysician providers may be similar. The care in other HSOs such as nursing facilities is more chronic and custodial, and only intermittent contact with a physician is necessary, even though contact with other LIPs and other caregivers such as registered nurses (RNs) and licensed practical nurses (LPNs) is frequent. Much care is provided by nonclinicians, even though that care has been ordered by members of the PSO, either by individual order or through standing orders that have been approved prospectively by the medical director or the PSO.

LEGAL STATUS

Nongovernmental (privately owned) HSOs are sole proprietorships, partnerships, or corporations. Many HSOs of various types are owned by state and local governments (county, city, or special tax district) and are established either by special enabling legislation or incorporated in the same manner as privately owned HSOs. A small number of HSOs are owned by the federal government. Their legal status is based on federal legislation, and the states may not regulate them. Examples are Department of Veterans Affairs hospitals; Army, Navy, and Air Force hospitals; and U.S. Public Health Service clinics.

Sole-proprietorship HSOs have no special legal status; the term simply describes a business owned by one person. A common example is a for-profit nursing facility.

Partnerships are voluntary contracts between two or more persons to engage in commerce or business. Partnerships may be general or limited. General partnerships are unlikely to have special legal status, but this depends on state law. A common example of a general partnership is a physician group practice. "General" means that each partner is liable for the debts and errors of other partners. Limited partnerships have one or more general partners who are jointly and individually responsible for the activities of the partnership and "limited" partners whose liability as to the partnership is limited to the assets they have invested. Limited partnerships are commonly found in joint ventures between HSOs and physicians. Examples are imaging centers or ambulatory surgery centers. Limited partnerships are established by filing papers with the state.

The most common legal status for HSOs is the corporation. States allow physicians and other types of LIPs to organize a special category of corporation, the professional corporation, in which case the letters "PC" follow its name. Some states use the word "limited," abbreviated Ltd.,to show the same status. Corporations are created by filing articles of incorporation with a state. When approved, a charter is issued to the corporation. Corporations may be incorporated as not for profit or for profit; the advantages and disadvantages of each depend on the tax laws. Charters are amended by application of the corporation and approval by the state. A corporation must develop bylaws that describe how it is organized to carry out its purposes, including definitions; meetings; elections; composition of the GB, committees, and officers; and the roles of the CEO and the PSO, if any. Bylaws are important because they guide governance and senior management. The charter and bylaws are the HSO's basic law, and all activities are subordinate to and must be consistent with them. An example is the PSO bylaws, which are approved by the GB.

The police power described in Chapter 2 is almost exclusively a state government domain, and HSOs are regulated by states. A common type of regulation is licensure; specific application of which is discussed below. State police power is delegated to local government, and HSOs are regulated just as are organizations carrying on functions such as storing, preparing, and serving food. Specialized regulatory activities apply to some types of HSOs. An example is control, storage, and use of radioactive materials, or disposal of hazardous wastes. Federal laws affect some of these areas, and regulation may occur through federal and state cooperation.

ORGANIZATIONAL STRUCTURE

Max Weber suggested that large-scale organizations must have a way to deal with the idiosyncrasies of individuals so that they do not interfere with the organization's ability to accomplish specific tasks.[3] One way to do this is to establish a bureaucracy in which each person has a place and a set of tasks. The typical bureaucratic structure is a pyramid, shown in Figure 7.1. This structure is based on a chain of command through which authority and responsibility are delegated downward. Historically, larger HSOs have been bureaucratically structured.

GOVERNING BODIES

The new environment for HSOs puts increasing pressure on GBs. The days when GB members were chosen because it was an honor or because they might make financial contributions are essentially gone. Members no longer have the luxury of casual participation. There is no doubt that pressures for GBs to be effective will increase. This means recruiting members who understand the health services field, are well prepared in business matters, and have a background in areas important to the HSO. Some acute care hospitals pay members to attend meetings—a common practice in business—and this practice may gain greater acceptance as demands on time and the need for expertise increase. In the future, many GB members will have no employment other than serving on GBs of noncompeting HSOs.

Role and Functions

The GB's first role is to set objectives and develop policy to guide the HSO in achieving its mission within the context of the organizational philosophy. The second is to determine whether the HSO has achieved its objectives. To do so, GB members should have a general understanding of the health services field at a level similar to that of HSO management.

The statement of GB role and functions developed by the American Hospital Association (AHA) applies to all HSOs. The governing body:

—Has the responsibility for organizing itself effectively, for establishing and following the policies and procedures necessary to discharge its responsibilities, and for adopting bylaws in accordance with legal requirements;
—Has the responsibility for selecting a qualified chief executive officer and for delegating to the chief executive officer the necessary authority to manage . . . effectively;
—Has the authority and responsibility for ensuring proper organization of the . . . (clinical) staff, and for monitoring the quality of care provided . . . ;
—Has the authority and responsibility for monitoring and influencing public policies concerning the establishment and maintenance of appropriate external relationships;
—Has responsibility and authority, subject to the . . . charter, for determining the . . . mission and for establishing a strategic plan, goals, objectives, and policies to achieve that mission;
—Is entrusted with resources . . . and with the proper development, utilization, and maintenance of those resources;
—Has the responsibility and authority for the organization, protection, and enhancement of . . . human resources; and
—Is responsible for the provision of health care education and research programs that further the . . . mission.[4]

Bylaws written, reviewed, and approved by the GB set out its organization and guide activities.

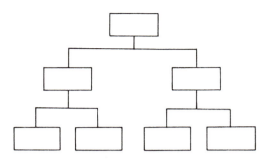

Figure 7.1. Typical bureaucratic pyramid.

Composition

Traditionally, many GB members of not-for-profit HSOs were drawn from the community and had special skills that the organization needed but often could not afford. Business and community leaders, attorneys, and clergy were commonly chosen. Data from hospitals suggest that this remains true. For-profit HSOs draw GB members from investors (owners), physicians on the PSO, and, to a lesser extent, from the same groups as not-for-profit HSOs. Data from hospitals suggest that the GBs of not-for-profit HSOs are likely to be considerably larger than those of for-profit HSOs.

Physicians on the staff of a not-for-profit hospital were often excluded from GB membership because it was feared they would have a conflict of interest. Decisions about resource allocation, equipment purchases, and the quality of clinical services provided by members of the PSO could cause clinicians to have interests and allegiances on both sides of a question. (Conflicts of interest were discussed in Chapters 3 and 4.) The current view is to encourage physician membership because it is believed that conflicts of interest are avoidable and that physicians bring vital clinical expertise to a GB. Hospital research cited below suggests that integrating physicians into management and governance enhances performance, a finding probably true in nonhospital HSOs, too.

GB members not employed by the HSO are known as external members; those who are employees are known as internal members. Internal members often include the CEO, medical director, and chief financial officer. The proportion of internal members seems to be increasing, probably because of the need for the specialized expertise these people bring to a board. The potential for conflicts of interest increases in such circumstances.

Committees

GBs have committees because of a need to specialize and because some GBs are large (sometimes 100 members), especially in not-for-profit HSOs. Large size greatly diminishes efficiency. Standing committees usually include executive, professional staff, human resources, quality assurance, finance, planning, public relations and development, investment, capital equipment and expenditure, and nomination. Committees on quality improvement and ethics are being added to many GBs. Special (ad hoc) committees are established as needed.

Two committees should be highlighted. The executive committee is the most powerful. Because meetings of the entire GB may be infrequent—quarterly or annual—the executive committee has continuing monitoring responsibility and authority over the HSO. Usually it receives reports from other committees, monitors policy implementation, and provides interim decision making. It may meet as often as weekly. Membership usually includes those who chair the standing committees. The person chairing the GB presides. It is very important that the CEO attend, but attendance is not universal. The executive committee's importance varies with size and frequency of GB meetings.

The second most important committee is the professional staff committee. It generally is concerned with PSO relations. It reviews PSO recommendations on membership and credentials for each applicant or member and makes a recommendation to the GB. It reviews performance of PSO members to determine if clinical privileges should be modified. To perform these tasks the committee must have access to clinical expertise, either through GB members who are experts or through consultants. There is increasing emphasis on the legal and ethical obligation of the HSO, through its GB, to protect patients from substandard care.

The need for management, PSO, and GB to communicate and coordinate is critical and may be achieved in several ways. One, the joint conference committee, is described in the section on acute care hospitals below. Other means are to include members from each of the three groups on one another's committees and to send copies of minutes and reports to other committees. Figure 7.2 shows the dual pyramid almost always found in hospitals and in other types of HSOs and suggests the difficulty of communicating and coordinating.

Relationship to the CEO

The GB's responsibility to recruit, select, and evaluate the CEO has been noted above. The CEO assembles and organizes resources and develops the systems to carry out programs and policies approved by the GB. The CEO also provides information to the GB so it can develop policy, monitor implementation, and oversee results. To do this, the CEO performs all functions of the manager.

The CEO's performance should be assessed regularly and systematically by the GB, and recommendations should result from this process. Performance is best measured against predetermined objective standards mutually identified and accepted by the CEO and GB. An example of a traditional scheme for assessing the CEO's performance is that developed by Harvey.[5] It uses specific accountabilities that are expected of the CEO, each of which has a performance level. This process requires negotiation and is a type of management by objectives with bilaterally established performance objectives. This is the preferred way, but more commonly the performance of senior managers is measured by negative developments rather than achievement of specific, positive goals. The GB should not set arbitrary goals that the CEO must attempt to meet.

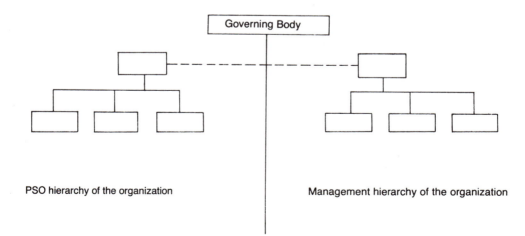

Figure 7.2. Dual pyramid of the typical hospital.

Employment contracts for CEOs are increasingly common in HSOs—a development that follows the pattern set in other sectors of the economy. These contracts set the terms of employment, including severance.

CEOs walk a narrow line as they focus GB members' expertise and encourage interest, dedication, and enthusiasm, but simultaneously discourage direct participation in internal operations. Historically, direct participation in operations has been especially problematic in not-for-profit HSOs. Figure 7.3 shows an appropriate GB–CEO/senior management relationship. If GB members deal directly in the HSO, CEO authority is undercut. This frustrates and confuses subordinates—conditions unlikely to enhance the HSO's effectiveness or efficiency. Interference can be forestalled by job descriptions for GB members. The CEO's role can also be clarified by GB member orientation and education.

CEOs are commonly members of the GB, a practice with advantages but also the potential for problems. The most important is conflict of interest (discussed in Chapters 3 and 4 and noted above regarding physicians), which was historically believed to disqualify a CEO from GB membership. The conflict occurs because an important GB function is selecting and monitoring CEO performance. As a voting member of the GB, the CEO's views about performance, salary, and retention may be at variance with objective interests of the HSO. This is lessened if CEOs absent themselves when issues in which they have a self-interest are considered. While minimizing the potential for conflict of interest, this practice does not eliminate it. Close professional and personal relationships between CEO and GB members lessen the objectivity of appraisals.

Conversely, there are advantages when the CEO is a voting member of the GB. Two of the

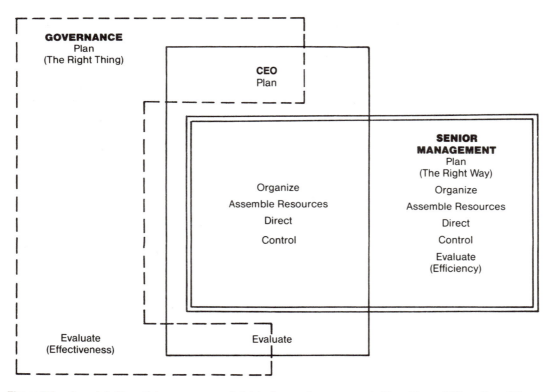

Figure 7.3. A model of hospital governance, administration, and management. (From Henry, William F., and Vernon E. Weckwerth. When corporate executives serve as hospital trustees. *Trustee* 34 [June 1981]: 30; reprinted by permission. Copyright 1981, American Hospital Publishing, Inc.)

most important are enhanced communication and participation in developing policies the CEO must implement. A measure of prestige accrues to the CEO, but this is more a personal than an organizational advantage.

MANAGEMENT

The work of HSO managers is unmatched. They are responsible for an organization that delivers a unique personal service to anxious persons in an extraordinarily complex, often emotionally charged, environment. In addition, many HSOs have relationships with a PSO that have no parallel in other types of enterprise.

Many different titles are used for chief managers in HSOs: administrator, director, CEO, president, and superintendent. This discussion uses the generic designation of chief executive officer (CEO), a title applicable to all types of HSOs. Comments about the CEO are usually applicable to all members of senior management.

Function

The CEO's basic task is to manage inputs of the HSO (human resources, material, technology, information, and capital) to achieve the outputs that are its goals. Except for the smallest HSO, CEOs delegate tasks and authority to subordinate managers. The responsibility for designing, changing, and operating an effective management structure to meet the HSO's objectives belongs to the CEO, however, and cannot be delegated. It is the CEO whom the GB will hold accountable for failure, and, perhaps, reward for success.

The CEO's job is to manage the entire HSO. Management has been defined in Chapter 1 as the process, composed of interrelated social and technical functions and activities (including roles), occurring in a formal organizational setting for the purpose of accomplishing predetermined objectives through the utilization of human and other resources. Inherent in this definition are four specific criteria that define the role of the CEO. The first is creation of and adherence to a set of objectives. Second, there must be input resources. Economic resources are by definition limited, and attaining goals (effectiveness) with optimal allocation is the CEO's responsibility. A third criterion is that there are other persons in the HSO. It is with and through people that the CEO and subordinate managers perform work. These human resources are also an input. Finally, the HSO must change over time, and this, too, defines the CEO's role. The theory and application of change are extensively treated in Chapter 16. Kovner noted the importance of change in the early 1970s when he said that, by reason of training, position, and responsibilities, the CEO is "the person most qualified and most likely to act as a change agent."[6] This is even more valid today.

Qualifications

The Joint Commission on Accreditation of Healthcare Organizations (Joint Commission) does not list requirements for education or experience for the position of hospital CEO, for example. It does state that the "chief executive officer is qualified by education and experience that is appropriate to the fulfillment of the responsibilities of the position."[7] Similar requirements are used in other types of HSOs accredited by the Joint Commission. The didactic and applied formal educational preparation of health services managers is described in Chapter 2, "The Health Care Delivery System."

Relationships

The relationships found in HSOs are unusually complex. This complexity stems from factors that include voluntary members of GBs in not-for-profit HSOs, lack of an employment relationship for most LIPs who do their work in hospitals and nursing facilities, and the highly skilled and specialized functions of most staff working in HSOs. Such complexity and interrelationships place special demands on managers.

Triad The GB selects and delegates authority to a CEO, who acts as its agent and exercises that authority to organize inputs to achieve organization objectives. The GB continues to be involved in the HSO in several ways, however. Since larger HSOs and all hospitals have PSOs, complexity increases greatly. The epitome of complexity is found in the academic medical center.

The CEO, GB, and PSO are known as a triad—group of three. The triad is common in acute care hospitals, but variations of it are found in other types of HSOs. Although the proportion of nonphysician LIPs is increasing, PSOs in acute care hospitals are overwhelmingly composed of physicians. Members of the PSO are likely to be independent contractors who use the HSO to treat their patients but have no employment relationship with it. This has major implications for the control function of management. The dual pyramid in Figure 7.2 suggests the triad.

From an organization theory perspective the triad is not very effective, and its problems have been described extensively. It is claimed to be incompatible with the demands on contemporary HSOs, especially acute care hospitals. Lack of a clear line relationship between the PSO and either the GB *or* the CEO confuses accountability. The triad remains pervasive, but there is a trend toward streamlining the structure and clarifying accountability. Ethical and legal pressures in that direction are irresistible, as is the imperative of common sense management.

CEO and Senior Management Larger HSOs are likely to divide the role of CEO into two parts. The CEO is primarily involved in GB and external relations, as well as planning, fundraising, and capital projects. PSO relations may be added to this list. The chief operating officer (COO) is responsible to the CEO for day-to-day operations. This useful division of responsibility helps meet increasingly complex demands. Universally found in larger HSOs is a chief financial officer. This position is an extension of the concept of controllership, with additional responsibilties for reimbursement, capital financing, and investment. In the near future, there likely will be a chief quality officer, a member of senior management responsible for the quality of services and their continuous improvement.

The presence of both a CEO and COO can cause problems if their spheres of responsibility and authority are not defined. Confusion is certain if the CEO intervenes directly in matters that are the responsibility of the COO; unless there are emergencies, lines of authority and responsibility should be followed. The COO must be cognizant of the upward reporting lines of responsibility so as not to bypass the CEO.

Below these senior managers are a number of management layers that ultimately lead to those who do the day-to-day work of the HSO. Data reported in 1991 show that the number of management layers in large health systems and major medical centers has declined dramatically since 1985 (Table 7.1).[8] It is especially noteworthy that in this study high-performing organizations had the fewest management layers. Reducing layers of management is consistent with the views of leading management theorists such as Peter Drucker[9] about the desirability of flattening organizations and reflects the move toward employee empowerment that is advocated by Deming and others and described in Chapter 11, "Quality and Productivity Improvement."

PROFESSIONAL STAFF ORGANIZATION

It is crucial to understand that the practitioners who treat and order treatment for patients are the engine that drives an HSO. In most HSOs, patients must be admitted before treatment can be ordered and begun. No medical treatment can be rendered without express orders or standing orders that were approved prospectively. Acute care hospitals want physicians and other practitioners who are independent contractors on their PSOs to admit patients, but once a patient is admitted the pressures of prospective payment (diagnosis-related groups) demand that treatment be efficient. Similarly, if an HSO's practitioners are salaried and an admission generates income,

Table 7.1. Layers of management in HSOs

	1985	1990	1990 (High performers)
Large health care systems	9	7.5	6.5
Major medical centers	6	5	4.5

Data from *Health Care Competition Week* 8 (May 20, 1991): 1.
Numbers are averages and are approximate.

the HSO encourages admissions. An HSO that receives no additional income when a patient is treated, however, will seek to minimize treatment consistent with patient needs.

HSOs with a PSO have a relationship unique by traditional organizational standards. The PSO is the third leg of the triad—a form most highly developed in acute care hospitals. A PSO is likely to have bylaws, officers, a committee structure, and other characteristics that reflect the autonomy of physicians and other LIPs who are often independent contractors in the HSO. Even when salaried, the clinical staff exhibit a high degree of independence and commonly have more allegiance to their profession than to the HSO. Because of the independence and the technical nature of clinical practice, in the past GBs have usually exercised little direct control over the PSO.

History

Acute care hospitals have the most complex and highly developed PSO structures. This development paralleled the concentration of medical technology in hospitals in the late 19th century as traditional physician–patient relationships were transferred to this new locus for delivering health services. These physician–patient relationships reflected the medical ethics of the American Medical Association (AMA), which was founded in 1847. The patient relationship was paramount, and AMA advocacy of fee-for-service practice reflected this philosophy. Thus, as physicians brought patients into hospitals, fee for service followed. The patient paid separately for services provided by the hospital. Any relationships or allegiances that interfered with physicians' judgments about what was best for their patients were unacceptable. Salaried arrangements for physicians were deemed unethical because employers might pressure physicians to act in ways contrary to the patient's best interests. Exceptions were allowed: military, government, and industrial medicine, and employment of physicians who were teachers, for example, in medical schools and teaching hospitals.

Treating private patients who paid a fee for service meant physicians were independent contractors with limited loyalty to the hospital. Furthermore, this independence caused them to believe they were accountable only to themselves, or at most, to colleagues. This reinforced a view that the functions of governance, management, and clinical practice were distinct. Convergence and control occurred at the GB level. This basic view continues today in HSOs with a PSO.

PSO Organization

Self-Governance As evidence of the strong tradition of physician independence, PSOs (historically known as medical staffs or medical staff organizations [MSOs]) in acute care hospitals continue to be largely self-governing. A similar situation is likely to exist in any HSO with a PSO. LIPs are part of the PSO whether they are salaried by the HSO or are fee-for-service LIPs. The PSO has its own bylaws, which must be approved by the GB. The bylaws are central to self-governance and identify officers, committees and their functions, categories of membership, the application process, the procedure for amending the bylaws, and a process for review of actions adverse to members. In addition, the PSO adopts rules and regulations that control clinical practice, which may be supplemented by even more detailed rules for clinical specialties, sub-specialties, and departments. Inferior (lesser) guidelines must be consistent with those that are superior.

Open or Closed The PSO may be open, closed, or a combination of the two. This concept is most highly developed in acute care hospitals, but may also affect nursing facilities, hospices, and ambulatory HSOs. If a PSO is open, any qualified LIP (as defined in the PSO bylaws) is granted clinical privileges (with or without PSO membership) and may treat patients. If a PSO is closed, qualified LIPs (as defined in the PSO bylaws) may or may not be granted clinical privileges (with or without PSO membership), depending on the parameters put on the PSO by the PSO itself, as approved by the GB. Such parameters may include absolute size of the PSO or limits on the numbers in various specialties or types of LIPs. Most hospitals, for example, have a combination of an open and a closed PSO in that they close some clinical departments, such as anesthesia, clinical and anatomical laboratories, emergency medicine, and radiology, but allow any qualified surgeon or physician to be granted privileges. Closing staffs and/or clinical departments is justified on the grounds that it improves quality of patient care and enhances efficiency. When departments are closed, the HSO usually has entered into an exclusive contract with a provider group—the concessionaires. All LIPs who function under the terms of the contract must have clinical privileges delineated consistent with their licenses.

Committees GB and PSO committee structures are parallel in many ways. The PSO is led by an executive committee that usually includes those who chair standing committees. Like its GB counterpart, the executive committee acts for the PSO and coordinates its activities. It provides continuity and enhances communication between the PSO and management. Major activities include implementing PSO policies, receiving and acting on reports and recommendations from PSO committees, making recommendations on PSO membership and clinical privileges, monitoring quality of care, and taking corrective action, including discipline. Subordinate committees are common, and these may include the following committees:

Credentials—reviews qualifications of clinicians for PSO membership and recommends specific privileges to executive committee. Reviews continuing appropriateness of privileges.

Surgical case review—reviews justification for surgery. Checks relationship between pre- and postoperative diagnoses.

Medical records—checks for timely completion of medical records. Reviews clinical usefulness and adequacy of record for quality of care.

Pharmacy and therapeutics—develops formulary and monitors drug use and other therapeutics policies. May have special interest in antibiotics use.

Utilization review—reviews resource use in providing care, with special attention given to length of patient stay and use of ancillary services.

Quality assessment—may be used instead of surgical case review and medical records committees, or may review pre- and postoperative reports, use of ancillary services such as radiology and laboratories, and condition of patient on discharge to determine appropriateness.

Other committees commonly found are infection control, blood use, risk management and safety, disaster planning, bylaws, and nominating. The CEO or a designee should attend all PSO meetings, including those of its committees.

In the future, PSOs will likely have a quality improvement committee. This committee will use the monitoring work of other PSO committees—their quality assessment activities—to focus the PSO's attention on process analysis and improvement (continuous quality improvement) in clinical areas. The new concept of continuous quality improvement is discussed in Chapter 11.

Clinical Departmentation

The extent and type of clinical departmentation (like its managerial counterpart) are determined by the HSO's activities and size. Nonhospital HSOs, such as health maintenance organizations and multispecialty group practices, have clinical departments. Nursing facilities and hospices have a medical director but are unlikely to have a PSO. Small hospitals have only departments of medicine and surgery in their PSO. Larger hospitals typically add obstetrics/gynecology, pediatrics, and family practice. Departmentation expands from there to include clinical specialties or subspecialties as separate departments or sections within departments. Figure 6.5 in Chapter 6, "Concepts of Organization Design," shows parallel managerial and clinical departmentation in a large general acute care hospital, among the most complex type of HSO.

Clinical department heads are clinicians who are elected or appointed. These clinical managers may be paid or unpaid, although larger units and greater demands on their managers increase the likelihood that the HSO will pay a salary to the clinician who is not already an employee. If specialization warrants, divisions and/or sections are established within departments. The upward chain of command goes to a physician, who may have the title chief of staff or medical director. Larger HSOs typically pay a salary to the medical director. Eventually, the line of authority reaches the GB. The medical director may report to the CEO, which is consistent with the accountability that the management structure should demand of the PSO. This reporting relationship is most likely to occur in an HSO where the CEO is also a clinician. It is least likely in a community hospital, where the CEO is rarely a clinician. A 1989 survey suggests that HSOs were not adequately developing their clinical manager resources; the survey found that two thirds of hospitals do not provide leadership training for PSO leaders or department heads.[10]

Managing the PSO

Control of the PSO was and is a problem regardless of HSO type, ownership, or size. The greatest potential for control is found in Department of Veterans Affairs and military facilities, where PSO members are employees and the CEO has line authority over them. Here, too, however, physicians especially have a great deal of independence. Historically, GBs were willing to accept assurances from the PSO that the quality in the HSO was acceptable. Changes in the tort system noted in Chapter 4, "Legal Considerations," however, and the tarnishing of medicine's image have changed HSO–patient relationships. This change has been most pronounced in the past several decades. Courts have determined and the public believes that HSOs, through GBs and managers, must be concerned about patient well-being and take steps to ensure the competence of clinicians.

The Credentialing Process

Background   Credentialing LIPs is crucial to the quality of care and is done by the HSO with the help of the clinical staff or PSO. It is especially important in the case of physicians because states grant them unlimited licenses to practice medicine and surgery. Only through the credentialing process are physician activities in HSOs made consistent with their actual skills. Nonphysician LIPs are issued limited licenses. Here, the credentialing process may narrow the range of clinical activities further, consistent with the practitioner's skills.

The credentialing process is divided into two parts. The first is determining the applicant's PSO membership category, if the applicant is eligible for membership. The second is assessing the level of *demonstrated current competence* to determine what the practitioner will be allowed (credentialed) to do—this is known as granting clinical privileges or privilege delineation. PSO membership (and category) and the clinical privileges the practitioner may perform in the HSO are separate. The two-part process applies to initial appointment and to reappointment, the specifics of which are different. PSO bylaws determine the content of the process and include due process safeguards for the applicant or reapplicant. PSO bylaws may provide that, in addition to physicians, all or only certain other types of LIPs may be members of the PSO. Or, the bylaws may have separate, nonmembership categories for nonphysician LIPs. Regardless, nonphysician LIPs may be precluded from serving on certain committees or holding PSO offices. Restrictions on committee membership and offices may apply to physicians in certain categories, too. Non-physician LIPs who are members of the PSO are credentialed only to perform certain clinical activities (privileges), just as are physicians. The nuances and variations are included in the by-laws, which have been developed by the PSO, subject to state law and approval by the GB.

Process   The credentialing process is usually organized and monitored by the CEO. Com-pleted files are referred to the PSO for credentials committee review, and this committee makes a recommendation to the PSO executive committee. The next level of review is the medical director and the president of the PSO. Final approval lies with the GB, through its committee structure. Previous actions were only recommendations. Historically, GBs have taken their responsibility to control PSO membership and credentialing more lightly than they should. Increased ethical and legal accountability, however, have forced HSOs to be more attentive and not delegate their re-sponsibility to the PSO.

PSO Membership

The application process for PSO membership should be thorough, detailed, and comprehensive. Information on an applicant should include undergraduate education; professional education; li-censure; postgraduate education (for physicians and many nonphysician LIPs these are internships [as applicable], residencies, and fellowships); continuing education, health status (including in-fectious diseases); other HSO affiliations; professional society memberships; specialty board/ organization fellowship and/or certification; and liability insurance coverage. It is prudent to re-quire photographs of applicants; these are sent to references to verify that applicants are who they claim to be. Specific questions should be asked about previous licensing, narcotics registration, disciplinary actions at other HSO/affiliations, and similar topics. The national data bank estab-lished by the Health Care Quality Improvement Act of 1986 (see Chapter 4) must be queried prior to both initial appointment and reappointment to determine if there are adverse reports concern-ing the practitioner. If the answers to such questions suggest a problem, investigations may be undertaken, as necessary.

It is imperative that the HSO put the burden of proof on applicants. This means they must complete the process to the HSO's satisfaction, including all the specific elements. *No assump-tions should be made*. Rather, the applicant must provide all information and documentation that the HSO requires. Character references may be chosen by the applicant. It is imperative, however, that the HSO choose professional references because only in this way can complete, objective information about clinical competence be obtained. Questions asked of references must be an-swered to the HSO's satisfaction. No one should be allowed to render care until the application is complete in all respects and has been reviewed *and* approved. Things are not always what they seem.

The PSO may have several categories of membership. This is always true for acute care hospitals. Typically, these range from most involved (active), to least involved (honorary). New members, except those in the honorary and consulting categories, often are given provisional appointments. This amounts to a probationary status and allows clinical performance to be re-viewed. In the future, the categories of PSO membership are likely to be fewer and include only "active" and "consulting."

In 1984, the Joint Commission on Accreditation of Hospitals, now the Joint Commission on Accreditation of Healthcare Organizations, adopted a new medical staff standard in its *Accredita-tion Manual for Hospitals*. It allowed hospitals to extend PSO membership to LIPs other than physicians and dentists. Prior to this time these LIPs could be granted only "clinical duties and responsibilities." The new standard was permissive, but was a major departure from previous philosophy and practice. Nonphysician LIPs are licensed and permitted by law to independently provide certain treatment. Caregivers not licensed to render care independently are dependent on the orders of a physician or a LIP and, absent such orders, may not treat patients. Some dependent caregivers, such as pharmacists and registered nurses, are licensed; others, such as phlebotomists and nurse aides, are unlicensed. As described in Chapter 2, many dependent caregivers are certified (an activity of a private group), but this does not substitute for licensure (recognition by a governmental regulatory body). Caregivers are dependent if their work depends on an order from an LIP. Without such an order, a pharmacist may not dispense a prescription drug, and a phlebotomist may not draw blood.

The 1984 accreditation standards changes were especially important for nonphysician LIPs such as podiatrists, clinical psychologists, and nurse-midwives, many of whom wish to treat patients in hospitals. Chiropractors, too, have benefited from this change, as well as the revisions in the AMA's Principles of Medical Ethics noted in Chapter 3. A 1989 AHA survey found that hospital PSO bylaws allowed nonphysician LIPs to apply for membership; 67% of hospital PSOs accept podiatrists, 43% accept clinical psychologists, and 5% accept chiropractors. These percentages are significant increases from a similar study done in 1984.[11] It bears repeating that, even if nonphysician LIPs cannot obtain PSO membership, they may have clinical privileges consistent with their license and demonstrated competence.

The Joint Commission accreditation standards for hospitals give physicians one last bastion—a majority of the PSO executive committee must be fully licensed physician members actively practicing in that hospital. In addition, a physician must be responsible for the general medical condition of patients admitted by a nonphysician LIP and must obtain a medical history and conduct a physical examination, unless the nonphysician LIP has been granted such privileges. Hospitals will be challenged to maximize the potential benefit from these changes. Doing so necessitates integrating the new categories of clinical staff into the delivery of services.

As noted, PSO membership is separable from clinical privileges. For example, someone appointed in the "honorary" category has no clinical privileges. In contrast, PSO members in the "active" category by definition will have significant clinical privileges, although they may be temporarily suspended because of a disciplinary action. Similarly, PSO bylaws may not allow nonphysician LIPs to be members; nonetheless, these LIPs may be granted clinical privileges.

Privileges

Clinical privileges must be delineated (individually or by category) for all LIPs delivering care in the HSO, whether or not they are PSO members. Prudence demands that clinical activities be limited to the skills and qualifications LIPs can initially demonstrate and continue to justify. In addition, what the LIP seeks to do must be compatible with the ability of the HSO to support the activities.

LIPs such as clinical psychologists, podiatrists, and nurse-midwives, are limited by their respective licensing statutes to performing certain activities. For example, podiatrists may medically and surgically treat the leg below the knee and prescribe certain medications. HSOs may further restrict what state licensing allows LIPs to do, but the HSO may not allow them to do more. Categories of LIPs may be granted privileges as a group in the HSO. Physicians and dentists are granted privileges individually.

Privilege delineation has two elements. The first is determination of specific content of clinical privileges. The second is ongoing and systematic review of care delivered to determine if changes in privileges, either increases or decreases, are justified. Clinical privileges should be specific to the HSO—for hospitals this is a Joint Commission requirement. Each procedure/

activity may be listed on the application or reapplication forms, or there may be a general reference such as "internal medicine" with whatever limitations are appropriate for the level of qualification held by the physician. The definition of a general term such as internal medicine must be found in the PSO bylaws or the PSO rules and regulations. Clinical privileges for nonphysician LIPs are handled similarly, although the privileges are more likely to be specifically listed. It is also common and desirable that any special relationships of nonphysician LIPs to physicians be described in the grant of privileges, or referenced in the PSO bylaws or the rules and regulations. Examples are nurse-midwives who work with (or are employed by) obstetricians or nurse-anesthetists who work with (or are employed by) surgeons.

PSO Discipline

Disciplinary action may be necessary against someone with clinical privileges. Often this results from minor infractions of the PSO bylaws or subsidiary rules and regulations. Sometimes, HSO policies are involved. Occasionally, the quality of care rendered by the practitioner is deficient. Regardless, it may be necessary to act to protect patients or find ways to encourage appropriate behavior. Almost always, this involves a recommendation by a PSO committee. Depending on the matter, recommendation, review, and approval by the GB may be necessary.

A common problem in hospitals is that clinical staff fail to complete medical records of discharged patients in the time limits set by the PSO rules and regulations. Such lapses do affect quality of care, but usually pose no danger to patients. Verbal or written warnings may be the first step in a disciplinary process. A continuing problem might require temporary suspension of admitting privileges, which means elective admissions are prohibited. Clinical staff whose admitting privileges are suspended usually take immediate steps to make records current.

PSO bylaws usually identify a variety of disciplinary options. In order of increasing severity, they are mandatory continuing or special medical education, letter of admonition, supervision, suspension of admitting and/or clinical privileges, censure, reduction of privileges, and termination of privileges. It may be appropriate to take two or more actions concurrently. The underlying motivation is to protect patients from inadequate or inappropriate clinical treatment. Depending on the action, the affected member may be entitled to due process as set out in the PSO bylaws. If so, the recommendation by the PSO is reviewed and the GB has the final decision. In situations in which there is risk of imminent harm to patients, the CEO, acting for the GB, must take whatever action is necessary. The Health Care Quality Improvement Act of 1986 requires that actions adverse to a physician's clinical privileges for a period longer than 30 days must be reported to a national data bank. Reporting requirements for other types of practitioners are likely to be added in the future.

Special Issues in Credentialing

Economic Credentialing   Competitive and reimbursement pressures are forcing HSOs to be more efficient. This suggests the importance of judging the economic performance of clinicians. Research shows wide variation in physician use of resources such as frequency of hospital admission and length of patient stay, use of diagnostic tests for outpatients, and types and duration of therapies ordered. Clinical decisions such as these have great cost and revenue implications for HSOs. With few exceptions, high-quality care is efficient care. Patients should receive needed services, no more and no less. Such care is both high quality and efficient. Health maintenance organizations were among the first to stress the economic dimension of health services.

Judging economic performance, often called economic credentialing, means that in addition to reviewing the quality of care clinical staff provide, data are collected as to their economic effect on the HSO. Two criteria are most important: volume of referrals (typical special HSO interests are admissions, generally, and admitting insured and private pay patients, if possible) and review

of practice patterns to determine whether resources are being used efficiently. Economic credentialing is possible because HSOs are increasingly able to link cost information and patient treatment information.[12] Although rare in the late 1980s and early 1990s, logic suggests economic
credentialing will become common. A 1991 survey of hospital CEOs found a split in predictions
of the 5-year future of economic contributions when considering reappointment: just over 40%
predicted that it would be used and almost 60% said it would not.[13]

Turf Conflicts Technology that permits new diagnostic and therapeutic procedures is
problematic in credentialing. HSOs must have a means by which clinicians claiming expertise in
new procedures are reviewed and receive (or are denied) clinical privileges to perform them. Self-
reported competence is inadequate; independent verification is necessary. In addition, Chapter 5,
"Health Services Technology," suggests the extent to which technology is blurring the lines that
have traditionally separated medicine and surgery and medical and surgical specialties and sub-
specialties. Such blurring causes turf conflicts that disrupt referral patterns and PSO relationships.[14] The results can be very negative for HSOs, especially acute care hospitals. The economic
dimensions of turf conflicts include duplication of equipment, space, and staff as a way to placate
both groups of clinicians, and the likelihood that disgruntled clinicians will sever their relationship with the HSO and treat their patients elsewhere. A preferred approach is to delay obtaining
technology until agreement about its use is reached.

Integration

Individual clinicians and the PSO as a whole perform technical services that must be integrated
into the total effort of the HSO to achieve organizational goals. Nonclinician managers cannot
deliver clinical services, nor can they independently judge quality. They can, however, obtain the
expert advice and technical assistance needed to make informed judgments about individual and
aggregate PSO practice. This effort is similar to what managers do when they judge the technical
aspects of pharmacy or data processing, for example.

Except when they are chiefs of clinical service, medical directors, or PSO officers, PSO
members have not historically participated in managing the HSO. In the past decade, however,
clinicians have increasingly been more a part of management decision processes. Such interactions are strongly recommended by the Joint Commission.

PSO members may be integrated into an HSO's managerial structure in several ways. They
may join PSO, management, or GB committees; management may informally or formally ask
them for advice; and those who manage clinical departments or units are part of the management
team. Clinical managers are a key element of HSO management. Even small PSOs are divided
into departments or sections based on clinical interest. Such relationships in a hospital are shown
in Figure 6.5 in Chapter 6. Clinical managers perform all the management functions. Medical
education and clinical practice teach physicians to think logically, to view problems systematically, and to consider their implications. These skills are useful, but do not adequately prepare
clinicians as managers. The HSO is responsible for so preparing them, and this is a matter of self-
interest because only competent clinical management can further organizational goals and objectives. The presence of full or part-time salaried clinical managers in an HSO allows even more
effective involvement in management. When clinicians and managers understand each other's
problems, enhanced communication and organizational effectiveness result.

Impaired Clinicians

PSOs, especially those in acute care hospitals, have an unenviable record of handling impaired
members of the clinical staff, especially physicians. The tendency has been for the clinical staff or
PSO to draw together and prevent patient and public scrutiny. This is a normal human tendency,
but it means the HSO and its clinical staff are ignoring ethical and legal duties to protect the

patients. HSOs are morally (and perhaps legally) obliged to try to rehabilitate all impaired staff, including physicians, whenever possible, but they may not do so in a way that puts patients at risk.

Impairment among caregivers is hard to document. It may be physical and/or mental because of aging or disease or may result from chemical abuse or dependency. Also impaired are those caregivers no longer competent because their clinical skills are outdated. Previous estimates suggest tens of thousands of physicians are impaired.[15] Estimates in the late 1980s ranged from 5% to 17% of all physicians and apply in Canada, as well as the United States.[16] The number of physicians impaired because of drug and alcohol addiction alone has been estimated at 15%.[17] Similar estimates of impairment of all types have been made for nonphysician caregivers. Regardless of the cause, however, it is ethically and legally incumbent on the HSO to identify the problem and act to protect the patients. Impairment may be detected through quality assessment and risk management, which are discussed in Chapter 12.

Both where clinical practice is clearly substandard and in marginal situations, HSOs often do not act. The reasons are unclear. Sometimes the HSO fears legal action by the impaired clinician; in other cases those who should act have an emotional dislike for the task. Members of the PSO should be even more interested in improving the quality of clinical practice than are management and the GB. Unless accountability mechanisms and authority available to management and the GB are defined *and* used, the problem will persist until a patient is harmed and legal action is brought against the HSO. Inaction is a luxury no HSO can afford.

Continuing Function of the PSO

Conclusions drawn by Guest in 1972, after reviewing the literature about structural relationships linking management, the GB, and the medical staff (clinical staff) are valid today and can be applied to PSOs. According to Guest, the main structural unit that links individual physicians to both management and the GB is the executive committee of the medical staff (now, the PSO). He also notes that the literature strongly supports the notion that there should be medical representation on the GB and that reciprocal representation with CEO and GB members present at medical staff (PSO) meetings is also important. The literature also suggests that the "dynamic links throughout the hospital organization are those forged through the informal day to day interactions, not by the periodic 'engineering' of structural arrangements."[18]

ORGANIZATION OF SELECTED HSOs

The preceding material is a background to discussing selected HSOs. Included in this discussion are acute care hospitals, hospices, managed care organizations, nursing facilities, ambulatory care organizations, birth centers, and home health agencies. These are the most dominant types, but the list is by no means exhaustive of the wide variety of different types that are, and will be, found in the health services system.

The discussion of each HSO uses the title most often given to the person that the HSO services. For example, hospitals use the word "patient." Managed care organizations use "enrollee" to describe the person served. Such titles are indicative of the relationship the organization and its staff have, or seek to have, with those served. The philosophical model that implicitly or explicitly underlies interactions with the person served is an important basis for the title chosen. Features of three models are discussed. They are shown in Table 7.2 and should be kept in mind as the various HSOs are discussed.

The *medical/hospital model* is driven by high technology, is physician directed, and is designed for persons with immediate acute health care needs. Treatment of disease is the principal goal. The *nursing home/social model* is driven by basic principles of the psychosocial disciplines, is directed by an interdisciplinary team, and is designed for persons with chronic, long-term physical and mental functional deficits. Quality of life is a major goal. The *hospitality/hotel model* is

Table 7.2. Basic models of HSO interactions with persons served

Model	Attributes
Medical/hospital model	Physician directed Acute care oriented High-technology setting Serves patient (curative)
Nursing home/social model	Interdisciplinary team directed Chronic long-term oriented Low-technology setting Serves resident (quality of life)
Hospitality/hotel model	Client directed Personal needs oriented No-technology setting Serves client (security/comfort)

Adapted from Stryker, Ruth. Characteristics of the residential care model. *Creative long-term care administration*, edited by George Kenneth Gordon and Ruth Stryker, 2d ed., 13. Springfield, IL: Charles C Thomas, 1988.

driven by marketing data that show client desires and satisfaction, is client directed, and is designed for persons with personal care needs. Security and comfortable living arrangements are major goals.[19]

Acute Care Hospitals

Background

History   Hospitals have been present in a variety of forms for millenia. Almost 5,000 years ago, Greek temples were the first, but similar institutions can be found in ancient Egyptian, Hindu, and Roman societies. These "hospitals" were very different than the hospitals of today, and over the span of time they have gone through a dramatic evolution from temples of worship and recuperation to almshouses and pesthouses and finally to sources of modern-day miracles.

The word "hospital" comes from the Latin *hospitalis*. Although well regarded earlier in history, hospitals in the Middle Ages and later had unsavory reputations and primarily served the poor. This reputation improved only slowly, beginning in the middle of the 19th century. Until well into the 20th century physicians provided charity care in hospitals but treated private (fee-for-service) patients at home. New medical technology made treatment efficacious, especially with surgical intervention, and this focused attention on acute care hospitals. Treatment of private patients brought acute care hospitals new prestige and acceptance. This evolution was well underway by the 1920s as acute care hospitals became differentiated and specialized to organize and deliver an expanded scope of services. Many acute care hospitals were small and owned by physicians as a convenient way to hospitalize their patients.

Definitions and Numbers   By convention of common use, a *community hospital* is an acute care hospital that treats the public for general medical and surgical problems. The title is used whether the hospital is not for profit or for profit. A community hospital provides permanent facilities, including inpatient beds, continuous nursing services, diagnosis, and treatment, through an organized PSO, for patients with a variety of surgical and nonsurgical conditions. This is in contrast to special hosptials, which admit only certain types of patients or those with specified illnesses or conditions.

In 1946, 6,125 hospitals were registered with the American Hospital Association (AHA). From a peak of 7,174 in 1974, the number declined to 6,649 in 1990.[20] This downward trend is likely to continue. Not all hospitals submit data or register with the AHA, but estimates are made for them and are included in the annual AHA publication *Hospital Statistics*, an important data source. The AHA reported that 761 hospitals of all types closed between 1980 and 1990, almost

75% of these were community hospitals.[21] It should be noted that these data count individual hospitals and do not, for example, delineate situations in which two hospitals merged and formed one corporate entity but continued to operate both facilities. The office of the inspector general of the Department of Health and Human Services (DHHS) found that a chain reaction triggered by rising costs, lagging revenues, and declining occupancy rates caused hospital closures in 1989.[22]

Table 7.3 shows the distribution of community hospitals by bed size; 45% have fewer than 100 beds. It is small hospitals that often need competent managers. They tend to be isolated and need linkages to other hospitals through networks and voluntary associations, as well as the multi-organizational systems described in Chapter 9.

Classification   Hospitals are classified in several ways: length of stay, type of control, and type of service. Length of stay is divided into short term and long term. Acute (of short duration or episodic) is a synonym for short term. Chronic (of long duration) is a synonym for long term. The AHA defines short-term stay hospitals as those with average lengths of stay shorter than 30 days, and long-term stay hospitals as those with average lengths of stay of 30 days or longer. More than 90% of hospitals are short term. Community hospitals are acute care (short term). Rehabilitation and chronic disease hospitals are long term. Psychiatric hospitals are usually long term. Some acute care hospitals have units to treat acute psychiatric illnesses.

Type of service denotes whether the hospital is "general" or "special." General hospitals provide a broad range of medical and surgical care, to which are usually added the specialties of obstetrics and gynecology; rehabilitation; orthopedics; and eye, ear, nose, and throat services. "General" can describe both acute and chronic care hospitals, but usually applies to short-term hospitals. "Special" hospitals offer services in one medical or surgical specialty (e.g., pediatrics, obstetrics/gynecology, rehabilitation medicine, or psychiatry) or in a discrete surgical procedure such as hernia repair. Although special hospitals are usually acute, they may also be chronic. A tuberculosis hospital is an example of the latter. In 1990 there were 477 long-term special hospitals.[23]

A third classification divides hospitals by type of control or ownership: not for profit, for profit (investor owned), or governmental (federal, state, local, or hospital authority). Figure 7.4 shows various types of hospital ownership. In 1990, of the 5,420 United States short-term general and special hospitals, approximately 59% were nongovernmental not for profit (also called voluntary), 14% were investor owned, and 27% were owned by state or local governments. The remaining 1,229 were either federally owned or psychiatric hospitals, tuberculosis and other respiratory

Table 7.3.   Distribution of community hospitals by bed size in 1980 and 1990[a]

Number of Beds	Number of hospitals		Percent change
	1980	1990	1980–1990
	5,830	5,384	−7.7
6–24	259	226	−12.7
25–49	1,029	935	−9.1
50–99	1,462	1,263	−13.6
100–199	1,370	1,306	−4.7
200–299	715	739	+3.4
300–399	412	408	−0.1
400–499	266	222	−16.5
500+	317	285	−10.1

Source: *American Hospital Association Hospital Statistics, 1991–1992,* xxxvii. Chicago: American Hospital Association, 1991.

[a]The AHA defines community hospitals as all nonfederal, short-term general and other special hospitals, excluding hospital units of institutions whose facilities are available to the public.

PRIVATE (NONGOVERNMENT) OWNERSHIP

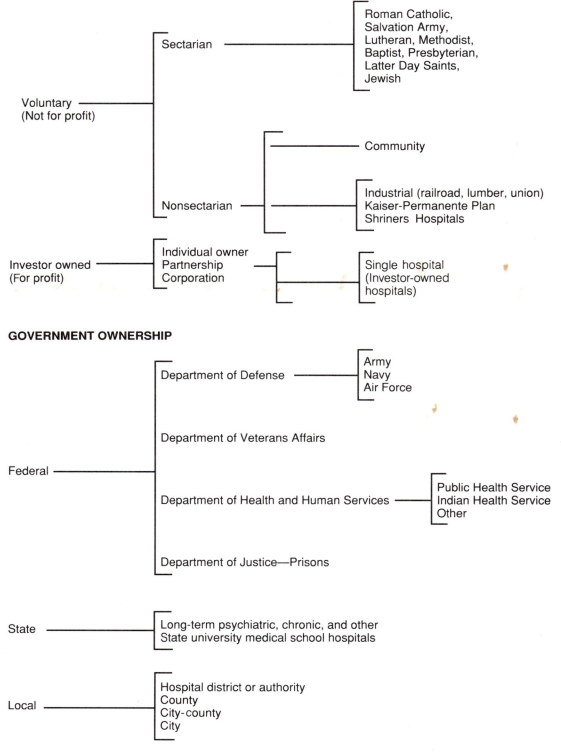

Figure 7.4. Hospital ownership.

hospitals, or long-term general and special hospitals, whether nongovernmental not for profit, investor owned, or owned by state or local government.[24] Table 7.4 shows short- and long-term hospitals by type of ownership for selected years.

The acute care hospital field has a strong tradition of voluntarism, and ownership is overwhelmingly not for profit. During the last part of the 19th and first part of the 20th centuries, acute care hospitals became larger and more complex and costly. In addition to voluntarism, the increase in not-for-profit acute care hospitals resulted from favorable tax treatment and the federal Hill-Burton program (begun in 1946), which provided money to build them.

Prior to passage of Medicare in 1965, the number of investor-owned acute care hospitals had been declining. After 1965, the number stabilized and in 1990, there were 749 investor-owned, acute care hospitals with 101,000 beds.[25] In addition, investor-owned companies have management contracts with a large number of hospitals.

In addition to privately owned hospitals, whether sectarian or nonsectarian or not for profit or investor owned, there are many acute care hospitals that are publicly owned. The 1991 *Hospital Statistics* reports that 1,469, or 27%, of community hospitals are owned by state and local government.[26]

New Types   Several states have blurred the traditional definition of acute care hospitals by licensing new types of facilities. The postoperative recovery center is neither a traditional inpatient acute care hospital nor an ambulatory HSO. Another name sometimes used is medical inn. It is estimated that 25% of postsurgical patients in acute care hospitals could recover uneventfully in such a facility.[27] Length of stay is limited, for example, to 48 hours in California. It is estimated that costs will be 25%–40% less than in an acute care hospital.[28] In addition, some states now license a category of facility whose level of service is between that of acute care hospital and that of a nursing facility. The difference lies in the emphasis on rehabilitation and the sophistication of medical care typically not found in a nursing facility.

Functions   Acute care hospitals diagnose and treat the sick and injured, and, sometimes, the worried well. The nature of a patient's illness determines the care received and, to some extent, the type of hospital in which it is provided. Care may be delivered on an inpatient or outpatient basis.

Table 7.4.   Short- and long-term hospitals with numbers of beds, according to type of ownership

Type of ownership	1960 Facilities	1960 Beds[a]	1970 Facilities	1970 Beds[a]	1980 Facilities	1980 Beds[a]	1990 Facilities	1990 Beds[a]
All ownership	6,876	1,658	7,123	1,616	6,965	1,365	6,649	1,213
Federal	435	177	408	161	359	117	337	98
Psychiatric	488	722	519	527	534	215	757	160
Tuberculosis and other respiratory diseases	238	52	101	20	11	2	4	0
Long-term general and other special	308	67	236	60	157	39	131	25
Short-term general and other special	5,407	639	5,859	848	5,904	992	5,420	929
Not for profit	3,291	446	3,386	592	3,339	693	3,202	657
Investor owned	856	37	769	53	730	87	749	101
State and local government	1,260	156	1,704	204	1,835	212	1,469	171

Source: *American Hospital Association Hospital Statistics, 1991–1992*, 2–6. Chicago: American Hospital Association, 1991.
[a]In thousands.

A second function is preventing illness and promoting health. Examples are instructing patients about self-care after discharge, referring them to other community services such as home health services, conducting disease screening, and holding childbirth and smoking cessation classes. The competitive environment has caused hospitals to mix illness prevention and health promotion with generous amounts of marketing.

A third function is educating health services workers. Physician education in residencies and fellowships is common. Acute care hospitals train staff such as nurse aides who will work in them. Acute care hospitals are a setting for many different types of health services workers who need clinical experience to receive a state license or professional society certification. Many health services management education programs require a residency, and it is common for managers to have spent time in an acute care hospital as an administrative resident or fellow.

A fourth function is research. Clinical trials for new drugs and devices come to mind first, but are the least common. Research such as assessing utilization of intensive care units and determining why staff ignore universal precautions when treating emergency room patients are more common. One type of nonclinical research focuses on improving hospital processes through quality improvement. This could include using patient satisfaction surveys, increasing efficiency in patient billing, and improving ways to deliver supplies to nursing units.

All acute care hospitals treat the sick and injured. Their emphasis on the other functions noted here depends on organizational objectives. Chapter 9 describes new relationships hospitals and other HSOs are developing to deliver services in unique and more effective ways.

Organizational Structure   The acute care hospital would be much less complex if it fit the usual organizational pyramid; however, this is not the case. Its organizational structure differs substantially from the bureaucratic model of other large organizations. These differences are caused by the unusual relationships between the formal authority of position represented by the managerial hierarchy and the authority of knowledge possessed by members of the PSO. In the typical community hospital, the members of the PSO do not fit into the pyramid, as do staff who work for and are paid by the hospital. The PSO includes physicians, dentists, and, increasingly, the other types of LIPs described in Chapter 2. Except for administrative work, PSO members are usually not paid by the hospital. As a result, the organizational pattern is a dual pyramid with the managerial hierarchy and the PSO hierarchy side by side, as shown in Figure 7.2. Adding governance to management and the PSO results in the triad described earlier in this chapter. Some acute care hospitals integrate the PSO into the organizational structure; in such cases most members of the PSO are salaried. Department of Veterans Affairs and military hospitals are examples.

A dual pyramid—two lines of authority—causes a management dilemma by violating the principle of unity of command. One line extends down from the GB to the CEO and from there into the managerial structure and hierarchy. The other extends from the GB to the PSO. These two intersect in departments such as nursing, where activities are both managerial and clinical. The complexity of this structure is illustrated by the fact that many hospital employees often have more than one immediate superior. Employees such as nurses who work in clinical areas are directed by their head nurse, who is part of management, and by members of the PSO, usually physicians, regarding specific patients. These directions may be contradictory because each group interprets objectives and the means of attaining them in terms of its own value systems and requirements.

Governance   Traditionally, hospital GBs have included business and financial leaders who were public spirited and engaged in community activities. A 1989 study shows that this pattern continues. According to this study, knowledge of business and finance is the most important criterion in selecting board members. Community activities, political influence, ideology and values, and time availability are next, in that order. Knowledge of health care ranks only sixth; clinical practice skills is eighth.[29] This ordering of criteria seems anachronistic and out of step with what is required of modern hospital GBs. Hospitals and business enterprises have similarities, but their differences are greater and require expertise that must be reflected in the GB.

About one half of GBs have no upper limit on the number of years a member may serve.[30] GBs are likely to be self-perpetuating, which means that current members nominate and select their replacements. Data from all hospitals show that only 48% set an upper limit on the number of years members may serve.[31] Unlimited lengths of service have both positive and negative aspects. Forty-three percent of hospital nominating committees include the chief executive officer (CEO).[32]

Data about the size of GBs show variation by type of ownership. The approximate average number of GB members in not-for-profit hospitals is 18, that in government hospitals is 8, and that in investor-owned hospitals is 10. The average GB size for all hospitals is approximately 15 members.[33]

The diverse and extensive changes in the external environment described in Chapter 2 have caused close scrutiny of the GB. Proposals to increase the competence of GB members have focused on specialized seminars and continuing education. Such approaches are inadequate, and many hospitals will be served best by adopting the business enterprise model in which directors are paid for their time and knowledge. In 1989, only 2% of hospitals paid GB members an annual fee; 7% paid a per-meeting fee, a significant decline from the 21% reported in 1985. Another 4% of hospitals paid GB members travel expenses plus a fee.[34] High-quality policy making is only a matter of chance if the GB is marginally or inadequately prepared.

To facilitate communication and coordination among the GB, management, and the PSO, many hospitals have a joint conference committee, which may be a standing committee of the GB or the PSO. The joint conference committee usually has few members and no line authority.

Management   Acute care hospitals are complex organizations with several levels of line management. Figure 7.5 shows the organization chart of a community hospital that uses corporate titles—a general trend. The dual hierarchy described above is suggested by showing the medical staff, the traditional term for the PSO, reporting to the board of trustees, also the traditional term. The senior vice president for medical affairs reports to the president of the hospital and has a number of responsibilities related to PSO functioning. The dotted lines connecting the president, the vice president for medical affairs, and the medical staff suggest a consultative relationship. The vice president for medical affairs may have the title "medical director." The line departments/activities that provide direct patient care, support, and administrative functions are readily identifiable from the titles. In addition, there are a number of staff departments/units, such as marketing, fund raising, certificate of need, and personnel services.

One of the most important roles of a GB is to select and evaluate the performance of the CEO. According to a 1989 study, only 66% of responding hospitals formally evaluate the CEO; written evaluation criteria/objectives and economic performance (97%) and medical staff relations (96%) are the most important criteria used. Personal qualities are used by 85% of responding hospitals, and quality of care by 77%.[35] The relative infrequency of using quality of care to evaluate a CEO suggests that many GBs fail to link management with quality of care, a view at best inappropriate and artificial.

Another important measure of the relationship between management and governance is whether the CEO is a voting member of the GB. In a 1989 study, 42% of hospitals had CEOs who were full voting members of the GB. Just over 45% reported that the CEO was an ex officio (by reason of the office) nonvoting member.[36] That same study reports that only 44% of hospital CEOs had an employment contract. In descending order, the elements most commonly found in employment contracts include compensation (91%), termination provisions (89%), job responsibilities (81%), terms of employment (63%), and performance standards (57%).[37] The relative infrequency of performance standards is surprising.

PSO   Members of the PSO, primarily the physicians, are critical to a hospital's economic success. This is true whether PSO members are independent contractors who charge patients a fee for service or are salaried. A community hospital, for instance, has a PSO whose members are

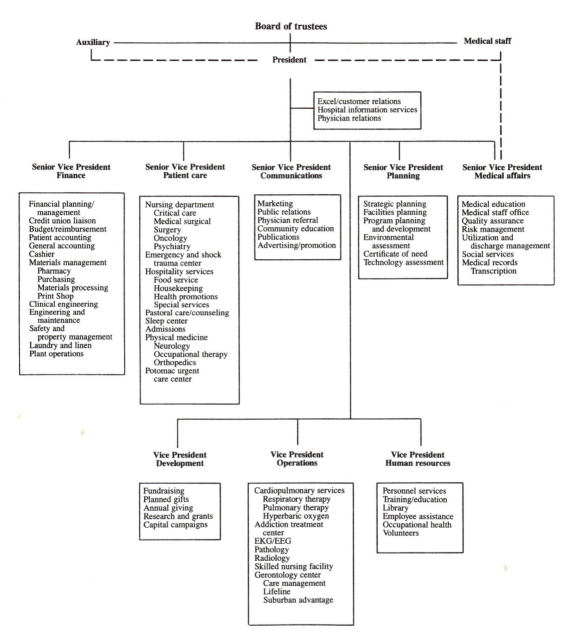

Figure 7.5.   Suburban Hospital, Inc., organization chart. (From Suburban Hospital, 8600 Old Georgetown Road, Bethesda, MD, December 1990; reprinted by permission.)

overwhelmingly independent contractors, and revenue is generated for the hospital only if they admit patients. It has been estimated that physicians control 73% of all hospital admissions and make the majority of decisions concerning which hospital services are used; a 1989 study found that an average physician generated annual revenue of $513,000 for inpatient admissions, a 15%

increase from 1988. The five specialties generating the most revenue were pulmonology, cardiovascular surgery, internal medicine, general surgery, and cardiology.[38]

Similarly, salaried practitioners increase a hospital's income if a patient admitted by them generates additional revenue. If the hospital is owned by an HSO that serves a capitated population (fixed payment per person), for example, an admission may be economically undesirable but is consistent with good medical treatment.

Accredited hospitals have a highly structured PSO (medical staff), and this is good practice regardless. As previously suggested, most hospital PSOs are largely self-governing. They have bylaws that set out how the PSO is organized and detail officers, committees, and various processes, including appointment of members, credentialing, and discipline.

The medical director is central to effective coordination, communication, and management of the PSO. This person is usually employed full time in larger hospitals and part time in smaller hospitals. Smaller hospitals may have a volunteer medical director who may be called the chief of staff. Other clinical managers include department chiefs or chiefs of service, who may or may not be paid depending on the demands on their time. Clinical managers have significant autonomy in managing those practicing in their departments, but they are ultimately accountable to the medical director for both clinical and administrative matters.

Numerous researchers have sought to understand, analyze, and describe physicians in hospitals: Georgopoulos and Mann studied 41 community general hospitals,[39] Roemer and Friedman studied the relationship between the medical staff organization (the PSO) and hospital performance,[40] Neuhauser studied the relationship between managerial activities and hospital performance,[41] and Shortell and Evashwick studied factors of medical staff organization (PSO) structures and their relationships to one another and certain hospital characteristics.[42] A general conclusion reached by these researchers is that increasing physician participation in hospital management will enhance effectiveness and efficiency and improve the quality of patient care. Later discussions of hospital–physician relationships continue this theme while recognizing the need for hospitals and physicians to be both competitors and collaborators.[43]

Perhaps no single organizational problem facing hospitals is more significant than the need to develop an effective relationship among the GB, management, and the PSO. Numerous means have been suggested. One is to include physicians on the GB. According to a 1989 study, the average GB has 2.24 physicians as members and physicians comprise 16% of GB membership overall.[44] Another means to create an effective relationship has been to appoint nonphysician GB members to PSO committees. According to the same 1989 study, GB members are appointed to the following PSO committees: quality assurance (44%); executive committee (25%); credentials committee (23%); and utilization review committee (22%).[45] Much effort, cooperation, and patience will be required to develop policies and practices that simultaneously maintain the prerogatives of clinical staff and the managerial integrity of the organization.

Caregiver and Support Staff   In 1990, 3.4 million full-time equivalent staff were employed in hospitals.[46] Numerous departments/units deliver clinical services: nursing, pharmacy, dietary services, radiology, and laboratories are common. In addition, there are numerous support departments, including housekeeping, maintenance, security, business office, and admitting. Figure 7.5 suggests the range and activity of these various departments/units. The ratio of staff to patients in community hospitals is more than 3 to 1; in teaching hospitals it is even higher. As treatment becomes more sophisticated, the types and numbers of specialized professional and technical staff increase. Chapter 17, "Personnel/Human Resources Management," notes that about 200 different types of positions are needed to staff a general acute care community hospital and more than 300 for a large teaching hospital, and the numbers are increasing.

Licensure and Accreditation   Hospitals are licensed in all states and must meet the regulations and requirements of their licensing states. In most states Joint Commission accreditation meets licensure requirements in whole or in part.

The Joint Commission hospital accreditation program accredited more than 5,400 U.S. hospitals in 1991.[47] Accreditation status is significant because it is required in order for the hospital to participate in certain programs and activities, such as postgraduate medical education (residencies). One of the most important links is with Medicare reimbursement. The original Medicare law in 1965 stated that hospitals accredited by the Joint Commission were "deemed" appropriate providers for purposes of reimbursement—this became known as deemed status. In 1972, a survey process and criteria known as the conditions of participation were developed by the Department of Health, Education, and Welfare (now DHHS) and are used in hospitals that are not Joint Commission accredited.

Future   Many acute care hospitals are organizing specialty activities that focus on diagnosing and treating specific diseases such as cancer or heart disease, or that focus on groups such as women or physical fitness and sports enthusiasts. These diagnostic and therapeutic services may be offered on either an inpatient or an outpatient basis. (The financing system has encouraged outpatient activities.) To some extent this is a competitive strategy that seeks to build centers of excellence. In addition, it reflects the trend toward boutique medicine. Other common efforts in acute care hospitals include joint risk taking, or joint ventures between hospitals and their PSOs, primarily physicians, and the effort to provide advances in patient convenience and patient-centered care.

Chapter 5 describes the increasing portability of technology and suggests some implications for hospitals. The most important is that members of the PSO will expand their nonhospital practices at the hospital's expense. Cooperating and competing with a PSO puts hospitals and managers in a difficult situation. Extrapolation of this trend of portability of technology suggests significant changes for the inpatient portion of hospital services.

In the future, hospitals may compete effectively with alternative providers such as health maintenance organizations and preferred provider organizations by contracting directly with employers to provide inpatient and outpatient services. Direct contracting means the hospital controls utilization and performance and eliminates the middle man, such as the preferred provider organization, thereby reducing costs by eliminating overhead.[48]

Despite the challenge from ambulatory health services providers, between 1984 and 1987 customer surveys showed that hospitals increased their share of outpatient care from 68.7% to 85.8%, at the expense of both freestanding centers and physicians' offices, whose market share declined.[49] Since 1988, however, customer surveys show that hospitals' market share of outpatient services declined to 81.8% in 1990 and 76.5% in 1991 and that most of the market share lost by hospitals went to freestanding surgical and diagnostic centers.[50] In terms of emergency services hospitals were clearly preferred, with 91% of those persons surveyed receiving care there.[51] Previous surveys of public perceptions about both emergency and outpatient care showed a strong preference for services delivered in hospitals,[52] but the decline in hospital market share suggests this preference may be changing. Such data suggest major problems and significant challenges for hospital managers.

There is speculation that in the future the inpatient portion of acute care hospitals will be large intensive care units because only the most acutely ill patients will require hospitalization. If true, this prediction means staff–patient ratios will increase, costs will increase, and the work of managers will be even more complex.

Nursing Facilities

Background

History   Saint Helena (250–330 A.D.) is credited with establishing one of the first homes for the aged (*gerokomion*). "She was a wealthy, intelligent, Christian convert and mother of Constantine the Great. Like other early Christian 'nurses' who devoted their lives to the sick and needy, she gave direct care herself."[53] Early American towns often operated almshouses—or poorhouses, poor farms, or workhouses, as they were also known—for those down on their luck and who needed a sheltered environment. In the early 1900s, privately owned "boarding houses" became available to the more affluent aged, and church-sponsored homes for the aged emerged.[54]

The Social Security Act of 1935 included an Old Age Assistance program with minimal requirements to be met by the states. States could not make payments to residents of public facilities, and this further stimulated growth of small private boarding houses. Most nursing-boarding homes were for profit and were operated by persons without special training.[55]

Definition and Numbers   HSOs that serve the frail elderly, the infirm, and other persons needing skilled care are commonly referred to as nursing homes. Only in 1950 were they licensed in every state.[56] In 1951, passage of the Kerr-Mills bill provided federal matching funds to states that met certain licensing and inspection requirements.[57]

Enactment of Medicare and Medicaid in 1965 placed major emphasis on delivery of skilled nursing care in nursing homes. The average size of nursing homes and the number of beds increased dramatically after 1965.[58] As Stryker notes, there are positive and negative effects of the law. Positive effects include mandated working relationships between hospitals and nursing homes and improved medical supervision and therapies for residents. Negative effects include: 1) defining extended care to mean time-limited, posthospital treatment rather than continued care of older adults with physical and mental disabilities; 2) basing the laws on the hospital/medical model, which emphasizes disease rather than functional competence, treatment rather than quality of living, and regulations viewing residents as a group rather than considering them as individuals; and 3) the greatest problem, the emphasis on physical rather than emotional and mental needs.[59] As a hybrid of the health care models discussed earlier to guide HSO interactions with the persons they serve, Stryker suggests the *residential model*:

> The residential model integrates certain qualities of all three models. Health care must be delivered, but it is delivered in a residential setting which incorporates resident driven decision making as much as possible in order to maintain the highest possible psychological and physical functioning. What is done for acute conditions in temporary settings is not appropriate for what is done for chronic conditions in long term settings. Provision of health care, attention to quality living environment, and as much resident decision making as possible characterize the residential model.[60]

Initially, federal regulations distinguished nursing homes by the nursing care provided. Skilled nursing facilities (SNFs) had the most nursing care—a licensed practical nurse (LPN) was on duty 24 hours a day and a registered nurse (RN) was on duty at least during the day shift 7 days a week. Intermediate care facilities (ICFs) provided nursing services in accordance with residents' needs. Nursing care was available to residents to achieve and maintain the highest degree of function, self-care, and independence. Residential care facilities (RCFs) had no nursing care and were only a sheltered environment for which there was no federal payment. Currently, states use a variety of titles for RCFs. It is common for various levels of care to be provided in different parts of the same facility.

The Nursing Home Reform Law, part of the Omnibus Budget Reconciliation Act of 1987, eliminated the distinction between SNFs and ICFs, and both were called nursing facilities (NFs) beginning in 1991. The nomenclature commonly used for "nursing homes" will continue to be confusing, however. The Nursing Home Reform Law also focused on quality of life and residents' rights and made numerous other changes.

In 1990, there were 15,607 NFs with more than 1.6 million licensed beds.[61] Well over half of NFs have fewer than 100 beds. Almost 6,000 have a capacity of 101–200 beds, for about 800,000 total beds.[62] In 1990, there were 8,688 Medicare-certified NFs.[63] NFs that do not provide skilled services cannot participate in Medicare. Nonetheless, they may serve Medicaid and private-pay residents.

Many acute care hospitals operate what were historically called extended care facilities.

They are known now as hospital-based NFs; in 1990, there were about 1,100.[64] They function like NFs, but a study reported in 1991 shows that they have fundamental differences. Hospital-based NFs have a much shorter length of stay, have double the number of staff per bed, and use 50% more RNs, LPNs, and nurse administrators than do freestanding NFs.[65] NFs that are part of a hospital are likely to be smaller; in 1990 2% of all NFs were part of a hospital.[66]

In 1990, almost two thirds of Medicare-certified NFs were investor owned.[67] In 1990, Medicaid covered 55.6% of all NF patients and accounted for 60.2% of NF revenues. Medicare accounted for 13.2% of revenue.[68] In 1989, the Health Care Financing Administration reimbursed NFs $99 per day per Medicare beneficiary.[69]

Functions   Federal regulations are important to NFs, even though most are *not* Medicare certified. Medicare-eligible NFs must meet four criteria:[70]

Residents must require and receive a skilled nursing or rehabilitative service provided directly by, or under the supervision of, an RN, LPN, or licensed therapist.
Services must be provided daily (with some exceptions).
Services must be reasonable and necessary in light of the resident's medical condition.
Services must need to be performed on an inpatient basis.

As early as 1970, Medicare regulations recommended 17 departments.[71] These include: clinical services, such as physician and dental care, nursing, and rehabilitation (occupational therapy, physical therapy, and speech therapy); clinical support services, such as laboratory, radiology, and pharmacy; and administrative services, such as housekeeping, laundry, and maintenance.[72] The work of committees in the clinical areas is likely to be coordinated by the medical director.[73] As of 1990, NFs certified for Medicare are deemed to meet Medicaid standards.[74]

Organizational Structure   Depending on their size, NF organizational structures may be pyramidal (tall), with several levels of management, or flat, with few levels of management. Most NFs are small and have few managers or levels of management between the administrator and staff. A large NF, however, may have several levels of managers between the administrator and staff, and these persons perform the typical line and staff functions such as general administration, financial management, and human resources administration. An organization chart for a medium-sized for-profit NF is shown in Figure 7.6.

Governance   Small NFs organized for profit are likely to be sole proprietorships or partnerships and will not have a board of directors. Governance and management functions will be combined.

Large for-profit or not-for-profit NFs are organized as corporations and have a board of directors. The functions of GBs of for-profit and not-for-profit corporations have few differences, and these GBs perform the generic functions discussed earlier. Traditionally, GB members of HSOs organized not for profit prefer to be called "trustees" whether or not there is actually a trust.

Management   All states require that NFs have a licensed administrator of record. There is wide variation in state requirements, however, and this limits reciprocity.[75] Other managers and special skills are present as size and activities require.

PSO   The PSOs of NFs receiving federal funds must have written bylaws and rules and regulations, just as do hospital PSOs. The content of such documents was described previously. It is likely that, in the future, nonfederally qualified NFs, especially the larger ones, will have a PSO such as that found in hospitals. PSOs may be open or closed, concepts described earlier. Fewer LIPs tend to be found in NFs compared with hospitals. As in hospitals, use of standing orders allows clinical activities to occur without a specific physician order.

Medicare requires a medical director; this is good practice regardless. The medical director may be full or part time and coordinates care to ensure that medical services are adequate and appropriate. This includes developing and implementing policies regarding primary physician

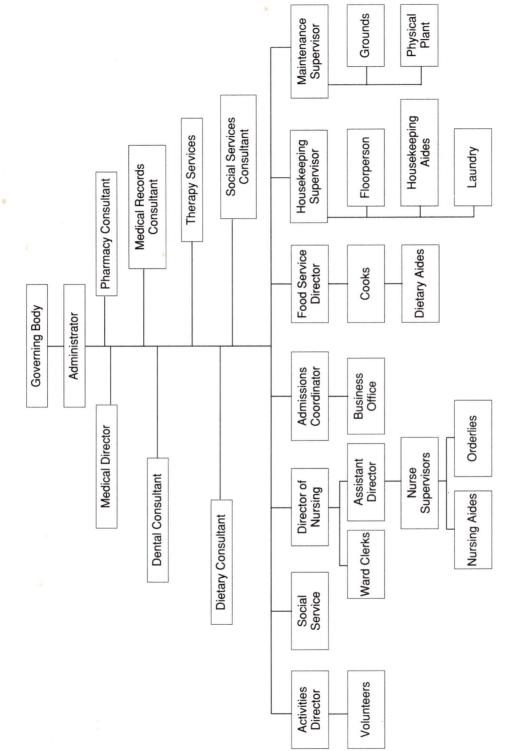

Figure 7.6. Tranquility Health Care Center organization chart. (From Brown, Richard. Capturing lost charges: Tranquility Health Care Center. In *Cases in long-term care management*, 157. Owings Mills, MD: National Health Publishing, 1989; reprinted by permission.)

272

credentialing, granting staff privileges, assuring compliance with regulations and disciplinary procedures, and reviewing and maintaining quality of care.[76]

Practitioners are credentialed as described previously. Because NF care is chronic and uses little technology, the resulting perception that patients are at low risk may suggest that a less demanding credentialing process is adequate. NFs should use the acute care hospital model and be rigorous in credentialing. Physician credentialing in NFs is a neglected area.[77]

Residents may be admitted by any licensed physician. Residents whose physicians have privileges may be attended by them. These physician services are paid by the resident, either directly or through insurance. Larger NFs may have salaried physicians on their staff to supplement the role of the resident's private physician and provide services, as needed.

Caregiver and Support Staff   The ideal in developing an effective treatment milieu in an NF is to have a multidisciplinary geriatrics team. The team concept presumes that participants have specialized expertise in gerontology, including clergy/ethics, clinical pharmacology, dental/oral hygiene, medical, nursing, nutrition support, ophthalmic/podiatric/surgical, psychiatry/psychology, rehabilitation therapy, and social work. All team members are expected to act as patient advocates.[78] These skills are likely to be found in larger NFs. Regardless of internal capacity, all these skills are available through consultants and volunteers.

In 1990, NFs employed 0.78 staff workers per set-up bed.[79] Medicare-certified NFs have a wide range of staff. Most are part of nursing service, including RNs, LPNs, and nursing assistants (who may be certified). Social service workers act as facilitators who allow residents to function at maximum capacities. They act as interviewers, therapists/counselors, case managers, and transition managers.[80] Individualized activities plans are prepared for each resident, and an activities coordinator develops programs that provide "opportunities for each resident to use existing abilities, build on past experiences, and to identify the motivations that will help each person to continue life's tasks."[81] The Nursing Home Reform Law (1987) requires that Medicare-certified NFs have an activities director and a dietitian. Depending on size, NFs may have other staff such as physical, occupational, and speech therapists, and pharmacists.

In 1985, more than 1.1 million full-time equivalent employees worked in NFs. On average, 5.5 employees providing administrative, medical, and therapeutic services and 43.4 nursing staff were employed per 100 beds in 1985.[82] Average turnover in Medicare-certified NFs in 1988 was just over 20% for RNs and LPNs, and ranged from 18% to more than 40% for nurse aides, dietary staff, activity staff, and nursing administration.[83]

Licensure and Accreditation   NFs are licensed in all states and must meet applicable regulations and requirements. The Joint Commission has an accreditation program for NFs, but they have no "deemed status" (as is the case with accredited hospitals under Medicare), and accreditation does not relieve NFs of federal Medicare certification inspections.

Future   Pessimistic predictions of the future for NFs suggest that inadequate reimbursement rates coupled with costly demands of new federal regulations and sicker residents may cause an economic crisis for these organizations. Those more optimistic believe that rising demand for NF beds and a more affluent elderly population will bring NFs a bright future.[84] Some states are considering applying certificate of need requirements to NFs to control unregulated growth and development.

Maintaining adequate staffing levels will challenge NFs. The demand for registered nurses and physical therapists will increase significantly in the 1990s.[85] Recruiting and retaining less skilled employees such as nursing assistants will continue to be a problem as well.

Nevertheless, the continued graying of America suggests that there will be a very strong demand for NFs in the decades ahead. A recent estimate shows that 43% of all Americans who reach the age of 65 in 1990—929,000 persons—will use an NF before they die.[86] The study also notes that by the year 2020, there will be 1.7 million Americans age 65 who will enter an NF before death.[87] Stated in another way, it is estimated that the NF population will increase from 2.3 million in 1988 to 4 million in 2018. During the same period, the costs for NF care will increase from $33 billion to $98 billion.[88] Data such as these suggest significant opportunities for clinical and managerial careers in NFs.

Ambulatory Health Services

Background Ambulatory care is not a recent development in health services delivery. Throughout history it has been the most common type. New, however, is the growing proportion of services that is delivered to persons who spend less than 24 hours in a facility. Ambulatory care may be defined as care delivered to persons who go to a physician's office (or other setting) under their own cognizance, at a time and place they determine, receive care, and return home. Physicians' offices are the most likely setting for ambulatory services. In addition, ambulatory services have been available for decades in the emergency departments and outpatient clinics of acute care hospitals. Chapter 5 describes how new technology increasingly allows significant diagnostic and therapeutic services to be provided to outpatients.

Ambulatory health services are specialized types of HSOs that are similar in several respects, but have different functions. Ambulatory HSOs provide a wide range of services. Comprehensive outpatient rehabilitation facilities, voluntary sterilization centers, renal dialysis centers, abortion clinics, family planning clinics, podiatry surgical centers, oral surgery centers, birth centers, health maintenance organizations, general purpose (same-day) ambulatory surgery centers, eye surgery centers, and dermatology surgery centers are examples of the myriad of different types.[89] Several of these are discussed in more detail below.

Many ambulatory health services operate as freestanding facilities. The definition of "freestanding" is elusive. The AHA defines it as a facility not on the hospital campus. The Joint Commission considers a facility to be part of a hospital when the hospital is legally responsible for its activities. The concept of freestanding is further complicated by state licensing practices, some of which give hospitals wide latitude to own and operate remote facilities under a single license. Others require hospitals to have licenses both for off-campus facilities and for separately administered units (separate part facilities) within the hospital building.[90] Complexities are heightened when these considerations are added to the extraordinarily wide range of business relationships, such as joint ventures, contractual relationships, and vertically and horizontally integrated systems, that might result in establishing an ambulatory HSO. The result is some uncertainty and disagreement about definitions and data.

Medical Group Practice A medical group practice may be defined as the application of medical services by three or more physicians who are formally organized.[91] The earliest evidence of such an arrangement is found in ancient Egypt around 2500 B.C. in the presence of a whole collegium of doctors, probably all specialists.[92] Throughout the latter half of the 19th century, American surgeons often worked as collaborators in hospital "clinics."[93] One of the first major American medical group practices was the Mayo Clinic, which was established in Rochester, Minnesota, after the American Civil War.

In 1988, 30% of the almost 500,000 nonfederal physicians in the United States were part of a single-specialty or multispecialty group, and the number of groups grew from 4,289 in 1965 to 16,579 in 1988.[94] By 1990, there were about 20,000.[95] The percentage of multispecialty groups remained stable from 1965 to 1980 at about 35% of all groups, but declined rapidly between 1984 and 1988 from 33.0% to 19.1%. From 1965 to 1988 the percentage of general practice groups decreased by one third, from 15.2% to 9.8%. Single-specialty group practices show recent strong growth, however. In 1965, single-specialty groups were approximately 50% of the total, and by 1980 they were 57.2%; between 1980 and 1988, however, they jumped to 70.6%.[96] These trends mirror the emphasis on specialization and the decline of general practice. The increase in formally linked physicians suggests that they recognize the many professional and economic advantages enjoyed by group practice.

The increase in health maintenance organizations is affecting group practice. A survey found that 50% of groups contract with one or more health maintenance organizations, 20% take their referrals, and 8% were established to provide services to a health maintenance organization.[97]

Freestanding Ambulatory Centers Freestanding ambulatory centers have evolved from emergency care centers and urgent care centers to be more involved in primary care. The 4,000 such facilities operating in 1988 served as walk-in alternatives for conditions such as respiratory tract infections, fractures, minor trauma, and colds and flu.[98] The typical freestanding ambulatory center treated about 13,500 patients in 1988.[99]

Ambulatory Surgery Centers Surgicenter and same-day surgical centers are names often applied to ambulatory surgery centers (ASCs). The first freestanding ASC in the United States was established in Phoenix in 1970,[100] but hospitals have provided this service for decades. In 1989, there were approximately 1,200 ASCs. Past growth and projections are shown in Table 7.5. It should be noted that ASCs grew over 25% between 1988 and 1989, as did the number of procedures performed in them.[101] The increase in ASCs, most of which are physician owned, is attributed to efforts to enhance income.[102] Four specialties—ophthalmology, gynecology, otorhinolaryngology, and orthopedics—accounted for 67% of all procedures.[103] Eighty percent of ASCs are operated independently of either hospitals or corporate chains.[104] Insurers and managed care providers encourage growth by contracting with ASCs, and about 60% of ASCs have business agreements with health maintenance organizations and nearly 50% contract with preferred provider organizations.[105] It is notable that, in 1990, 82% of outpatient surgery was performed in hospitals.[106]

In 1980, Medicare was amended so that Part B covered surgery performed at ASCs; the regulations identified approximately 100 covered procedures. Over the years, the Medicare list has been updated and expanded. Currently, the Health Care Financing Administration (HCFA) has established groups of procedures and pays ASCs in a manner similar to that by which hospitals are paid under diagnosis-related groups.[107]

Diagnostic Imaging Centers In 1990 there were approximately 1,500 diagnostic imaging centers; it is estimated there will be 1,800 by 1991.[108] Greater portability of technology means that

Table 7.5. Number of surgery centers and admissions

Year	Number of facilities[a]	Total admissions	Admissions per facility[b]
1983	239	377,266	1,578
1984	330	517,851	1,569
1985	459	783,864	1,708
1986	592	1,033,604	1,746
1987	865	1,383,540	1,712
1988	964	1,722,367	1,787
1989	1,221	2,162,391	1,771
1990[c]	1,386	2,527,000	1,823
1991[c]	1,510	2,870,000	1,901
1992[c]	1,643	3,200,000	1,948

From Henderson, John A. Surgery centers continue making inroads. *Modern Healthcare* 20 (May 21, 1990): 98–100 (data source: SMG Marketing Group); reprinted by permission.

[a]Open as of December 31.

[b]Centers open 1 year or more.

[c]Projections.

imaging centers will continue to increase in number. More than 75% offer ultrasound and 63% offer mammography.[109] Magnetic resonance imagers and positron emission tomography scanners are increasingly common, and mammography systems and color-flow ultrasound are two technologies that will improve the capability of imaging centers.[110]

Organizational Structures   The various types of ambulatory HSOs are organized similarly, although the specifics vary widely.

Governance   Ambulatory HSOs are almost always corporations that can be organized for profit or not for profit. Physicians are commonly involved as owners-investors, and this suggests that many ambulatory HSOs will be organized for profit. Regardless of ownership, the GBs of ambulatory HSOs set policy and evaluate performance of management and, ultimately, the practitioners. GB composition and size is a function of whether the ambulatory HSO is organized for profit or not for profit.

Management   Managers include a CEO, whose title is likely to be administrator, director, or clinic manager. It is common in ambulatory HSOs that CEOs are physicians who may have special preparation in management. In such cases a nonphysician administrator or business manager is hired to assist them. Ambulatory HSOs are likely to have flat organizational structures with few levels of managers. Larger organizations will have intermediate-level managers as required. Depending on specific activities, the HSO may employ marketing and contract specialists who interact with a managed care organization if the ambulatory HSO is a preferred provider, for example. There may be a medical director or chief of staff who is responsible for clinical matters and who in many instances also may be the CEO.

PSO   Ambulatory HSOs are unlikely to have the number of LIPs that would necessitate a PSO such as found in hospitals. In addition, because physicians are both owners and employees, they are unlikely to see the need for a PSO. The physician-owners employ other LIPs who are likely to be screened and credentialed in a less formal process than in a hospital. There may be a committee that evaluates performance.

Caregiver and Support Staff   Caregiver staff may include a variety of types depending on the specific activities of the organization. RNs, LPNs, nurse aides, surgical assistants, laboratory technologists, and radiology technicians are common. Support staff include secretaries, receptionists, transcriptionists, billing and collections clerks, medical records technicians, and supervisory staff. Some nonphysician employees may have employment contracts.

Licensure and Accreditation   Licensure requirements for ambulatory HSOs vary widely, especially as to which types must be licensed and how affiliation with a hospital affects licensure and regulation. The Joint Commission accredits ambulatory HSOs, which may include ambulatory surgery centers, emergency and urgent care centers, family practice centers, and multispecialty group practices.

The Accreditation Association for Ambulatory Health Care (AAAHC) also accredits ambulatory HSOs. Its program includes medical and dental group practices, surgery centers, managed care organizations, urgent and immediate care centers, community and college health centers, occupational health services, and hospital-sponsored ambulatory care clinics.[111] AAAHC member organizations include groups such as the American Society of Outpatient Surgeons, the Federated Ambulatory Surgery Association, the American College Health Association, and the Association of Freestanding Radiation Oncology Centers. The AAAHC began its accreditation program in 1979 and in 1990 accredited more than 350 ambulatory health services organizations.[112]

Future   Ambulatory HSOs have become a major force in health services and have challenged more traditional providers for market share. Hospitals responded by developing on-campus outpatient centers rather than pursuing off-campus sites. Off-campus sites proved difficult to operate and manage and often were in conflict with hospitals' ongoing inpatient and outpatient operations.[113]

It has been suggested that the rapidly growing home health market offers excellent opportunities for multispecialty group practices, primarily because of the continuity of care they can offer and the potential for significant new referrals.[114] Portability of technology and an increasingly competitive relationship between hospitals and their practitioners, especially physicians, means that ambulatory services are likely to grow in range and medical complexity.

Hospices

Background

History   The modern hospice concept was developed in England by Cicely Saunders, M.D., in the early 1960s, but its progenitors were found in India in the time before Christ.[115] Dr. Saunders's work was stimulated by the very unsatisfactory conventional treatment of the terminally ill. Her work led to the establishment of St. Christopher's Hospice near London in 1967.[116] The first United States hospice program was established in New Haven, Connecticut, in 1974.[117] Dr. Elisabeth Kübler-Ross is credited with stimulating the acceptance of the hospice concept in the United States.[118]

Function and Numbers   Hospice care has a unique philosophy. Most HSOs seek to intervene dramatically and in ways that return a patient to maximum functioning. Hospice care, however, does not include therapeutic (curative) intervention even though there is attention to maximizing a patient's quality of life. Hospice care follows five principles:

—Dying is a normal part of living;
—Palliation (comfort or treating symptoms, not the underlying disease) is the major treatment goal;
—Both patients and their closest companions—family and friends—constitute the unit of care;
—The spectrum of care should include support for survivors throughout their bereavement; and
—An interdisciplinary team, including volunteers, is best able to provide the spectrum of necessary care.[119]

This sharply contrasts with the medical model. Historically, the hospice provided no artificial medical support, including hydration and nutrition. The philosophy is broader today, however, and the focus is commonly on doing what needs to be done to enhance the quality of a patient's life without therapeutic (curative) intervention. Treatment in a hospice is appropriate only when the patient is terminally ill and has only weeks, or several months, to live. Hospice care stresses patient autonomy and family involvement.

After a trial period beginning in 1983, hospice care has been covered by Medicare since 1986. As with other Medicare-reimbursed services, conditions of participation must be met. These include a core of services available at all times: skilled nursing, medical social services, physician services, and counseling. In addition, the hospice must provide, as needed, either directly or under arrangement, the following: physical and occupational therapy and speech-language pathology; services of home health aides; homemaker services; medical supplies, including outpatient drugs and biologicals for palliation, and medical appliances; and short-term inpatient care, including respite care limited to periods of not more than five consecutive days.[120] A physician must certify that the medical prognosis is such that the individual's life expectancy is 6 months or less.[121]

Once these requirements and others found in the conditions of participation are met, Part A of Medicare will pay for hospice care without limit. The previous maximum of 210 days was eliminated in 1990.[122] Both home care and inpatient hospice care are covered. Payments are made on a per diem basis, but are capped for each beneficiary treated in a hospice program. In 1990 the amount was $9,787.[123] Few beneficiaries reach the cap, and the per diem payment is the more important. In addition to Medicare, hospice care is covered by Medicaid in some states, private insurance, and some health maintenance organizations. Unreimbursed hospice care is dependent on community charitable support and the work of volunteers.[124]

It has been argued that the hospice concept was evolving when it became reimbursed under Medicare, that the rules and regulations result in a rigid, overly restrictive organizational model that is impractical in many communities, and that there are incentives for hospices to underserve patients, which could lead to a reduction in the quality of care and profiteering.[125] The Medicare requirement to employ nurses adds to the impracticality of establishing Medicare-certified hospices in less densely populated areas.[126]

In 1989, only 703 hospice programs (approximately 50%) were participating providers under Medicare's hospice certification program.[127] By 1990, there were more than 1,450 programs offering comprehensive hospice care in the United States. (Comprehensive is defined as combined care of the physical, sociological, emotional, and spiritual needs of the patient/family unit.[128]) Another 250 were working to become comprehensive hospices. Hospice programs served about 230,000 terminally ill patients and their families in 1991.[129]

Models   There are several models of the organization and provision of hospice care:[130]

1. *Hospital-based hospice*—the defining characteristic is that supervision, budgeting, cash flow, and major administrative decisions are made by the hospital; hospice care is a program or department. Care may be provided in the hospital and/or in the patient's home.
2. *Home health agency–based hospice*—the two may be separately staffed and managed teams, or the hospice program may be integrated into the home health agency as a concept of care in which some or all of the agency's nurses participate.
3. *Independent community-based hospice*—governed by community board. These hospices usually are associated with small, volunteer-intensive agencies, but this need not be the case.
4. *Coalition-based hospices*—provide coordination and administrative support to a coalition of HSOs such as home health agencies and hospitals. These hospices may directly provide volunteers, ancillary services, and/or professional services. In theory, this system provides the most economical use of resources, but coordination may be a problem.
5. *Other hospice models*—types such as hospice teams; hospice units within NFs; hospices owned by religious groups, health maintenance organizations, or Blue Cross; or a combination of the models described above.

Contracts can be used to expand the types of relationships. For example, although hospices are rarely based in NFs, independent hospices have begun to contract with NFs to provide a residence for their patients when there is no caregiver to allow the patient to remain at home.

Organizational Structure   Hospice services may be offered in the home or on an inpatient basis. The hospice may be freestanding or it may be part of another organization such as a hospital, a home health agency, or, in rare cases, a NF. In addition, it may be a for-profit corporation or a not-for-profit corporation, although the former are very rare. It must be stressed that hospice care is a program, an institution or building, and this is apparent from the National Hospice Organization's definition: "Hospice is a coordinated interdisciplinary program of supportive services and pain and symptom control for terminally ill people and their families. Hospice is primarily a concept of care, not a specific place of care."[131]

The hospice organizational structure is very flat and there are few management levels. Few managers or levels are needed because the hospice tends to be small and there are few staff, as compared with acute care hospitals or NFs, for example. Below the director are a few supervisory personnel and the staff. A large hospice has managers between the director and staff. These persons perform the typical line and staff functions such as general administration, financial management, and human resources administration. Because reimbursement and patient service depend on the staff providing direct services, hospices seek to minimize management staff.

Governance   The type of governance depends on whether the hospice is independent or dependent. Independent hospices have a GB like that of any freestanding organization. This means the GB has full authority and accountability and performs the generic functions described earlier. A dependent hospice may have a committee that provides guidance, or guidance may simply be the responsibility of a member of the parent organization's management team. In the latter case, the usual organizational relationships would be present.

Management   Because there are few staff, the hospice has few managers. Typically, there is a director, who may be a nurse or social worker, although persons with master's level management preparation are increasingly present. As the hospice movement continues to grow in number and size, opportunities for managers will increase.

Caregiver and Support Staff   The hospice care concept uses an interdisciplinary team that is described by McDonnell.[132] The core team consists of the patient's family; attending physician; oncologist (as appropriate); psychiatrist; nurse; social worker; various therapists, such as physical, speech, occupational, and respiratory therapists; patient care coordinator; volunteer coordinator; pharmacist; nutritionist; and clergy. Not all types of staff are available daily. Other special services should be available: enterostomal therapy, specialty medical evaluations, mental health counseling, bereavement counseling, art therapy, music therapy, pastoral counseling, and assistance by volunteers.

> Every member of the hospice interdisciplinary patient care team recognizes the value of his or her own particular level of expertise, in either a professional or personal capacity, for meeting at least one aspect of a patient and family's needs with the awareness that each discipline relates with other disciplines in the delivery of the overall plan of care to the patient. This results in what is often referred to as "role blurring." . . . The strength of the interdisciplinary team . . . is that all members of the team have a common commitment to meet the patient's and family's needs, and this commitment supersedes the boundaries of their own disciplines."[133]

Hospices make heavy use of volunteers.

Dependent hospices (part of another HSO) may find that staffing problems are less significant than independent hospices. Using staff from an acute care hospital or home health agency, for example, may raise problems of compatible philosophy, however, because it must be remembered above all that the philosophy of hospice care is palliation, not treatment.

Licensure and Accreditation   About 30 states license hospices, and the requirements vary widely. Absent licensure requirements, many hospices have chosen to be licensed in other categories, usually as home health agencies or health facilities.[134] The Joint Commission accredited hospices from 1984 to July 1, 1990, when the program was ended because of lack of participation and an inability to become financially self-supporting.[135] It plans to more fully address the needs of dying patients in its standards manual and not simply focus on hospices.[136]

The National League for Nursing's Community Health Accreditation Program (CHAP) accredits a wide variety of home care and community health programs, such as clinics and community nursing centers, home health agencies, infusion therapy programs, home medical equipment programs, and home pharmacy services. In 1989, CHAP began surveying hospices. Their accreditation process is similar to that of the Joint Commission and includes application for survey, self-study, site visit, and board review of the self-study and site visit. Standards emphasize the organization's structure and function, quality of services, resources, and long-term viability.[137]

Future   Given the demographics of the United States population, as well as the likelihood of increased acceptance of hospice care for the terminally ill, it is certain there will be significant growth in hospice programs in the next several decades. Table 7.6 shows the growth of hospice

Table 7.6. Hospice program data

Fiscal year	Admissions	Days per admission	Cost per hospice day	Cost per admission	Total cost (outlays of millions)
1984	2,200	29	$62	$1,800	$4
1985	11,000	33	66	2,200	25
1986	28,012	37	66	2,442	68
1987	68,721	41	74	3,034	208
1988	84,770	44	74	3,256	276
1989	89,008	48	74	3,470	309
1990[a]	102,359	51	85	4,245	435
1991	112,595	53	93	4,828	544
1992	120,477	55	98	5,270	635
1993	126,501	57	103	5,749	727
1994	132,826	59	108	6,258	831
1995	139,467	61	114	6,811	950

From Committee on Ways and Means, U.S. House of Representatives. *Overview of Entitlement Programs, 1990 Green Book: Background Material and Data on Programs within the Jurisdiction of the Committee on Ways and Means,* 147. Washington, D.C.: U.S. Government Printing Office, 1990 (data source 1984–1989: CBO estimates; 1990–1995: CBO baseline projections, January, 1990).

[a]Figures from 1990 to 1995 are projections.

programs. Bereavement support and respite care may be increasingly important future services provided by hospices.

Coverage of hospice care under Medicare (and Medicaid in many states) was a significant step. It is likely that benefits provided by third-party payors will be expanded. This is not only cost effective, it is also both clinically appropriate and in the patient's best interests.

Managed Care

Background

History The first "managed care" programs can be traced to health maintenance organizations (HMOs), which earlier had been called prepaid group practice plans. The term *health maintenance organization* was coined in the early 1970s during the Nixon administration. HMOs resulted from efforts to provide an alternative delivery system based on a unique philosophy about health services. The HMO philosophy stresses a close relationship among patients and their physicians and a financial arrangement and preventive measures (compared with the acute treatment emphasized by traditional third-party coverage), and provides incentives to both insureds and providers to minimize expensive inpatient (hospital) treatment. Prepaid group practice plans and early HMOs usually had salaried physicians. Enrollees paid a fixed premium that covered all services provided.

A unique aspect of early HMOs was that they were not conventional HSOs. An HMO grouped hospitals, physicians, and other health personnel into an "organization"—more accurately, an arrangement—that provided a full range of medical services to an enrolled population for a fixed fee, paid in advance. Thus, it may have been only a set of contracts—a paper HSO—or a true organization. It was clearly a forerunner of the preferred provider organization. According to Zelten, "the feature which most clearly differentiates HMOs from existing health delivery and financing systems is the combination of delivery and financing within one organized system."[138] Two thirds of all plans are organized as for-profit corporations, but over half of all enrollees are in plans organized as not-for-profit corporations.[139]

Definitions and Models By 1990, managed care was a $26 billion business.[140] HSOs (including HMOs) that provide "managed care" are commonly called "managed care plans." Managed care organizations:[141]

> Offer one or more products that integrate financing and management with delivery of health services to an enrolled population
>
> Are responsible for delivering services (using their HSOs or through contractual arrangements) and (as a network or as individual providers) either share financial risk and/or have some incentive to deliver efficient services
>
> Use an information system capable of monitoring and evaluating patterns of utilization and financial outlays

This broad definition can include managed care Blue Cross/Blue Shield plans and managed indemnity insurance plans, as well as HMOs.

The organizations and arrangements that meet this definition run a wide gamut:[142]

> *Staff-model HMOs*—employ physicians and pay them a salary. Physicians work only for that HMO and generally care only for that HMO's patients.
>
> *Group-model HMOs*—contract with one or more multispecialty medical group practices to provide services. The HMO pays the group a monthly amount, and the group pays physicians, who may treat fee-for-service patients as well as HMO patients.
>
> *Open-ended HMOs*—remove lock-in, which requires that enrollees receive services only from the HMO's providers. Enrollees may receive services without referral outside the HMO network. Nonplan coverage is like traditional indemnity insurance; the coverage includes deductibles, copayments, and/or co-insurance.[143]
>
> *Independent practice association (IPA)-model HMOs*—differ from the staff- and group-model HMOs mainly in how physicians are paid and organized. IPA-model physicians are independent and practice singly or in groups. IPA physicians may treat nonplan patients, who may be a majority of their practice. The IPA determines how physicians are paid; financial incentives are used to control utilization.
>
> *Open-panel IPA-model HMOs*—a variation of the IPA model. Physicians are even less formally organized than in the usual IPA model. The HMO contracts directly with individual physicians or small groups of physicians who are paid a fee for service; financial incentives are used to control utilization.
>
> *Preferred provider organizations (PPOs)*—patients are directed to selected physicians or providers who discount their fees to plan members. Patients who go out of the PPO network pay deductibles and copayments. (Shouldice argues that PPOs should be called preferred provider arrangements because they are brokered arrangements between providers and purchasers of health services, the terms and conditions of which are specified by contract.[144])
>
> *Exclusive provider organizations (EPOs)*—similar to PPOs but restrict enrollees to the list of preferred providers. EPOs may operate similarly to HMOs, but typically have more flexibility in benefit design and pricing structure.[145]
>
> *Multiple option plans*—often called dual- or triple-option plans. Two or more plans, such as an HMO, a PPO, and/or an indemnity insurance plan, are combined into one plan and offered by a single carrier. Enrollees are permitted numerous choices.

HMOs and PPOs are most clearly different in how they reimburse providers.[146] PPOs are likely to pay physicians a fee for service, perhaps with a discounted fee schedule based on a relative value scale. Hospitals may be paid on a discounted basis, a per diem, or using diagnosis-related groups.[147] Group- and staff-model HMOs often use salary and/or capitation payments; IPA-model HMOs may use combinations of individual and group capitation and/or modified fee-for-service arrangements. PPOs are moving toward more risk sharing with hospitals.[148] It should be noted that an HMO may be a PPO and offer a PPO product through its provider network as the delivery system for both types of managed care.[149] HMOs may also offer indemnity plans. Competition continues to blur the distinctions between managed care plans and traditional indemnity insurers. Figure 7.7 shows how various characteristics compare in different types of indemnity and managed care plans.

The evolution of managed care began in the late 1980s, and HMOs and PPOs have already established their importance among providers, payors, and employers eager to control health care costs.[150]

HMOs   The genesis of HMOs was in prepaid group practice plans in the late 1920s and the early 1930s. Their numbers increased slowly for several reasons: indemnity and service insurance coverage is widespread, people are reluctant to give up their choice of physician, organized medicine opposed HMOs, and physicians have traditionally preferred fee-for-service payment. Opposition by organized medicine resulted in the landmark antitrust case described in Chapter 4.

In 1972, there were only 72 HMO plans with 4.5 million enrollees. The federal government

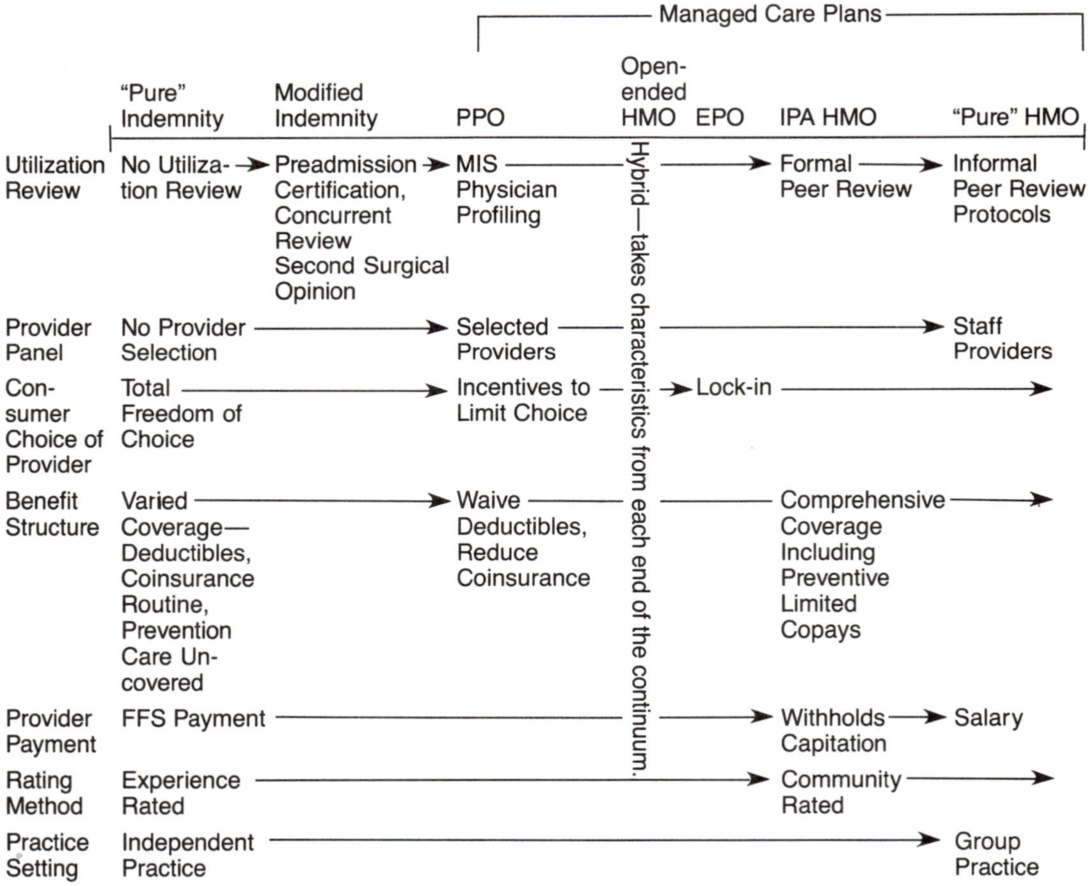

Figure 7.7. Managed care continuum. (EPO, exclusive provider organization; MIS, management information systems; FFS, fee for service.) (From Hale, Judith A., and Mary M. Hunter. *From HMO movement to managed care industry: The future of HMOs in a volatile healthcare market,* 13. Minneapolis: Interstudy Center for Managed Care Research, 1988; reprinted by permission.)

recognized the potential of HMOs in 1973 and enacted legislation to assist plans in starting. By 1982, 265 plans had almost 11 million enrollees. In 1990, there were 35 million members in 615 HMO plans, a decline of 41 plans from 1988.[151] The average enrollment of 50,000 per HMO is a level that analysts consider profitable; approximately 75 plans have 100,000 or more members.[152] Nationwide HMO penetration in 1990 was 14.4%, an increase from 1989.[153] Prepaid group practices (both staff- and group-model HMOs) include a quarter of all plans, but 42% of enrollment.[154]

IPAs The first of what are known as IPAs was begun in 1954 when the San Joaquin Foundation for Medical Care was established by fee-for-service physicians who were competing with the Kaiser-Permanente prepaid group practice plan. In 1991, IPAs comprised 61% of all plans, with 43% of all HMO enrollees.[155] IPAs, a distinct type of managed care organization, are usually developed to deliver services in conjunction with HMOs or PPOs. An IPA-model HMO is a common example. Some IPAs were established as a way for physicians to offer their services as a PPO to purchasers such as insurers or employers. This type predominantly includes solo practitioners, but multispecialty group practices may participate.[156] Utilization patterns are reviewed when physicians apply to the IPA to determine whether those physicians are efficient users of resources. Such review continues throughout the relationship.

PPOs PPOs are a development of the 1980s. Even more than an HMO, a preferred provider is a concept, not a specific type of HSO. A PPO may be an insurance company, an HMO, a hospital, a medical group practice, an ASC, or an IPA. Regardless, it is an organization that is usually an HSO and that contracts with employers or enrollees. In turn, it may provide services or contract with independent physicians (and other HSOs, such as hospitals) to provide services. The PPO concept is broad enough that an employer that offers its employees medical services from specific providers with which it has contracts would meet the definition.

As a group, PPOs are growing faster than HMOs (which may also be PPOs) because they are seen as a lower cost alternative.[157] By the end of 1988 there were 691 PPOs with an estimated 18.3 million members. With 50 plans and 4.4 million members, Blue Cross and Blue Shield Associations sponsored the most PPOs.[158] In 1991 it was estimated that there were more than 800 PPOs with 60–65 million eligible members.[159]

Organizational Structures Managed care organizations are so varied in how they may be organized that a comprehensive discussion is not possible here. What follows is information generally applicable to managed care organizations, including specific examples.

Governance Managed care organizations are corporations that can be organized for profit or not for profit. Both have boards of directors to set policy and evaluate overall performance. Figures 7.8 and 7.9 are examples of organization charts for a staff-model HMO and a PPO, respectively.[160]

Management Managers include a CEO, whose title is likely to be executive director, administrator, or president. It is common in managed care organizations that CEOs are physicians who may be trained in management. Managed care organizations are likely to have flat organizational structures with few levels of managers.

Other managers include those at the intermediate level, as required. Among the most important of these is the medical director, who will be employed either part or full time. As in other HSOs with medical directors, this position in managed care has clinical and administrative responsibilities. Monitoring efficient use of medical and hospital services (utilization review) is a primary activity. Other activities include quality assurance, recruiting clinicians, credentialing, disciplinary action, and developing and implementing policies and procedures related to medical services. The medical director also has a role in negotiating and managing provider contracts and in enrollee relations.[161]

PSO Managed care organizations have a wide variety of approaches to organizing profes-

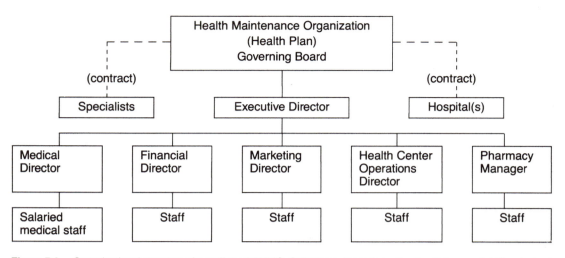

Figure 7.8. Organizational structure of a staff-model HMO. Solid lines, direct lines of authority/accountability; dashed lines, contractual relationships between the HMO and another party. (From Shouldice, Robert G. *Introduction to managed care,* 98. Arlington, VA: Information Resources Press, 1991; reprinted by permission.)

sional staff. They are unlikely to use the PSO model found in hospitals. The most tightly controlled is the staff-model HMO, where physicians and other LIPs are employed and are screened and credentialed similarly to hospitals. The least controlled are managed care organizations with characteristics of an IPA. In the past, HMOs often did not perform their own credentialing of physicians, but relied on the credentialing done by their affiliated hospitals. The disadvantages of this approach are such that the HMO now must do its own credentialing.[162] Furthermore, potential malpractice liability caused this policy to be reconsidered.[163]

Relationships with physicians are established through contracts, which may be employment contracts or service contracts, depending on the type of managed care organization. (Such contractual relationships should be contrasted with hospitals, where physicians are unlikely to be

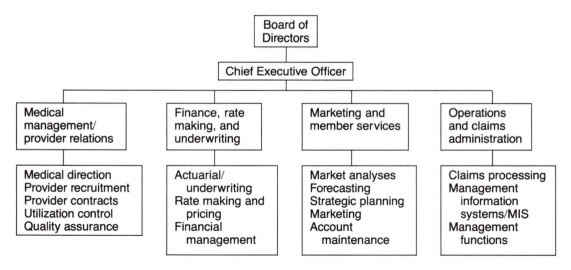

Figure 7.9. Typical PPO organizational chart. (From Shouldice, Robert G. *Introduction to managed care,* 69. Arlington, VA: Information Resources Press, 1991; reprinted by permission.)

employees, and use a hospital only to treat patients and have no financial relationship with it.) The least complex contract is found in a staff-model HMO, where the plan hires practitioner and support staff in all categories and is their employer.[164] Nonphysician LIPs who are employees are likely to have employment contracts that specify duties and compensation. Support staff are unlikely to have contracts.

Caregiver and Support Staff   Figures 7.8 and 7.9 suggest the variety of personnel and skills that may be found in managed care organizations. The staff-model HMO employs the widest range of staff, from RNs and other staff who support the work of physicians and other LIPs to marketers and contract specialists. The ratio of prepaid group practice staff to physicians is from four to five direct paramedical personnel per physician, with the average usually on the lower side.[165] Table 7.7 shows data on nonphysician full-time equivalent staff per full-time equivalent physician.

Some PPOs achieve delivery of clinical services to enrollees through contracts with providers and employ no clinicians. The staff of such PPOs is concerned with finances, marketing, underwriting, and recruiting new enrollees. Utilization review is central to maintaining financial viability and is likely to be found in all managed care organizations. Few managed care organizations, however, have staff and programs with the same characteristics.

Licensure and Accreditation   There is no specific licensure for managed care organizations, except to the extent that they must be licensed to perform an activity, such as delivering medical services as a specific type of HSO, or as the states regulate the writing of insurance. The Joint Commission accredits managed care organizations as part of its ambulatory care accreditation program.

Future   Despite their early presence in American health services and the boost given by federal legislation, the number of HMOs has grown slowly. Contributing factors include consumer reluctance to give up choice of physicians and physician reluctance to relinquish autonomy and fee-for-service payment. Major efforts by employers (and to a lesser extent beneficiaries) to control costs will likely eliminate this reluctance in the 1990s, however. It is estimated that, by the year 2000, nearly 90% of health care services will be provided through managed care.[166]

Successful managed care organizations will have excellent management, will be diversified, and may or may not be legally constituted as HMOs. Many will be product lines of larger health management companies. It is suggested that there is an emerging fourth generation of managed care, and that no single definition exists for this concept. In it, providers (hospitals and physicians) will control the organization and there will be peer review and utilization review, quality control with computerized monitoring of patient care data, cost control measurement, high standards of practice by physicians and paramedical personnel, and efficient administration in the operation of the medical facility as a business.[167] Figure 7.10 suggests the content of this new model. "Total managed care organizations" will emerge to manage employers' total health care dollars.[168]

The plans of the 1980s such as HMOs and PPOs will lose their usefulness.[169] Winners in the 1990s and beyond will be those health care plans—whatever their structure or acronym—that can document delivery of high-quality care in an efficient manner.[170]

Birth Centers

Background

History   As late as 1900, less than 5% of births occurred in hospitals.[171] It was not until 1940 that half of births occurred in hospitals, and by 1960 almost all births occurred in hospitals.[172] About 1940, the movement toward "natural childbirth" began.[173] This was the beginning of a small but determined effort to take normal childbirth out of the high-technology setting.

> By the 1970s the thrust for natural childbirth, which had been a loosely organized cultural movement among middle-class women, aimed at enhancing their experience in birth, acquired a social and polit-

Table 7.7. Number of full-time equivalent (FTE) employees per FTE physician by managed care revenue percentage of total net revenue for multispecialty groups[a]

Employee category	No managed care		Managed care revenue percentage of total net revenue					
			10% or less		11%–50%		51%–100%	
	Count	Median	Count	Median	Count	Median	Count	Median
Total FTE employees per FTE physician	80	4.09	113	4.03	132	4.34	32	4.99
Administrative staff	76	.17	108	.16	122	.19	29	.16
Business office	74	.65	111	.62	122	.67	29	.67
Information services	43	.15	65	.16	78	.16	23	.15
Housekeeping/maintenance/security	53	.16	78	.11	86	.16	22	.12
Other administrative support staff	26	.11	54	.14	70	.12	23	.18
Registered nurses	63	.35	99	.47	108	.49	26	.34
LPNs, medical assistants, etc.	73	.82	100	.62	113	.76	27	1.05
Medical receptionists	70	.45	108	.53	118	.67	27	.74
Medical secretaries/transcribers	73	.27	103	.27	112	.21	24	.20
Medical records	62	.29	101	.31	104	.32	27	.40
Nonphysician providers	40	.14	61	.09	66	.13	23	.17
Laboratory	66	.31	88	.33	99	.33	25	.36
Radiology/imaging	58	.18	87	.18	100	.20	26	.25
Physical therapy	15	.17	19	.08	34	.13	13	.12
Optical	13	.08	27	.05	28	.05	14	.09
Certified registered nurse-anesthetists	0	*	0	*	14	.09	0	*
Other medical/ancillary service staff	30	.31	54	.14	68	.15	21	.15

From Medical Group Management Association. *The Cost and Production Survey Report: 1990 Report Based on 1989 Data,* 28. Englewood, CO, 1990; reprinted by permission from The Medical Group Management Association, 104 Inverness Terrace East, Englewood CO, 80112; telephone (303) 397-7879.

[a]An asterisk in a median column indicates that data are suppressed when the count (number of responding groups) is less than 10. A zero in a count column indicates that the count is less than 10. Data for university- and government-affiliated groups are excluded from this table.

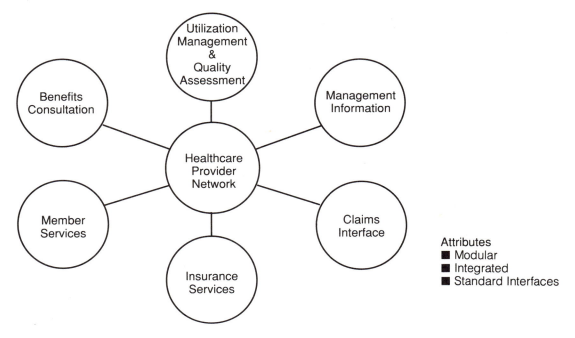

Figure 7.10. Fourth-generation managed health care organization. (From Berry, Howard R. Managed care's 4th generation. *Group Practice Journal* 38 [July/August 1989]: 48; reprinted with permission.)

ical cast; women of all classes began to organize, to educate one another, and to try to change or avoid the professional and institutional structures that exerted such dominance over birth.[174]

In 1975, the Maternity Center Association of New York City opened a birth center that offered obstetrical and nurse-midwife care during labor and delivery in a homelike setting. This created a furor among obstetricians, and their professional organization issued a strong statement opposing out-of-hospital delivery as unsafe for mother and child.[175] Despite this opposition, birth centers flourished.

Definition and Numbers   Birth centers provide prenatal, intrapartum, and postpartum care for normal pregnancies. They are not ambulatory surgery centers. Surgical procedures are limited to those needed during normal, uncomplicated births, such as episiotomy and repair, and do not include operative obstetrics and cesarean sections. Surgical procedures such as tubal ligation and abortion are performed in birth centers if the centers are licensed to do them. Routine laboratory tests are usually done on site, and food service should be available. Mothers and infants are expected to be discharged within 24 hours.[176]

The criteria for belonging to the professional association for birth centers, the National Association of Childbearing Centers, also suggest their nature. Membership is limited to centers that meet certain standards of care and safety, agree to nonintervention in the process of natural childbirth, use a personalized approach with families, eliminate unnecessary cost, and use qualified nurse-midwives and physicians.[177]

Despite the significant opposition described above, there were 150 birth centers nationwide by 1988; approximately 28% were physician owned and managed.[178] The goal is natural childbirth, but women using birth centers do not avoid all interventions. About 40% receive some analgesia or tranquilizing medication, 38% have artificial rupture of the amniotic membranes, and about 15% are transferred to a hospital.[179]

Of the approximately 39,000 births that occur outside hospitals annually (about 1% of all births), about 9,000 are attended by physicians; 10,000 by certified nurse-midwives (some at birth centers); 7,000 by lay midwives, both licensed and unlicensed; and 13,000 by others, including fathers and policemen.[180] Less than 0.5% of all deliveries occur in birth centers.[181]

Throughout the United States, deliveries in birth centers are lower cost than in a hospital. In 1989, the average cost for a 1-day birth center stay was $2,111, versus a 1-day hospital stay cost of $3,233.[182]

Organizational Structure

Governance   Birth centers may be organized as for-profit or not-for-profit corporations. The significant involvement of physicians as owners suggests that many will be for profit. The composition and number on the GB will vary by type of ownership, as suggested above.

Management   Birth centers are small and have a flat organizational structure. The CEO is almost certain to be a clinician, whether a certified nurse-midwife or a physician. Supervisory personnel will depend on the number of staff and range of services.

PSO   Clinical staff may include obstetricians, whose presence may be required by state law but who will be on call as backup, regardless. Certified nurse-midwives are the primary caregivers. They are registered nurses with advanced training in midwifery, are certified by the American College of Nurse-Midwives, and are licensed as midwives in many states. In 1991 there were more than 4,000 certified nurse-midwives in the United States,[183] a large increase from the approximately 1,500 in 1988.[184] Some states license midwives, who are trained laypersons but not RNs.[185] Licensed midwives are unlikely to be on a birth center staff.

The PSO should have bylaws that include requirements for membership, delineation of privileges, and organization. Consulting obstetricians should have hospital privileges.

Caregiver and Support Staff   Compared with other types of HSOs, staffing in a freestanding birth center is of limited scope and complexity. Nurse aides (who may be certified) assist the certified nurse-midwives. Support staff include clerical personnel, laboratory technologists, and housekeepers. Backup services are provided by a hospital emergency department, but are needed infrequently since only low-risk pregnancies are treated in freestanding birth centers. Volunteers are common in birth centers and are important to the centers' mission and philosophy.

Licensure and Accreditation   Most states regulate birth centers through licensure.[186] Birth centers are accredited by the Commission for the Accreditation of Freestanding Birth Centers, which was established in 1985 by the National Association of Childbearing Centers.[187]

Future   Although birth centers have developed a presence in many areas of the United States, they have apparently achieved limited acceptance. This is regrettable because the National Birth Center Study concluded that:

> Few innovations in health service promise lower cost, greater availability, and a high degree of satisfaction with a comparable degree of safety. The results of this study suggest that modern birth centers can identify women who are at low risk for obstetrical complications and can care for them in a way that provides these benefits.[188]

Birth centers have an uncertain future. Despite modern origins, they remain few in number and provide services to a limited group of pregnant women. Birth centers will not disappear as a source of care for uncomplicated deliveries, but they are likely to provide care to fewer patients than their potential suggests.

Home Health Agencies

Background

History   A program similar to a contemporary visiting nurse association (VNA) provided home health services in Philadelphia as early as 1842.[189] The first sustained effort for home health care in the United States, however, dates from 1893, when Lillian Wald established the Visiting Nurse Service of New York City, as part of the Henry Street Settlement services to the city's poor.

By 1909, she had persuaded the Metropolitan Life Insurance Company to begin a home nursing service for its policyholders in New York City. The pilot project was so successful that it was adopted in many communities by other insurance companies in the 1920s.[190] Home health care services in rural communities were pioneered as a visiting nurse service through the Red Cross.[191]

The first European program to provide services in the home was organized in Frankfurt, Germany, in 1892. A similar program for "home helps" followed in London in 1897.[192] Home help paraprofessional groups did not appear in U.S. health care until the middle of the 20th century. Homemakers were the first; they were often financed by welfare funds for the poor and were available through some VNAs. Home health aides as a group were first included in the Kerr-Mills Medical Assistance for the Aged act in 1960. They were defined as health caregivers (similar to hospital aides) and were separate from homemakers.[193]

In 1947, the first hospital-based home care program was established at Montefiore Hospital in the Bronx, New York, to serve patients just discharged from hospitals. It expanded traditional home nursing and used an interdisciplinary team that coordinated physicians, therapists, aides, and social workers.[194]

Before Medicare (1965), most home care was delivered by voluntary (not-for-profit) VNAs. Few were organized for profit. Except in rural areas, few public agencies provided home care. Nursing was the main service offered; homemakers and home health aides were sometimes available.[195] Medicare covered home care under both Parts A and B, and it sought to substitute home care for extended and costlier hospitalization. The mainstay of pre-Medicare home care agencies, the VNAs, decreased after 1965 because of the expense and risk to small entities of building the care components needed for Medicare eligibility.[196]

Definition and Numbers Home health agencies (HHAs) are defined as public or private organizations primarily engaged in providing skilled nursing services by RNs and LPNs; physical therapy (PT), occupational therapy (OT), and speech therapy; and home health aides. Home health services are defined by Medicare as skilled, intermittent, part-time services ordered by a physician and provided in the residence of the homebound client. The hospital insurance (Part A of Medicare) and the supplementary medical insurance (Part B of Medicare) programs cover home health services without a deductible or co-insurance charge. If the beneficiary needs the care, there is no limit on the number of home health visits covered and there is no prior hospitalization requirement. Reimbursement to home health agencies is based on Medicare rules for reasonable cost reimbursement.[197]

Medicare changed home health care dramatically. It is now a medical adjunct to acute care, and despite their lack of skill and interest in this care, it is physicians who nominally direct the system. This has added greatly to the cost of care.[198] Since the introduction of the prospective pricing system (diagnosis-related groups) for hospital reimbursement under Medicare in 1983, the home care program has been the fastest growing segment of the Medicare program and the top growth area for hospital diversification.[199]

At the end of 1990, there were 9,270 HHAs in the United States, an increase of 14% since mid-1989.[200] In 1989, 5,546 HHAs participated in Medicare, a decline from 1988 (5,769) and 1987 (5,887).[201] In 1988, approximately 40% of HHAs were not-for-profit organizations, 34% for profit, and 26% government owned.[202] More than 2,000 acute care hospitals offer home care services, and there are an estimated 8,000 durable medical equipment (DME) providers.[203] Medicare (Parts A and B) home health benefit payments were $2.6 billion in 1989 and are projected to reach $4.4 billion by 1995.[204] Total expenditures for home health from all sources were $8.4 billion in 1990.[205] In 1990, 60 million home health visits were reimbursed by Medicare.[206]

It was estimated that the total revenue for all home health care would exceed $10 billion by 1991.[207] In 1990, 21% of HHAs had revenues of more than $1 million.[208] Medicare reimbursements accounted for 59.8% of HHA revenue in 1990, and Medicaid reimbursements for 11.2%.[209]

Despite these very significant expenditures, a 1987 study found that a total of 4.6 million elderly people with functional difficulties received no formal services, compared with a total of 2.3 million who received at least one service.[210] Contemporary home care no longer refers only to provision of skilled nursing services. It means a wide array of products and services that can be offered in the home.

Functions

Skilled Care   Skilled nursing is the only service required in a Medicare-qualified home care program. In addition, at least one other therapeutic service (PT, OT, speech therapy, medical social services, or home health aide services) must be offered.[211] Nonskilled home care providers include homemakers, home health aides, chore workers, and personal care aides; this group accounts for the majority of money spent on home care services. Other services may include supplies and equipment.[212] Most providers use Medicare eligibility guidelines because a large percentage of their clients are Medicare-reimbursable beneficiaries.[213] Medicare requirements continue to be made more stringent. For example, as of January 1, 1990, HHAs may not employ as home health aides persons who are not licensed to furnish a covered service unless they have successfully completed a state-approved training and/or a competency evaluation program for that service.[214] This will increase costs.

The care given by skilled caregivers is usually categorized as intermittent, compared with the nonskilled, continuous service provided by homemakers. Skilled services are available as needed. Home health aides spend approximately two hours per visit, two to three times a week. The average duration of a case is 60 days and includes 16–18 visits.[215] Demand is strongest for home health aides, followed by RNs, LPNs, and PTs. The average HHA made 266 visits per week in 1990, an increase of 7.7% from 1988.[216]

The client in the skilled segment is referred directly by or with the concurrence of the attending physician. This referral is often through hospital discharge planning. The nurse or social worker may identify a need for skilled services and assist the physician with the referral. Approximately two thirds of those clients referred to skilled care come directly from hospitals. This causes freestanding providers to be concerned that hospitals will dominate the market.[217]

Private or Demand Services   Home care clients may also engage services that are private-duty or demand services. The private-duty HHA may offer a full range of services: RNs, LPNs, PTs, OTs, homemakers, companions, household assistants, and household aides. In practice, major activities are to provide home health aides, homemaker services, and companions.[218] The client usually requires assistance because of disability, illness, or the infirmities of age and generally does not meet the criteria that clients of a Medicare-certified provider must meet. Care may be desired rather than required.[219] However, many persons require assistance in the activities of daily living, and such services are unlikely to be covered either by public or private payment; it is estimated these needs are significant.[220] This type of client is referred from a variety of sources.

DME   Another use of home care services involves durable medical equipment (DME). Typical products include ambulatory and comfort aids such as wheelchairs, canes, commodes, and hospital beds; home oxygen therapy, including respirators, ventilators, and other inhalation therapy equipment; prosthetic devices; nutritional support equipment, including pumps, solutions, and tubing; ostomy supplies and devices; medical supplies; and health-related items such as bandages, pads, and personal assistance and convenience items that help debilitated persons function more independently.[221] Third-party financing of DME generally requires a physician's order, and the recipient is subject to qualification guidelines. The Medicare program often imposes specific criteria for services, especially those that have been abused.[222]

Organizational Structure   The HHA may be organized in several ways. It may be an independent organization, incorporated either for profit or not for profit. It may be in a dependent relationship with an acute care hospital (or other provider), either as a department or freestanding. Each has advantages and disadvantages.

The organizational structure is likely to be flat, with a CEO, perhaps an associate, and department heads for various specialized activities such as skilled care (provided by RNs, LPNs, speech therapists, OTs, and PTs) and unskilled services such as those provided by home health aides. The management team will also include specialized personnel such as a financial officer, billing staff, and data processers. There is increasing attention to marketing the HHA's services, so there likely will be a marketing staff. Foci of this effort include insurers, employers, and private physicians, who are an important source of referrals, especially for non–hospital-affiliated home care agencies. Figure 7.11 is an example of the organization of an HHA.

Governance   Not-for-profit HHAs that are not hospital affiliated will have a separate GB. An HHA organized for profit may or may not have a GB. If an HHA is a sole proprietorship or a partnership, the owner(s) make(s) policy decisions.

Hospital-affiliated HHAs may be freestanding, in which case they have a separate GB. If integrated as a hospital department, the HHA will not have a separate GB but will report through the hospital hierarchy to the hospital GB. Vertically integrated health services systems or diversified HSOs may have a variety of relationships with the HHA, including overlapping GB membership.

Management   As is typical in small HSOs, small HHAs have few managers beyond the CEO, who often has the title "administrator."[223] In small HHAs the CEO is usually responsible for operations and is also the clinical leader.[224] Larger HHAs have an administrator educated in management, who may have a clinical background. Large HHAs have characteristics and scalar relationships similar to those of large HSOs, and specialized functions are provided by staff; clinical coordinators, a financial officer, and marketing specialists are common. Attention to reimbursement is important because home care has distinct reimbursement and regulatory constraints.

Home care is very different from the services that most HSOs deliver. It is unique because practitioners work without direct supervision to provide services at many individual sites. This necessitates specialized mechanisms for organizing staff and ensuring quality of care.

PSO   HHAs have no PSO as such, but skilled care is ordered by and is under the direction of the attending physician. Orders for all services must be in writing and must be renewed every 62 days.[225] This regulation reflects the requirements of Medicare and is often applied to all clients of certified HHAs. Academic medical education programs specific to home care are rare, and few faculty are experienced in teaching or research in home care. The result is that physicians tend to be unaware of the significant advances in home care, and this is undoubtedly a limiting factor in its effective use.[226] Some family practice residencies include home care experiences.

Medicare-certified HHAs must have a group of professional personnel—at least one practicing physician, one RN, and appropriate representation from other professional disciplines—to establish and review annually the HHA's policies governing scope of services offered, admission and discharge policies, medical supervision and plan of care, emergency care, clinical records, personnel qualifications, and program evaluation. At least one member of the group must be neither an owner nor an employee of the HHA.[227]

Caregiver and Support Staff   The types of services provided suggest the staff. Medicare requires only skilled nursing, which includes RNs and LPNs. In addition, OTs, PTs, speech therapists, and social service workers are typically found in a HHA. A variety of home care providers, including homemakers, home health aides, chore workers, and personal care aides, is required to offer a full range of services. These staff have little formal education and may not be high school graduates. Their activities are largely unskilled in a clinical sense, but they are a very important source of interaction with clients. They receive job-specific training.

Licensure and Accreditation   Most states license HHAs, in which case they must meet legal and regulatory requirements. Two organizations accredit HHAs, the Joint Commission and the National League for Nursing's subsidiary, the Community Health Accreditation Program

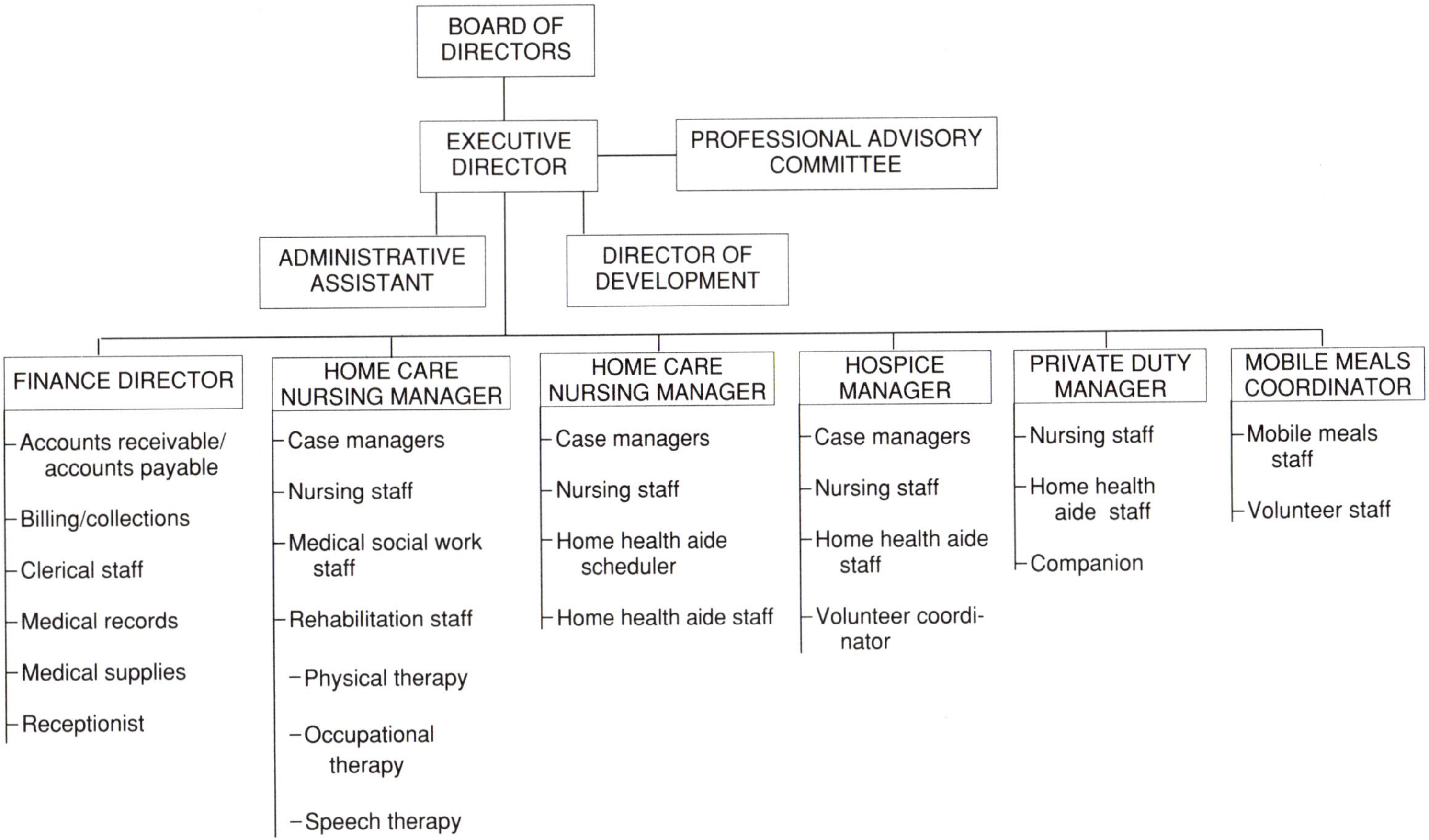

Figure 7.11. Home health agency organization chart.

```
BOARD OF
DIRECTORS
    |
PROFESSIONAL ADVISORY
COMMITTEE
    |
EXECUTIVE
DIRECTOR
    |
    ├── DIRECTOR OF DEVELOPMENT
    ├── ADMINISTRATIVE ASSISTANT
    |
    ├── FINANCE DIRECTOR
    │       ├─ Accounts receivable/accounts payable
    │       ├─ Billing/collections
    │       ├─ Clerical staff
    │       ├─ Medical records
    │       ├─ Medical supplies
    │       └─ Receptionist
    |
    ├── HOME CARE NURSING MANAGER
    │       ├─ Case managers
    │       ├─ Nursing staff
    │       ├─ Medical social work staff
    │       ├─ Rehabilitation staff
    │       ├─ Physical therapy
    │       ├─ Occupational therapy
    │       └─ Speech therapy
    |
    ├── HOME CARE NURSING MANAGER
    │       ├─ Case managers
    │       ├─ Nursing staff
    │       ├─ Home health aide scheduler
    │       └─ Home health aide staff
    |
    ├── HOSPICE MANAGER
    │       ├─ Case managers
    │       ├─ Nursing staff
    │       ├─ Home health aide staff
    │       └─ Volunteer coordinator
    |
    ├── PRIVATE DUTY MANAGER
    │       ├─ Nursing staff
    │       ├─ Home health aide staff
    │       └─ Companion
    |
    └── MOBILE MEALS COORDINATOR
            ├─ Mobile meals staff
            └─ Volunteer staff
```

292

(CHAP). CHAP's organization and activities were discussed in the section on hospices. The National Homecaring Council does not accredit HHAs, but its standards assist HHAs to improve quality.

As previously indicated, only certified HHAs are eligible to receive Medicare reimbursement. The certification process is conducted on behalf of Medicare by state health departments.

Future   Although home care expenditures were only 3.8% of total Medicare expenditures in 1987, home care is a rapidly growing segment of Medicare.[228] Physicians tend to prescribe therapies they know and use in their work. Therefore, home care, which was historically low technology and low cost, under Medicare has become a service filled with high-cost care. It is not unusual for a physician to order a battery of expensive blood tests rather than make a home visit.[229]

Opportunities for diagnostic and therapeutic activities in home care seem almost limitless. Intravenous drug therapy and total parenteral nutrition are common, as are wound management (pressure sores, surgical wounds with healing complications, and ulcers) and gastrointestinal drainage systems management. Electrocardiography, blood and urine collection, oximetry, glucometry, and portable kits for drug levels are available. Even portable radiology and ultrasound services are in use.[230]

The future for HHAs is bright, and significant growth is expected. It is estimated that about 70% of acute care hospitals participate in some form of home care. Coupled with aggressive discharge planning, the availability of an HHA, whether hospital owned or not, allows acute care hospitals to reduce lengths of stay and maximize their income from diagnosis-related groups. Eleven percent of hospitals report that their medical staffs have home care programs that compete with them.[231]

It is estimated that in 1988 Americans spent $8.6 billion on home care and that by 2018 expenditures will increase to $21.9 billion, and that the number of elderly persons using home care will increase by 60% during this period from 4 to 6.4 million.[232] One example of the staffing implications of this growth is suggested by U.S. Department of Labor estimates that show that by the year 2000 the number of home health aides will increase between 137,000 and 173,000, or an increase of 58%–73% from the 236,000 employed in 1988.[233] Opportunities for managers will increase proportionately.

SUMMARY

This chapter begins by providing a basic, generic background about how HSOs are established and organized. The components of governance, management, and clinical staff are detailed. The roles and relationships among these three elements of the triad are described and analyzed, as are the difficulties this unique organizational structure presents for managing the many types of HSOs that have it. Other special problems addressed include credentialing PSO members and dealing with impaired practitioners.

The chapter continues by describing several types of HSOs in detail, including background; definitions and numbers; organizational structure, including governance, management, PSO, and caregiver and support staff; licensure and accreditation; and their future. Space is insufficient to identify and describe the myriad of current HSOs or to suggest the potential new HSOs and organizational patterns that may be developed to meet future demands of health services delivery. Those presented run the gamut of the types of organizations that provide health services. They are paradigmatic and assist in understanding management and the organizational principles that apply.

DISCUSSION QUESTIONS

1. Identify the typical legal status of various types of HSOs. Why are most organized as corporations?

2. Describe the generic roles and activities of the GB, management, and PSO. Relate these roles and activities to HSO ownership.
3. Describe the triad. Identify the types of problems the triad causes using management terms and concepts. Suggest means to eliminate or minimize the problems.
4. Refer to the discussion of conflicts of interest found here and in Chapters 3 and 4. How do conflicts of interest arise in the roles and relationships of persons in the triad?
5. Most types of HSOs have physicians and other LIPs whose credentials are reviewed before their membership on the PSO is approved and clinical privileges are delineated. Describe the credentialing process. How does it differ for an acute care hospital, NF, and an IPA-model HMO? Why?
6. What are the functions of a general acute care hospital? It has been defined as a health team. What other definitions are appropriate?
7. How does the typical general acute care hospital differ organizationally from the usual bureaucratic form? Why? Are these differences necessary?
8. How does the organizational structure of a NF differ from that of a general acute care hospital? Relate these differences to the ease or difficulty of managing each.
9. How can relationships between members of the typical PSO (or physicians and other LIPs, if there is no PSO) and management be improved to enhance organizational effectiveness? Why is this important?
10. Federal reimbursement for medical services provided in several types of HSOs was referenced in this chapter. Identify why federal reimbursement is important *and* the implications it has for managing these HSOs, generally.

CASE STUDY 1: THE CLINICAL STAFF

You are the CEO of Bradley Hospital, a 400-bed voluntary, general acute care hospital. The recently elected president of the PSO has just told you that many members, but especially the physicians, are unhappy because they believe you are trying to control their activities. She stated, "We feel that hospital management should take care of the nonmedical areas and leave the practice of medicine where it belongs—in the hands of professionals."

Questions

1. How would you respond to the president of the PSO?
2. What arguments should you use to support your position?
3. Sketch an outline showing the appropriate relationship between GB, management, and PSO.

CASE STUDY 2: THE EMERGENCY DEPARTMENT

You are the CEO of Holbrook Hospital, which has an active emergency department (ED) with more than 60,000 visits annually. Historically, the department has been organized like that of most hospital EDs. Nursing staff report to nursing service; registration clerks, cashiers, and other clerks report to the admissions department; security officers report to the security department; house staff physicians who provide medical services report to various chiefs of departments such as internal medicine and surgery; and the crisis intervention social workers report to the department of social work.

You have just employed a full-time salaried physician as ED director. He has informed you that changes must be made if he is to do the job properly. The basic change is that all nursing service employees must report to him instead of nursing service. He has considerable experience in emergency medicine and has told you that this change will help employees feel a greater *esprit de corps* since they would all be in one department rather than dividing their loyalties between the

ED and their "home" department. The director believes this change will promote efficiency, boost morale, and make coordinating work in the ED easier.

The director of nursing service is not pleased with the proposal. She has told you that if the change is approved the ED director should not expect nursing service to provide staff even in an emergency. For example, if an ED nurse does not report because of illness the director will have to call in other ED nurses, rather than expect nursing service to move nurses from elsewhere in the hospital. At present, when ED needs more nurses, either because of absenteeism or sudden increased activity, nurses are pulled from various floors.

The director of nursing pointed out, too, that in the past nursing service, with help from the human resources department, has been responsible for recruiting and training ED nursing staff. If the change is made she thinks the ED director should be responsible for these activities, as well.

Currently, operating room (OR) nurses report to nursing service even though a salaried chief of surgery heads the department. The same is true in the intensive care unit (ICU), where nurses report to nursing service even though a salaried physician is head of ICU. These physicians are unconcerned that nursing employees report to nursing service because they retain responsibility for directing the nurses' professional activities.

Questions

1. Why does the ED director want nursing personnel to have a line relationship to him?
2. What advantages and disadvantages would this have when compared with the pattern in OR and the ICU?
3. Will this change accomplish the things the ED director claims (better *esprit de corps,* efficiency, morale, coordination)? Why? Why not?
4. What decision would you, as the CEO, make? Why?

CASE STUDY 3:   AUTHORITY RELATIONSHIPS

You were recently appointed CEO of Green Acres, a 300-bed NF, after your predecessor retired. You found many problems. Your predecessor refused to delegate authority, and all 17 department heads report to you. You have been unable to determine the quality of their performance, but you believe most will not meet your expectations. One reason for this belief is that the former CEO didn't delegate and department heads could not develop their managerial skills. As a result, they come to you for every decision and you are constantly bombarded with requests for permission to do the smallest things.

In contrast, the medical director functioned with such freedom that you are concerned the facility will not be able to pass the next Joint Commission survey. Patient records are poorly organized and often unavailable and there are no minutes of PSO committee meetings. Your philosophy is that members of the PSO should have considerable autonomy, but the GB is legally responsible for the facility, and management and the PSO must be a team if organizational objectives are to be met.

Questions

1. As a new CEO, what would you do? (Resigning is not an option!)
2. What priorities would you establish? Why?
3. What major problems do you face in making changes?
4. Would it be easier to solve these problems in a for-profit or in a not-for-profit organization? Why?

CASE STUDY 4:   THE ORTHOPEDIC SURGERY GROUP PRACTICE

Your executive assistant prepared the following data about the 15-member orthopedic surgery group practice where you were recently appointed administrator.

1. *Membership status* in the PSOs at the four community hospitals where members of the group admit patients for surgery:
    Active members: 6
    Associate members: 9
    TOTAL: 15
2. *Board certification:*
    Board certified: 8
    Eligible to take boards: 3
    Failed boards twice: 4
3. *Age distribution:*
    Average age: 59
    Range: 34–68
4. *Surgical procedures performed:*

| | Year | | | | |
Type	1989	1990	1991	1992	1993 (proj.)
Major	3,351	2,801	2,922	2,545	2,300
Minor	3,911	4,265	4,198	4,077	4,100
Total	7,262	7,066	7,120	6,622	6,400

Questions

1. Prepare an analysis of these data that will be given to the management committee of the group practice.
2. What recommendations will you make?
3. What additional data should you request?

CASE STUDY 5:   THE RIGHT THING TO DO*

Mr. Sterling, CEO of University Hospital, leaned back in his chair and contemplated the document in his hands with mild disbelief. The "Executive Summary of the Hospice Inpatient Unit Feasibility Study" was concise and emphatic. All committee members had individually summarized their reasons for recommending establishment of a discrete inpatient hospice unit at the hospital. The summary noted, too, that if the hospital and/or its physicians failed to provide, or foreclosed, the hospice option to terminally ill patients, such action might constitute a harm that could be unethical or illegal. Failing to inform terminally ill patients about the option of hospice, whether located in or out of the hospital, was unacceptable to the committee.

Professional perspectives included:

Hospital legal counsel—Foreclosing the hospice option may be a tort in negligence because it fails to meet the duty owed by physicians to inform patients of alternative forms of treatment. It could also be actionable as a breach of physicians' fiduciary duty to give patients information that is in their best interests to know.

Hospital physician-ethicist—Failing to disclose the hospice option could be judged as ma-

*Used with permission of the author, Carolyn H. Longest.

nipulating information, an external constraint on autonomous decision making. Failing to seek the greater balance of good over harm for the patient, as seen by the patient, is unethical.

Member, board of trustees—Institutional policies and mission statements affirm the patient's right to self-determination. University Hospital is in an academic medical center and well positioned for hospice care. Interorganizational relationships offer well-developed referral patterns; patient volume is sufficient to fill a hospice unit; and the trustees take pride in community perceptions that the hospital, and their role in it, is to provide innovative medical and nonmedical *care*.

Physician director, ICU—On reflection, recent increases in ethics consultations for ICU patients and their families were largely attributable to the many terminally ill patients inappropriately referred to ICU. Availability of an in-house hospice as a resource for patients, families, *and* physicians would reduce inappropriate referrals.

Mr. Sterling considered the recommendations. From his viewpoint there was financial risk in creating a discrete inpatient hospice unit, as well as in changing from income-generating, high-technology care to low-technology, palliative care with a possible reduction in some types of reimbursement. However, he also realized that even if the hospice lost money, benefits might outweigh losses: as part of the hospital, the hospice would provide charitable or altruistic services to the community, thereby justifying its valuable tax-exempt status.

Mr. Sterling realized he had an opportunity to do something that made sense medically, reduced legal risks, and met high ethical standards. He wondered, however, about the economic implications for the hospital and for some PSO members, especially those who treated many terminally ill patients. What was the right thing to do?

Questions

1. A large academic medical center might be able to invest in an inpatient hospice unit. Could a medium-size community hospital do so? What are the implications of enhanced fund-raising and/or public relations in this decision?

2. Even if a hospital lost money on an inpatient hospice unit, what noneconomic factors are important? Can an HSO overlook the ethical and legal implications of foreclosing this option to terminally ill patients?

3. Would your decision be different if ethical, legal, and medical factors supported establishing an inpatient hospice unit, but a number of physicians saw it as an economic threat to their practices?

NOTES

1. Geisel, Theodor Seuss (Dr. Seuss). *If I ran the zoo*, 1. New York: Random House, 1950.
2. Joint Commission on Accreditation of Healthcare Organizations. *Accreditation manual for hospitals, 1992*, 255. Oakbrook Terrace, IL: 1991.
3. Weber, Max. *The theory of social and economic organizations*, translated by A.M. Henderson and Talcott Parsons, 151–157. New York: The Free Press, 1947.
4. American Hospital Association. *Role and functions of the hospital governing board*, 1–4. Chicago, 1990.
5. Harvey, James D. Evaluating the performance of the chief executive officer. *Hospital & Health Services Administration* 23 (Spring 1978): 5–21.
6. Kovner, Anthony R. The hospital administrator and organizational effectiveness. In *Organization research on health institutions*, edited by Basil Georgopoulos,

373. Ann Arbor: Institute for Social Research of the University of Michigan, 1972.
7. Joint Commission, *Accreditation manual, 1992*, 43.
8. *Health Care Competition Week* 8 (May 20, 1991): 1.
9. Drucker, Peter F. The coming of the new organization. *Harvard Business Review* 66 (January–February 1988): 45–53.
10. More non-MDs eligible for med staffs. *Trustee* 43 (November, 1990): 26.
11. More non-MDs eligible, 26.
12. Ewell, Charles M. Economic credentialing: Balancing quality with financial reality. *Trustee* 44 (March 1991): 12.
13. Koska, Mary T. Hospital CEOs divided on use of economic credentialing. *Hospitals* 65 (March 20, 1991): 42.

14. An excellent treatment of the issues of physician domain and turf conflicts is found in Bloom, Stephanie Lin. Hospital turf battles: The manager's role. *Hospital & Health Services Administration* 36 (Winter 1991): 590–599.

15. Council on Mental Health of the American Medical Association. The sick physician: Impairment by psychiatric disorders, including alcoholism and drug dependence. *Journal of the American Medical Association* 223 (February 5, 1973): 684–687; Teich, Jeffrey. How to bring the impaired physician to treatment. *Hospital Medical Staff* 11 (September 1982): 8–14.

16. Jacyk, William. Impaired physicians: They are not the only ones at risk. *Canadian Medical Association Journal* 141 (July 15, 1989): 147; Talbott, G. Douglas, and Karl V. Gallegos. The pilot impaired physicians epidemiologic surveillance system. *QRB* 14 (April 1988): 133.

17. Fugedy, James. Should hospitals test doctors for drugs? *Washington Post,* Health Section (July 16, 1991): 14.

18. Guest, Robert H. The role of the doctor in institutional management. In *Organization research on health institutions,* edited by Basil Georgopoulos, 296. Ann Arbor: Institute for Social Research of the University of Michigan, 1972.

19. Stryker, Ruth. Characteristics of the residential care model. In *Creative long-term care administration,* edited by Kenneth George Gordon and Ruth Stryker, 2d ed., 13. Springfield, IL: Charles C Thomas, 1988.

20. *American Hospital Association Hospital Statistics, 1991–1992 Edition,* 2. Chicago: American Hospital Association, 1991.

21. Green, Jeffrey. 50 community hospitals closed, 43 opened in 1990. *AHA News* 27 (March 18, 1991): 1.

22. "Chain reaction" blamed for closure of 76 hospitals in 1989. *AHA News* 27 (February 18, 1991): 2.

23. AHA *Statistics,* 10–11.

24. AHA *Statistics,* 4–6.

25. AHA *Statistics,* 5.

26. AHA *Statistics,* 6.

27. Overnight recovery care facilities getting more attention from hospitals. *FASA Update* 7 (September/October 1990): 20.

28. Steinman, Joni M. Postsurgical recovery centers: A service option worth considering. *FASA Update* 8 (January/February 1991): 6–7.

29. Alexander, Jeffrey. *The changing character of hospital governance,* 8. Chicago: The Hospital Research and Educational Trust, 1990.

30. Alexander, *Changing character,* 8.

31. Alexander, *Changing character,* 8.

32. Alexander, *Changing character,* 7.

33. Alexander, *Changing character,* 4.

34. Alexander, *Changing character,* 25.

35. Alexander, *Changing character,* 15–16.

36. Alexander, *Changing character,* 13.

37. Alexander, *Changing character,* 13–14.

38. Coker, Jackson, and Steven Robbins. Providing competitive physician benefits within the law. *Trustee* (February 1990): 22; Cerne, Frank. Inpatient revenue per physician jumps 15%: Study. *AHA News* 26 (December 17, 1990): 1.

39. Georgopoulos and Mann, 1962. Cited in Shortell, Stephen M. Hospital medical staff organization: Structure, process, and outcome. *Hospital Administration* 19 (Spring 1974): 104.

40. Roemer and Friedman, 1971. Cited in Shortell, Stephen M. Hospital medical staff organization: Structure, process, and outcome. *Hospital Administration* 19 (Spring 1974): 104.

41. Neuhauser, Duncan. *The relationship between administration activities and hospital performance.* Research Series No. 28, Chicago: University of Chicago Center of Health Administration Studies, 1971; Shortell, Stephen M. Hospital medical staff organization: Structure, process, and outcome. *Hospital Administration* 19 (Spring 1974): 104.

42. Shortell, Stephen M., and Connie Evashwick. The structural configuration of U.S. hospital medical staffs. *Medical Care* 19 (April 1981): 419.

43. Shortell, Stephen M. The medical staff of the future: Replanting the garden. *Frontiers of Health Services Management* 1 (February 1985): 3–48; Shortell, Stephen M. Revisiting the garden: Medicine and management in the 1990s. *Frontiers of Health Services Management* 7 (Fall 1990): 3–32.

44. Alexander, *Changing character,* 17.

45. Alexander, *Changing character,* 19.

46. AHA *Statistics,* xlvi.

47. Joint Commission on Accreditation of Healthcare Organizations. *Facts about Joint Commission accreditation.* Oakbrook Terrace, IL. 1991.

48. Solovy, Alden. Cutting out the middlemen. *Hospitals* 62 (November 20, 1988): 52–57.

49. Where consumers go for outpatient care. *AHA News* 25 (December 4, 1989): 7.

50. Robertson, E. Marie. Hospitals, doctors losing ground to diagnostic centers for outpatient care. *Health Care Competition Week (Suppl.)* 8 (March 25, 1991): 1–2, 7–8.

51. Robertson, Hospitals, doctors losing.

52. Robertson, E. Marie. Hospitals still hold the lead in emergency and outpatient care. *Health Care Competition Week (Suppl.)* 6 (December 11, 1989): 7–10.

53. Stryker, Ruth. Historical obstacles to management of nursing homes. In *Creative long-term care administration,* edited by George Kenneth Gordon and Ruth Stryker, 2d ed., 5. Springfield, IL: Charles C Thomas, 1988.

54. Stryker, Historical obstacles, 6.

55. American Nursing Home Association. *Nursing home fact book, 1970–1971,* 3. Washington, D.C., n.d.

56. American Nursing Home Association, *Nursing home fact book,* 3.

57. American Nursing Home Association, *Nursing home fact book,* 4.

58. American Nursing Home Association, *Nursing home fact book,* 5.

59. Stryker, Historical obstacles, 7.

60. Stryker, Characteristics, 14.

61. Marion Merrell Dow, Inc. *Marion Merrell Dow managed care digest: Long term care edition* (pamphlet), 5. Kansas City, MO, 1991.

62. Marion Merrell Dow, Inc., *Managed care digest: Long term care* (1991), 7.

63. Division of Information Analysis, Office of Statistics and Data Management, Bureau of Data Management and Strategy, Health Care Financing Administration,

U.S. Department of Health and Human Services. *1990 HCFA statistics* (pamphlet), 19. Washington, D.C., 1990.

64. AHA *Statisics,* xliii.

65. Eubanks, Paula. Skilled-nursing services in hospitals v. freestanding facilities: There's a difference. *AHA News* 27 (May 27, 1991): 6.

66. Marion Merrell Dow, Inc., *Managed care digest: Long term care* (1991), 12.

67. Division of Information Analysis, *1990 HCFA statistics,* 19.

68. Marion Merrell Dow, Inc., *Managed care digest: Long term care* (1991), 14, 15.

69. Office of Research and Demonstrations, Health Care Financing Administration, U.S. Department of Health and Human Services. Unpublished data, 1991.

70. Cogen, Raymond. Medicare coverage in the skilled nursing facility. *Journal of Long-Term Care Administration* 17 (Fall 1989): 18–19.

71. Allen, James E. *Nursing home administration,* 74. New York: Springer Publishing Company, 1987.

72. Allen, *Nursing home,* 66–69.

73. Stryker, Ruth. Medical care and the role of the medical director. In *Creative long-term care administration,* edited by George Kenneth Gordon and Ruth Stryker, 2d ed., 178. Springfield, IL: Charles C Thomas, 1988.

74. Office of Information Analysis, *1990 HCFA Statistics,* 19.

75. Warzinski, Katherine V., and Ann Ward Tourigny. Nursing home administration licensure: A history. *Journal of Long-Term Care Administration* 15 (Spring 1987): 8–9.

76. Stryker, Medical care, 178.

77. Jewell, Kay E. Legal, policy, and regulatory issues. In *Medical direction in long term care: Clinical and administrative guide,* edited by Steven A. Levenson, 308. Owings Mills, MD: Rynd Communications, 1988.

78. Rogers, Elizabeth L. Physicians and the long-term care team. In *Medical direction in long term care: Clinical and administrative guide,* edited by Steven A. Levenson, 175. Owings Mills, MD: Rynd Communications, 1988.

79. Marion Merrell Dow, Inc., *Managed care digest: Long term care* (1991), 25.

80. Abrahamson, Joan. Social services in long-term care. In *Creative long-term care administration,* edited by George Kenneth Gordon and Ruth Stryker, 2d ed., 203. Springfield, IL: Charles C Thomas, 1988.

81. Eggleston, Judy, and Ruth Hastings. Activities: Life means living. In *Creative long-term care administration,* edited by George Kenneth Gordon and Ruth Stryker, 2d ed., 220, 224. Springfield, IL: Charles C Thomas, 1988.

82. Strahan, Genevieve. Nursing home characteristics: Preliminary data from the 1985 National Nursing Home Survey. *NCHS Advancedata* 131 (March 27, 1987): 6.

83. Marion Laboratories. *Marion Long-term care digest: Nursing home edition* (booklet), 28. Kansas City, MO, 1989.

84. Nursing homes see little relief in coming years. *Hospitals* 64 (April 20, 1990): 109, 112.

85. Griffin, Kathleen M., Robert A. Leftwich, Jr., and Sara A. Smith. Current forces shaping long-term care in the 1990s. *Journal of Long-Term Care Administration* 17 (Fall 1989): 8.

86. Murtaugh, Christopher M., Peter Kemper, and Brenda C. Spillman. The risk of nursing home use in later life. *Medical Care* 28 (October 1990): 959.

87. Murtaugh, Kemper, and Spillman, Risk of nursing, 959.

88. Rivlin, Alice M., and Joshua M. Weiner. *Caring for the disabled elderly: Who will pay?,* 42–43. Washington, D.C.: The Brookings Institution, 1988.

89. Duggar, Benjamin C. Ambulatory surgery facilities: Definition and identification. *Journal of Ambulatory Care Management* 13 (February 1990): 2–3.

90. Duggar, Ambulatory surgery facilities, 2–3.

91. Havlicek, Penny L. *Medical groups in the U.S.,* 1. Chicago: American Medical Association, 1984.

92. Sigerist, Henry E. *A history of medicine.* Vol. I, *Primitive and archaic medicine* 320. New York: Oxford University Press, 1951.

93. Madison, Donald L. Notes on the history of group practice: The tradition of the dispensary. *Medical Group Management Journal* 37 (September/October 1990): 54.

94. Havlicek, Penny L. *Medical groups in the U.S.: A survey of practice characteristics,* 34. Chicago: American Medical Association, 1990.

95. Shouldice, Robert G. *Introduction to managed care,* 2d ed., 181. Arlington, VA: Information Resources Press, 1991.

96. Havlicek, *Medical groups* (1990), 34.

97. Charting trends in medical groups. *Medical Staff Leader* 20 (February 1991): 7.

98. Henderson, John A. Healthcare providers will face critical issues in 1990's. *FASA Update* 7 (May/June 1990): 14.

99. Henderson, Healthcare providers, 14.

100. Congratulations to Surgicenter on its 20th anniversary. *FASA Update* 7 (March/April 1990): 19.

101. Henderson, John A. Surgery centers continue making inroads. *Modern Healthcare* 20 (May 21, 1990): 98.

102. Larkin, Howard. Physicians turning to surgery centers. *American Medical News* 33 (October 26, 1990): 12.

103. Henderson, Surgery centers, 100.

104. Henderson, Surgery centers, 99.

105. Henderson, Healthcare providers, 13.

106. Anderson, Howard J. Outpatient planning: Still more art than science. *Hospitals* 64 (December 20, 1990): 31.

107. Durant, Gail D. Ambulatory surgery centers: Surviving, thriving into the 1990s. *MGM Journal* 36 (March/April 1989): 18, 20.

108. Henderson, Healthcare providers, 18.

109. Alternate care. *Hospitals* 64 (November 20, 1990): 23.

110. Henderson, Healthcare providers, 18.

111. Accreditation Association for Ambulatory Health Care, Inc. *Facts about accreditation for health care organizations* (pamphlet). 1990.

112. AAAHC news. *FASA Update* 7 (May/June 1990): 31.

113. Henderson, Surgery centers, 99.

114. Studin, Ira, Barbara Grenell, and Debbie Brandel. Home health care. *Group Practice Journal* 38 (May/June 1989): 44.

115. An excellent history of the development of hospice care is found in Manning, Margaret. *The hospice alterna-*

tive: Living with dying. London: Souvenir Press Ltd, 1984.

116. Davidson, Glen W., ed. *The hospice: Development and administration,* 2nd ed., 2. Washington, D.C.: Hemisphere Publishing Corporation, 1985.

117. Mor, Vincent, David S. Greer, and Robert Kastenbaum, eds. *The hospice experiment,* 11. Baltimore: The Johns Hopkins University Press, 1988.

118. McDonnell, Alice. *Quality hospice care: Administration, organization, and models,* 4. Owings Mills, MD: National Health Publishing, 1986.

119. Davidson, *The hospice,* 3.

120. Davis, Feather Ann. Medicare hospice benefit: Early program experiences. *Health Care Financing Review* 9 (Summer 1988): 100.

121. Part 418—Hospice Care, Subpart C—Conditions of Participation. 42 CFR, Chapter IV.

122. News at deadline. *Hospitals* 65 (January 20, 1991): 10.

123. Simione, Robert J. and Jean F. Preston. Hospice management: Operational, reimbursement, and financial issues. *Caring* 9 (November 1990): 80–81.

124. Beresford, Larry. Private communication, January 25, 1991.

125. Hoyer, Robert G. Public policy and the American hospice movement: The tie that binds. *Caring* 9 (March 1990): 30.

126. Hoyer, Public policy, 33.

127. Committee on Ways and Means, U.S. House of Representatives. *Overview of entitlement programs, 1990 green book: Background material and data on programs within the jurisdiction of the Committee on Ways and Means,* 136. Washington, D.C.: U.S. Government Printing Office, 1990.

128. Kilburn, Linda H. *Hospice operations manual: A comprehensive guide to organizational development, management, care planning, regulatory compliance, and financial services,* 93. Arlington, VA: National Hospice Organization, 1988.

129. National Hospice Organization. *Hospice facts.* Arlington, VA, 1990.

130. Beresford, private communication.

131. National Hospice Organization. *The basics of hospice* (pamphlet). Arlington, VA, 1988.

132. McDonnell, *Quality hospice care,* 38–39.

133. McDonnell, *Quality hospice care,* 39.

134. Beresford, private communication.

135. Beresford, Larry. Growing pains for hospices. *Business & Health* 8 (September 1990): 62.

136. Quality watch. Hospitals 64 (July 20, 1990): 18.

137. The Community Health Accreditation Program, Inc. CHAP accreditation (information sheet). New York, 1990.

138. Zelten, Robert A. *Alternative HMO models.* Issue Paper No. 3, 2. Philadelphia: National Health Care Management Center of the University of Pennsylvania, 1979.

139. Gold, Marsha. Health maintenance organizations: Structure, performance, and current issues for employee health benefits design. *Journal of Occupational Medicine* 33 (March 1991): 289.

140. Kenkel, Paul J. Improving managed care's management. *Modern Healthcare* 20 (May 14, 1990): 27.

141. Hale, Judith A., and Mary M. Hunter. *From HMO movement to managed care industry: The future of HMOs in a volatile healthcare market,* 18. Minneapo-

lis, MN: Interstudy Center for Managed Care Research, 1988.

142. Hale and Hunter, *From HMO movement,* Appendixes A and B.

143. Hale and Hunter, *From HMO movement,* 14.

144. Shouldice, *Introduction to managed care,* 60.

145. Hale and Hunter, *From HMO movement,* 15–16.

146. Hale and Hunter, *From HMO movement,* 23.

147. Hale and Hunter, *From HMO movement,* 23.

148. Hale and Hunter, *From HMO movement,* 21.

149. Hale and Hunter, *From HMO movement,* 14.

150. Henderson, Healthcare providers, 15.

151. Marion Merrell Dow, Inc. *Managed care digest: Update edition* (booklet), 7. Kansas City, MO, 1990.

152. Henderson, Healthcare providers, 15.

153. Marion Merrell Dow, Inc., *Managed care digest: Update,* 6.

154. Gold, Health maintenance, 289.

155. Gold, Health maintenance, 289.

156. Shouldice, *Introduction to Managed Care,* 111.

157. Henderson, Healthcare providers, 15.

158. Henderson, Healthcare providers, 18.

159. Shouldice, *Introduction to Managed Care,* 58.

160. These models are described in Chapters 3 and 4 of Shouldice, *Introduction to Managed Care.*

161. Shouldice, *Introduction to Managed Care,* 187.

162. Shouldice, *Introduction to Managed Care,* 191.

163. Shouldice, *Introduction to Managed Care,* 248.

164. Shouldice, *Introduction to Managed Care,* 98–99.

165. Shouldice, *Introduction to Managed Care,* 203.

166. Berry, Howard R. Managed care's 4th generation. *Group Practice Journal* 38 (July/August 1989): 50.

167. Berry, Managed care's, 46.

168. Berry, Managed care's, 48.

169. Hale and Hunter, *From HMO movement,* ii.

170. Hale and Hunter, *From HMO movement,* iii.

171. Wertz, Richard W., and Dorothy C. Wertz. *Lying-in: A history of childbirth in America,* 133. New Haven, CT: Yale University Press, 1989.

172. Wertz and Wertz, *Lying-in,* 135.

173. Wertz and Wertz, *Lying-in,* 178.

174. Wertz and Wertz, *Lying-in,* 179.

175. Wertz and Wertz, *Lying-in,* 285.

176. Guidelines for licensing and regulating birth centers. *American Journal of Public Health* 73 (March 1983): 333.

177. National Association of Childbearing Centers. Pamphlet. Perkiomenville, PA, 1991.

178. Wertz and Wertz, *Lying-in,* 285.

179. Wertz and Wertz, *Lying-in,* 285.

180. Wertz and Wertz, *Lying-in,* 292.

181. Minor, A.F. *The cost of maternity care and childbirth in the United States, 1989* (pamphlet), 7. Washington, D.C.: Health Insurance Association of America, 1989.

182. Minor, *Cost of maternity,* 8.

183. American College of Nurse-Midwives. *Today's certified nurse-midwives* (pamphlet). Washington, D.C., 1991.

184. Wertz and Wertz, *Lying-in,* 285.

185. Minor, *Cost of maternity,* 7.

186. Rooks, Judith P., Norman L. Weatherby, Eunice K.M. Ernst, Susan Stapleton, David Rosen, and Allan Rosenfield. Outcomes of care in birth centers: The National Birth Center Study. *New England Journal of Medicine* 321 (December 28, 1989): 1804.

187. The Commission for the Accreditation of Freestanding Birth Centers. *Accreditation for freestanding birth centers* (pamphlet). Perkiomenville, PA, n.d.

188. Rooks, Weatherby, Ernst, Stapleton, Rosen, and Rosenfield, Outcomes of care, 1810.

189. Deloughery, Grace L. *History and trends of professional nursing*, 8th ed., 102. St. Louis: The C.V. Mosby Co., 1977.

190. Mundinger, Mary O'Neil. *Home care controversy: Too little, too late, too costly*, 37. Rockville, MD: Aspen Systems Corporation, 1983.

191. Mundinger, *Home care controversy*, 38.

192. Spiegel, Allen D. *Home healthcare: Home birthing to hospice care*, 10. Owings Mills, MD: National Health Publishing, 1983.

193. Mundinger, *Home care controversy*, 18.

194. Lerman, Dan, ed. *Home care: Positioning the hospital for the future*, 1. Chicago: American Hospital Publishing, Inc., 1987.

195. Mundinger, *Home care controversy*, 39.

196. Mundinger, *Home care controversy*, 43.

197. Committee on Ways and Means, *Overview of entitlement*, 143.

198. Mundinger, *Home care controversy*, 42.

199. Lerman, *Home care*, 1.

200. Marion Merrell Dow, Inc., *Managed care digest: Long term care* (1991), 30.

201. Committee on Ways and Means, *Overview of entitlement*, 136.

202. Marion Laboratories, Inc. *Marion long-term care digest: Home health care edition* (booklet), 3. Kansas City, MO, 1989.

203. Church, Louis. Home health care: New challenges, new solutions. *Hospitals* 63 (January 5, 1989): 80.

204. Committee on Ways and Means, *Overview of entitlement*, 144–145.

205. Henderson, Healthcare providers, 19.

206. HHAs advised to review interim payment rates. *NAHC Report* 383 (October 19, 1990): 2.

207. Church, Home health care, 80.

208. Marion Merrell Dow, Inc., *Managed care digest: Long term care* (1991), 29.

209. Marion Merrell Dow, Inc., *Managed care digest: Long term care* (1991), 47.

210. Short, Pamela Farley, and Joel Leon. *Use of home and community services by persons ages 65 and older with functional difficulties*, 5. Washington, D.C.: Agency for Health Care Policy and Research, Public Health Service, Department of Health & Human Services, 1990.

211. Health Care Financing Administration, Department of Health and Human Services. Medicare program, home health agencies: Conditions of participation and reduction in recordkeeping requirements. Interim Final Rule. 42 CFR 484. *Federal Register* 54 (August 14, 1989): 33369.

212. Fanale, James E. Home health care: What's available and what Medicare pays for. *Geriatrics* 43 (August 1988): 16.

213. Lerman, *Home care*, 19.

214. Grimaldi, Paul L. New law changes Medicare home health regulatory system. *Nursing Management* 19 (April 1988): 16.

215. Lerman, *Home care*, 19.

216. Marion Merrell Dow, Inc., *Managed care digest: Long term care* (1991), 32.

217. Lerman, *Home care*, 18.

218. Lerman, *Home care*, 22.

219. Lerman, *Home care*, 23.

220. Blanchard, Leah, Margaret M. Guenveur, and Wanda Ryan. Long-term home care: Does it really work? *Caring* 7 (March 1988): 8.

221. Lerman, *Home care*, 26.

222. Lerman, *Home care*, 27.

223. Marion Laboratories, Inc., *Marion long-term care digest*, 19.

224. Anderson, Tim. Priorities of expertise: What home care agencies look for in managers. *Caring* 8 (February 1989): 53.

225. Health Care Financing Administration, Medicare program, 33371.

226. Keenan, Joseph M., and James E. Fanale. Home care: Past and present, problems and potential. *Journal of the American Geriatrics Society* 37 (November 1989): 1078.

227. Health Care Financing Administration, Medicare program, 33370–33371.

228. Short and Leon, *Use of home*, 4.

229. Mundinger, *Home care controversy*, 42.

230. Keenan and Fanale, Home care, 1077.

231. Lutz, Sandy. Despite its pitfalls, home care keeps growing. *Modern Healthcare* 18 (June 24, 1988): 24.

232. Rivlin and Weiner, Caring for, 41–42.

233. Bureau of Labor Statistics, U.S. Department of Labor, *Monthly Labor Review* 112 (November 1989): 55.

BIBLIOGRAPHY

Alexander, Jeffrey. *The changing character of hospital governance*. Chicago: The Hospital Research and Educational Trust, 1990.

Allen, James E. *Nursing home administration*. New York: Springer Publishing Company, 1987.

American Hospital Association. *Role and functions of the hospital governing board*. Chicago, 1990.

Beresford, Larry. Growing pains for hospices. *Business & Health* 9 (September 1990): 52, 54, 56, 58, 60, 64.

Berry, Howard R. Managed care's 4th generation. *Group Practice Journal* 38 (July/August 1989): 46–51.

Carpenter, Letty. Medicaid eligibility for persons in nursing homes. *Health Care Financing Review* 10 (Winter 1988): 67–77.

Cogen, Raymond. Medicare coverage in the skilled nursing facility. *Journal of Long-Term Care Administration* 17 (Fall 1989): 18–20.

Committee on Ways and Means, U.S. House of Representatives. *Overview of entitlement programs, 1990 green book: Background material and data on programs within the jurisdiction of the Committee on Ways and Means*. Washington, D.C.: U.S. Government Printing Office, 1990.

Davidson, Glen W., ed. *The hospice: Development and administration*, 2nd ed. Washington, D.C.: Hemisphere Publishing Corporation, 1985.

Davis, Feather Ann. Medicare hospice benefit: Early program experiences. *Health Care Financing Review* 9 (Summer 1988): 99–111.

Deloughery, Grace L. *History and trends of professional nursing*, 8th ed. St. Louis: The C.V. Mosby Co., 1977.

Drucker, Peter F. The coming of the new organization. *Harvard Business Review* 66 (January–February 1988): 45–53.

Duggar, Benjamin C. Ambulatory surgery facilities: Definition and identification. *Journal of Ambulatory Care Management* 13 (February 1990): 1–9.

Durant, Gail D. Ambulatory surgery centers: Surviving, thriving into the 1990s. *MGM Journal* 36 (March/April 1989): 14, 16–18, 20.

Gordon, George Kenneth, and Ruth Stryker. *Creative long-term care administration,* 2d ed. Springfield, IL: Charles C Thomas, 1988.

Griffin, Kathleen M., Robert A. Leftwich, Jr., and Sara A. Smith. Current forces shaping long-term care in the 1990s. *Journal of Long-Term Care Administration* 17 (Fall 1989): 8–11.

Hale, Judith A., and Mary M. Hunter. *From HMO movement to managed care industry: The future of HMOs in a volatile healthcare market.* Minneapolis: Interstudy Center for Managed Care Research, 1988.

Havlicek, Penny L. *Medical groups in the U.S.: A survey of practice characteristics.* Chicago: American Medical Association, 1990.

Health Care Financing Administration, Department of Health and Human Services. Medicare program, home health agencies: Conditions of participation and reduction in record-keeping requirements. Interim Final Rule. 42 CFR 484. *Federal Register* 54 (August 14, 1989): 33354–33373.

Hoyer, Robert G. Public policy and the American hospice movement: The tie that binds. *Caring* 9 (March 1990): 30–35.

Jacyk, William. Impaired physicians: They are not the only ones at risk. *Canadian Medical Association Journal* 141 (July 15, 1989): 147–148.

Joint Commission on Accreditation of Healthcare Organizations, *Accreditation manual for hospitals, 1992.* 1991.

Keenan, Joseph M., and James E. Fanale. Home care: Past and present, problems and potential. *Journal of the American Geriatrics Society* 37 (November 1989): 1077.

Kilburn, Linda H. *Hospice operations manual: A comprehensive guide to organizational development, management, care planning, regulatory compliance, and financial services.* Arlington, VA: National Hospice Organization, 1988.

Lerman, Dan, ed. *Home care: Positioning the hospital for the future.* Chicago: American Hospital Publishing, Inc., 1987.

Levenson, Steven A., ed. *Medical direction in long term care: A clinical and administrative guide.* Owings Mills, MD: Rynd Communications, 1988.

Madison, Donald L. Notes on the history of group practice: The tradition of the dispensary. *Medical Group Management Journal* 37 (September/October 1990): 52–54, 56–60, 86–91.

Marion Laboratories, Inc. *Marion long-term care digest: Home health care edition* (booklet). Kansas City, MO, 1989.

Marion Laboratories. *Marion long-term care digest: Nursing home edition* (booklet). Kansas City, MO, 1989.

Marion Merrell Dow, Inc. *Managed care digest: Update edition* (booklet). Kansas City, MO, 1990.

Marion Merrell Dow, Inc. *Marion Merrell Dow managed care digest: Long term care edition* (pamphlet). Kansas City, MO, 1991.

McDonnell, Alice. *Quality hospice care: Administration, organization, and models.* Owings Mills, MD: National Health Publishing, 1986.

Mor, Vincent, David S. Greer, and Robert Kastenbaum, eds. *The hospice experiment.* Baltimore: The Johns Hopkins University Press, 1988.

Mundinger, Mary O'Neil. *Home care controversy: Too little, too late, too costly.* Rockville, MD: Aspen Systems Corporation, 1983.

Murtaugh, Christopher M., Peter Kemper, and Brenda C. Spillman. The risk of nursing home use in later life. *Medical Care* 28 (October 1990): 952–962.

Neuhauser, Duncan. *The relationship between administration activities and hospital performance.* Research Series No. 28, Chicago: University of Chicago Center of Health Administration Studies, 1971.

Part 418—Hospice Care, Subpart C—Conditions of Participation. 42 CFR, Chapter IV.

Rivlin, Alice M., and Joshua M. Weiner. *Caring for the disabled elderly: Who will pay?* Washington, D.C.: The Brookings Institution, 1988.

Rooks, Judith P., Norman L. Weatherby, Eunice K.M. Ernst, Susan Stapleton, David Rosen, and Allan Rosenfield. Outcomes of care in birth centers: The National Birth Center Study. *New England Journal of Medicine* 321 (December 28, 1989): 1804–1811.

Rorem, C. Rufus. *Non-profit hospital service plans.* Chicago: American Hospital Association, 1940.

Short, Pamela Farley, and Joel Leon. *Use of home and community services by persons ages 65 and older with functional difficulties.* Washington, D.C.: Agency for Health Care Policy and Research, Public Health Service, Department of Health & Human Services, 1990.

Shortell, Stephen M. Hospital medical staff organization: Structure, process, and outcome. *Hospital Administration* 19 (Spring 1974): 104.

Shortell, Stephen M. The medical staff of the future: Replanting the garden. *Frontiers of Health Services Management* 1 (February 1985): 3–48.

Shortell, Stephen M. Revisiting the garden: Medicine and management in the 1990s. *Frontiers of Health Services Management* 7 (Fall 1990): 3–32.

Shortell, Stephen M., and Connie Evashwick. The structural configuration of U.S. hospital medical staffs. *Medical Care* 19 (April 1981): 419–430.

Shouldice, Robert G. *Introduction to Managed Care,* 2d ed. Arlington, VA: Information Resources Press, 1991.

Sigerist, Henry E. *A history of medicine.* vol. I, *Primitive and archaic medicine.* New York: Oxford University Press, 1951.

Spiegel, Allen D. *Home healthcare: Home birthing to hospice care.* Owings Mills, MD: National Health Publishing, 1983.

Studin, Ira, Barbara Grenell, and Debbie Brandel. Home health care. *Group Practice Journal* 38 (May/June 1989): 44–48.

Talbott, G. Douglas, and Karl V. Gallegos. The pilot impaired physicians epidemiologic surveillance system. *QRB* 14 (April 1988): 133–136.

Torrens, Paul R., ed. *Hospice programs and public policy.* Chicago: American Hospital Publishing, Inc., 1985.

Warzinski, Katherine V., and Ann Ward Tourigny. Nursing home administrator licensure: A history. *Journal of Long-term Care Administration* 15 (Spring 1987): 6–10.

Weber, Max. *The theory of social and economic organizations,* translated by A.M. Henderson and Talcott Parsons, 151–157. New York: The Free Press, 1947.

Wertz, Richard W., and Dorothy C. Wertz. *Lying-in: A history of childbirth in America.* New Haven, CT: Yale University Press, 1989.

IV

Strategic Planning and Interorganizational Linkages for Health Services Organizations

8

/ # Strategic Planning and Marketing

> *"Cheshire Puss, . . . would you tell me,*
> *please, which way I ought to go from here?"*
> *"That depends a good deal on where you*
> *want to get to," said the Cat.*
> *"I don't much care where— " said Alice.*
> *"Then it doesn't much matter which way*
> *you go," said the Cat.*
> *"—so long as I get* somewhere," *Alice*
> *added as an explanation.*
> *"Oh, you're sure to do that," said the*
> *Cat.*
>
> Lewis Carroll, *Alice's Adventures in*
> *Wonderland[1]*

As the opening quotation indicates, Alice did not know where she wanted to get to and the Cheshire Cat responded, "then it doesn't much matter which way you go." Without planning, where a health services organization (HSO) is to get to (objectives to be accomplished) is unclear and the way to get there (to achieve the objectives) is unknown or at best haphazard. Planning provides direction and order for HSO activities. If they do not know where they are going, HSOs will usually end up somewhere they don't intend to go.

In Chapter 1, "The Management Process and Managerial Roles," planning was described as a technical managerial function that enables HSOs to deal with the present and anticipate the future. It involves deciding what to do; when, where, and how to do it; and for what purpose. It was also described as a primary function because the other management functions of organizing, staffing, directing, controlling, and decision making are predicated upon the most important outcomes of planning: objectives, strategies, and operational programs. Thus, planning has been appropriately termed "the fundamental function of management."[2]

Strategic planning and one of its elements, marketing, are the primary focus of this chapter. Through an understanding of the strategic planning process, it is possible to answer questions such as: How can the HSO anticipate future demands and adapt to its environment, whether accommodating or hostile? How are objectives (i.e., desired outputs) of an HSO established, and what influences their formulation? How does the HSO develop and choose specific strategies and operational programs to accomplish objectives? How should the HSO make structure, tasks/technology, and people arrangements, and allocate resources to meet present and future demands?

This chapter begins with foundation material, including a definition of planning, planning characteristics, and planning outcomes. The HSO planning environment and health services marketing follow. An HSO strategic planning model that integrates marketing is presented and analyzed. Finally, a model for interacting with stakeholders in a strategic context is presented.

PLANNING DEFINED

Planning has been described in various ways. Pearce and Robinson consider it to be "determining the direction of a business by establishing objectives and by designing and implementing strategies necessary to achieve those objectives."[3] Planning is an orderly process that gives organizational direction, helps the organization prepare for change, and helps it cope with uncertainty. Planning involves deciding what to do and how to do it, as well as anticipating the future, which implies contending with the environment[4] and preparing for the future.[5]

Each description of planning incorporates at least one distinct attribute of planning. First, planning can be considered futuristic since it deals with anticipating future events, determining what will be required of the HSO in the future, and how this will be accomplished. Second, it involves decision making, because determining what is to be done, and when, where, how, and for what purposes it is done, requires that alternatives be evaluated, decisions made, and resources allocated. Finally, planning is dynamic and continuous—planned organizational activities are affected by future events and internal and external environmental forces. Consequently, continuous environmental surveillance and adaptive change are attributes of planning.

Incorporating these attributes, planning is defined as *anticipating the future, assessing present conditions, and making decisions concerning organizational direction, programs, and resource deployment.* This process results in answers to questions of what to do and when, where, how, and for what purposes it is to be done. The process of planning—how it is done—consists of a series of activities that include assessing present information about the organization and its environment; making assumptions about the future; evaluating present objectives and/or developing new ones; and formulating organization strategies and operational programs that, when implemented, will accomplish objectives.

PLANNING AND THE MANAGEMENT MODEL

When related to the management model (see Figure 1.6), the importance of planning becomes evident. Planning enables HSOs and managers to deal with their external environment—their immediate health care environment and the larger macroenvironment. Thus, planning reduces uncertainty, ambiguity, and risk.[6] By anticipating trends, and at times proactively influencing environmental forces, HSOs are more prepared for and able to respond to the myriad forces that affect them. Environmental forces that affect HSOs and the planning process are presented in Part II (The Health Services Environment).

Planning forces managers to focus on outputs. All organizational activity is directed toward accomplishing objectives. As a product of planning, objectives are the ends, desired results, or outputs to be attained by the HSO and its units. From them, input needs are determined.

Planning enables managers to develop priorities and make better decisions about conversion design as well as allocation and use of resources. It is through integration of structure, tasks/technology, and people that inputs are converted to outputs. By identifying and focusing on objectives and formulating strategies and operational programs, managers can design appropriate conversion processes and systems. These include some of the organizational arrangements presented in Chapters 6 and 7 and initiatives such as continuous quality improvement and work process design, to be described in Chapter 11. The function of decision making and its importance to the HSO's planned conversion of inputs to outputs is presented in Chapter 10.

As managers implement planned organizational activity for the purpose of accomplishing predetermined objectives through chosen strategies and operational programs, they do so through people. The four chapters in Part VI and the two chapters in Part VII focus on this important input resource—people.

Finally, planning is the foundation for resource allocation and control. It enables HSOs to measure progress and determine whether expected results are being achieved. The control process, which is described in Chapter 12, involves establishing standards for resource use and monitoring HSO activity. Criteria for measuring progress are ultimately based on objectives derived through planning.

PLANNING CHARACTERISTICS

Planning is often characterized by type and time frame, the individuals who plan, and the various approaches used in planning. A typology of these characteristics is presented in Figure 8.1.

Type of Planning

Type of planning refers to level (strategic/operational) and scope (broad/narrow). Strategic planning in HSOs is performed at the senior management level with input from other organization members, including those of the professional staff organization who hold leadership positions.[7] It is broad, all encompassing in scope, and particularly concerned with environmental assessment; it addresses the elements of organization objective and strategy formulation. Conversely, operational planning in HSOs is more narrow and limited than strategic planning and is performed at lower levels of the organization. Operational planning is subservient to, derived from, and must be in harmony with strategic planning. Included are establishing subobjectives along with operational programs, policies, and procedures in major differentiated units of the organization that may encompass groups of departments or individual departments.

Time Frame of Planning and Who Plans

Time frames of planning vary. Strategic planning is long range and encompasses multiple years. Operational planning is usually short term, with a time frame of one year or less. The governing body and senior management are responsible for strategic planning in HSOs. The governing body is responsible for setting the HSO's direction and its mission and objectives. Senior management has significant input in formulating organization objectives and is charged with developing and implementing organization strategies to accomplish them. The governing body's role does not include originating strategy.[8] It is responsible, however, for ensuring that proposals brought before it by senior management are properly prepared and are consistent with the HSO's mission and culture and its responsibilities to stakeholders.

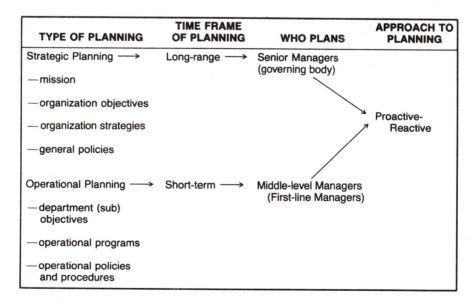

Figure 8.1. Planning characteristics.

Middle-level managers also plan. Generally, they are concerned with short-term operational planning and design and implementation of programs, policies, and procedures in their area of responsibility. This most often occurs at the level encompassing multiple departments. Finally, department managers and first-line supervisors also plan, usually in relation to specific operations or activities such as estimating work load, scheduling work activity, and allocating resources.

Approach to Planning

There are many approaches to planning, and here they are described as opposites. The names of such approaches as individual-committee, systematic–ad hoc, and quantitative-nonquantitative describe how planning is done and are self-explanatory. There are others, such as developmental-incremental and proactive-reactive, that merit further attention.

Developmental-incremental planning refers to the degree of autonomy in the planning process. Organizational settings or environments with fewer constraints, precedents, restrictions, and conventions are particularly conducive to the use of developmental planning by HSOs or individual managers. Developmental planning is characterized by bold, new, innovative, and nontraditional planning outcomes, especially organization strategies. An industrial sector associated with developmental planning is personal computers. Here, product lines are not yet frozen, markets and uses are evolving, conventions and traditions are not fixed, and organizational rigidity is minimal. As a generalization, investor-owned, multiorganizational systems have led the way in HSO developmental planning, in part because there are fewer restrictions on the governing body and senior management in setting organization direction and greater autonomy in developing strategy. Many contemporary not-for-profit HSO organizational structures, vertical integration and diversification strategies, and interorganizational linkages had their genesis in these systems. As some restrictions and conventions have been ameliorated in the health services sector, particularly through deregulation and more emphasis on competition as public policy, not-for-profit HSOs have experienced greater autonomy and consequently are now more developmental in their planning.

Incremental planning is the opposite of developmental planning. It is characterized as less bold, less innovative, and more traditional. It may occur because of internal or external restrictions or because limited managerial autonomy has been granted by the governing body. Some settings may be conducive to developmental planning, but incremental planning may still occur when managerial perspective is characterized by a limiting mindset, emphasis on short-term goals, narrow assumptions, and desire to avoid risk. Incremental planning involves marginal versus major changes in direction, thrust, and strategy. It can be characterized as mechanistic, versus the more creative developmental planning,[9] or as "satisficing"—doing well enough but not necessarily as well as possible.

Another planning approach is *proactive-reactive*. Proactive planning is overt, systematic, formalized, and anticipatory. It involves not only anticipating the future but also intervening and influencing environments—making things happen and shaping events in the best interest of the HSO. Reactive planning, as the opposite of proactive, is default planning. It responds to events, is nonsystematic, and certainly is not anticipatory.

Often, proactive planning takes on some of the attributes of developmental planning. Those who are proactive will make things happen, do things differently—perhaps innovate boldly. Reactive planners are followers. They tend to have the attributes of incremental planning—doing things differently on the margin yet very much the same, altering and modifying activities because of the actions of others (competition) or environmental forces rather than shaping forces and causing others to react. More importantly, proactive-reactive planning is a major element in strategic planning relative to process and perspective. The treatment of HSO strategic planning here advocates and presumes a proactive approach.

PLANNING OUTCOMES

Items traditionally considered to be outcomes of planning—determining what to do and where, when, how, and for what purpose to do it—are organization mission, objectives, strategies and operational programs, and policies and procedures (see Figure 8.1).

Mission

All organizations have a mission, which is almost always explicitly stated. Missions are generally statements that identify, in broad terms, the purposes for which the organization exists.[10] The mission specifies the unique aim of the organization and differentiates it from other organizations. For example, an HSO's mission is significantly different from that of an automobile manufacturer. Generally, elements embodied in an HSO mission statement are: Who are we? What are we? Why do we exist? Who is our constituency?[11] The statement reflects a philosophy about the organization and its role in health services delivery. The mission is the foundation for all organizational planning and is determined by the governing body. Table 8.1 is an example of a hospital system mission statement.

Objectives

Objectives are statements of the results that the HSO seeks to accomplish. In the context of the management model in Figure 1.6 they are also HSO outputs. They are the ends, targets, and desired results toward which all organizational activity is directed. Most objectives are explicit, but some are implied. There are primary and secondary organization objectives—those to be accomplished by the organization as a whole—and subobjectives for particular differentiated units (i.e., divisions or departments of the organization). This relationship is presented in Figure 8.2.

Organization objectives give direction to the entire HSO and are established by the governing body. Often expressed in broad terms, organization objectives, when accomplished, result in mission fulfillment. Thus, they are derived from and reflect the mission. In their classic study of hospitals, Georgopoulos and Mann describe organization objectives as follows: "The chief objective of the hospital is, of course, to provide adequate care and treatment to its patients. . . . A hospital may, of course, have additional objectives including its own maintenance and survival, organizational stability, and growth."[12]

Typical HSO organization objectives are listed in the management model presented in Chapter 1 (see Figure 1.6). Included are patient care and customer service, high-quality care and quality improvement, appropriate costs relative to quality, growth and survival, fulfilling the HSO's social responsibility and being responsive to stakeholders, education/training/research, and reputation/image. They are the outputs of the input-conversion process. Organization objectives seldom change, but emphasis does. In that way, a particular objective that was once secondary may become primary. Survival becomes the foremost organization objective for an HSO facing deteriorating market share, declining census and clinical staff, and insolvency.

Table 8.1. Mission statement for Community Hospital Association

Community Hospital Association is a not-for-profit corporation. Its mission and the purposes for which the corporation is formed are:
  (1) To establish, maintain, and operate hospitals;
  (2) To carry on educational activities related to care of the sick and injured, or promotion of health;
  (3) To promote and carry on scientific research related to care of the sick and injured, or promotion of health; and
  (4) To engage in any activity designed to promote the general health of the community.

Subobjectives are ends and results to be accomplished by various HSO units. They provide direction for managers and employees and are subsidiary to overall organization objectives. Figure 8.2 shows the hierarchical relationship between organization overall objectives and subobjectives. The latter are typically jointly formulated by middle-level and senior managers, or they may be established by first-line managers subject to approval. They are derived from and must be consistent with primary and secondary organization objectives. Accomplishment of subobjectives throughout the organization results in accomplishing overall organization objectives. Table 8.2 presents examples of both.

Objectives that state realistic, attainable, and measurable results are critical to HSOs. First, they enable the organization and managers at various levels to focus attention on and initiate work toward specific ends. Second, they provide prioritizing criteria for decision making about services and programs.[13] Third, they facilitate efficiency, particularly in allocating and using resources. Fourth, they give employees a uniform sense of direction that results in greater organization stability. Fifth, knowledge of intended results is critical to formulating strategies to accomplish organization objectives and operational programs to achieve subobjectives. Finally, they become criteria to be used in the control process.

Organization Strategies and Operational Programs

Organization strategies are broad, general programs designed by an HSO to accomplish organization objectives. They are long-term major patterns of activity requiring a substantial commitment of resources. Traditionally, "strategy" is the term reserved to describe the means (way) of accomplishing organization objectives. Examples of organization strategies include changing the scope of services, perhaps by specializing (adding a catheterization laboratory or open heart surgery unit); diversification (establishing a for-profit medical office building subsidiary); and forward or backward integration (expanding service area through a satellite family practice center or convert-

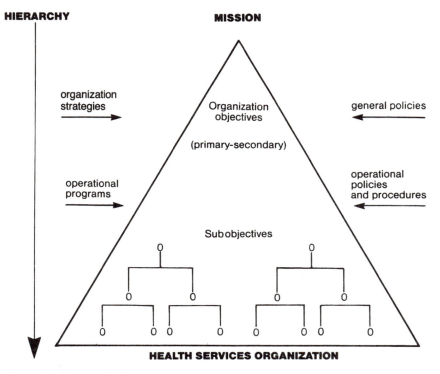

Figure 8.2. Operationalizing an HSO's mission.

Table 8.2. Examples of primary, secondary, and departmental objectives

Primary objectives	An HSO may have primary objectives of *providing quality patient care and a wide range of services to meet community needs.*
Secondary objectives	Secondary objectives could consist of *providing a sound medical education program and maintaining organizational stability.*
Departmental (sub)objectives	1. A subobjective for nursing service (which would be subsidiary to organization primary/ secondary objectives) might be to *provide quality nursing care to all patients in a manner consistent with professional standards and ethics.* 2. Subobjectives of the dietary department might be to *serve to patients, personnel, and guests food that is tasty, is at the proper temperature, and meets nutritional requirements in a cost-effective manner.* 3. Subobjectives of the medical records department might be to *provide and maintain an efficient system in which patient records are kept safe from loss or destruction, protected from unauthorized use, adequately indexed, and readily accessible to authorized personnel, while also ensuring that medical records practices and procedures comply with legal requirements.*

ing acute care beds to rehabilitation beds). Strategy formulation is the responsibility of senior management in HSOs.

Conversely, operational programs are the specific, planned activities of individual HSO units; their scope is less broad and global than that of organization strategies and they are subsidiary to them. Just as all HSOs have a hierarchy of objectives, they also have a hierarchy of ways to accomplish them. As indicated in Figure 8.2, organization strategy is the means to accomplish the HSO's primary and secondary objectives, and operational programs are the subcomponents of strategies that accomplish HSO unit (departmental) subobjectives.

Policies and Procedures

Policies are officially expressed or implied guidelines for behavior, decision making, and thinking within the organization. They set boundaries of permissible activity, behavior, and decision making within which managers and employees may act.[14] They help organizations attain objectives and thus must be consistent with them and the HSO's mission. Policies are classified as general and operational. The former apply to the entire organization and are formulated by senior management; the latter apply to a specific unit or department and may be formulated by department managers so long as they are consistent with general policy.

General and Operating Policies The general policies most familiar are those governing the personnel/human resource management function: compensation, terms of employment, and on-the-job behavior. Examples are: We are an equal opportunity employer; whenever possible promotion will be from within; and our organization's compensation levels are competitive with those in the community. Other examples of general policies are: All patients will receive care regardless of ability to pay; capital equipment expenditures over $20,000 must have prior senior management approval; and life support for the terminally ill will be maintained unless the patient has an advance directive.

Operational policies that govern particular departments are subsidiary to general policies and must be consistent with them. A personnel/human resource department operational policy might be to continuously update the compensation system's pay grades and rate ranges to remain competitive with similar HSOs in the area. A nursing service policy might be replacing licensed practical nurses with registered nurses to increase the intensity of nursing care as vacancies occur through attrition.

Procedures are guides to action. Unlike policies, which are guidelines to thinking, behavior, and decision making, procedures suggest actions for specific situations. They are generally expressed as a preestablished sequence of steps involved in performing a task. Formal procedures give direction to employees in performing their duties. For example, there are procedures for patient admission and discharge, requisition of supplies, ordering tests, sterilizing equipment, and processing patient records.

Characteristics of Good Policies   Good policies are not easy to develop and implement. To be effective, a policy must be clear and appropriate and must serve to guide the ways in which organizational activities are carried out. Good policies have several characteristics.[15]

First, policies must be well thought out before they are formalized and must be in harmony with objectives. Policies whose effects have not been considered can be detrimental. For example, a professional staff formal or informal policy of ordering a full laboratory workup for all newly admitted patients may have a noble (or defensive) purpose, but may be inconsistent with the organization's objectives of quality care at reasonable costs.

Second, policies must be flexible so they can be applied to normal *and* abnormal situations. Inflexible policies diverge from their intended purpose of providing guidelines for behavior and decision making. Situations may be encountered by a department head, supervisor, or employee that require judgment and atypical action. At times, managers appropriately deviate from policy.

Third, to be effective a policy must be communicated, understood, and accepted by those to whom it applies. Acceptability implies that HSO members consider the policy to be reasonable, legitimate, and fair. Policies that display unwarranted favoritism toward certain employee groups or those that appear to be arbitrary and with no sound purpose will be resisted or possibly even ignored.

Fourth, to serve their purpose policies should be consistent with each other. Inconsistency among policies and in their application and enforcement is confusing and can cause disharmony, employee dissatisfaction, and frustration and will detract from accomplishing objectives. Inconsistencies generally occur among operational policies of various departments. Finally, to serve their intended purpose, policies must be continuously reevaluated and changed if necessary.

HSO PLANNING ENVIRONMENT

HSO planning, especially strategic planning, must occur in the context of its environment. Not only are HSOs and their managers affected by the external environment, but they must anticipate, predict, or make assumptions about its future configuration and the resulting effect on them. Several environmental forces affecting HSOs are shown in the management model in Figure 1.6. The macroenvironment includes ethical/legal, political, cultural/sociological, economic, and ecological forces. The HSO's health care environment includes public planning and policy (regulation, licensure, and accreditation), competition, health care financing (public and private), technology, health research and education, health status, and public health activities. For good or ill these forces will continue to affect HSOs—what HSOs do, where, how, and for what purpose.

Despite federal initiatives to increase access to health care through Medicare and Medicaid, alternative delivery systems, and cost containment, the post–World War II health services environment was rather unobtrusive until the early 1980s. It was an era of expansion in capacity and growth in demand. The environment was stable and predictable. Role clarity existed for HSOs. Risk was low. Proactive HSOs grew, those that were efficient thrived, and even the inefficient survived.

Since the mid-1980s, the HSO environment has changed rapidly and become more turbulent and hostile. Most important, however, it is less certain. Today, HSOs are less insulated. They are buffeted by fast-paced and changing external forces. The changes wrought by high technology and new diagnostic and treatment procedures are breathtaking. Societal, consumer, and third-party payor assertiveness and demands for greater accountability are accelerating, and power is shifting from providers to purchasers and consumers of care.[16] Public and private sector initiatives to control costs are intensifying, and this heightens financial risk for HSOs. These forces, in addition to the federal government's philosophy of less regulation, are contributing to intense, and at times cut-throat, competition among providers. One of the results has been the formation of new delivery arrangements, such as health maintenance organizations (HMOs), preferred provider organizations (PPOs), joint ventures, mergers and consolidations, and multiorganizational systems. HMOs and PPOs are described in Chapter 7, "How HSOs Are Organized." The others are discussed in Chapter 9, "Interorganizational Relationships."[17]

As environmental turbulence gained momentum in the late 1980s and accelerated into the 1990s, HSOs pursued initiatives to contain forces, decrease uncertainty, and lessen risk. Recognizing that the rules of the game have changed, senior managers of HSOs realize that their organizations no longer have guaranteed demand for their services from traditional constituencies, nor are they guaranteed a right to survive.[18] The first major sign of a proactive response to environmental forces was for more HSOs to engage in marketing and to undertake formalized, systematic strategic planning to a greater extent. The remainder of this chapter presents these two subjects. Health services marketing is cast as an environmental link to and integral part of strategic planning.

HEALTH SERVICES MARKETING—AN ENVIRONMENTAL LINK

HSOs have engaged in marketing-type activities for years.[19] Examples include public relations, liaison with and information dissemination to patients and other stakeholders, promoting the HSO's image and services, donor/fund development, addition of new services to meet patient needs, aggressive recruitment and retention of physicians and other staff, and patient origin studies and patient satisfaction surveys.[20]

Marketing in HSOs has changed significantly in the past 2 decades. It is no longer viewed as a segregated, stand-alone activity that consists of disseminating information about types of products and services and their quaility, or gathering information about patient/customer satisfaction. Informed individuals do not construe it only as advertising and selling with the implication that physicians and patients will only utilize the HSO's facilities when there is a substantial promotional effort. It is not the artificial creation of demand for services.[21] While marketing in HSOs is properly consumer focused,[22] the contemporary perspective of marketing is that it is a designed process, integrated with other HSO activities, in which the HSO seeks to identify and satisfy the needs and wants of stakeholders—who may be patients, clinical staff, and the community at large—so that the HSO can accomplish its objectives and fulfill its mission. Kotler and Clarke, for example, observe that marketing is "a central activity of modern organizations. To survive and succeed, organizations must know their markets, attract sufficient resources, convert these resources into appropriate products, services, and ideas, and effectively distribute them to various consuming publics."[23]

Marketing is an integral part of strategic planning.[24] In fact, it is impossible to plan strategically without including an assessment of the market (external) environment, through a marketing audit, and integrating both the information obtained and the marketing function with strategic planning.[25] The link between health services marketing and strategic planning is best understood with a base of knowledge in the marketing concept, marketing audit, and elements of marketing.

Marketing Concept

Authorities agree that the central concept of marketing is that of a voluntary exchange of something of value. The buyer receives something of value (a product or service) from the seller—the HSO—in exchange for something of value.[26] Consummation of exchange requires that sellers/providers create and make available, and that buyers/consumers locate and choose, products and services.[27] Extended, this notion of exchange results in the marketing concept—a process by which HSOs seek to determine the wants and needs of prospective consumers and satisfy them with products or services.[28] Applying the basic marketing concept, health services marketing can be defined as "the analysis, planning, implementation, and control of carefully formulated programs designed to promote voluntary exchanges of values with target markets with the purpose of achieving organizational objectives."[29]

Marketing involves designing the HSO's products and services in response to the target market's needs and desires and using effective pricing, communication, and distribution to provide better service. Figure 8.3 shows several important components of this definition. First, identifying needs, wants, and desires of target markets implies that HSOs know who their customers are. Second, identifying wants and needs leads to creating new or realigning existing products and services rather than creating products and services first and then searching for customer needs. Third, the HSO must engage in certain activities to facilitate exchange of products and services. These are identified in Figure 8.3 as the elements of marketing. Information that leads to development of HSO marketing programs and activities is derived from the marketing audit.

Marketing Audit

The marketing audit is the systematic evaluation of the HSO's marketing situation.[30] It includes: 1) environmental surveillance to identify target markets and their needs, along with identifying opportunities and assessing competition; 2) evaluating present product line or service mix[31] rela-

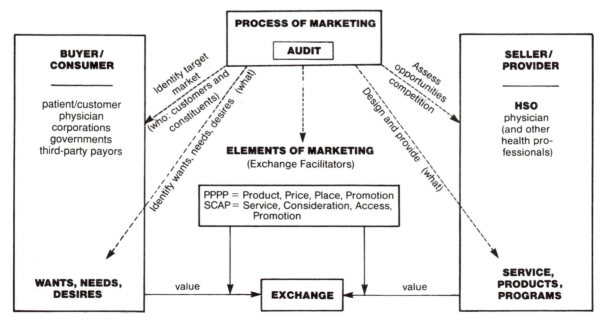

Figure 8.3. Health services marketing.

tive to identified target market needs; and 3) modifying exchange facilitators so they are consistent with HSO strengths and weaknesses and facilitate exchange.[32] Table 8.3 presents informational elements typically addressed in the marketing audit.

Target Market   Environmental assessment identifies present and potential target markets for HSOs, its constituents and purchasers of services, and those who influence purchase decisions. Included is identification of their present and future needs, wants, and desires. In health services, the ultimate consumer in the exchange process is the patient. However, there are others who may intervene and influence who buys what, for how much, and where. For example, physicians not only control patient access to hospitals and nursing facilities but determine the services provided. Third-party payors, in particular government and large corporations, influence the price charged for services. Regulation influences directly or indirectly the type and intensity of service an HSO provides through accreditation, licensure, quality assessment, and reimbursement mechanisms. Self-insured corporations influence where customers receive service by advocating alternatives such as HMOs and PPOs and can, through purchasing power, also influence the type, scope, and price charged for services. Consequently, HSO marketing must seek to satisfy wants and needs of patients and also identify, recognize, address, and satisfy the wants and needs of others who influence the purchase decision. Facility and staff support are important in building and retaining clinical staff. Cost and quality control are important in satisfying governmental and corporate payors. Depth and breadth of service are important in satisfying community needs.

Product Line/Service Mix   A marketing audit identifies the extent of an HSO's service area and evaluates its attributes, the needs of specific target markets, and the extent of competition. Such information allows the product lines or service mix (scope and intensity) to be expanded, reduced, realigned, or focused. Service areas can be large or small and are defined geographically. A general acute care hospital is likely to have a service area encompassing the community and its environs. A tertiary hospital service area may encompass a large region. Target markets can be classified by type of care (preventive, acute/short term, chronic/long term, rehabilitative); service (medical and surgical, obstetrics and gynecology, oncology); age (gerontology, pediatrics); income level; or type of payor (private, commercial, public). Assessment information from the marketing audit reveals gaps in product line or service mix, potential target markets, competitive and other threats to the HSO, and whether special opportunities exist.

As target markets change, as health service needs, preferences, and attitudes shift and change, and as competition and technology intensify, HSOs must evaluate and realign their mix of products, services, and programs. Such realignment must be consistent with the HSO's capabilities and strengths and may include expansion or elimination of services under conditions of downsizing.[33] For example, a competitor's introduction of an urgent care center or formation of an HMO in the service area may require reassessment of the target market, planning how to reach that market, and changes in services. Decline in birth rates may mean reevaluating the scope of the obstetrics service with the possible aim of redirecting resources to other services. New technology may suggest the need to introduce services such as coronary bypass, neonatal care, and nuclear medicine. Identified opportunities may lead to a hospital offering wellness and employee assistance programs to large corporations, pharmacy services to nursing facilities, and home health services to discharged patients.

Elements of Marketing (PPPP and SCAP)

Figure 8.3 presents the elements of marketing that facilitate and make possible the exchange between consumer and seller. The marketing literature identifies them as the four Ps: product, price, place, and promotion.[34] A more appropriate classification for health services is SCAP: service, consideration, access, and promotion.[35]

Table 8.3. Questions for an HSO marketing audit

I. Marketing Environment

A. Constituents

   1. What are the organization's major constituents, and which should be targets of marketing activities?
   2. What are the geographic, demographic, psychosocial and usage/participation characteristics of each target market?
   3. Should the various markets be segmented and, if so, how?
   4. What are the needs that each market and segment is seeking to satisfy?
   5. What attitudes do the markets and segments have toward the organization and its competitors (i.e., what do they know and how do they feel)?
   6. What is the level of satisfaction of each user/supporter group? What factors contribute to satisfaction and dissatisfaction?
   7. How do people in the various target markets make the decision to use or support the organization?
   8. Does the health organization utilize resources and expertise available in the community, such as universities and business leaders?

B. Competition

   1. Who are the organization's direct and indirect competitors?
   2. What are the product/service, price, distribution, and promotion strategies of the competition?
   3. What are the marketing strengths and weaknesses of each competitor (i.e., in terms of price, products and services offered, distribution, promotion, image, rate of growth, and relationships with markets)?
   4. What is the objective position of the organization vis-à-vis the competition (i.e., how is it similar and different)?

C. Social, Technological, Professional, and Legal Constraints

   1. How are developments and trends in the following areas affecting the organization's activities:

      State of the economy?

      Demography of the marketing territory?

      Activities of consumer groups?

      Reimbursement policies of third-party payors?

      Technological innovations?

      Professional educational and certification requirements?

      Planning, regulatory, and support activities of the local, state, and federal government?

      Changes in human values and life-styles?

II. Marketing Mix

A. Services

   1. What are the core services offered by the organization? What ancillary or peripheral services are provided?
   2. Are the employees and volunteers who deliver the services properly trained, motivated, and evaluated?
   3. What is the cost, revenue, and demand situation of each service? Are some services over- or underutilized?
   4. What are the strengths and weaknesses of each program? Are there services that should be changed, eliminated, or added?
   5. How are quality and effectiveness evaluated?
   6. Are there satisfactory procedures for handling complaints?
   7. Are the names given to different services or programs appropriate, descriptive, and appealing?

B. Access and Delivery

   1. Are services offered at appropriate geographic locations (i.e., at a fixed site, temporary or mobile facilities, or in-home)?

(continued)

Table 8.3. *(continued)*

    2. Would it be advantageous to the public and to the health organization to offer a service in a different or additional location?

    3. Are services offered at times of the day, week, and year that are compatible with user needs?

    4. Are facilities easily reached by public and private transportation? Is there sufficient parking? Access for the handicapped?

    5. Does the environment in which a service is offered convey a suitable atmosphere (e.g., of relaxation, warmth, efficiency)?

    6. Does the organization cultivate referral agents?

C. Price

    1. What considerations determine pricing policies? Cost? Demand? Return on investment? Competition? Reimbursement requirements?

    2. What is the elasticity of demand for different services?

    3. Is price used as a competitive weapon? Is it used to manipulate demand (i.e., to increase or decrease service usage)?

    4. How does the organization's pricing structure compare with the competition?

    5. Do users see price as a cue for quality? Do they see price as being in line with value?

    6. What groups are most sensitive to price (users, referral agents, third-party payors, physicians, regulators, competitors)?

    7. Are quantity, seasonal, prompt payment, or other discounts offered? If price is adjusted to consumer income, does the sliding scale need revision?

    8. What are the psychological costs of using each service (e.g., in terms of anxiety, travel and waiting time, disruption of routine, red tape, coping with unfamiliar people and procedures, physical pain, personal abuse, loss of face or self-image, loss of control over one's life, demand for commitment, physical or mental exertion)?

D. Promotion

    1. Public Relations

       a. Is there a formal public relations program?

       b. Are there annual statements of goals, objectives, and strategies for the public relations program?

       c. Are public relations efforts appropriately distributed among various internal and external target publics, including employees, volunteer groups, the medical staff, referral agents, patients, donors, the community, and the media?

       d. Does the organization have a policy for dealing with negative publicity?

       e. How is the effectiveness of the public relations effort measured?

       f. Is the public relations function adequately coordinated with other marketing activities?

    2. Advertising and Incentives

       a. Does the organization use paid or public service advertising for recruiting, fund raising, or promoting services?

       b. How big is the advertising budget and how is it set?

       c. Are specific objectives set for the advertising program, and is it evaluated in terms of those objectives?

       d. Are the advertising media appropriate in terms of the organization's resources and coverage of the target market?

       e. Does the advertising copy communicate effectively?

       f. Is the tone of the advertising congruent with the organization's desired image?

       g. Does or should the organization use a paid or volunteer advertising agency?

       h. Does the organization make effective use of such incentives as pre-

(continued)

Table 8.3. *(continued)*

          miums or gifts, health fairs, diagnostic screenings, contests, etc.? Are
          the incentives compatible with the image of the organization?

  3. Personal Selling

    a. Does the organization use a paid or voluntary sales force for fund rais-
       ing or selling services?

    b. If so, is this sales force properly organized, trained, motivated, re-
       warded, and evaluated?

    c. Is the sales force large enough to achieve the organization's objectives?

    d. Is management utilized effectively to sell the organization?

Adapted from Schlinger, Mary Jane. Marketing audits for health organizations: A practical guide. *Hospital & Health Services Administration* 26 (Special Issue II, 1981): 38–41; used by permission. © 1981, Foundation of the American College of Healthcare Executives.

Service   As HSOs plan and implement programs designed to bring about voluntary exchange between customer and provider, it is presumed that target markets and their needs and wants have been identified and the present service mix has been evaluated through the marketing audit. Such information causes HSOs to respond. Services are realigned (existing services are modified, or new ones introduced) to satisfy consumer and/or stakeholder needs, preferences, and expectations. Included in the bundle of services are not only actual care rendered or product delivered, but amenities, physical decor and comfort, and patient satisfaction with staff. In the context of continuous quality improvement, all aspects of the customer's interaction with the HSO are included in the concept of service.

Consideration   Consideration is the value (price) given for the product or service.[36] When price is paid directly by consumers, it may be a barrier to service. When price is not paid directly by consumers, they may be indifferent to cost and it may not be an important variable in the exchange decision. In fact, consumers may choose higher priced service (hospital inpatient care) that is third-party reimbursed rather than similar, lower priced care in a setting not qualifying for third-party coverage. However, the trend toward deductibles and copayments for those with third-party coverage has made patients (consumers) more price conscious. Also, in competitive environments some HSOs are recognizing the price sensitivity of large self-insured corporate customers and are bundling and pricing services nontraditionally; PPOs are an example. Beyond actual dollar price, consideration also includes intangibles such as patient anxiety, inconvenience, waiting time, and the psychological value of service based on image and reputation, which affect the purchase-exchange decision.[37]

Access   In exchange, access is important—where service is provided and the ease of obtaining it, including location and hours of operation. Freestanding or satellite ambulatory care and family practice centers and mobile screening units are examples of methods to enhance access and expand geographic market area. Group practices that extend weekday hours and are open on weekends do so to enhance access as well as competitive position.

Promotion   Awareness is an important component in facilitating exchange in HSO marketing. Customers or their intermediaries must be made aware of and informed about services (type, scope, quality) that are offered, where and when, and for what consideration. Through promotion, HSOs not only convey such information but suggest a reputation or image that is analogous to brand identification in the corporate sector.

Most of the criticism about health services marketing has been directed at promotion; some view advertising as artificially creating demand. This criticism is inconsistent with the marketing concept and the ethics of health services management.[38] Promotion *is* the legitimate and necessary dissemination of information about service, consideration, and access so that consumers can make more informed purchase decisions.

Ethics and marketing as related to the issue of service expansion or contraction is addressed in Chapter 3, "Ethical Considerations." Certainly HSOs must be responsive to stakeholders, especially patients and payors. HSOs are social enterprises with explicit and implicit responsibilities, however; they can only carry out their mission if they remain solvent. As stated in Chapter 3, "No money, no mission!" The marketing audit gathers information about target market and stakeholder needs, external environment, and the HSO's circumstances relative to the environment and competition. Choice of organization strategies that may result in expanding or contracting products and services are recommended by senior management and approved by the governing body just as are decisions about price, which may include the amount of uncompensated care the HSO will absorb. These decisions must include ethical considerations and be consistent with the HSO's mission and its responsibility to society.

HSO STRATEGIC PLANNING

Strategic planning is overt, anticipatory, and long term. Its perspective embraces the whole HSO rather than single departments or units. It is both externally and internally oriented and involves assessment of the HSO vis-à-vis its environments. An integral part of strategic planning is health services marketing, particularly the marketing audit, which facilitates environmental linkage. Strategic planning is the process concerned with: 1) formulating HSO primary and secondary objectives, and 2) developing organization strategies and the derived operational plans to achieve them. It is an ends-means process in which objectives are ends to be achieved and strategies are means—the ways to accomplish them.[39]

Objectives (primary, secondary, and subsidiary) were previously defined and examples were given. Organization strategies were described as the HSO's long-range, major patterns of activity requiring a substantial commitment of resources. It is appropriate to expand that definition here and add that strategies are the unified, comprehensive plans (means) that capitalize on the HSO's strengths, take advantage of external opportunities, seek to reduce and/or overcome threats, and mitigate weaknesses. Organization strategies are the means to achieve objectives. The discussion that follows is linked to the HSO strategic planning model presented in Figure 8.4 and addresses each element in turn. Components are referenced by number.[40]

The components of strategic planning presented in Figure 8.4 are formulating objectives [I], strategic assessment [II], and strategy choice [III]. Subsequent to choosing one or more strategies, program implementation [IV] occurs through operational planning, resource allocation, and conversion. Finally, HSO managers control [V] by monitoring and evaluating HSO outputs to determine if the strategies chosen and implemented result in objectives being accomplished. Discussion here focuses on the first three components of Figure 8.4. The latter two are treated in other chapters.

I: Formulating Objectives

All HSOs have objectives; some are primary, others secondary. Occasionally, objectives are reprioritized and new ones added. As the ends, targets, and desired outputs, they are the focus of organization activity. As presented in Figure 8.4, objectives [I] influence selection criteria for strategy choice [IIIc]. If specific strategies, when implemented, are likely to accomplish objectives, several of the choice criteria have been met.

The governing body formulates HSO objectives. In doing so, it is affected by other forces: organizational culture, influence of stakeholders, and values/ethics of the choice makers.[41]

Organizational Culture As discussed in Chapter 1, organizational culture is the ingrained pattern of shared beliefs, values, and assumptions acquired by organization members over time. Culture is the legacy—what the HSO is and what it stands for—that permeates the HSO. It is known to and, it is hoped, shared by all. Culture shapes acceptable behavior of members and

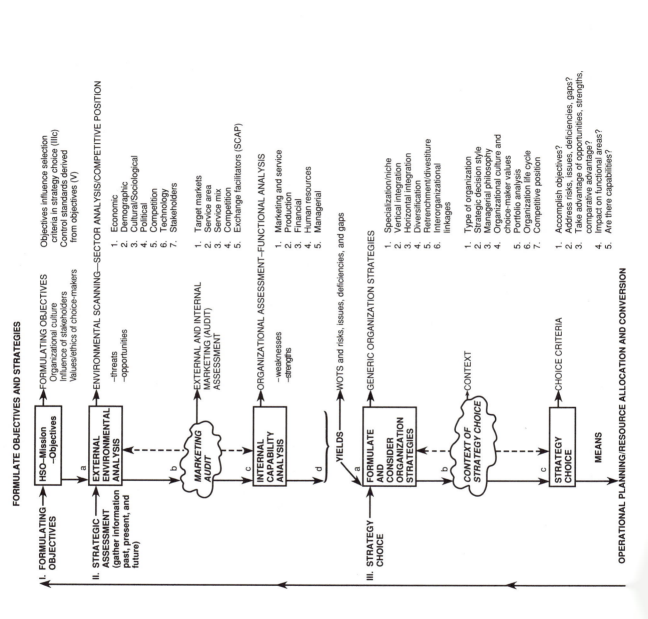

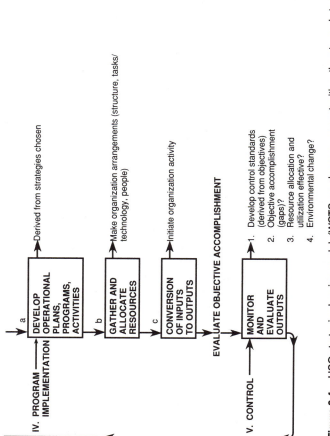

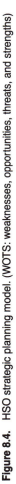

Figure 8.4. HSO strategic planning model. (WOTS: weaknesses, opportunities, threats, and strengths)

depicts the desired nature of relationships between the HSO and its stakeholders, including customers and employees. Objectives must be consistent with mission, culture, and the derived relationship with others as reflected by the culture. If the culture is incompatible with mission and mission-oriented objectives, it must be changed. If objectives are inconsistent with mission and mission-oriented culture, the objectives must be changed.

Stakeholders   Stakeholders are those constituents with a vested interest in the affairs, actions, and objectives of the HSO. They are individuals, groups, or organizations affected by the HSO who may seek to influence it and its objectives. In Chapter 1, three types of stakeholders were identified: internal stakeholders, such as employees; interface stakeholders, such as patients and members of the professional staff organization; and external stakeholders, such as third-party payors, government, and the community at large. Figure 8.5 shows the multiple stakeholders and the nature of their relationships for a large U.S. hospital—most of whom would be stakeholders for other forms of HSOs.*

Each stakeholder group and subgroup may have interests and demands that conflict with those of others and may seek to influence the HSO's priorities and objectives. As new objectives are established by the governing body or the emphasis on existing objectives is changed, these stakeholders will seek to influence the outcome. It is the governing body's responsibility to balance stakeholder demands and ensure that they are compatible with the HSO's mission. Balancing requires maintaining ethical values and social responsibility and preventing inappropriate stakeholder demands from predominating.[42]

Values and Ethics   Establishing new objectives or modifying present objectives requires choice—a decision by one person or a group. Almost always it is the governing body that makes this choice. Just as culture and stakeholders influence objectives, so, too, do the values and ethics of those who make the choice.

Final Comments   HSO objectives change for many reasons. New governing body members with different values influence the organization's direction. Other influences include emergence of new, more powerful stakeholders, change brought about internally or imposed externally, or regulation. The primary objectives of Chrysler Corporation in the mid-1980s were profitability and market share; in the early 1990s its objective was survival. Given the turbulent, high-risk environment in which HSOs function, survival is now a primary objective for some. Finally, accomplishing objectives or a change in mission results in a need to reformulate objectives. Eradication of polio caused the mission of the March of Dimes and its objectives to change. Similarly, new medications and treatment for tuberculosis closed many sanitariums and altered the mission of those remaining.

II: Strategic Assessment

Strategic assessment [II] is the heart of strategic planning. Essentially, it involves gathering and evaluating information about the past and present and making assumptions about the future. The two major elements shown in Figure 8.4 include external environment analysis [IIa] and internal capability analysis [IIc]. The marketing audit [IIb] facilitates both. The "yields" or results of assessment [IId] include identifying external environmental threats and opportunities, organizational strengths and weaknesses (called WOTS-UP† analysis), and risks, issues, and deficiencies confronting the HSO. As observed by others in the business sector, principal assessment activities in strategy formulation include:

---

*This figure is also used in Chapter 15, "Communication," to illustrate the complexity of HSO interorganizational communication networks (see Figure 15.6).

†WOTS means weaknesses, opportunities, threats, and strengths. The UP is added only to emphasize the acronym. Some refer to it as SWOT analysis.

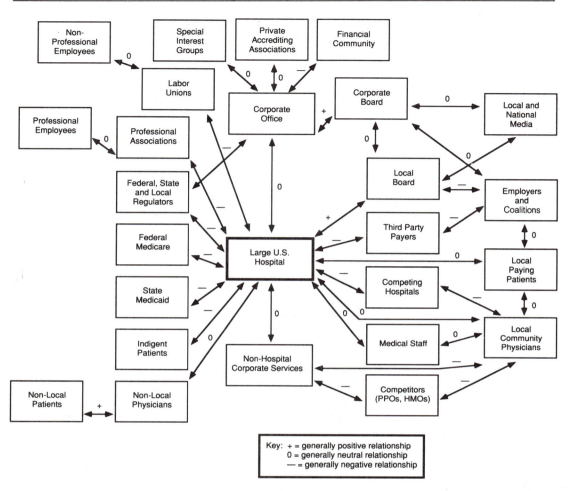

Key: + = generally positive relationship
0 = generally neutral relationship
— = generally negative relationship

Figure 8.5. Stakeholders in a large hospital. (From Fottler, Myron D., John D. Blair, Carlton J. Whitehead, Michael D. Laus, and Grant T. Savage. Assessing key stakeholders: Who matters to hospitals and why? *Hospital & Health Services Administration* 34 [Winter 1989]: 530; reprinted by permission. © 1989, Foundation of the American College of Healthcare Executives.)

identifying opportunities and threats in the company's environment and attaching some estimate of risk to the discernible alternatives. Before choice can be made, the company's strengths and weaknesses should be appraised together with the resources on hand and available. Its actual or potential capacity to take advantage of perceived market needs or to cope with attendant risks should be estimated as objectively as possible.[43]

External Environmental Analysis [IIa]   Environmental scanning to identify external threats and opportunities is critical to strategy formulation and choice. Threats in the environment are events that may adversely affect the HSO. Examples include competition and alternate forms of delivery; change in third-party reimbursement; change in target market demographics and health status; new technologies; changes in accreditation, regulation, and licensure; and status of the economy.

Opportunities are favorable or advantageous circumstances in the external environment that may benefit the HSO. They include changing demographics and service patterns; decline in primary care physicians in a rural area, which enables a hospital to open a family practice center; altering of a reimbursement policy to cover preadmission testing; and changes in federal law. In part, opportunity evaluation includes a market assessment of present services and gaps (heart disease, trauma, perinatology) in service and clientele served.

Sector analysis is one way in which systematic environmental analysis can be peformed and threats and opportunities identified.[44] Among the important sectors are:

Economic: recession, business cycle, capital availability, unemployment (with loss of third-party health insurance), business flight

Demographic: changes in service area or target market numbers, age, income, location, health status, public health, rise of communicable disease

Cultural/sociological: respect or disrespect for authority, attitudes of employees about work, sexual mores, personal ethics

Political: health care as an actual or perceived right, public policy and federal fiscal responsibility for health care, regulation

Competition: barriers to entry or exit, new providers, financial incentives, new delivery arrangements

Technology and support: health personnel, medical education and research, cost and pace of technological development

Stakeholders: their power and influence, their relative importance to the HSO, and their demands

Competitive position is also part of external environmental assessment. While not focusing on global sectors such as the state of the economy or public policy, it focuses on the HSO's position relative to competitors. Components evaluated include:[45]

Nature of competition Is it docile/cooperative or aggressive/uncooperative in nature?

Threat of potential entrants Are other competitors likely to expand products and services in the service area, or are there are barriers to entry? Barriers to entry are economies of scale, switching costs for consumers, capital requirements, access to important factors of production such as physicians and staff, and the image/reputation (i.e., brand identification) of existing HSOs.

Threat of substitute products New technologies such as magnetic resonance imaging may surpass an HSO's existing technology (computed tomography). New organizational forms, such as a managed care organization that uses preferred providers, may cause an HSO to take a defensive posture or come under severe economic pressure.

Power of suppliers and buyers An HSO (supplier of health services) has power if it is dominant in a market with barriers to entry, its services are specialized, and there are few substitute products or services. A buyer (customer or third-party payor of care) is powerful if it purchases in large volumes, such as a managed care organization; the services it purchases are undifferentiated (lab tests); or the cost of switching to another provider (supplier) is low.

The degree to which external environmental analysis—composed of sector analysis and competitive position—identifies threats and opportunities significantly influences the scope and quality of organization strategies the HSO considers and ultimately chooses. Absence of such analysis amplifies the HSO's risk.

Marketing Audit [IIb] The marketing audit is a systematic evaluation of target markets and their needs. It is an environmental link, and such evaluation facilitates strategic planning environmental analysis. To examine target markets means using many of the environmental components of sector analysis. Consequently, information pertaining to service area, target market, competition, and appropriateness of exchange facilitators (SCAP) is an integral part of strategic planning.

Internal Capability Analysis [IIc]   Internal capability analysis[46] concerns assessing the HSO's strengths and weaknesses, and drawing inferences about comparative advantage or, as some have called it, distinctive competence. Organization strengths include referral patterns, reputation for quality, cost efficiency, qualifications and stature of clinical staff and other professionals, resource (financial) availability, the range and types of products and services provided, a cohesive culture, and proactive management. Weaknesses may include shortage of capital, outdated physical plant and equipment, hostile labor environment, poor reputation, aging or decreasing numbers of physicians, or reactive management.

Functional area analysis is one method by which systematic internal capability analysis can be performed to identify strengths and weaknesses.[47] Among those functional areas analyzed are:

Marketing and service: includes service area, target markets, reputation, specialization, image, barriers to market entry, breadth and depth of service, market share, access, and clinical staff

Production: composed of work processes and methods, cost of production, tasks-technology relationships, and equipment and facility size, capacity, and age

Financial: patient-payor mix, capital structure, leverage, reserves, accounting and billing systems, and earnings

Human resources: quality of personnel skills, attitudes, compensation, stability of employment, productivity, and labor relations

Managerial: quality, skills, perspective, experience, values, ethics, philosophy, and effectiveness

Awareness of an HSO's strengths in all functional areas permits conclusions about comparative advantage. Some of these conclusions specify its particular skills, where it excels compared to other HSOs, and how it can be differentiated. Is the HSO the lowest cost producer? Does it have the best reputation? Is it on the cutting edge of technology application? Comparative advantage is a barrier to entry that other HSOs must overcome in order to compete. Information about comparative advantage, strengths, and weaknesses allows consideration of organization strategies that capitalize on the first two and mitigate the latter.

Yields [IId]   The systematic appraisal and evaluation of an HSO through external environmental analysis [IIa] and internal capability analysis [IIc] identifies external threats and opportunities facing the HSO as well as internal strengths and weaknesses and comparative advantage. WOTS-UP analysis enables managers to identify risks facing the HSO, issues confronting it, organizational deficiencies, and gaps in objectives. Gaps in objectives are the difference or discrepancy between actual and desired results[48] and are partially derived from the control [IV] portion of Figure 8.4. Are objectives being met, and will they be met in the future? The degree to which a gap exists, or is likely to exist, along with identification of WOTS, risks, issues, and deficiencies, influences what strategies are considered and chosen.

III: Strategy Choice

Figure 8.4 indicates that strategy choice includes formulation of organization strategies for consideration [IIIa] and choice of one or more strategies relative to criteria [IIIc]. Both are done within a particular context [IIIb].

Formulate and Consider Strategies [IIIa]   At any given time, an array of organization strategies can be identified, evaluated, chosen, and concurrently implemented by HSOs to achieve objectives. Seldom does an HSO implement only one strategy; it usually implements a combination. Strategies are extensively discussed in the literature, which uses several typologies.[49] The generic organization strategies discussed here appear in Figure 8.4 [IIIa]:

Specialization/niche by product/service and/or market

Vertical integration, both forward and backward

Horizontal integration

Diversification, both concentric (related or complementary) and conglomerate (unrelated)

Retrenchment (downsizing) or divestiture

Interorganizational linkages (joint ventures, mergers and consolidations, and multiorganizational arrangements)

In order to categorize and describe organization strategies, two important points must be made. First, the categorization of strategy is always relative to the frame of reference of the HSO—that is, its core products and services. For example, adding a full-line family practice center would be categorized as related diversification for an acute care hospital (if the center were freestanding in a different geographic or market area it would also be categorized as vertical integration), but adding a related service to become a full-line family practice center would be horizontal integration in the case of a physician group practice. The second point is that HSOs seldom choose and implement only one strategy; it is common for multiple organization strategies to be implemented concurrently.

Specialization/Niche   Specialization is an organization strategy in which HSOs focus on or emphasize selected products or services, often based on disease or acuity of illness. Some hospitals, for example, are known for their specialization in oncology, organ transplantation, and cardiac surgery; nursing facilities specialize in chronic care; hospices specialize in care of the dying. A niche strategy involves focusing on a service area, such as the inner city, or target market, such as ambulatory outpatients. Both strategies are usually implemented in tandem—as in the case of a pediatric hospital that specializes by type of care (neonatal) and has a niche in a specific target market (children)—and may involve differentiation based on low-cost, high-technology leadership.

Vertical Integration   The organization strategy of vertical integration occurs when an HSO operates at more than one point on a chain of production and/or distribution.[50] Conrad and Dowling describe vertical integration as a "broad range of patient care and support services operated in a functionally unified manner."[51] Brown and McCool define vertical integration as adding upstream or downstream services.[52] The concept of vertical integration may also be based on the patient's acuity of illness, which can range from acute to chronic. Examples of forward integration for an acute care hospital would be ambulatory care, satellite family practice clinics, and wellness promotion.[53] Backward integration includes long-term care and rehabilitation.

Integration may also occur in nonservice areas—that is, in factors of production that involve make/buy decisions.[54] In this instance it is backward integration. Examples are the development or acquisition of businesses that provide contracted housekeeping or data processing services for the HSO, or those that supply or manufacture generic pharmaceuticals, prosthetic devices, and intravenous solutions used by a hospital.[55]

Horizontal Integration   Horizontal integration in health services, in contrast to vertical integration, is an organization strategy in which an HSO expands its core products or services at the same point in the production process and in the same part of the industry. This is usually done to round out product/service lines and to enter new markets. Horizontal integration may be achieved through internal development, acquisition, or merger. An acute care hospital that adds coronary bypass surgery to its existing surgical services or that builds a suburban acute care facility is horizontally integrating. Multihospital systems and nursing facility chains, in which member facilities offer the same core products/services, are horizontally integrated, and they most often use this strategy to reach new markets and to achieve economies of scale for support and management services, enhance access to capital, and lower overall corporate risk. Horizontally linked HSOs may be closely coupled through ownership or loosely coupled through affiliations.

Diversification Diversification is an organization strategy in which HSOs add new products/services and/or enter new markets.[56] Diversification is usually defined relative to 1) the organization's traditional main line of business and/or core services, and 2) whether the activity is related or unrelated.[57] For acute care hospitals, diversification includes adding new non–inpatient-care products/services,[58] such as industrial medicine, women's medicine, and wellness programs, and/or non–acute-care activities, such as rehabilitation and substance abuse treatment.[59]

There are two types of diversification: concentric and conglomerate. *Concentric* diversification occurs when different *but related* health care products/services are added to the existing core of services. This may be done to increase revenues[60] or to enhance competitive position and reach new target markets. Depending on frame of reference (i.e., the HSO's core services and position on the "stage of illness" scale), concentric diversification may *also* constitute forward or backward integration. For example, an acute care hospital that diversifies into long-term care by converting acute care beds is also engaging in backward integration;[61] establishing a freestanding diagnostic center is forward integration.

The second form of diversification is *conglomerate* diversification. Here an HSO produces non–health-related products or services that are *unrelated* to the HSO's principal business or core services. An example is a hospital providing laundry or computer services to other organizations; investing in real estate, such as shopping centers, homes, apartments; or providing catering services. Concentric diversification is the most common form for HSOs; few engage in conglomerate diversification.

Retrenchment/Divestiture A strategy of retrenchment, or downsizing, involves reducing the scope or intensity of products and services, partial withdrawal from a market area, or decreasing capacity in terms of facilities, equipment, or staff. A divestiture is eliminating products or services, withdrawing from a market area, or closing facilities. In highly competitive markets in which the HSO has no comparative advantage or in instances in which demand has decreased, an HSO may implement a strategy of retrenchment—in extreme cases, divestiture. The more commonly implemented strategy is retrenchment. This reduces losses, permits reallocation of resources to more promising services, and, in extreme cases, enables the HSO to survive. Declining birth rates caused some hospitals to downsize obstetrics; high levels of uncompensated care led others to close (divest) trauma centers; low inpatient occupancy rates caused others to reduce the number of acute care beds (retrenchment) while simultaneously increasing beds in long-term or rehabilitative care (diversifying).

Interorganizational Linkages Joint ventures, mergers and consolidations, and multiorganizational systems have become prevalent arrangements in health services delivery. For the most part these interorganizational relationships are of recent origin and represent an organization strategy that is usually coupled with one or more of those previously described: joint ventures can be coupled with vertical and horizontal integration and/or diversification strategies; multiorganizational system arrangements can be coupled with specialization, integration, and even retrenchment strategies. Chapter 9 focuses on voluntary and involuntary forms of interorganizational relationships.

Context of Strategy Choice [III b] The range of alternative organization strategies considered and those eventually selected is greatly influenced by the context in which choice is made. While there are other classifications of context, the focus here is on those identified in Figure 8.4 [III b] and Figure 8.6.

Type of organization
Strategic decision style
Managerial philosophy
Organizational culture and choice-maker values
Portfolio analysis

Organizational life cycle
Competitive position

Type of Organization   Type of organization refers to self-image and how the HSO adapts. Organization types may be described as defender, prospector, or reactor.[62] A defender organization seeks to maintain the status quo and stability and is not innovative. Generally, such HSOs vigorously protect what they have, such as a niche or specialized product/service domain.[63] Prospector organizations occasionally redefine markets, seek new target markets, seize the initiative and capitalize on opportunities, and are proactive. They tend to be innovative and at the forefront of applying new technologies. Reactor organizations may not have a clear sense of direction and are "seriously out of stride with environmental or competitive change."[64] They are passive and usually only stir to action in a crisis or when external environmental forces can no longer be ignored.

Strategic Decision Style   Strategic decision style describes the process by which organization strategic alternatives are formulated and evaluated and decisions are made. It can be classified as systematic, entrepreneurial, or incremental.[65] A systematic strategic decision style is pro-

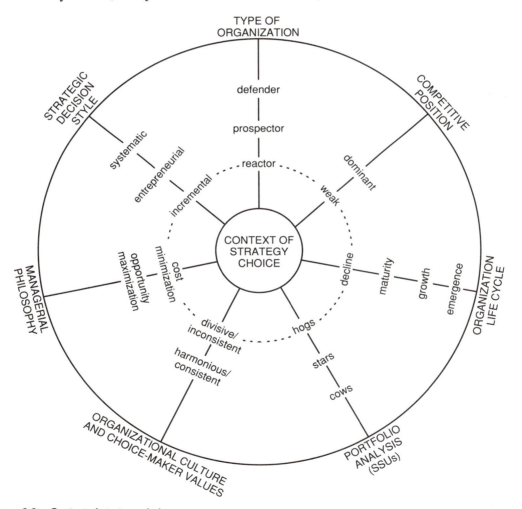

Figure 8.6.   Context of strategy choice.

active. It involves comprehensive external and internal analysis; understanding interrelationships of threats, opportunities, strengths, and weaknesses; considering all strategic alternatives; and selecting an organization strategy on the basis of rational criteria. Entrepreneurial strategic decision style has been described as "gut feel," hunch, or intuition. It generally does not include full and comprehensive strategic assessment, only selected review; thus, it is more accurately described as a style in which strategic decisions are made carefully but quickly. In mature HSOs and industries, entrepreneurial decision style is generally inappropriate. However, it may be appropriate for emerging HSOs or mature HSOs in a turbulent, fast-changing environment, especially if windows of opportunity rapidly close, thus making quick decision making an imperative. Incremental strategic decision style is generally reactive and usually involves change at the margin. Sometimes it means simply muddling through. It is a piecemeal approach to strategy choice and does not include comprehensive, systematic strategic assessment or reviewing and evaluating a full range of strategies.

Managerial Philosophy   Managerial philosophy in the context of strategy choice is best described as a continuum ranging from opportunity maximization to cost minimization. The former is a proactive, prospector, systematic/entrepreneurial perspective. It implies that organization strategies are chosen to take advantage of opportunities and capitalize on strengths. Cost minimization as a philosophy implies conservatism. It may be consistent with a defender HSO, but certainly is so with a reactor HSO. It implies a focus on "how we can save a buck" without considering opportunity costs. While no organization is entirely at one end of the continuum, organizations can generally be located somewhere between the ends of the dichotomy, usually closer to one end or the other. Other similar descriptive terms are aggressive-innovative versus lethargic-conservative or risk taking versus risk averse. HSOs that are opportunity maximizers, aggressors-innovators, and risk takers usually consider and choose different strategies than those at the other end of the continuum.

Organizational Culture and Choice-Maker Values   Organizational culture and the values of decision makers (choice makers) are contextual variables from which the choice of strategies cannot be divorced. Organizational culture is a continuum from harmonious to divisive, and the values of choice makers can be consistent or inconsistent with culture. Cultural disarray— perhaps caused by splintered factions, internal hostility, and a lack of cohesion, mutual support, and shared beliefs—leads to divisiveness in the HSO. In such circumstances, it may be impossible to gain the commitment of participants to implement complex strategies and weather the resulting organizational change.[66] Mismatching culture and strategy translates into implementation difficulties.[67] This restricts the range of realistic strategies.

As Bower and colleagues observe, "strategy is a human construction; it must in the long run be responsive to human needs. It must ultimately inspire commitment. It must stir an organization to successful striving against competition. People have to have their hearts in it."[68] HSOs with strong, cohesive cultures and values shared by managers and staff can prospect, be more opportunistic, and successfully implement a wider range of organization strategies than those with a divisive culture and managerial values at variance with the culture. As Digman observes, "What a business is able to accomplish may be determined as much, if not more, by its culture than its strategic plan. Strategies are only as good as the culture that exists to encourage and support them."[69]

Portfolio Analysis   Portfolio analysis is borrowed from marketing and describes and categorizes resource-producing or resource-consuming products and services. The typical nomenclature is cows, hogs, and stars.[70] Cows are product lines or services that yield more than they consume; hogs consume more than they yield; and stars, if fed, will evolve from embryonic resource consumers into cows. Portfolio analysis of product line or service could determine that pharmacy and radiology are cows, obstetrics is a hog, and sports medicine is a star. HSOs with a preponderance of cows and stars are in a better position to prosper and have greater latitude in strategy choice than those with a preponderance of hogs. Portfolio analysis is important to strategy formulation and choice because it allows choice makers to recognize the cows, hogs, and stars of their HSOs and how alternative strategies may change the ratio of these three categories.

Another variable that affects the context of strategy choice is strategic business unit or, as applied in health services, strategic service unit (SSU) analysis.[71] This type of segmentation is like portfolio analysis except that SSU generally refers to identifiable, relatively autonomous organizational units with distinct product lines and services that are offered to distinct target markets.[72] SSUs have reasonable control over their activities, are separate from other SSUs, compete with external groups for market share, and have their own revenues and costs.[73] Each hospital in a multiorganizational system is a separate SSU. Pegels and Rogers observe that an HSO that owns two hospitals, an HMO, and a nursing facility could segment them into four SSUs.[74] SSUs are important to the context of strategy choice because distinct and even different strategies may be chosen and implemented for each.

Organization Life Cycle   Organization life cycle refers to the stage of development of an organization. Conceptually, organization life cycle borrows from theories of aging for human beings and product life cycle as applied in marketing. All organizations go through stages of emergence, growth, maturity, decline, and perhaps regeneration, although the time span varies. Figure 8.7 presents this concept graphically, and Table 8.4 describes the stages of the organization life cycle as applied to industrial organizations.

It is important to note that external or internal events (changing technology, competition) can increase or decrease the slope of the life cycle curve, lengthen its line, and enable the HSO to regenerate from one stage (maturity) to another (growth) or accelerate from one stage (maturity) to another (decline). Depending on where the HSO is in its life cycle, the context of strategy choice differs. Those in the growth stage may choose aggressive, expansionary-type strategies such as forward and horizontal integration and concentric diversification. They are likely to be prospectors and opportunity maximizers. Those in decline will likely be forced to retrench and minimize cost.

Competitive Position   The feasible set of organization strategies that an HSO can consider is partially predicated on its competitive position. Barriers to market entry, threat of new entrants (competitors), availability of substitute products or services, and the HSO's strength as a seller or buyer are attributes of competitive position. Table 8.5 presents a competitive position/product life cycle matrix that suggests strategic behavior for each cell. These behaviors are determined by the strength of the HSO's competitive position and the position of its products/services in the product life cycle.[75] An HSO with a mature service in a dominant position, such as acute inpatient care, would seek to hold its market share and grow with the industry. One in a weak competitive position, but with a growth service such as cardiac surgery, could choose to make a substantial resource commitment (turnaround) to strengthen competitive position or abandon that service and redirect those resources.

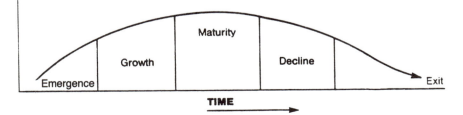

Figure 8.7. Life cycle of an HSO.

Table 8.4. Life cycle of an organization

Emergence	There is almost invariably a shortage of liquid cash, a need to create consumer demand, and a need to expand production to meet this demand. Administrative processes are loosely defined and a flexible use of labor reduces dependence on more costly specialized personnel.
Growth	A point is reached where major refinancing becomes necessary and there may be some acquisitions as well. Extensions are made to the basic product line and overseas markets are evaluated. At the same time as new plants and machinery are purchased, control systems are strengthened and formal personnel policies instituted.
Maturity	Initially investments produce high returns, but over time higher unit production costs and overhead cut in. There is a tendency to become very conservative in marketing and to sacrifice opportunities. Unit production costs are increasingly affected by declining economies of scale and obsolescence of equipment. Conformity rather than individuality is rewarded and labor problems increase.
Regeneration	If regeneration occurs, it may be internal or external. Internally a company may divest itself of unprofitable subsidiaries, sell off assets, resort to rigid cost cutting, reduce labor use, and close some production lines. There is an attempt to reverse the decline in sales and profits of existing products and introduce new, profitable products. External regeneration may involve sacrificing a controlling interest, merger, being completely acquired, or government assistance.
Decline	As internal reserves are depleted, external financing becomes more difficult. The company is selling products that few want at excessive prices. Equipment becomes obsolete, production costs skyrocket, key personnel leave, and labor becomes increasingly militant.

Reprinted by permission of Macmillan Publishing Company from *Management policy and strategy* by George A. Steiner, John B. Miner, and Edmund R. Gray. Copyright © 1986 Macmillan Publishing Co.

Table 8.5. Competitive position/product life cycle matrix

Strength of competitive position	Life-Cycle Stage			
	Embryonic	Growth	Maturity	Aging
Dominant	Hold position All-out push for share	Hold position Hold share	Hold position Grow with industry	Hold position
Strong	Attempt to improve position All-out push for share	Attempt to improve position Push for share	Hold position Grow with industry	Hold position or harvest
Favorable	Selectively attempt to improve position Selective or all-out push for share	Attempt to improve position Selective push for share	Custodial or maintenance Find niche and attempt to protect it	Harvest Phased withdrawal
Tentative	Selectively push for position	Find niche and protect it	Find niche and hang on Phased withdrawal	Phased withdrawal or abandon
Weak	Up or out	Turnaround or abandon	Turnaround or phased withdrawal	Abandon

As adapted from Peter Patel and Michael Younger, "A Frame for Strategy Development," *Long-Range Planning II* (April 1978) p. 8. From Digman, Lester A. *Strategic management: Concepts, decisions, and cases*, 2d ed., 221. Homewood, IL: BPI/Irwin, 1990.

Strategy Choice [IIIc] In choosing organization strategies, the major context variables that influence choice are type of organization, strategic decision style, managerial philosophy, organizational culture and choice-maker values, portfolio analysis, organization life cycle, and competitive position. Specific criteria used in selecting strategies are presented in Figure 8.4 [IIIc]. Some of these are: Will the organization strategy accomplish objectives? Will the strategy address risks, issues, and deficiencies? Will the strategy take advantage of opportunities in the environment and capitalize on HSO strengths and comparative advantage? Will the strategy lessen threats and overcome weaknesses? In addition, attention must be given to the effect the organization strategy selected will have on functional areas of the HSO. That is, considering strengths and weaknesses, is it feasible? Does the HSO have the capacity, financial resources, managerial system and human resources, and productivity and conversion processes necessary to successfully implement the strategy? If so, implementation is the next step. This is depicted in Figure 8.4 [IV].

Once organization strategies are chosen, operational plans, programs, and activities are developed for units or segments of the organization [IV,a]. They are derived from the strategies and must be consistent with them. It is necessary to gather and allocate resources and make organizational arrangements concerning structure, tasks/technology, and people so that, when all are integrated, inputs are converted to outputs [IV,b,c]. Finally, after implementing the strategy or strategies, it is necessary to control. Results must be monitored and evaluated (see Figure 8.4 [V]) to determine if objectives are being accomplished and if resource allocation and utilization are effective. If not, the process begins again (Figure 8.4 [I]). In fact, strategic planning is a process that never ends. There is a reciprocal relationship between strategy formulation and implementation. Both are concurrent and continuous. Even though present strategy(ies) may result in an HSO achieving its objectives, strategic assessment must continue in order to monitor environments—whether and how they are changing and whether and how the HSO should respond.

STAKEHOLDERS AND STRATEGIC PLANNING

Stakeholders, such as those identified in Figure 8.5, can affect HSO strategic planning in two ways: 1) they can influence formulation of organization objectives, and 2) they can be important, even critical, to successful implementation of strategy. Relative to the latter, Blair, Savage, and Whitehead have developed a useful model that suggests tactics for interacting and negotiating with stakeholders based on two conditions: the potential threat to the HSO and the potential for cooperation.[76]

Figure 8.8 presents the HSO tactics of *collaborate, subordinate, compete,* and *avoid negotiating.* They are predicated on: 1) whether the "substantive outcome," such as implementing a diversification or forward integration strategy, is or is not important; and 2) whether the HSO's "relationship outcome" with stakeholders, such as maintaining friendly relations and cooperation, is or is not important. Depending on the HSO's priorities for these outcomes, interaction tactics with stakeholders are suggested. These four tactics appear in the "organizational contingencies" part of the expanded model in Figure 8.9. Adding the element of "stakeholder contingencies" expands the possible HSO tactics for interacting with stakeholders. Questions such as, "Can HSO management ensure stakeholder acceptance?" and "Will likely stakeholder coalitions be acceptable to the organization?" must be answered. For example, if a substantive outcome such as vertical integration is important to the HSO and the relationship outcome with the PSO stakeholder is important, a collaborative tactic (C1) is suggested. Furthermore, if HSO management can ensure stakeholder acceptance of the strategy and the stakeholder is *not* likely to form a coalition that is acceptable to the HSO, then either a cautious collaborative tactic (C2) or respectful competitive tactic (P2) is suggested.

This model assists strategic planning in two ways. First, it allows HSO senior management

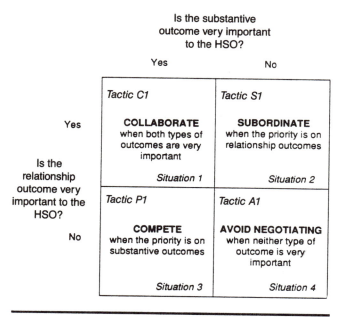

Figure 8.8. Selecting outcome-focused negotiation tactics. (Adapted from Blair, John D., Grant T. Savage, and Carlton J. Whitehead. A strategic approach for negotiating with hospital stakeholders. *Health Care Management Review*, Vol. 14, No. 1, p. 17, with permission of Aspen Publishers, Inc., © 1989.

to assess systematically the potential threat or the potential for cooperation with the myriad of HSO stakeholders. Second, it indicates how the HSO should interact with stakeholders who may have an impact on implementing these strategies.

SUMMARY

This chapter discusses planning with specific focus on strategic planning and its integral component, marketing. Planning is a managerial function defined as anticipating the future, assessing present conditions, and making decisions concerning organizational direction, programs, and resource deployment. The results of planning answer questions of what to do, when, where, how, and for what purpose. Planning is linked to the management model. It helps HSO managers cope with environments; reduce uncertainty, ambiguity, and risk; focus on outputs, develop priorities, design conversion processes, and allocate resources; and control to ensure that organization objectives are accomplished.

Planning characteristics addressed include type of planning, time frame and who plans, and approaches to planning. Figure 8.1 details these classifications. Outcomes of planning are discussed. Included are mission, organization objectives (primary, secondary, and subobjectives), strategies and derived operational programs, and policies and procedures. Figure 8.2 presents their relationships.

Another major section of the chapter focuses on health services marketing and its link to strategic planning. The concept of marketing means determining the needs, wants, and desires of target markets and designing programs, products, and services to satisfy them. The marketing audit is instrumental in identifying and assessing target needs and wants along with elements of marketing to facilitate exchange between buyer/consumer and seller/provider. The traditional elements of marketing (product, price, place, and promotion) are recast and presented in the health service context as service, consideration, access, and promotion (SCAP).

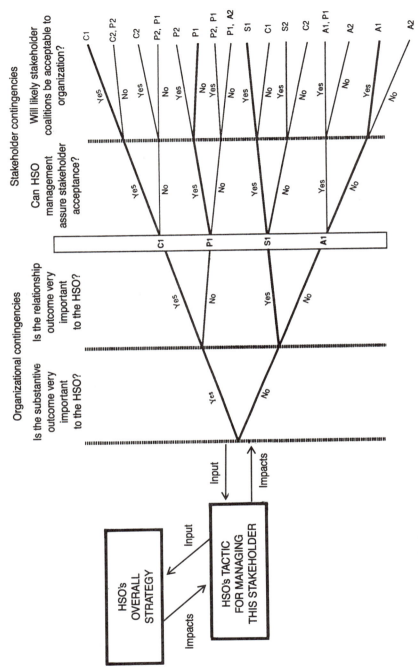

Figure 8.9. Selecting and refining stakeholder negotiation tactics. (Adapted from Blair, John D., Grant T. Savage, and Carlton J. Whitehead. A strategic approach for negotiating with hospital stakeholders. *Health Care Management Review*, Vol. 14, No. 1, p. 19, with permission of Aspen Publishers, Inc., © 1989.

The final section focuses on HSO strategic planning: 1) formulating HSO objectives, and 2) identifying, evaluating, choosing, and implementing organization strategies and operational programs to accomplish objectives. Organization strategies are defined as long-term patterns of activities requiring substantial commitment of resources; they are the means by which organization objectives are accomplished. Organizational culture and values of choice makers are discussed.

An HSO strategic planning model is presented in Figure 8.4. The strategic assessment component includes external environmental analysis, which identifies threats and opportunities; internal capability analysis, which identifies weaknesses and strengths; and the marketing audit, which links them. The results of strategic assessment yield information about the HSO's WOTS, risks, issues, deficiencies, and objective gaps.

The strategy choice component of the strategic planning model addresses three elements: formulation and consideration of strategies, strategy choice, and the context of strategy choice. The generic organization strategies discussed are classified as specialization/niche, vertical and horizontal integration, diversification, retrenchment/divestiture, and interorganizational linkages. In review of the context of strategy choice, the following components are examined: type of organization, strategic decision style, managerial philosophy, organizational culture and choice-maker values, portfolio analysis, organization life cycle, and competitive position.

DISCUSSION QUESTIONS

1. Define planning. How is it related to the management model (see Figure 1.6)?
2. Identify and describe the characteristics of planning.
3. Identify the outcomes of planning and discuss how they are interrelated.
4. What is health services marketing? What is the difference between contemporary health services marketing and that of 2 decades ago?
5. Identify and discuss the elements of marketing.
6. Define strategic planning. Be prepared to discuss the strategic assessment components identified in Figure 8.4. How does the marketing audit relate to strategic assessment?
7. Identify and give examples of generic organization strategies for HSOs. How does context of strategy choice affect consideration and selection of strategy? Give examples.
8. Identify an HSO. Describe a situation in which the substantive and relationship outcomes were important to the HSO, and a CI tactic with a stakeholder was suggested (refer to Figures 8.8 and 8.9).

CASE STUDY 1:   HOSPITAL MARKETING EFFECTIVENESS RATING INSTRUMENT[77]

The following instrument is to be completed by you. Choose a hospital. Circle the one most appropriate answer (A, B, or C) for each question below.

Customer Philosophy

1. How does the organization view its markets?
   A. Hospital management thinks in terms of serving patient needs based on the facilities and clinical staff currently available.
   B. Management attempts to offer a broad range of hospital services, performing all of them well.
   C. Management thinks in terms of serving the needs of well-defined patient and physician segments that offer to the hospital the best prospect for long-term growth and financial return.

2. What is the status of the hospital's publicity, promotion, and community education programs?
   A. There is limited activity in this area.
   B. The hospital has a number of programs in this area, but coordination among them is limited.
   C. The hospital has a well-coordinated program of information and community outreach efforts, all under the guidance of one staff member.
3. How does the hospital attract and retain the clinical staff?
   A. Primary responsibility for selection and attraction of staff resides with current staff members.
   B. The hospital relies essentially on specific incentives such as high salaries or special equipment to attract new members.
   C. As part of the planning and coordination process, the hospital has developed a comprehensive system to determine and influence the factors affecting the PSO affiliation decision.

Integrated Marketing Organization

4. Is there a vice-president or director of marketing responsible for planning, executing, and coordinating the marketing functions?
   A. No such individual exists.
   B. Yes, but there is little integration of this individual within the planning/decision-making process. This individual primarily provides marketing services.
   C. Yes, and the individual participates in hospital policy making as well as providing marketing services.
5. To what extent are marketing-oriented functions (e.g., planning, public relations, marketing research, advertising, promotion and fundraising) coordinated in the hospital?
   A. Not very well. There is sometimes unproductive conflict among these functions.
   B. Somewhat. There is some formal integration, but less than satisfactory coordination and control.
   C. Very well. There is effective coordination and control of these functions.
6. Is there a formal systematic procedure for evaluating potential new services and technologies?
   A. There is no formal procedure.
   B. A procedure exists, but it does not include heavy inputs from marketing.
   C. The procedure is well developed, and includes heavy inputs from marketing.

Marketing Information System

7. Does the hospital conduct patient exit interviews and other surveys of patient satisfaction and suggestions?
   A. Rarely or never
   B. Occasionally, but not on a formal basis
   C. Yes, systematically, on a formal basis
8. Does the hospital collect information regarding trends in demand for various types of treatments and the availability in the market of competitive services?
   A. Rarely or never
   B. Occasionally
   C. Yes, on a systematic, continuous basis
9. Does the hospital have an information system containing relevant and up-to-date marketing data?

A. Such information is limited, and is not maintained on an ongoing basis.
B. Adequate records are maintained and updated on a routine basis, essentially in hard-copy form.
C. An extensive, computer based information system is provided for systematic storage, maintenance, update and analysis of marketing data.

Strategic Orientation

10. Does the hospital regularly monitor and evaluate patient services in order to identify potential new services to offer and current services to curtail or drop?
    A. The hospital does not evaluate the marketing viability of its various services.
    B. The hospital occasionally evaluates its current services and studies potential new services.
    C. The hospital regularly evaluates its current services and systematically studies potential new services.
11. Does the hospital carry out strategic market planning as well as annual marketing planning?
    A. Strategic market planning is only initiated under special circumstances such as when considering facility expansion or debt financing.
    B. Strategic market planning is carried out regularly but is not done very well.
    C. Strategic market planning is carried out regularly and is done very well.
12. Does the hospital prepare contingency plans?
    A. No
    B. Contingency plans are occasionally developed to meet a major threat.
    C. Contingency plans are routinely developed as part of the normal planning process.
13. Does hospital management know the costs and profitability of its various services?
    A. Such information is not available.
    B. Limited information is available.
    C. Hospital management knows the costs and profitability of its various services.
14. Are marketing resources utilized effectively on a day-to-day basis?
    A. Such resources are either not available or are inadequately utilized.
    B. The resources are adequate and utilized to a significant extent, but not in an optimal manner.
    C. Yes. Such resources are employed adequately and effectively.
15. Does management examine the results of its marketing expenditures to know what it is accomplishing for its money?
    A. No
    B. To a limited extent
    C. Yes

Scoring

For all of the 15 questions, indicate the number of:

A responses   _____ × 0 = _____
B responses   _____ × 1 = _____
C responses   _____ × 2 = _____

Total Score   _____

The following scale shows the hospital's level of marketing effectiveness:

0– 5 = None
6–10 = Poor

$11-15$ = Fair
$16-20$ = Good
$21-25$ = Very good
$26-30$ = Superior

Question

1. How does the HSO you evaluated score on the marketing effectiveness rating instrument? If it was low, please explain why.

CASE STUDY 2:   HSO STRATEGIC ASSESSMENT

Assume you are the chief executive officer of an HSO such as a hospital, nursing facility, or HMO. It may be one in your present locale or elsewhere, if details about it are known. Using the strategic planning model as a guide (see Figure 8.4), conduct a strategic assessment including: 1) external environmental analysis, 2) marketing audit, and 3) internal capability analysis.

Questions

1. Compile a detailed list of "strategic assessment" considerations (factors, items, etc.) that are relevant to the HSO selected.
2. List the "yields" (risks, issues, deficiencies, and gaps) confronting the HSO.
3. Attempt to identify and describe past and present generic (and other) organization strategies the HSO has implemented or is implementing.
4. Are you aware that any of the "context of strategy choice" variables are present in the situation? If so, describe them and discuss the reasons that they are applicable.

CASE STUDY 3:   CLOSING PEDIATRICS

Your hospital has a pediatric department with 35 beds. For the past several years the occupancy has varied between 40% and 60%. There is a definite downward trend, but it appears to be stabilizing at about 45% occupancy. The low occupancy has caused a financial strain. Other area hospitals are experiencing a similar situation. As a result, several hospitals have proposed forming a community task force to study the situation and determine whether one or more pediatric departments should be closed, thereby increasing occupancy for those remaining. It is hoped that this will reduce costs and increase quality.

Although this proposal may benefit the community as a whole, it raises questions for your hospital. Among them is the effect on two objectives: to provide a full range of quality services and to offer a full range of graduate medical education, including residencies in pediatrics.

Questions

1. What effect would the retrenchment strategy have on your objectives?
2. Who are the stakeholders who influence the decision?
3. Are there other strategies that can be considered by the HSO?
4. Argue against the closure. What reasons support your position?

CASE STUDY 4:   NATIONAL HEALTH INSURANCE

Yesterday, the president signed a bill passed by Congress establishing universal-comprehensive health insurance. It will cover all residents for medically necessary hospital inpatient and outpatient services, physician and other licensed independent practitioner services, and nursing facility care. The National Health Insurance (NHI) program becomes effective 12 months from yesterday.

Funding for the NHI program will be through a national value-added tax. All residents, whether employed or unemployed, are covered by the NHI program from birth to death and there are no beneficiary deductibles or co-payments. State government State Health Insurance Boards (SHIBs) will be the fiscal intermediaries. Private health insurance for covered services will be barred when the NHI program takes effect.

Delivery of services will be private, as before, and will be done through existing providers (e.g., hospitals, nursing facilities, private practitioners). Institutional providers' services and capacities will be frozen in place the day the NHI program begins. They may only be changed (added to or deleted) subject to SHIB approval based on the SHIB's assessment of area needs. Start-up and facility expenditures for approved expansions in services and capabilities will be fully funded by the federal NHI Board through the SHIB.

Amounts paid to all independent providers such as physicians for care rendered to beneficiaries will be fee-for-service. National rates for all services will be determined by the federal NHI Board and will vary in amount only by geographic area based on a market-basket consumer price index. Institutional providers will not be reimbursed on fee-for-service, but will receive annual global budgets that are fixed. These budgets will be determined by each SHIB and will be largely based on capacity, such as type and number of beds. Providers will not be allowed to extra bill patients. Since uninhibited access is an objective of the NHI program, all providers will be required to service all customers who present themselves.

Questions

1. Is the NHI program a threat or an opportunity for providers? Why?
2. If you were a hospital chief executive officer, what organization strategies would you recommend for implementation before the start of the NHI program? What strategies after it begins?
3. Once NHI becomes effective, what changes in stakeholder relations would you predict?

CASE STUDY 5: VIOLATION

Bill Richardson, purchasing department storeroom clerk at Parks Manor, a 200-bed nursing facility, spotted a fire in a difficult-to-reach air shaft. He ran to the nearest call box, turned in the alarm, and asked a nearby employee to stay at the box and direct the fire department to the fire location in shaft No. 2 when they arrived. After grabbing a soda-acid fire extinguisher, he crawled into the air shaft and at considerable risk to himself, because the fire was near electrical wiring, put out the fire. When the fire department arrived, 3 minutes after the alarm was sounded, a smoke-befuddled Richardson was crawling out of the shaft.

Richardson was congratulated and his department head said he would write a commendation report to be attached to his personnel record. Their conversation had scarcely ended when another fire broke out in the vicinity of the air shaft. Acidulated water from the extinguisher had seeped down into a high-voltage junction box, and within moments a severe electrical fire, worse than the one Richardson had put out, was raging. The fire department, with some difficulty, brought the fire under control.

Richardson was censured by the director of maintenance for using the wrong type of fire extinguisher. On the clip that held the soda-acid extinguisher was a large, color-coded placard stating that the extinguisher was not to be used on electrical fires. A carbon dioxide extinguisher, approved for electrical fires, was located near the one Richardson used. "You should leave things to trained personnel!" yelled the maintenance director. "There is a policy that, in case of fire, employees are to activate the nearest alarm, notify their supervisor, see to the safety of patients, and not attempt to extinguish the fire themselves unless specifically trained to do so. Now you have created a real mess!"

Questions

1. Did Richardson violate a policy or a procedure? What is the difference between them?
2. Is something wrong with this (policy) (procedure)? If so, what is it and how can it be corrected?
3. When is it appropriate to deviate from (policy) (procedure)? Can one be ignored with less potential damage to the organization than the other?
4. Should Richardson have been reprimanded? Why or why not?

NOTES

1. Carroll, Lewis. *Alice's adventures in wonderland*, 57. New York: Delacorte Press/Seymour Lawrence, 1978.
2. Higgins, James M. *The management challenge: An introduction to management*, 141. New York: Macmillan Publishing Company, 1991.
3. Pearce, John A., II, and Richard B. Robinson, Jr. *Management*, 12. New York: Random House, 1989; see also Ivancevich, John M., James H. Donnelly, Jr., and James L. Gibson. *Management principles and functions*, 4th ed., 68. Homewood, IL: BPI/Irwin, 1989.
4. Kaluzny, Arnold D., D. Michael Warner, David G. Warren, and William N. Zelman. *Management of health services*, 8. Englewood Cliffs, NJ: Prentice Hall, Inc., 1982.
5. Higgins, *Management challenge*, 141.
6. Pearce and Robinson, *Management*, 167–168.
7. Ashmos, Donde P., and Reuben R. McDaniel. Physician's role in hospital strategic decision making. *Health Texas* 45 (December 1989): 7; Clemenhagen, Carol, and Francois Champagne. Medical staff involvement in strategic planning. *Hospital & Health Services Administration* 29 (July/August 1984): 82; Kovner, Anthony R., and Martin J. Chin. Physician leadership in hospital strategic decision making. *Hospital & Health Services Administration* 30 (November/December 1985): 73.
8. McManis, Gerald L. The board's role in strategic planning. *Healthcare Executive* 5 (September/October 1990): 22.
9. Peters, Joseph P. *A strategic planning process for hospitals*, 36. Chicago: American Hospital Publishing, Inc., 1985.
10. Scotti, Dennis J. Cultural factors in choosing a strategic posture: A bridge between formulation and implementation. In *Strategic management of the health care sector: Toward the year 2000*, edited by Farhad Simyar and Joseph Lloyd-Jones, 152. Englewood Cliffs, NJ: Prentice Hall, 1988.
11. Gibson, C. Kendrick, David J. Newton, and Daniel S. Cochran. An empirical investigation of hospital mission statements. *Health Care Management Review* 15 (Summer 1990): 35.
12. Georgopoulos, Basis S., and Floyd C. Mann. *The community general hospital*, 5. New York: Macmillan Publishing Co., Inc., 1962.
13. American Hospital Association. *Evaluating diversification strategies: Management advisory*, 3. Chicago: American Hospital Association, 1990.
14. Pearce and Robinson, *Management*, 249–250.
15. See Ivancevich, Donnelly, and Gibson, *Management principles*, 87–88.
16. Shortell, Stephen M., Ellen M. Morrison, and Susan Hughes. The keys to successful diversification: Lessons from leading hospital systems. *Hospital & Health Services Administration* 43 (Winter 1989): 472.
17. For an excellent tabular presentation of a contemporary typology for hospitals, ambulatory group practices, nursing facilities, and health departments relative to thirteen attributes including external environment, mission and goals, technology, complexity of structure, task specialization, and nature of manager-physician relations, see Stephen M. Shortell, and Arnold D. Kaluzny. *Health care management: A text in organization theory and behavior* 16. New York: John Wiley & Sons, 1988.
18. Kaiser, Leland R. Survival strategies for not-for-profit hospitals. *Hospital Progress* 64 (December, 1983): 43.
19. MacStravic, Robin E. The end of health care marketing. *Health Marketing Quarterly* 7 (1990): 3.
20. Winston, William J. *How to write a marketing plan for health care organizations*, 2. New York: The Haworth Press, 1985.
21. For myths about marketing in HSOs, see Kotler, Philip, and Roberta N. Clarke. *Marketing for health care organizations*, 2d ed., 22–25. Englewood Cliffs, NJ: Prentice Hall, Inc., 1987.
22. Cooper, Philip D. Marketing from inside out. In *Health care marketing: Issues and trends,* edited by Philip D. Cooper, 2d ed., 109. Rockville, MD: Aspen Systems Corporation, 1985.
23. Kotler and Clarke, *Marketing for health*, 4.
24. Seidel, Lee F., John W. Seavey, and Richard J.A. Lewis. *Strategic management for healthcare organizations*, 36. Owings Mills, MD: National Health Publishing/AUPHA Press, 1989.
25. Kotler and Clarke, *Marketing for health*, 90.
26. Keith, Jon G. Marketing health care: What the recent literature is telling us. In *Health care marketing: Issues and trends,* edited by Philip D. Cooper, 2d ed., 16. Rockville, MD: Aspen Systems Corporation, 1985.
27. Kotler and Clarke, *Marketing for health*, 45–53; MacStravic, Robin E. *Marketing health care*, 4. Germantown, MD: Aspen Systems Corporation, 1977.
28. Cooper, Philip D. *Health care marketing: issues and trends,* 2d ed., 6. Rockville, MD: Aspen Systems Corporation, 1985.
29. Kotler and Clarke, *Marketing for health*, 5. For similar definitions of the marketing concept, see Cooper, Philip D. What is health care marketing? In *Health care marketing: Issues and trends,* edited by Philip D. Cooper, 3. Rockville, MD: Aspen Systems Corporation, 1985; Keith, Marketing health, 15–16; MacStravic, Robin E. *Marketing religious health care*, 1. St.Louis: The Catholic Health Association of the United States, 1987; and Winston, *How to write*, 3.
30. See Berkowitz, Eric N., and William A. Flexner. The

marketing audit: A tool for health services organizations. In *Health care marketing: Issues and trends,* edited by Philip D. Cooper, 2d ed., 130–131. Rockville, MD: Aspen Systems Corporation, 1985; Schlinger, Mary Jane. Marketing audits for health organizations: A practical guide. *Hospital & Health Services Administration* 26 (Special Issue II, 1981): 32–50; MacStravic, Robin E. *Marketing by objectives for hospitals,* chpt. 1. Germantown, MD: Aspen Systems Corporation, 1980.

31. Zelman, William N., and Deborah L. Parham. Strategic, operational, and marketing concerns of product-line management in health care. *Health Care Management Review* 15 (Winter 1990): 29.

32. The literature refers to these activities as strategic marketing. See Hillestad, Steven G., and Eric N. Berkowitz. *Health care marketing plans: From strategy to action,* chpt. 3. Homewood, IL: Dow Jones-Irwin, 1984; MacStravic, *Marketing by objectives,* chpts. 5 and 6; Malhotra, Naresh K. Hospital marketing in the changing health care environment. *Journal of Health Care Marketing* 6 (September 1986): 38–41; Zelman and Parham, Strategic, 29–35.

33. Cooper, Philip D., and James W. Cagley. Elimination of services? A possible model for health care services. In *Health care marketing: Issues and trends,* edited by Philip D. Cooper, 2d ed., 373–379. Rockville, MD: Aspen Systems Corporation, 1985. For an excellent review of downsizing, see Fottler, Myron D., Howard L. Smith, and Helen J. Muller. Retrenchment in health care organizations: Theory and practice. *Hospital & Health Services Administration* 31 (September/October 1986): 29–43; and McLaughlin, Curtis P. Strategic planning under current cutback conditions. *Health Care Management Review* 7 (Summer 1982): 7–17; and of downsizing relative to systems, see Brown, Montague, and Barbara P. McCool. Health care systems: Predictions for the future. *Health Care Management Review* 15 (Summer 1990): 90–91. For a discussion of demarketing, in which an HSO seeks to lessen the demand for a service that may be unprofitable, see Breindel, Charles L. Marketing in the academic health center. *Health Care Strategic Management* 5 (January 1987): 8–10.

34. Mobley, Mary F., and Ralph E. Elkins. Megamarketing strategies for health care services. *Health Marketing Quarterly* 7 (1990): 13.

35. Keith, Marketing health, 17.

36. For pricing tactics, see Pointer, Dennis D., and Jack Zwanziger. Pricing strategies and tactics in the new hospital marketplace. *Hospital & Health Services Administration* 31 (November/December 1986): 5–18.

37. MacStravic, Robin E. Price of services. In *Health care marketing: Issues and trends,* edited by Philip D. Cooper, 2d ed., 232–234. Rockville, MD: Aspen Systems Corporation, 1985.

38. Kotler and Clarke, *Marketing for health,* 25.

39. For varying definitions and discussions of strategic planning in health services, see Abendshien, John. *A guide to the board's role in strategic business planning,* 15–24. Chicago: American Hospital Publishing, 1988; Breindel, Charles L. External influences and constraints on organizations in the health care sector. In *Strategic management in the health care sector: Toward the year 2000,* edited by Farhad Simyar and Joseph Lloyd-Jones, 85–100. Englewood Cliffs, NJ: Prentice Hall, 1988; Desai, Harsha B., and Charles R. Margenthaler. A framework for developing hospital strategies. *Hospital & Health Services Administration* 32 (May 1987): 237; Files, Laurel A. Strategy formulation in hospitals. *Health Care Management Review* 13 (Winter 1988): 9–15; Luke, Roice D., and James W. Begun. The management of strategy. In *Health care management: A text in organization theory and behavior,* edited by Stephen M. Shortell and Arnold Kaluzny, 2d ed., 4–65. New York: John Wiley & Sons, 1988; Pegels, C. Carl, and Kenneth A. Rogers. *Strategic management of hospitals and health care facilities,* 57–68. Rockville, MD: Aspen Publishers, Inc., 1988; Rakich, Jonathon S., and Kurt Darr. Outcomes of hospital strategic planning. *Hospital Topics* 66 (May/June 1988): 23–27; Sheldon, Alan, and Susan Windham. *Competitive strategy for health care organizations,* chpt. 2. Homewood, IL: Dow Jones-Irwin, 1984; Shortell, Stephen M., Ellen M. Morrison, and Shelley Robbins. Strategy making in health care organizations: A framework and agenda for research. *Medical Care Review* 42 (Fall 1985): 220; Simyar, Farhad, Joseph Lloyd-Jones, and Denis H.J. Caro. Strategic management: A proposed framework for the health care services industry. In *Strategic management in the health care sector: Toward the year 2000,* edited by Farhad Simyar and Joseph Lloyd-Jones, 6–17. Englewood Cliffs, NJ: Prentice Hall, 1988; and Zuckerman, Alan. The impact of DRG reimbursement on strategic planning. *Hospital & Health Services Administration* 29 (July/August 1984): 42.

40. For further reading on the strategic planning process and models, see Abendshein, *Guide to the board's,* 12–13; Desai and Margenthaler, Framework, 235–243; Luke and Begun, Management of strategy, 464–486; Pegels and Rogers, *Strategic management,* 23–40; Peters, *Strategic planning,* chpt. 9; Pratt, John R. Strategic planning in long-term care organizations. *Journal of Long-Term Care Administration* 18 (Fall 1990): 22–25; Shortell, Morrison, and Robbins, Strategy making, 224–225; Shortell, Stephen M., Ellen M. Morrison, and Bernard Friedman. *Strategic choices for America's hospitals: Managing change in turbulent times,* chpt. 2. San Francisco: Jossey-Bass Publishers, 1990; Seidel, Seavey, and Lewis, *Strategic management,* 11–16; Smith, David P. One more time: What do we mean by strategic management? *Hospital & Health Services Administration* 32 (1987): 219–233; Webber, James B., and Joseph P. Peters. *Strategic thinking: New frontier for hospital management,* 10–18. Chicago: American Hospital Association, 1983.

41. Pointer, Dennis D. Offering-level strategy formulation in health services organizations. *Health Care Management Review* 15 (Summer 1990): 18; Rakich and Darr, Outcomes, 23–24.

42. For an exhaustive treatment of stakeholder analysis, see Blair, John D., and Myron D. Fottler. *Challenges in health care management: Strategic perspectives for managing key stakeholders.* San Francisco: Jossey-Bass Publishers, 1990. For a model suggesting ways to assess stakeholders' potential for threat, potential for cooperation, and relevance to the HSO as well as negotiation approaches to use, see Blair, John D., Grant T. Savage, and Carlton J. Whitehead. A strategic approach for negotiating with hospital stakeholders. *Health Care Management Review* 14 (Winter 1989): 13–23; Savage, Grant T., and John D. Blair. The importance of relationships in hospi-

tal negotiation strategies. *Hospital & Health Services Administration* 34 (Summer 1989): 231–253.

43. Bower, Joseph L., Christopher A. Bartlett, C. Roland Christensen, Andrall E. Pearson, and Kenneth R. Andrews. *Business policy: Text and cases*, 7th ed., 109. Homewood, IL: Irwin, 1991.

44. Zentner, Rene D. Scenarios: A planning tool for health care organizations. *Hospital & Health Services Administration* 36 (Summer 1991): 213.

45. Sheldon and Windham, *Competitive strategy*, 30; Christensen, C. Roland, Kenneth R. Andrews, Joseph L. Bower, Richard G. Hamermesh, and Michael E. Porter. *Business policy: Text and cases*, 6th ed., 231–243. Homewood, IL: Irwin, 1987.

46. Reeves, Philip N. Organizational competence analysis for strategic planning. In *Strategic management in the health care sector: Toward the year 2000*, edited by Farhad Simyar and Joseph Lloyd-Jones, 65–84. Englewood Cliffs, NJ: Prentice Hall, 1988.

47. Desai and Margenthaler, Framework, 238.

48. Reeves, Philip N. Strategic planning for every manager. *Clinical Laboratory Management Review* 4 (July/August 1990); 272.

49. See Alexander, Jeffrey A. Diversification behavior of multihospital systems: Patterns of change, 1983–1985. *Hospital & Health Services Administration* 35 (Spring 1990): 83–87; Brown, Montague, and Barbara P. McCool. Vertical integration: Exploration of a popular strategic concept. *Health Care Management Review* 11 (Fall 1986): 8–9; Clement, Jan P. Vertical integration and diversification of acute care hospitals: Conceptual definitions. *Hospital & Health Services Administration* 33 (Spring 1988): 100–101; Coddington, Dean C., Lowell E. Palmquist, and William V. Trollinger. Strategies for survival in the hospital industry. *Harvard Business Review* 63 (May-June 1985): 129–130; Conrad, Douglas A., and William L. Dowling. Vertical integration in health services: Theory and managerial implications. *Health Care Management Review* 15 (Fall 1990): 9–11; Fottler, Myron D., Robert L. Phillips, John D. Blair, and Catherine A. Duran. Achieving competitive advantage through strategic human resource management. *Hospital & Health Services Administration* 35 (Fall 1990): 352; Haglund, Claudia L., and William L. Dowling. The hospital. In *Introduction to health services*, edited by Stephen J. Williams and Paul R. Torrens, 3d ed., 193–195. Albany, NY: Delmar Publishers, Inc., 1988; Mick, Stephen S. and Douglas A. Conrad. The decision to integrate vertically in health care organizations. *Hospital & Health Services Administration* 33 (Fall 1988): 347–349; Pointer, offering-level strategy, 19; Reynolds, James X. Using DRGs for competitive positioning and practical business planning. *Health Care Management Review* 11 (Summer 1986): 39; Rosenstein, Alan H. Hospital closure or survival: Formula for success. *Health Care Management Review* 11 (Summer 1986): 29–35; Shortell, Morrison, and Hughes, Keys, 472–473; and Vraciu, Robert A. Hospital strategies for the eighties: A mid-decade look. *Health Care Management Review* 10 (Fall 1985): 15.

50. Clement, Vertical integration, 99; Luke and Begun, Management of strategy, 481.

51. Conrad and Dowling, Vertical integration, 9–10.

52. Brown and McCool, Vertical integration, 7.

53. Haglund and Dowling, The hospital, 194.

54. Conrad and Dowling, Vertical integration, 10; Harrigan, Kathryn Rudie. Vertical integration and corporate strategy. *Academy of Management Journal* 28 (June 1985): 397.

55. Flexner, William A., Eric N. Berkowitz, and Montague Brown. *Strategic planning in health care management*, 15. Rockville, MD: Aspen Systems Corporation, 1981.

56. Shortell, Morrison, and Hughes, Keys, 472.

57. Alexander, Diversification, 84.

58. Shortell, Stephen M., Ellen M. Morrison, Susan L. Hughes, Bernard S. Friedman, and Joan L. Vitek. Diversification of health care services: The effects of ownership, environment, and strategy. In *Advances in health economics and health services research: A research annual*. Vol. 7, Mergers in health care: The performance of multi-institutional organizations, edited by Richard M. Scheffler and Louis F. Rossiter, 3–40. Greenwich, CT: JAI Press Inc., 1987.

59. Sabatino, Frank. Home health, diagnostic centers were financial winners in 1990. *Hospitals* 65 (January 20, 1991): 27.

60. American Hospital Association, *Evaluating diversification* 1.

61. For a good discussion of hospital diversification into long-term care, see Giardina, Carole W., Myron D. Fottler, Richard M. Shewchuk, and Daniel B. Hill. The case for diversification into long term care. *Health Care Management Review* 15 (Winter 1990): 71–82.

62. See Ginn, Gregory O. Strategic change in hospitals: An examination of the response of the acute care hospital to the turbulent environment of the 1980s. *Health Services Research* 25 (October 1990): 569–571; Shortell, Morrison, and Friedman, *Strategic choices*; Scotti, Cultural factors, 156.

63. Scotti, Cultural factors, 156.

64. Scotti, Cultural factors, 156.

65. Scotti (Cultural factors, 148) uses the terms "formal planning," "entrepreneurial," and "adaptive strategic decision modes."

66. Craig, Tim T. Formulating patterns of strategic behavior. In *Strategic management in the health care sector: Toward the year 2000*, edited by Farhad Simyar and Joseph Lloyd-Jones, 193. Englewood Cliffs, NJ: Prentice Hall, 1988.

67. Scotti, Cultural factors, 144.

68. Bower, Bartlett, Christensen, Pearson, and Andrews, Business policy, 341.

69. Digman, Lester A. *Strategic management: Concepts, decisions, cases*, 2d ed., 335. Homewood, IL: BPI/Irwin, 1990.

70. Craig, Formulating patterns, 182–183; Desai and Margenthaler, Framework, 242–245.

71. Sheldon and Windham, *Competitive strategy*, 118.

72. Harrell, Gilbert D., and Matthew F. Fors. Planning evolution in hospital management. *Health Care Management Review* 12 (Winter 1987): 12; Malhotra, Hospital marketing, 38. For application of strategic business unit analysis by diagnosis-related group, see Reynolds, Using DRGs.

73. Pegels and Rogers, *Strategic management*, 98.

74. Pegels and Rogers, *Strategic management*, 98.

75. A matrix using financial strength and profit/price of service is found in Cleverley, William O. Promotion and pricing in competitive markets. *Hospital & Health Services Administration* 32 (August 1987): 329–333. An in-

teresting growth and nongrowth opportunity matrix is presented by Breindel, Charles L. Nongrowth strategies and options for health care. *Hospital & Health Services Administration* 33 (Spring 1988): 37–45.

76. Blair, Savage, and Whitehead, A strategic approach, 17–20.

77. From Kotler, Philip, and Roberta N. Clarke. *Marketing for health care organizations*, 2d ed., 32–35. Englewood Cliffs, NJ: Prentice Hall, Inc., 1987; reprinted by permission. This instrument was prepared by Rick Heidtman under the supervision of Professor Philip Kotler.

BIBLIOGRAPHY

Abendshien, John. *A guide to the board's role in strategic business planning.* Chicago: American Hospital Publishing, 1988.

Alexander, Jeffrey A. Diversification behavior of multihospital systems: Patterns of change, 1983–1985. *Hospital & Health Services Administration* 35 (Spring 1990): 83–102.

Berkowitz, Eric N., and William A. Flexner. The marketing audit: A tool for health services organizations. In *Health care marketing: Issues and Trends,* edited by Philip D. Cooper, 2d ed., 128–135. Rockville, MD: Aspen Systems Corporation, 1985.

Blair, John D., and Myron D. Fottler. *Challenges in health care management: Strategic perspectives for managing key stakeholders.* San Francisco: Jossey-Bass Publishers, 1990.

Blair, John D., Grant T. Savage, and Carlton J. Whitehead. A strategic approach for negotiating with hospital stakeholders. *Health Care Management Review* 14 (Winter 1989): 13–23.

Bower, Joseph L., Christopher A. Bartlett, C. Roland Christensen, Andrall E. Pearson, and Kenneth R. Andrews. *Business policy: Text and cases,* 7th ed. Homewood, IL: Irwin, 1991.

Breindel, Charles L. External influences and constraints on organizations in the health care sector. In *Strategic management in the health care sector: Toward the year 2000,* edited by Farhad Simyar and Joseph Lloyd-Jones, 85–100. Englewood Cliffs, NJ: Prentice Hall, 1988.

Breindel, Charles L. Marketing in the academic health center. *Health Care Strategic Management* 5 (January 1987): 8–10.

Breindel, Charles L. Nongrowth strategies and options for health care. *Hospital & Health Services Administration* 33 (Spring 1988): 37–45.

Brown, Montague, and Barbara P. McCool. Health care systems: Predictions for the future. *Health Care Management Review* 15 (Summer 1990): 87–94.

Brown, Montague, and Barbara P. McCool. Vertical integration: Exploration of a popular strategic concept. *Health Care Management Review* 11 (Fall 1986): 7–19.

Christensen, C. Roland, Kenneth R. Andrews, Joseph L. Bower, Richard G. Hamermesh, and Michael E. Porter. *Business policy: Text and cases,* 6th ed. Homewood, IL: Irwin, 1987.

Clemenhagen, Carol, and Francois Champagne. Medical staff involvement in strategic planning. *Hospital & Health Services Administration* 29 (July/August 1984): 79–94.

Clement, Jan P. Vertical integration and diversification of acute care hospitals: Conceptual definitions. *Hospital & Health Services Administration* 33 (Spring 1988): 99–110.

Cleverley, William O. Promotion and pricing in competitive markets. *Hospital & Health Services Administration* 32 (August 1987): 329–339.

Coddington, Dean C., Lowell E. Palmquist, and William V. Trollinger. Strategies for survival in the hospital industry. *Harvard Business Review* 63 (May-June 1985): 129–138.

Conrad, Douglas A., and William L. Dowling. Vertical integration in health services: Theory and managerial implications. *Health Care Management Review* 15 (Fall 1990): 9–22.

Cooper, Philip D. *Health care marketing: Issues and trends.* 2d ed. Rockville, MD: Aspen Systems Corporation, 1985.

Cooper, Philip D. Marketing from inside out. In *Health care marketing: Issues and trends,* edited by Philip D. Cooper, 2d ed., 109–111. Rockville, MD: Aspen Systems Corporation, 1985.

Cooper, Philip D. What is health care marketing? In *Health care marketing: Issues and trends,* edited by Philip D. Cooper, 2d ed., 1–8. Rockville, MD: Aspen Systems Corporation, 1985.

Cooper, Philip D., and James W. Cagley. Elimination of services? A possible model for health care services. In *Health care marketing: Issues and trends,* edited by Philip D. Cooper, 2d ed., 373–380. Rockville, MD: Aspen Systems Corporation, 1985.

Craig, Tim T. Formulating patterns of strategic behavior. In *Strategic management in the health care sector: Toward the year 2000,* edited by Farhad Simyar and Joseph Lloyd-Jones, 179–202. Englewood Cliffs, NJ: Prentice Hall, 1988.

Desai, Harsha B., and Charles R. Margenthaler. A framework for developing hospital strategies. *Hospital & Health Services Administration* 32 (May 1987): 235–248.

Digman, Lester A. *Strategic management: Concepts, decisions, cases,* 2d ed. Homewood, IL: BPI/Irwin, 1990.

Files, Laurel A. Strategy formulation in hospitals. *Health Care Management Review* 13 (Winter 1988): 9–16.

Flexner, William A., Eric N. Berkowitz, and Montague Brown. *Strategic planning in health care management.* Rockville, MD: Aspen Systems Corporation, 1981.

Fottler, Myron D., Robert L. Phillips, John D. Blair, and Catherine A. Duran. Achieving competitive advantage through strategic human resource management. *Hospital & Health Services Administation* 35 (Fall 1990): 341–363.

Fottler, Myron D., Howard L. Smith, and Helen J. Muller. Retrenchment in health care organizations: Theory and practice. *Hospital & Health Services Administration* 31 (September/October 1986): 29–43.

Georgopoulos, Basis S., and Floyd C. Mann. *The community general hospital.* New York: Macmillan Publishing Co., Inc., 1962.

Giardina, Carole W., Myron D. Fottler, Richard M. Shewchuk, and Daniel B. Hill. The case for diversification into long-term care. *Health Care Management Review* 15 (Winter 1990): 71–82.

Gibson, C. Kendrick, David J. Newton, and Daniel S. Cochran. An empirical investigation of hospital mission statements. *Health Care Management Review* 15 (Summer 1990): 35–45.

Ginn, Gregory O. Strategic change in hospitals: An examination of the response of the acute care hospital to the turbulent environment of the 1980s. *Health Services Research* 25 (October 1990): 566–591.

Haglund, Claudia L., and William L. Dowling. The hospital. In *Introduction to health services,* edited by Stephen J.

Williams and Paul R. Torrens, 3d ed., 160–211. Albany, NJ: Delmar Publishers, Inc., 1988.

Harrell, Gilbert D., and Matthew F. Fors. Planning evolution in hospital management. *Health Care Management Review* 12 (Winter 1987): 9–22.

Harrigan, Kathryn Rudie. Vertical integration and corporate strategy. *Academy of Management Review* 28 (June 1985): 397–425.

Higgins, James M. *The management challenge: An introduction to management*. New York: Macmillan Publishing Company, 1991.

Hillestad, Steven G., and Eric N. Berkowitz. *Health care marketing plans: From strategy to action*. Homewood, IL: Dow Jones-Irwin, 1984.

Ivancevich, John M., James H. Donnelly, Jr., and James L. Gibson. *Management principles and functions*, 4th ed. Homewood, IL: BPI/Irwin, 1989.

Kaluzny, Arnold D., D. Michael Warner, David G. Warren, and William N. Zelman. *Management of health services*. Englewood Cliffs, NJ: Prentice Hall, Inc., 1982.

Keith, Jon G. Marketing health care: What the recent literature is telling us. In *Health care marketing: Issues and trends* edited by Philip D. Cooper, 2d ed., 13–25. Rockville, MD: Aspen Systems Corporation, 1985.

Kotler, Philip, and Roberta N. Clarke. *Marketing for health care organizations*, 2d ed. Englewood Cliffs, NJ: Prentice Hall, Inc., 1987.

Kovner, Anthony R., and Martin J. Chin. Physician leadership in hospital strategic decision making. *Hospital & Health Services Administration* 30 (November/December 1985): 64–79.

Luke, Roice D., and James W. Begun. The management of strategy. In *Health care management: A text in organization theory and behavior*, edited by Stephen M. Shortell and Arnold Kaluzny, 2d ed., 463–491. New York: John Wiley & Sons, 1988.

MacStravic, Robin E. *Marketing by objectives for hospitals*. Rockville, MD: Aspen Systems Corporation, 1980.

MacStravic, Robin E. *Marketing health care*. Rockville, MD: Aspen Systems Corporation, 1977.

MacStravic, Robin E. *Marketing religious health care*. St. Louis: The Catholic Health Association of the United States, 1987.

MacStravic, Robin E. Price of services. In *Health care marketing: Issues and trends*, edited by Philip D. Cooper, 2d ed., 230–235. Rockville, MD: Aspen Systems Corporation, 1985.

Malhotra, Naresh K. Hospital marketing in the changing health care environment. *Journal of Health Care Marketing* 6 (September 1986): 37–48.

McLaughlin, Curtis P. Strategic planning under current cutback conditions. *Health Care Management Review* 7 (Summer 1982): 7–17.

McMillan, Norman H. *Marketing your hospital: A strategy for survival*. Chicago: American Hospital Association, 1981.

Mick, Stephen S., and Douglas A. Conrad. The decision to integrate vertically in health care organizations. *Hospital & Health Services Administration* 33 (Fall 1988): 345–360.

Pearce, John A., II, and Richard B. Robinson, Jr. *Management*. New York: Random House, 1989.

Pegels, C. Carl, and Kenneth A. Rogers. *Strategic management of hospitals and health care facilities*. Rockville, MD: Aspen Publishers, Inc., 1988.

Peters, Joseph P. *A strategic planning process for hospitals*. Chicago: American Hospital Publishing, Inc., 1985.

Pointer, Dennis D. Offering-level strategy formulation in health services organizations. *Health Care Management Review* 15 (Summer 1990): 15–23.

Pointer, Dennis D., and Jack Zwanziger. Pricing strategies and tactics in the new hospital marketplace. *Hospital & Health Services Administration* 31 (November/December 1986): 5–18.

Pratt, John R. Strategic planning in long-term care organizations. *Journal of Long-Term Care Administration* 18 (Fall 1990): 22–25.

Rakich, Jonathon S., and Kurt Darr. Outcomes of hospital strategic planning. *Hospital Topics* 66 (May/June 1988): 23–27.

Reeves, Philip N. Organizational competence analysis for strategic planning. In *Strategic management in the health care sector: Toward the year 2000*, edited by Farhad Simyar and Joseph Lloyd-Jones, 65–84. Englewood Cliffs, NJ: Prentice Hall, 1988.

Reynolds, James X. Using DRGs for competitive positioning and practical business planning. *Health Care Management Review* 11 (Summer 1986): 37–55.

Rosenstein, Alan H. Hospital closure or survival: Formula for success. *Health Care Management Review* 11 (Summer 1986): 29–35.

Savage, Grant T., and John D. Blair. The importance of relationships in hospital negotiation strategies. *Hospital & Health Services Administration* 34 (Summer 1989) 231–253.

Schlinger, Mary Jane. Marketing audits for health organizations: A practical guide. *Hospital & Health Services Administration* 26 (Special Issue II 1981): 32–50

Scotti, Dennis J. Cultural factors in choosing a strategic posture: A bridge between formulation and implementation. In *Strategic management in the health care sector: Toward the year 2000*, edited by Farhad Simyar and Joseph Lloyd-Jones, 143–161. Englewood Cliffs, NJ: Prentice Hall, 1988.

Seidel, Lee F., John W. Seavey, and Richard J.A. Lewis. *Strategic management for healthcare organizations*. Owings Mills, MD: National Health Publishing/AUPHA Press, 1989.

Sheldon, Alan, and Susan Windham. *Competitive strategy for health care organizations*. Homewood, IL: Dow Jones-Irwin, 1984.

Shortell, Stephen M., and Arnold D. Kaluzny. *Health care management: A text in organization theory and behavior*. New York: John Wiley & Sons, 1988.

Shortell, Stephen M., Ellen M. Morrison, and Bernard Friedman. *Strategic choices for America's hospitals: Managing change in turbulent times*. San Francisco: Jossey-Bass Publishers, 1990.

Shortell, Stephen M., Ellen M. Morrison, and Susan Hughes. The keys to successful diversification: Lessons from leading hospital systems. *Hospital & Health Services Administration* 43 (Winter 1989): 471–492.

Shortell, Stephen M., Ellen M. Morrison, Susan L. Hughes, Bernard S. Friedman, and Joan L. Vitek. Diversification of health care services: The effects of ownership, environment, and strategy. In *Advances in health economics and health services research: A research annual*. Vol. 7., *Mergers in health care: The performance of multi-institutional organizations*, 3–40. Greenwich, CT: JAI Press Inc., 1987.

Shortell, Stephen M., Ellen M. Morrison, and Shelley Robbins. Strategy making in health care organizations: A framework and agenda for research. *Medical Care Review* 42 (Fall 1985): 219–266.

Simyar, Farhad, and Joseph Lloyd-Jones, eds. *Strategic Management in the health care sector: Toward the year 2000*. Englewood Cliffs, NJ: Prentice Hall, 1988.

Simyar, Farhad, Joseph Lloyd-Jones, and Denis H.J. Caro. Strategic management: A proposed framework for the health care services industry. In *Strategic management in the health care sector: Toward the year 2000*, edited by Farhad Simyar and Joseph Lloyd-Jones, 6–17. Englewood Cliffs, NJ: Prentice Hall, 1988.

Smith, David P. One more time: What do we mean by strategic management? *Hospital & Health Services Administration* 32 (May 1987): 219–233.

Vraciu, Robert A. Hospital strategies for the eighties: A mid-decade look. *Health Care Management Review* 10 (Fall 1985): 9–19.

Webber, James B., and Joseph P. Peters. *Strategic thinking: New frontier for hospital management*. Chicago: American Hospital Association, 1983.

Williams, Stephen J., and Paul R. Torrens. *Introduction to health services*. Albany, NY: Delmar Publishers, Inc., 1988.

Winston, William J. *How to write a marketing plan for health care organizations*. New York: The Haworth Press, 1985.

Zelman, William N., and Deborah L. Parham. Strategic, operational, and marketing concerns of product-line management in health care. *Health Care Management Review* 15 (Winter 1990): 29–35.

Zentner, Rene D. Scenarios: A planning tool for health care organizations. *Hospital & Health Services Administration* 36 (Summer 1991): 211–222.

Zuckerman, Alan. The impact of DRG reimbursement on strategic planning. *Hospital & Health Services Administration* 29 (July/August 1984): 40–49.

9

Interorganizational Relationships

*The scope and size of an organization help
determine its ability to control both internal and
external environments. Large, integrated
systems are less vulnerable to changes in the
external environment and have the resources to
control and adequately direct the internal
environment. The reverse is true for single
institutions.*
B. Jon Jaeger, Arnold D. Kaluzny, and
Kathryn Magruder-Habib[1]

Survival is the major challenge facing health services organization (HSOs) during the 1990s; it will require them to be economically efficient and to organize effectively. To flourish, however, will mean working with and through other organizations, both HSOs and non-HSOs. Establishing and maintaining interorganizational linkages will be a central element in any strategic plan. This chapter begins with a conceptual framework for interorganizational linkages and describes the ways HSOs can work with one another and with regulators. Voluntary and involuntary interorganizational relationships are the two primary types. Success in either will be determined by effective strategies and managerial negotiating skills.

Corporate restructuring is a common way to create interorganizational linkages, and this organization strategy came to health services after being applied for decades in business enterprise. Acute care hospitals have been among the most enthusiastic users, but after rushing headlong into this organization strategy, many have paused to reconsider. One result of corporate restructuring has been multiorganizational arrangements. These may include multihospital systems or a great many combinations of various types of HSOs that may be vertically integrated. Such systems are common in both the for-profit and not-for-profit sectors. This chapter examines the advantages and disadvantages of vertical integration.

Diversifying into health services–related and –unrelated activities may be part of corporate restructuring or may follow from it. The impetus for, as well as the advantages and disadvantages of, this organization strategy are examined. Acute care hospitals have been especially aggressive in developing collateral revenue streams as reimbursement from traditional sources has become less generous. Joint ventures are one way in which HSOs can generate new streams of revenue. In addition, they can be used as a way to bond members of the clinical staff, especially physicians, to the HSO. Acute care hospitals have undertaken numerous joint ventures with their physicians, sometimes with disastrous results.

Regardless of the precise strategies used by managers to make their HSOs flourish in the 1990s, it is virtually certain they will include increasing use of interorganizational linkages. Skill in the use of these linkages will be a key to success.

LINKAGES AMONG ORGANIZATIONS[2]

There are two reasons why effective interorganizational linkages are important to the success of HSOs. First, many may be stakeholders of the HSO. Second, interorganizational linkages, such as joint ventures, are an organization strategy that can be used by an HSO to accomplish its objectives. Often, these interorganizational relationships involve a high degree of interdependence because at least one of the organizations does not completely control the conditions necessary to achieve its objectives or purposes. For a particular focal HSO, other organizations that can affect, or that are affected by, the achievement of its purposes are interdependent with it.[3] Figure 9.1 shows how an organization in the health sector—a hospital or a health maintenance organization (HMO), for example—might maintain relationships with "interdependent others" (stakeholders) as diverse as consumer groups, government agencies, or suppliers of inputs it needs. Furthermore, a focal HSO can simultaneously choose as an organization strategy involvement in systems, joint ventures, partnerships, or any of a host of affiliations, consortia, and confederations, all of which entail interdependent relationships.

The multiplicity of potential interorganizational linkages suggests the need for a typology of the basic types available to health services managers. For example, some linkages are the simple market exchanges needed to acquire resources or assure markets for outputs. Some are more complex interorganizational linkages, voluntarily established and ranging from loosely structured couplings to tight bureaucracies. Still others are involuntary arrangements (from the focal HSO's perspective) that guide relationships with regulators, fiscal intermediaries, or utilization management companies. Increasingly, an important element of success for HSOs is the ability of their managers to develop and maintain effective interorganizational linkages as a means of managing

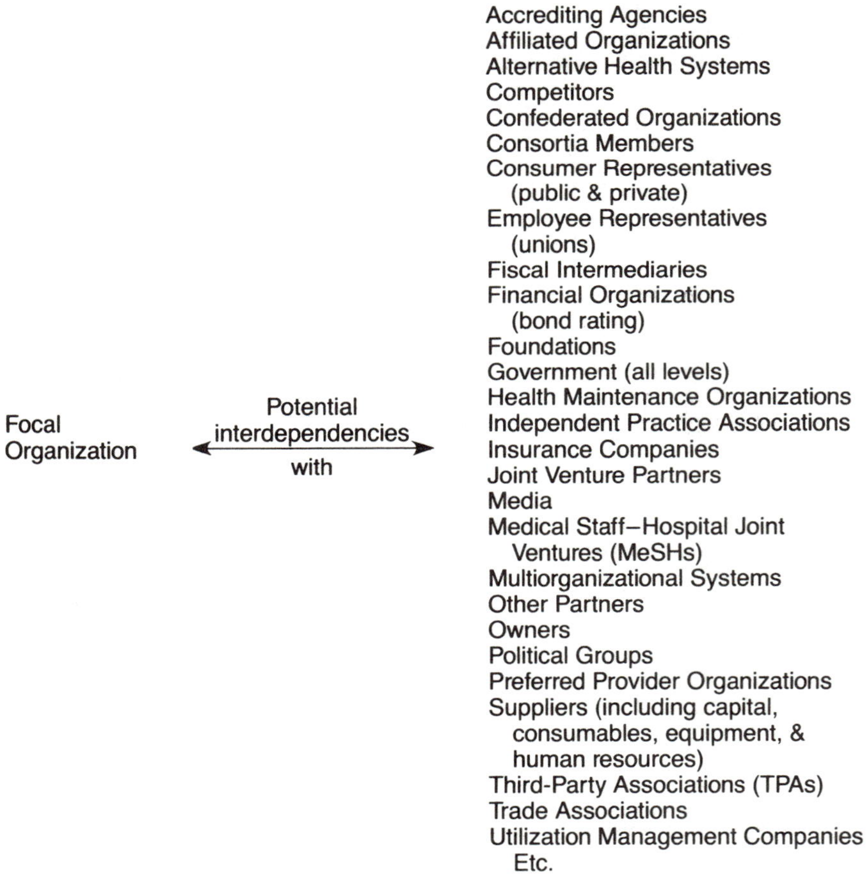

Focal Organization ←→ Potential interdependencies with

Accrediting Agencies
Affiliated Organizations
Alternative Health Systems
Competitors
Confederated Organizations
Consortia Members
Consumer Representatives
    (public & private)
Employee Representatives
    (unions)
Fiscal Intermediaries
Financial Organizations
    (bond rating)
Foundations
Government (all levels)
Health Maintenance Organizations
Independent Practice Associations
Insurance Companies
Joint Venture Partners
Media
Medical Staff–Hospital Joint
    Ventures (MeSHs)
Multiorganizational Systems
Other Partners
Owners
Political Groups
Preferred Provider Organizations
Suppliers (including capital,
    consumables, equipment, &
    human resources)
Third-Party Associations (TPAs)
Trade Associations
Utilization Management Companies
    Etc.

Figure 9.1.   Interdependencies among organizations in the health sector.

their organizations' interdependencies. Three general types of mechanisms enable HSOs to manage interdependencies with other organizations: market transactions, voluntary interorganizational relationship transactions, and involuntary interorganizational relationship transactions. These categories of linkage mechanisms, each with a place in the management of interdependence between and among organizations in health services, are summarized in Table 9.1 and more fully elaborated below.

MARKET TRANSACTIONS

Market transactions are the most prevalent type of linkage with interdependent others for HSOs. Usually, they are the simplest as well. In market transactions, HSOs buy inputs and sell outputs. These transactions also occur between a focal organization and persons such as nonunionized employees and some patients. Transactions between a focal organization, as shown in Figure 9.1, and its customers (and their advocates and representatives), suppliers, and employees, including physicians, are usually straightforward market exchanges.

Applying exchange principles (most notably that HSOs calculate rewards and costs of exchanges) results in development of contracts that, even if implicit, govern most market transactions by defining the parameters of exchanges among all parties. "This economic view of exchange relations, often criticized as overly calculative when applied to interpersonal relations, is highly applicable to the analysis of interorganizational relations, where the corporate entities have well-established mechanisms for monitoring rewards and costs."[4]

Contracts, which were described in Chapter 4, "Legal Considerations," are widely used to manage linkages in a variety of interorganizational relationships. They are usually *negotiated* agreements between parties for the exchange of future performance. Contracts can rest simply on the faith and belief that each party will perform as agreed or, more rigorously, on specific terms that can be evaluated by third parties and that are the basis for penalties if performance by either or both of the parties to the contract is unsatisfactory.

Table 9.1.   Categories of linkage mechanisms in the health sector

Market Transactions
Many, but not all, interdependent relationships stem from the necessity for a focal organization to enter economic exchanges with other organizations to obtain resources needed to conduct its affairs or a market for its outputs. These exchanges are market transactions. They, like market exchanges among all organizations in market economies, are governed by certain basic exchange principles. These principles hold that organizations engaging in exchange transactions seek exchanges that are mutually beneficial or rewarding. Furthermore, they hold that the organizations are calculative; that is, they make assessments of both relative rewards and costs. Relationships that produce greater utility by going beyond market transactions, as well as those that cannot be achieved through market transactions, are candidates for management through voluntary or involuntary interorganizational relationship transactions.

Voluntary Interorganizational Relationship Transactions
As relationships with other interdependent organizations become more important and sustained, there may be advantages to extending the relationship beyond a straightforward market transaction. In these situations, interdependent organizations can voluntarily seek to manage their interdependence through a variety of interorganizational relationship transactions. The voluntary dimension of these transactions is their most important distinguishing feature. It implies that the participating organizations have other choices as to how they manage their interdependence. They can simply continue to handle it through market transactions, they can choose to shift the interdependence to other organizations that are better able to meet their requirements or more amenable to meeting them, or they can seek to become independent of other organizations along a particular dimension.

Involuntary Interorganizational Relationship Transactions
This class of mechanisms is a unique function of the necessity to interact with certain organizations involuntarily. Some relationships with interdependent others are precluded from market transactions, and the choice of interorganizational relationship transactions is limited or fixed by the interdependent other. These include relationships with government regulatory agencies, utilization management companies, or intermediaries, such as Blue Cross/Blue Shield, in their roles as fiscal intermediaries for Medicare reimbursement.

Exchange relationships based on contracts may entail only an agreement for products or services, or they may be a complex agreement between a hospital and an HMO, for example, to provide certain services to a defined population. Contracts permit HSOs to establish stable and predictable (but interdependent) relationships with federal and state governments and commercial insurers for various types of reimbursement. They also permit employment and utilization of a work force and orderly acquisition of other inputs.

The most important skills in managing organizational interdependencies through market transactions are negotiating skills. Negotiation (also called bargaining) is "the process whereby two or more parties attempt to settle what each shall give and take, or perform and receive, in a transaction between them."[5] In negotiating, the parties seek agreement on a mutually acceptable outcome in a situation in which their preferences about outcomes are usually negatively related. Indeed, if preferences for outcomes are positively related, agreement is easily reached. This is rare among interdependent organizations. More typically, at least two sources of conflict must be resolved: 1) dividing resources—the so-called tangibles of negotiation, such as which organization will receive how much money, goods, or services in exchange for what considerations; and 2) resolving psychological dynamics and satisfying personal motivations of the leaders of organizations involved in the negotiations. The latter aspects are so-called intangibles of negotiation and can include such variables as appearing to win or lose, competing effectively, or cooperating fairly. Negotiations between interdependent organizations, such as contract negotiations between a Blue Cross plan and a hospital, sometimes hinge more on the intangibles than the tangibles.

Negotiations between interdependent organizations usually follow one of two strategies:* 1) cooperative, win/win; or 2) competitive, win/lose. The negotiating strategy is a function of several variables. Optimal conditions for cooperative and competitive negotiating strategies include:[6]

Cooperative Negotiating Strategies

- Tangible goals of both [sides] are to attain a fair and reasonable settlement.
- Resources in the environment are sufficient for both sides to attain their tangible goals, more resources can be attained, or the problem can be redefined so both sides can actually "win."
- Each side believes it is possible for both [sides] to attain their goals through negotiating.
- Intangible goals of both [sides] are to establish a cooperative relationship and work toward a settlement that maximizes joint outcomes.

Competitive Negotiating Strategies

- Tangible goals of both [sides] are to attain a specific settlement or to get as much as possible.
- There are insufficient resources for both [sides] to attain their goals, or their desires to get as much as possible makes it impossible for one or both to attain their goal(s).
- Both [sides] perceive it is impossible for both to attain their goals.
- Intangible goals of both [sides] are to beat the other, keep the other from attaining [its] goals, humiliate the other, or refuse (for various reasons) to make concessions in negotiating position.

Phases of Negotiation

Whether interdependent organizations are engaged in cooperative or competitive negotiation, the process tends to proceed in distinct phases.[7] First is *preparation*, during which both assess the conflict, establish their goals and priorities and try to guess those of their opponents, and devise a

---

*The use of the word "strategy" in this context means behavior—a plan of action or tactic—and is different from the term "organization strategy" as used in Chapter 8.

negotiating strategy. Second is *entry*, during which they make initial contact, establish an agenda and the rules and procedures for the negotiation, and present initial goals and priorities. The third phase, *elaboration and education*, is characterized by learning more about the other's stated goals and priorities and elaborating initially stated goals and priorities based on what is learned. Fourth, *bargaining*, is the heart of negotiating and entails attempts by both parties to challenge their opponent's goals and logic, defend their own, search for compromises and trade-offs, and develop alternative solutions. The final phase of negotiating is *closure*, during which both parties seek to arrive at a basic agreement, consolidate issues, record the agreement in mutually satisfactory language, and plan implementation.

Table 9.2 outlines tactics that can be used in each phase of the process for both cooperative and competitive negotiating strategies. Negotiations are usually neither purely cooperative nor purely competitive and require a mixture of tactics for success.

VOLUNTARY INTERORGANIZATIONAL RELATIONSHIP TRANSACTIONS

Voluntary interorganizational relationship transactions are common as managers secure and stabilize the place of their HSO in a turbulent and hostile environment. Vertically integrated systems, joint ventures, partnerships, and various affiliations, consortia, and confederations are pervasive and illustrate the range of voluntary interorganizational relationship transactions—an organization strategy—that HSO managers use to better manage their organizations' interdependencies.

Table 9.2. Tactics in competitive and cooperative negotiations

Phase of negotiation	Competitive tactics	Cooperative tactics
Preparation	Set specific goals, bottom lines, and opening bids; develop firm positions and competitive tactics to attain those goals at the expense of the other.	Develop general goals and broad objectives; cultivate good options; cultivate good relations of trust and openness with opponent to promote effective problem solving.
Entry-problem identification	State the problem in terms of the organization's preferred solution; publicly disguise or misrepresent organization needs and goals; don't let the other side know what's really important.	State the problem in terms of the underlying needs of both sides; represent organization needs accurately to the other side; listen carefully to understand their needs.
Elaboration or education	Disclose only that information necessary to support the organization's position and have the other side understand it; hide possible vulnerabilities and weaknesses.	Disclose all information that may be pertinent to a problem, regardless of whose position it supports; expose vulnerabilities in order to protect them in the joint solution.
Bargaining	Include false issues, dummy options, or options of low priority in order to trade them away for what your side wants; make an early public commitment and stick to it.	Minimize the inclusion of false or dummy issues and stick to the major problems and concerns; avoid early and public commitments to preferred alternatives in order to give all options full consideration.
Closure	Maximize own utility while not caring about the other's; overvalue concessions to other; undervalue achieved gains; use "nibbling" strategy of taking issues off the table as favorable settlements are achieved.	Maximize solutions that have joint utility; be honest and candid in disclosing preferences; use "nothing is ever final until all issues are settled" strategy.

Adapted from Greenberger, David, Stephen Strasser, Roy J. Lewicki, and Thomas S. Bateman. Perception, motivation, and negotiation. In *Health care management: A text in organization theory and behavior*, 2nd ed., by Stephen M. Shortell and Arnold D. Kaluzny and Associates, Delmar Publishers Inc., Albany, NY, Copyright © 1966; used by permission.

Voluntary interorganizational relationship transactions are of four types. Thompson calls two of these linking mechanisms *co-opting* and *coalescing*.[8] Pointer, Begun, and Luke,[9] building on the earlier conceptualization of Eccles,[10] added a third type, the *quasi firm*. *Ownership* is a fourth type of interorganizational transaction. Here, interdependencies that cannot be managed through market transactions or one of the other forms of interorganizational transaction are brought within the boundaries of the focal organization through ownership. "Consumption" is an apt synonym for ownership.[11] Each type of linkage represents relationships through which interorganizational interdependencies can be managed; each has advantages and disadvantages; and each successive type mentioned is more complex.

Co-opting

Co-opting involves absorbing leadership elements from other organizations into the focal organization. Other than market transactions, co-opting is most flexible and easiest to implement, two advantages that make it pervasive. In health services this mechanism takes one of two forms: 1) management contracts, or 2) placing representatives of interdependent organizations on the focal organization's governing body (GB). Management contracts are described by Starkweather as an example of co-opting.[12] They permit one organization to supply senior management to another. Management in these arrangements includes at least the chief executive officer (CEO), who reports to the governing body of the managed organization *and* to the managing organization. The *management contract* contrasts with the practice prevalent in HSOs of having *contract management* for departments such as housekeeping, food service, or respiratory therapy. A study reported in 1991 found that 43% of hospitals used contract management.[13] Clinical services were most commonly managed, followed by "hotel" and business services.[14]

Another common co-opting mechanism is to appoint representatives from external organizations to positions in the focal organizations, usually its GB. For example, a hospital system needing access to capital can get expertise in financial markets by putting an investment banker on its GB. Similarly, an HMO may find advantages in putting members of the clinical staff on its governing body.

Coalescing and Loose Coupling

The health sector is replete with the coalescing type of linkage in joint ventures, partnerships, consortia, and federations. Its central feature is the *partial* pooling of resources by two or more organizations to pursue defined goals.[15] Glassman calls this interorganizational relationship "loose coupling."[16] Loosely coupled interorganizational relationships link interdependent and mutually responsive organizations in ways that preserve their legal identities and most of their functional autonomy.[17] These relationships are bound by stronger ties than those in market transactions, but are less binding and extensive than those in ownership arrangements.

Loosely coupled (coalesced) organizational relationships differ on dimensions such as importance, permanence, and directionality:[18]

> First, loosely coupled relationships differ in terms of their relative *importance* to the success and viability of participating organizations.[19] HSOs are part of many interorganizational relationships; importance differentiates those that are strategic and those that are not.
> Second, loosely coupled relationships can be distinguished by degree of *permanence*. Some interorganizational relationships are of short duration, others are long term. Enduring relationships are necessary if organizations are to achieve shared strategic purposes.[20]
> Third, loosely coupled relationships vary in terms of *directionality*. Organizations can be linked vertically, horizontally, or symbiotically.[21]

Horizontal combinations entail interrelationships among similar organizations operating in the same industry, which serves geographic markets with roughly equivalent products. Vertically integrated combinations occur among organizations that operate along a chain of production in which the output of one is the input of another. Such relationships are developed to secure inputs or dispose of outputs. In symbiotic combinations, organizations complement each other in the provision of services to customers and/or achieve joint competitive advantage in other areas (shared marketing or management, or both). They occur between organizations operating in different segments of the same industry or in totally different industries. In either case, no significant amount of input/output is exchanged, and competition among such organizations is limited or nonexistent.

Joint ventures, an increasingly prevalent organization strategy in health services, "can be predicted by considerations of resource interdependence, competitive uncertainty, and conditions that make various forms of interdependence more or less problematic."[22] Joint ventures between hospitals and members of their clinical staffs are commonplace. As Shortell notes:

> Hospitals and physicians are exploring new kinds of relationships through a variety of joint ventures. These range from highly formal activities such as hospital-sponsored group practices, health maintenance organizations sponsored by hospitals and their medical staffs, and preferred provider organizations (PPOs), to somewhat less formal arrangements involving leasing of space and equipment or providing ancillary services, computerized billing, financial analyses, and medical records services.[23]

As Blair et al. point out:

> Facing increasingly complex financial circumstances, hospitals in the 1980s sought to increase market share, channel referrals, and erect competitive barriers. As a result of these complexities, hospitals have sought to link physicians to their facilities. Although many different methods have been tried, the hospital-physician joint venture has perhaps the greatest potential for success. Thus, hospitals have entered into many joint ventures with physicians, such as physician practice purchase, surgicenters, urgicenters, and many others.[24]

Large, loosely coupled networks of health services providers such as the Voluntary Hospitals of America and the American Healthcare Systems can joint venture with health insurance carriers to develop a range of alternative delivery system products. Trade associations are a particularly prevalent form of loosely coupled, or coalesced, structures. For example, the American Hospital Association has more than 5,000 member organizations and mounts a sophisticated political/lobbying activity on their behalf. Similarly, there are regional and state hospital associations that base affiliation on a geographic or state community of interests. As states have become more involved in regulatory and control activities, state hospital associations have undertaken aggressive lobbying efforts on behalf of member hospitals.

Quasi Firm

The quasi firm is an interorganizational transaction that lies between market relationships and ownership arrangements. A quasi firm has been defined as "a loosely coupled, enduring set of interorganizational relationships that are designed to achieve purposes of substantial importance to the viability of participating members."[25] Such arrangements have many characteristics of a true firm (shared goals, mutual dependency, task subdivision and specialization, bureaucratic structures, and formal coordinating and control mechanisms), but they lack ownership linkages.

An example of a quasi-firm arrangement is where an acute care hospital, a large multi-speciality group practice, a nursing facility, and an insurance carrier collaborate to design, produce, and market a managed care product. In such an arrangement, the four organizations continue to operate independently of one another in accomplishing other, perhaps mutually exclusive, objectives. However, the collaborative activity may have significant strategic importance to the participating organizations, including survival.[26] In this example, the interdependencies among participating organizations are managed neither through purely market transactions nor through the bureaucratic mechanisms characteristic of ownership arrangements. Instead, the quasi-firm configuration accomplishes strategic purposes that do not lend themselves to market transactions, while avoiding the restrictions and diminution of autonomy and identity associated with acquiring or merging with other interdependent organizations.

Ownership

The final type of voluntary interorganizational transaction for managing interdependencies is ownership. Thus far in the health services field most ownership arrangements have been voluntary. However, hostile acquisitions and takeovers are more likely in the future. For now, this type of relationship is more appropriately put in the voluntary category. For example, a focal HSO, as an organization strategy, might choose to voluntarily participate with other organizations in owning a new, special-purpose entity; in reality, this mechanism may be only a small step beyond the quasi firm. Or, it could voluntarily merge with, acquire, or be acquired by an HSO with which it is interdependent.

It is not unusual for HSOs to create a new entity, sometimes called an "umbrella" organization, to span but *not* replace the organizations forming it. Starkweather describes two important subtypes of the umbrella corporation with regard to hospitals. One subtype gives the umbrella corporation limited authority within which its decisions are final. In the other, the umbrella corporation has more general authority that is usually exercised through unified management, policy, and fiscal control.[27]

Restructuring   Extreme and complex voluntary interorganizational transactions occur in mergers and consolidations. A merger results when one (or more) HSO corporation is absorbed by another, which retains its own name and identity. Consolidation occurs when two or more HSO corporations dissolve and are unified in a new legal entity. As interorganizational linkage mechanisms, both merger and consolidation involve restructuring organizational interdependence.

Organization Strategies   Restructuring may involve other organization strategies, such as vertical integration, in which a hospital acquisition of a nursing facility (NF) facilitates discharge to an appropriate level of care and provides referrals to the NF. Restructuring may involve a specialization/niche strategy in which one HSO acquires another to achieve a different capacity/service configuration or to target a specific market. Finally, restructuring may result in diversifying into health services–related or –unrelated activities, such as acquiring a retail pharmacy chain or a hotel, respectively.

Vertical Integration   The most complex restructuring scheme is vertical integration. As a general organization strategy, vertical integration is "the combination, under single ownership, of two or more stages of production or distribution (or both) that are usually separate."[28] As Clement notes, " a vertically integrated firm links the stages of production and distribution of its product into a chain spanning all or part of the distance from ownership and procurement of raw materials to the distribution channels that get the goods or services to the consumer."[29] Vertical integration in health services usually "involves linking together different levels of care and assembling the human resources needed to render that care."[30] As Conrad and Dowling note, "the primary purposes of vertical integration in health care are to enhance the comprehensiveness and continuity of patient care and to control the sources of patients or other users of a delivery system's services."[31] Vertical integration has advantages and disadvantages:[32]

> Advantages
>   Reduced buying and selling costs
>   Assurance of supply and raw materials and/or patients
>   Improved coordination
>   Enhanced technological capabilities
>   Higher entry barriers for competitors

Disadvantages
High capital requirements
Potential for unbalanced throughput
Reduced flexibility and increased risk
Loss of specialization

The most important consideration is often sufficient to override the possible disadvantages of vertical integration: enhanced competitive position through the improved coordination available to interdependent organizations linked in this way. This type of linkage is not suited to all HSOs. For example, using one hospital as the focal organization, there are two important aspects of vertical integration:

> integration forward into the patient acquisition chain to achieve greater control of health plans and primary care physicians, or integration backward toward control of the continuum of care (long-term care, home health care, and so on). In our view, opportunities for successful forward integration are limited to a few players who begin with substantial market power. Opportunities for successful backward integration, however, are available to many health care systems in both large and small markets.[33]

Effective Linkages

Each ownership form of interorganizational transaction carries significant burdens. Varying degrees of autonomy are sacrificed, and interdependencies among participating HSOs, although locked together by the bonds of ownership, must still be managed if relationships are to serve their purposes. Achieving effective linkages among various units of such arrangements is a demanding management task. Porter suggests ways to develop effective linkages among participants in diversified configurations:[34]

> *Structural features* that cross unit lines, such as partial centralization and interunit task forces or committees that facilitate communication.
> *Management systems* with cross-unit dimensions in planning, control, incentives, capital budgeting, and management information systems.
> *Human resource practices* that facilitate unit cooperation, such as cross-unit job rotation, management forums, and training.
> *Conflict resolution processes* that resolve conflicts and settle disputes among units.

In systems with different GBs for some or all units, effective linkages are particularly important and difficult. Here, the most efficacious mechanism may be interlocking GBs because they provide a stable structure to coordinate activity and communication.

An important consideration for HSOs contemplating any of the voluntary linking mechanisms described above is the degree of *goal congruence* they share with other organizations with which they might link. As Luke notes, "Goal congruency, which has to do with the degree to which organizations share similar goals, organizational objectives, missions, and cultures, enhances trust and thereby facilitates the pursuit of cooperative relationships among organizations."[35]

INVOLUNTARY INTERORGANIZATIONAL RELATIONSHIP TRANSACTIONS

Some interdependencies among organizations in the health services sector cannot be managed through market transactions or through voluntary interorganizational relationship transactions. Most notably these involve relationships with regulatory agencies, but they may also include interactions with fiscal intermediaries and utilization management companies. The strategies outlined are specific to interactions with regulatory bodies, but they can be modified and applied to other involuntary interorganizational relationship transactions.

Regulatory Agency Relationships

Despite all the deregulation rhetoric and some limited action in the 1980s, organizations in the health sector remain highly regulated. For example, regulation of HSOs includes fiscal and utilization controls and controls on facilities and services, human resources, and quality.[36] Similarly, insurance carriers and their products are highly regulated by the states.

Regulated HSOs have an interdependent relationship with the organizations that regulate them. Such interdependencies cannot be legally managed through market transactions, which, by definition, involve economic exchanges. Furthermore, the nature of the interdependent relationship between a regulated HSO and its regulator means that the relationship is not subject to the voluntary types of interorganizational transactions described above. These involuntary relationships lead to unique ways of managing interdependence. For example, a primary reason for some coalescing activities among HSOs with a common regulatory agency is to share expertise and thus gain a stronger hand in dealing with the regulator and its regulations.

Managing Interdependence

Regulation of any industry encourages consolidation among the regulated in order to develop counterregulatory expertise and power. The focus here, however, is mechanisms to manage interdependence between an individual regulated organization and its regulator.

Popular Mechanisms Ingenious strategies for managing interdependence have been devised. Some of the more common ones have been described by Altman, Greene, and Sapolsky.[37]

The Litigation Strategy An important mechanism is litigation. Most regulatory decisions can be appealed in the courts, which are sensitive to procedural errors or infringement of due process rights. Regulators who overlook requirements for notice, public hearings, or the opportunity for full consideration of issues invite litigation. Regulators may lack resources for proper legal representation, or sometimes must rely on state legal staffs without expertise in health matters. Another factor that facilitates the litigation strategy is that some standards used by regulators are not substantiated by analysis or fact and thus are vulnerable to judicial scrutiny. Antitrust law as a regulatory mechanism in interorganizational relationships was discussed in Chapter 4.

The Political Intervention Strategy While distasteful to many, cultivating supportive relationships with the executive and legislative branches and with state and federal regulatory agencies can be effective protection against overly enthusiastic or even dutiful regulators. It is no accident that hospitals routinely place prominent public officials and politically connected private citizens on their GBs, that physicians are among the most generous political campaign contributors, or that well-connected consultants flourish in and around Washington, D.C., and state capitals.

The Loaf-and-a-Half Strategy This strategy is drawn from textbooks on negotiating. In it, a regulated organization initially seeks more than it expects to get. For example, by enlarging a project for which a certificate of need is sought, the regulated HSO gives the regulator the opportunity to "play hardball" and force a scaling back of a project without actually jeopardizing what the HSO really wants. A common variation of this strategy is to offer regulators something they want (e.g., a commitment to provide care for indigent patients) in order to obtain approval.

The Constituency Strategy Regulated organizations with the support of a politically powerful constituency are less vulnerable to adverse regulatory decisions than others. The constituency may be based on religion, ethnicity, geography, or another common bond. Regulated HSOs sometimes are each other's constituents, and they trade regulatory approval opportunities.

Less Ethical Mechanisms In addition, there are strategies for managing interdependence that are unethical and/or illegal. While uncommon, they have been used by regulated organizations.

The Data Overload Strategy   An advantage HSOs have over their regulators is their technical expertise and the ability to assemble and manipulate large volumes of data. When challenged, regulated HSOs may flood the agency with technical data that justify their position or simply obscure the issues.

The Open Job Offer Strategy   A well-worn but effective strategy is to "buy off" regulators with promises of attractive jobs. U.S. Patent Office examiners often become patent attorneys. A few years of experience with the Federal Communications Commission are excellent training for lawyers seeking positions with law firms specializing in communications law. Organizations in health services know this strategy, too. Regulators, particularly those in state agencies, often go to work for state hospital associations or large hospitals. Usually, these are legitimate and appropriate transfers of knowledge and experience. However, sometimes they repay a debt incurred in transactions between regulators and the regulated.

The Deception Strategy   Clearly illegal and unethical, deception is possible in relationships between regulators and the regulated. The cost and scope of projects can be understated. Pertinent data can be fabricated or falsified. Projects can be altered after approval. The complexity of projects, long lead times, turnover of regulatory staff, and the difficulty government agencies have in coordinating their programs can prevent close scrutiny of regulated organizations and encourage cheating.

MANAGING INTERORGANIZATIONAL LINKAGES

Cutting across market, voluntary, and involuntary interorganizational relationship transactions is the matter of the managerial skills needed to establish efficacious and efficient linkages with interdependent organizations. These skills include: 1) discerning the necessity of linkages with interdependent others, and 2) choosing from among possible linking mechanisms the one most appropriate for a situation.

As a starting point, managers must realize that all interdependencies are not equally important, nor are the interorganizational relationships developed to manage them. Some relationships have strategic purposes, some do not; distinguishing them is crucial. Relationships with greater effect on the financial condition and/or competitive position of participating organizations and that are relatively more permanent (or intended to be permanent) are more strategic than those less important or not expected to be permanent.[38] Managers must be more concerned with relationships that have a strategic purpose than with those that do not.

Types of Interdependence

When judging importance, managers should remember there are several types of interdependence: pooled, sequential, or reciprocal.[39] *Pooled interdependence* occurs when related organizations have no close connection; they contribute separately to a larger whole. A group of geographically dispersed NFs owned by one corporation are linked in that each contributes to total performance, but they have little functional interdependence. *Sequential interdependence* occurs when organizations have a close and sequential connection. The relationship between an HSO and Blue Cross or some other fiscal intermediary is sequential in that the HSO's cash flow depends on the intermediary to process reimbursement for health services. *Reciprocal interdependence* occurs when HSOs have a close relationship and interdependence goes in both directions. A vertically integrated health care system with acute and long-term care units exhibits reciprocal interdependence. Long-term care beds are occupied by referrals from acute care beds; the acute care organization depends on the long-term care organization to discharge certain patients. The acute care unit suffers if the long-term care unit cannot accept a referral. Conversely, the long-term care unit suffers if patients are not discharged to it from the acute care unit.

As interdependence moves from the pooled to the sequential to the reciprocal form, effective management is more important,[40] and the need for managerial attention to effective linkages increases as well. Sequential and reciprocal linkages are more complex because they involve issues such as the nature of exchange relationships between participating organizations, which will have the most power, the terms of resource transactions, and how innovations will be developed and diffused.[41]

Managers must understand that the situation affects the choice of linking mechanisms. Selecting an option is among the most important and difficult decisions managers face. Continuing a straight market transaction when a voluntary interorganizational relationship transaction could produce greater benefits may be a costly mistake. Conversely, managing interdependence through a complex ownership arrangement in which important legal and functional autonomies are sacrificed when a simple market transaction would suffice may be even more costly. Hence, great care must be exercised in choosing and implementing an option for linking interdependent organizations.

Linkage Costs

In choosing from among alternatives, it must be remembered that interorganizational linkages have costs; most obvious are the time, personnel, and money needed to support the linkage mechanism. The potential to lose some autonomy is omnipresent. Less obvious but important costs include what Porter calls the cost of compromise and the cost of inflexibility.[42] Compromise has costs because linking across organizational boundaries may require that an activity be performed consistently, but in a way that is suboptimal for individual participants. The cost of compromise can be reduced if an activity is *designed* for sharing. Participants in a merger may find that developing a management information system specifically for the new organization is better than using the existing system at either organization or than linking the two separate systems and fixing the gaps in them.

The cost of inflexibility is not a continuing cost of interorganizational linkages. It arises when there is need for flexibility. It often occurs when there is a need to respond to a competitor's move or a market opportunity. It occurs because linkages to manage interorganizational interdependencies add complexity and, often, inflexibility. Managers must weigh these costs against the benefits.

HSOs are moving toward more complex and pervasive interorganizational linkages. This suggests that a vital skill for managers will be judging the desirability of linkage mechanisms with interdependent others and choosing the most appropriate.

CORPORATE RESTRUCTURING

In the 1970s and well into the 1980s, it was common for HSOs, especially acute care hospitals, to redesign traditional organizations and organizational relationships. Corporate restructuring is defined as creating two or more corporate entities to perform medical and nonmedical functions previously performed by one corporation—a multiorganizational arrangement. Diversification, which may be a result of or a cause of corporate restructuring, is discussed below. Figure 9.2 shows two examples of restructuring. In one type a hospital corporation forms a related charitable foundation whose purpose is to benefit the hospital by engaging in health– and nonhealth–related activities. In another common type a holding company is established that holds controlling interest in a hospital and other corporate entities, some of which are engaged in nonhealth-related activities.

Such corporate restructuring models vary widely, but generally each seeks to overcome problems inherent in the traditional way hospitals are organized. Hospitals restructured in the mid-1970s to establish foundations that sheltered endowment funds from Medicare. During the late 1970s and early 1980s, many hospitals established subsidiaries to bypass certificate-of-need

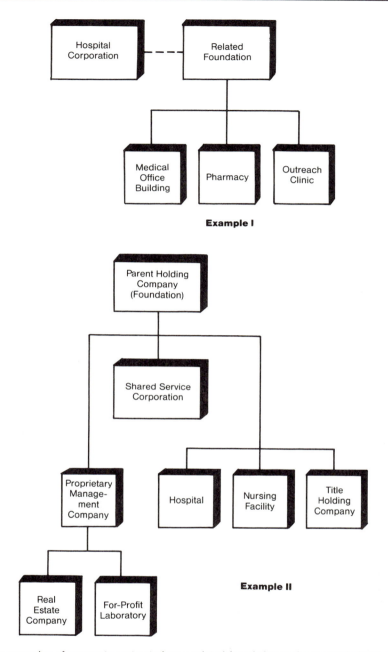

Figure 9.2. Two examples of corporate restructuring; a related foundation and a parent holding company. (From Coopers and Lybrand. A *layman's guide to hospitals III: Hospital corporate reorganizations.* New York, 1981; reprinted by permission.)

regulations. In the mid- to late 1980s, hospitals used the organization strategy of diversification to offset declining state and federal reimbursement.[43] During the 1980s, 42% of hospitals had restructured; almost two thirds of those restructurings occurred between 1985 and 1989.[44] Figure 9.3 shows the types of restructuring in which hospitals engaged in the 1980s.

In the late 1980s and early 1990s, hospitals began to reconsider their rush to restructure and

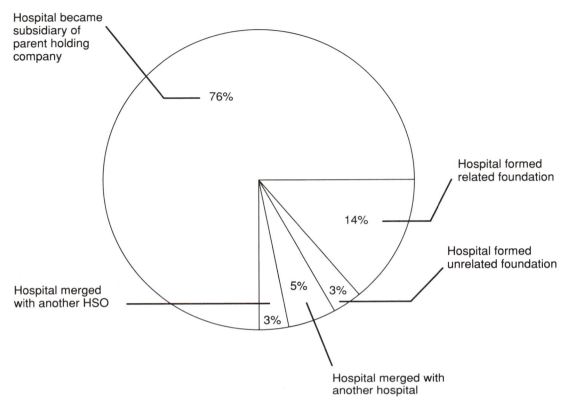

Hospital became subsidiary of parent holding company

76%

Hospital formed related foundation

14%

Hospital formed unrelated foundation

Hospital merged with another HSO

5%   3%

3%

Hospital merged with another hospital

Figure 9.3.   Structure of the most recent reorganization for hospitals, 1980–1989. (Data source: Alexander, Jeffrey A. *The changing character of hospital governance*, 10. Chicago: The Hospital Research and Educational Trust, 1990; data are based on a 1989 survey. Percentages total to more than 100 because of rounding.)

moved to simplify corporate organizations and relationships. This reflected a changed environment, but several other factors were important: excessive complexity, confused lines of authority, management that was often ill prepared for the demands of a restructured organization, diffuse views of vision and goals, high overhead costs, diversification into activities that did not support the mission, risk to tax-exempt status (discussed in Chapter 4), and community image.[45]

Hospitals believe they will gain several advantages by simplifying corporate structures:

Reduce the administrative expenses that come with multiple corporations and multiple boards;
Cut subsidiary losses that are draining hospital assets;
Divest businesses that don't further an organization's strategic goals;
Focus on the hospital's core business; and
Avoid challenges to the hospital's tax-exempt status.[46]

The effort to get back to basics will continue into the 1990s.

MULTIORGANIZATIONAL ARRANGEMENTS

Organizations in the health sector are in flux, and relationships between or among hospitals and other HSOs are changing. A multiorganizational arrangement is defined as two or more HSOs owned, leased, sponsored, or managed under contract by one organization. Multihospital systems have attracted the most attention, but more important and far more pervasive changes are found in a wide variety of multiorganizational arrangements. The concept of multihospital systems is limited; this discussion treats the more generic concept of multiorganizational arrangements, which includes a broad array of relationships between or among HSOs.

Types of Arrangements

The numbers and types of multiorganizational arrangements are virtually limitless. Figure 9.4 suggests a continuum conceptualization. The divisions between the categories are permeable, and multiorganizational arrangements may include elements of more than one of them.

Arrangements on this continuum fall into two categories: between or among one type of HSO exclusively, and between or among various types of HSOs such as acute care hospitals, NFs, and ambulatory HSOs. Combinations in which there are linkages among organizations at the same point in the production process and in the same part of the industry, such as among two or more hospitals or two or more NFs, are horizontal interrelationships. Linkages among organizations at different points in the production process, such as between an acute care hospital, an NF, and a hospice, constitute vertical integration.

HSOs may be located anywhere on the continuum with regard to multiorganizational activities and may enter a variety of arrangements. Multiple arrangements of HSOs are called "networking."[47] A hospital that networks may establish several affiliations, share a variety of services, belong to one or more consortia, manage other HSOs under contract, or merge. Conclusions reached by Berman in 1982 continue to be applicable:

> There are many free standing hospitals in this country whose communities want them to retain their independent identity and unique community roots. These hospitals will not merge nor will their community allow them to give up their identity to a multihospital system.
>
> Yet to prosper, to continue to be able to serve, these hospitals will have to link together with other institutions—they will have to form networks. And in fact may become part of several networks.
>
> The networks will be characterized by a hub organization and then links of cooperative arrangements between institutions. In some instances the hub organization will be a hospital which will acquire or merge into itself other hospitals. However, the key is going to be a series of cooperative arrangements—not direct control.[48]

The HSO multiorganizational arrangements in Figure 9.4 cover a continuum from pluralism to fusion. Informal affiliations (1) are joint undertakings without written agreement. An example is joint sponsorship of a health fair or screening for a disease or medical condition. Formal affiliations (2) occur when two or more HSOs formally undertake limited activities together. An example is an affiliation for purposes of medical education. Shared or cooperative services (3) are managerial, clinical, or service functions common to two or more HSOs and used jointly or coop-

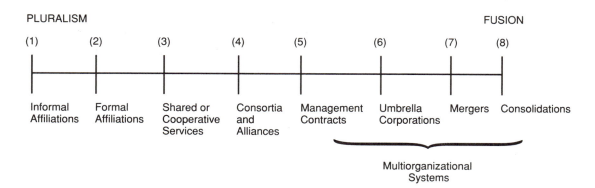

Figure 9.4. Continuum of multiorganizational arrangements.

eratively by them. An example is a shared laundry facility or joint purchasing. Consortia and alliances (4) are voluntary associations of HSOs that may be located in the same geographic area. Consortia and alliances are formed for specific, usually limited purposes. Examples are access to capital and consulting services in specialized areas such as labor relations and management information systems.

In multiorganizational arrangements that involve management contracts (5), one HSO supplies senior management to another; managers include the CEO, who reports to the GB of the managed organization *and* to the managing organization, and often the chief financial officer. The differences between contract management and management contracts were noted earlier. Umbrella organizations (6) exist when a new corporation is formed to span, but not replace, existing HSOs. As noted earlier, Starkweather describes two important subtypes of umbrella corporations:

> One is where only limited authorities are granted to the new corporation, but in these realms the umbrella corporation's authority is final. These arrangements often deal with planning or allocation of services among otherwise distinct hospitals [for example]. There is usually no central management or central fiscal control. In the other subtype the umbrella corporation's authority is more general and complete, usually exercised through unified management, policy, and fiscal control. This type is akin to the parent-subsidiary form found commonly in the business world. In this arrangement the participating hospitals are required to turn over all assets to the new corporation, and it in turn assumes their liabilities. New assets that are developed are typically owned by the umbrella corporation. Services which are combined in this arrangement include hospital support and administration activities as well as professional services. In addition to these aspects of horizontal integration, the new corporation may engage in vertical integrations by developing or acquiring diagnostic clinics, group practices, home health services, extended care facilities, etc.[49]

Mergers (7) and consolidations (8) are at the fusion end of the continuum of arrangements (Figure 9.4). In both, at least one corporation is dissolved. A merger results when one (or more) HSO corporation is absorbed by another, which retains its own name and identity. Consolidation occurs when two or more HSO corporations dissolve and are unified in a new legal entity. Starkweather notes that "The prerogatives of the successor organization (in both merger and consolidation) are enumerated in formal agreements which assume permanence and which prohibit autonomous activity by prior-existing entities."[50] These definitions suggest that the four arrangements closest to the fusion end of the continuum presented in Figure 9.4 are forms of multiorganizational systems.

Growth and Extent of Multiorganizational Arrangements

Among the most dramatic developments in health services delivery during the 1970s and 1980s was the emergence of the multiorganizational arrangements shown in Figure 9.4. The forms are varied, but the arrangements share a common trait: they reflect the health services industry's move away from its historical structure of autonomous, independent organizations.[51]

Hospital participation in one or more of these types of arrangements is extensive. As early as 1975, more than 60% of United States community hospitals shared one or more services. In 1979, 26% of community hospitals with 31% of beds were part of a system—they occupied at least one of the last four positions at the fusion end of the continuum in Figure 9.4. Barrett noted that the number of hospitals and hospital beds in multiorganizational systems grew even more in 1980 and 1981.[52] Brown and co-workers produced a comprehensive set of statistics on the extent of multihospital systems activities, based on the American Hospital Association's annual hospital survey.[53]

Reasons for Growth Knowing the reasons for the growth of multiorganizational arrangements is vital to understanding the changing health services system. Noteworthy is that growth occurred with no hard evidence of real benefits.[54] Longest theorizes that:

Participation in multihospital arrangements is part of a stabilization strategy elaborated by many hospital managers. Such strategies are often seen in organizations . . . when they face environments similar to those faced by hospitals during the past decade [1970s]. . . .[D]ecision makers in participating hospitals believe that the formation of multihospital arrangements makes possible the achievement of a higher level of organizational stability than is available . . . when their organizations remain completely autonomous and independent. It has been demonstrated in other industries that formal, multiorganization arrangements represent methods for extending organizational control over vital exchanges that participants must enter into (1) for increasing the participating organizations' power in these exchanges and reducing uncertainty caused by competition and (2) for reducing the participating organizations' dependence on other dominant organizations.

[T]his view of multihospital arrangement growth [makes] it . . . [un]necessary to search for the "evidence" that they will produce efficiencies or quality improvements for those organizations participating in them as the explanatory factor in the growth pattern. Rather, it is only necessary to understand the relationship between the external environment facing a hospital and the strategies elaborated for it. This view does not mean that efficiency or quality goals do not partially explain the increase in participation in multihospital arrangements, or that if there is mounting evidence of efficiency or quality improvements, the evidence will not spur additional growth. This view does, however, provide a framework within which to explain why the growth in these arrangements [has] *preceded* all but the most preliminary and mixed evidence of their efficacy.[55]

Multihospital Systems and Alliances

In 1989, more than one third (36%) of United States hospitals belonged to a multihospital system, defined as two or more hospitals that are owned, leased, or sponsored by one administrative entity.[56] Shortell predicts that by the year 2000, "Upwards of 80 percent of America's hospitals will then be formal members of systems, with the remaining 20 percent or so representing a combination of affiliated networks, alliances, quasi firms, and some freestanding hospitals filling in the niches and crevices."[57] Figure 9.5 illustrates Shortell's projection.

Alliances were conceived in the 1970s and are a type of multiorganizational arrangement that involves not-for-profit (tax-exempt, charitable) acute care hospitals. Alliances were identified by leaders in the not-for-profit sector as a way to counter the rapid growth of for-profit (investor-owned) chains that were developing into supermeds, multiorganizational arrangements that it was believed would soon dominate the United States hospital field.[58] In addition to growing pains, alliances in the mid-1980s had to adjust to changing conditions and began meeting the needs of hospitals and systems competing in regional markets. They concentrated on serving a wide range of needs for a narrowly defined set of hospitals, or they concentrated on providing a few services to a large number of diverse HSOs. Experience suggested that doing both well was not possible.[59] Shared purchasing is ubiquitous to alliances. Other activities are likely to include financial and management consulting, access to capital, managed care and contracting, physician recruitment and bonding services, insurance and risk management, data exchange, shared services and personnel, and technology and research.[60] Among the largest and most prominent alliances are Voluntary Hospitals of America, American Healthcare Systems, and SunHealth Network. Specialized alliances include Premier Hospitals Alliance (community teaching hospitals) and University Hospital Consortium.[61]

Most of the literature about multiorganizational arrangements in health services suggests that growth occurred on the assumption that benefits would accrue: possible improvement in efficiency of health services delivery—through economies of scale and reducing duplicative services—and possible improvement in quality, comprehensiveness, and continuity of patient care. However, as Barrett concluded in the early 1980s, "as the novelty wears off, tough questions will be asked concerning their performance as well as their promise."[62] As noted below, this prediction has proved correct.

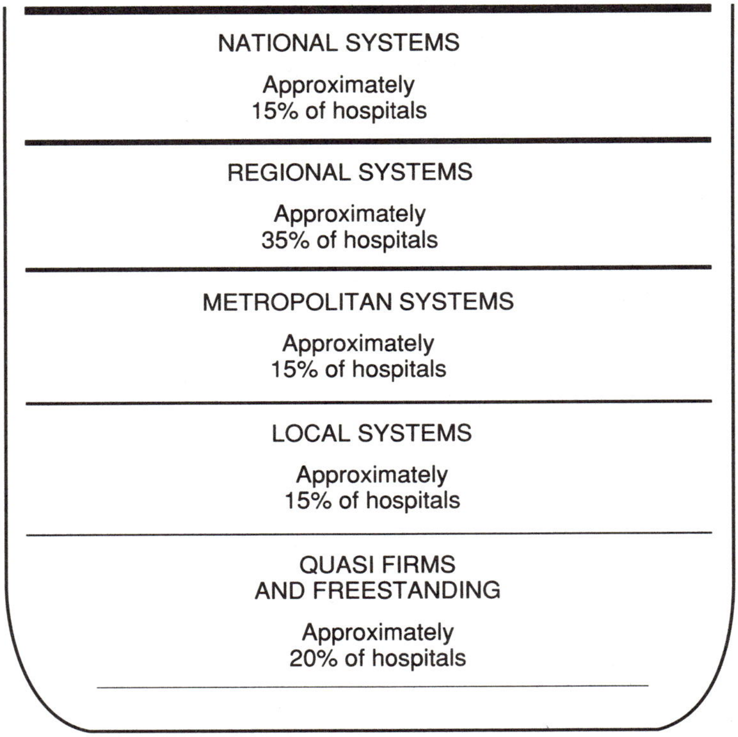

Figure 9.5. The hospital industry as organizational strata in the year 2000. (From Shortell, Stephen M. The evolution of hospital systems: Unfulfilled promises and self-fulfilling prophesies. *Medical Care Review* 45 [Fall 1988]: 191; Health Administration Press, Ann Arbor, MI. Reprinted by permission. Copyright © 1988, Foundation of the American College of Healthcare Executives.)

Problems and Benefits

Significant problems occur in multiorganizational holding companies that have multiple GBs. Despite the presence of one CEO, these GBs have differences in philosophies that create dynamic tension between them, often with the CEO caught in the middle. The parent GB is likely to have a futuristic vision, while the operating company (hospital) GB focuses on operational effectiveness and efficiency.[63] These conflicts occur despite the fact that approximately 50% of hospital GB members also serve on the system's corporate GB.[64] CEOs may be able to avoid this conflict and the discontinuities it causes by insisting that their GBs help them develop a shared vision through the strategic plan.[65]

Potential benefits of multiorganizational arrangements are considerable, even though evidence about the reality of performance is mixed and must be interpreted with caution. One source of information is a survey that found that successful systems seem to share certain characteristics:[66]

Regional focus

Common strategy, with emphasis on differentiation and uniqueness

Commonality of organization, with a clear organizational structure, centralization and consolidation of staff functions and decentralization of patient care, assured economies of scale, and an organizational structure matched to the system's overall strategy

Focused corporate culture, with a strong performance orientation

Emphasis on rewards for employees, with top executives earning more than the national average and greater use of incentives and wider participation in incentive plans

In addition, total quality management (a synonym for continuous quality improvement, discussed in Chapter 11, "Quality and Productivity Improvement") was pervasive in leading hospital systems. The survey also found that top performers spend less time on finance, planning, and development functions and emphasize strategy implementation rather than strategy formulation.[67]

The potential benefits of multiorganizational arrangements may be of several types and accrue at different levels. Zuckerman developed a framework to assess potential benefits, categorized them as economic, human resources, and organizational, and suggested that they may accrue to the organizations involved or to the community—those served.[68] Zuckerman's conceptualization is somewhat oversimplified but is useful (Table 9.3). For example, organizations are not homogeneous; potential benefits for a large teaching hospital may be quite different from those for a small community hospital. Similarly, benefits of a multiorganizational arrangement for citizens of a community with an extensive array of health services might be very different compared with those for persons in a rural or poorly served urban area.

DIVERSIFICATION[69]

Diversification is a process in which organizations add to existing product/service mixes and/or enter new markets with existing and/or new products/services. Diversification has become a common organization strategy for HSOs in the past 20 years, especially in acute care hospitals. In fact, one of the most identifiable trends in the health services field in the 1970s and 1980s was the propensity of many HSOs, most often acute care hospitals, to diversify. Diversification is such a basic aspect of the strategic behavior of United States hospitals that it has been suggested that

Table 9.3. Summary of potential benefits of multiorganizational arrangements

Type of benefit	Level of benefit	
	Institutional	Community

Economic	Cost savings via economies of scale:
	Operating advantages—
	  increased productivity
	  improved utilization of resource capacity
	  lower staffing requirements
	  reduced unit costs from joint activities
	Financial advantages—
	  access to capital markets
	  improved credit standing
	  reduced borrowing costs
		Lower prices
		Reduced duplication and excess capacity of facilities
		Improved resource allocation

Human resources	Improved recruitment of health occupations and managers Improved retention of health occupations and managers Strong clinical and management capability	Greater access to and availability of breadth and depth of health occupations and managers Improved distribution of health occupations
Organizational	Organizational growth (e.g., extend referral networks, penetrate new markets, expand existing markets) Organizational survival (e.g., financial improvements, accreditation standards) Greater political power	Improved access to care Increased availability of services Broader, more comprehensive scope of services

Adapted from Zuckerman, Howard S. Multiinstitutional systems: Promise and performance. *Inquiry* 16 (Winter 1979): 294, used by permission.

"diversification must be a part of each hospital's strategy regardless of its specific strategic orientation."[70]

Impetus for Hospital Diversification

Fundamentally, the attractiveness of new sources of revenue for HSOs—indeed, their necessity for many—results from changes in traditional revenue sources. Almost without exception, acute care hospitals that have diversified in the past decade have done so in the hope that these activities would provide new income to offset declines in revenue from inpatient activities. Once generous hospital reimbursement policies based on actual costs have been supplanted largely by capitation, negotiated rates, and fixed payment schemes. This slowed the rate of growth or actually reduced hospital revenues. Furthermore, hospitals and, increasingly, other HSOs, face unrelenting cost control pressures from the public and private sectors, often through schemes to monitor and manage utilization of services.

Among the direct consequences of stringent policies has been a precipitous decline for many hospitals in production of inpatient days—their traditional core product/service and their more important source of revenue. The magnitude of this decline is critical to understanding the appeal of diversification. After years of steady growth, inpatient days began to decline in the early 1980s. The average daily census of inpatients in U.S. hospitals has decreased about 20% since 1982.[71] Reflecting this decline in volume, almost 60% of community hospitals had negative net patient margins (i.e., they lost money on patient care services) by the late 1980s.[72]

Utilization declines and resultant revenue problems made it more difficult, and in some cases impossible, to maintain state-of-the-art physical plant and technology, compete for a dwindling pool of skilled labor, or provide uncompensated care. Not surprisingly, hospitals aggressively chose diversification into activities that offered opportunities for new revenue and expanded markets. They pursued diversification as a way to support core activities in the face of reduced demand and declines in profitability of traditional activities. Favorite diversification options include freestanding outpatient surgery centers, women's health centers, various outpatient programs, industrial medicine programs, and a variety of services for the elderly, including home health care.

Diversification has been a strategic response to the less munificent environment that has faced hospitals since the early 1980s. For many, this organization strategy has been a matter of survival. Between 1980 and 1990, 761 United States hospitals closed.[73] Seeing this as the beginning of a Darwinian winnowing of those least able to withstand a harsh environment, many hospital managers believe that survival depends on their institution's successful diversification into profitable new products/services and/or markets.

Revenue enhancement and profitability are the most important reasons to diversify, but there are other motives. Some are only indirectly economic, but they may be important to hospital survival and well-being in the future. For example, some hospitals have viewed diversification as "a means of building an integrated health care system" that would enhance the quality of each phase of care.[74] In theory, the synergies gained provide a significant competitive advantage for the systems and their components. Coddington and Moore offer a more elaborate set of possible motives for diversification by HSOs:

Community service—Health care needs might go unmet without an HSO diversifying to respond to the need.

Innovation—Being at the cutting edge of new products/services gives HSOs an advantage in identifying emerging business opportunities.

Risk management—HSOs can minimize financial risk by spreading it among several activities and markets.

Clinical staff relations—Diversifying into services that the clinical staff want to provide or have available to patients (e.g., substance abuse treatment) is a way to improve relationships with them. [75]

These and other factors contributed to the impetus for diversification. It must not be forgotten, however, that diversification by hospitals came primarily from a need to improve their bleak financial picture, which resulted from relying on traditional revenue sources.

Context of Hospital Diversification

Hospitals had few constraints as they diversified into new products/services and new markets, and this was a stimulus. Hospitals have a large stock of technology, human resources, and management and patient care expertise, and this encouraged managers to deploy these assets in diversified endeavors, especially those closely related to core patient care activities. Furthermore, much diversification is programmatic—it needs no expensive space—and it avoids regulatory constraints that focus on brick and mortar projects.

Hospitals that diversify are not completely unfettered, however. They face the same capital, competitive, and market opportunity constraints that any firm faces. In addition, HSOs have unique constraints. Two deserve comment because they explain some choices managers make in diversifying.

A long-standing constraint on diversification lies in the fact that voluntary (i.e., private, not-for-profit) ownership and control predominate in the hospital industry. In 1990, of the 5,420 community hospitals in the United States, 3,202 were voluntary, 1,469 were controlled by state or local government, and only 749 were investor owned. [76] Thus, of the total number of community hospitals only a relative few—typically the investor owned—are able to diversify products/services or expand into new markets without regard to nonmarket issues that accompany ownership and control. Even among investor-owned hospitals, which may have more flexibility in strategic decisions, many are the sole providers in their communities and can ill afford to make product/service mix or market adjustments that disregard community preferences.

Hospitals under public or voluntary control are locked into some courses of action and precluded from others. A publicly sponsored hospital is subject to a public agenda that may bear little relationship to the need to reshape its product/service mix or redefine markets. A voluntary hospital is a social charity that has been granted tax exemption, a privilege carrying the responsibilities and obligations described in Chapter 4. These burdens limit the freedom managers have to make diversification decisions on financial grounds.

A more recent constraint on diversification options is found in *Key Enterprises of Delaware, Inc. v. Venice (FL) Hospital* (919 F.2d 1550 [11th cir. 1990]). This ruling puts hospital subsidiaries at risk of an antitrust action by competitors. [77] The court ruled that Venice Hospital's medical supply business (a diversification) had an unfair competitive advantage in gaining customers compared with businesses not directly associated with the hospital. The decision could affect common types of hospital diversification (e.g., home care services, durable medical equipment services, rehabilitation units, and hospices) because managers and clinical staff in hospitals that have diversified into these activities can influence or direct potential customers to them. Additional information on the legal aspects of antitrust is found in Chapter 4.

Obviously, diversification that produces antitrust actions will be unpopular. This does not mean all diversification is threatened, however. In fact, vulnerability to antitrust action requires a market-by-market analysis. In many circumstances it may be possible to avoid antitrust challenges simply by giving patients and physicians a choice to select from services that compete with a hospital's diversified activities, avoiding disparaging competitors, and making no unsubstantiated claims for hospital services. Conversely, it is likely that this ruling, which resulted from the unique relationship between hospitals and their customers, could have a chilling effect on hospital diversification.

Types of HSO Diversification Activities

As an organization strategy, hospital diversification can be categorized in two ways: concentric and conglomerate. Concentric diversification is that in which different *but related* and complementary products/services are added to the HSO's existing set of products/services. Conglomerate diversification is that in which products/services that are *unrelated* to the HSO's principal business or core products/services are added to the portfolio.

Concentric (Related and Complementary) Diversification Concentric diversification generally entails developing or acquiring products/services to complement existing ones, expanding sales to current markets, and/or penetrating new markets. Characteristically, in pursuing this strategy the HSO remains close to its competencies.[78] Because health services involve unique competencies that are often protected by licensure and professional dominance and are rarely substitutable, it is not surprising that most diversification in HSOs is concentric. This proclivity for concentric diversification distinguishes HSOs from organizations elsewhere in the economy, where diversifying within present competencies may be less important.

Most of the diversification that has occurred in the health services field is clearly concentric because it revolves around a core of technologies inherent in health services. Even when diversifying into services that do not involve direct patient care and that are unrelated to their principal business, HSOs tend to perform activities that capitalize on their competencies. For example, hospitals may diversify by providing computer or laundry services to other organizations or by food catering.

Sometimes, HSOs undertake complex and extensive forms of concentric diversification. One example is that of a hospital that collaborated with a large multispecialty group practice, an NF, and an insurance carrier to design, produce, and market a managed care program.[79] They formed a quasi firm, which was described earlier.[80] The arrangement permitted each to continue operating independently to accomplish other objectives while simultaneously adding a new concentric diversified product (the managed care program) to their product/service mix. These HSOs diversified without the expense, restrictions, or possible diminution of autonomy and identity that would have resulted from acquiring or merging with the other organizations involved.

Related diversification can be achieved by expanding into new product/service lines through internal development or acquisition. Opportunities for product/service diversification through internal development or acquisition are limited only by the products/services the diversifying hospital does not offer. Prominent examples of product/service diversification by acute care hospitals in the 1980s were outpatient therapeutic services such as chemotherapy and radiation therapy, outpatient diagnostic services such as computed tomography and magnetic resonance imaging, and outpatient health promotion services such as health screening and fitness centers. In addition, hospitals can add an array of inpatient services to expand their products/services. Examples are rehabilitation, psychiatric, obstetric, pediatric, or trauma services.

Often the objective of concentric diversification is to enter new markets for existing and/or new products/services. Many of the product/service diversifications noted above allow this. For example, adding obstetrics or pediatrics may open new population groups to other hospital services. Services that target the elderly, such as geriatric day care, home-delivered meals, durable medical equipment, and in-home skilled nursing services, are examples of the opportunities derived by serving a new population group.

Diversification to reach new markets often means establishing satellite primary care or urgent care centers to serve as sources of new customers, both for the new center and through referral to existing services. In this instance vertical integration is coupled with diversification.

Diversification also may include establishing new patient referral patterns for existing services in order to enhance market share. This widely used strategy is based on redefining markets. One such redefinition involves the flow of patient referrals, which in the past went almost exclusively from routine care to specialty care. This meant teaching hospitals were the prime beneficiaries. As consumers become more price sensitive, however, high-cost providers must refer routine cases to less expensive settings. HSOs that recognize this change and develop appropriate referral arrangements can expand markets for current and new products/services.

Conglomerate (Unrelated) Diversification Conglomerate diversification entails the development or acquisition of products/services that are unrelated to the HSO's core mix of products and services. Some HSOs, for example, have undertaken real estate development to a limited extent. However, in that unrelated diversification does not generally revolve around HSO competencies or core technologies, it is much less prevalent than concentric diversification. A common criterion for conglomerate diversification is whether the newly acquired or developed unit can meet stringent standards of profitability when controlled by the diversifying HSO.[81] Profitability is considered quite important because HSOs enter into these types of diversification as means of generating income that can be used to support the HSO's core mission.

Outcomes of Hospital Diversification

The frequency of health services diversification during the past decade does not mean it was always successful. This is especially true at the level of individual institutions, where a large volume of diversification seems linked to failure. There is evidence that *less* diversification improves the probability of success for that which is undertaken, regardless of type. It has been shown, for example, that hospitals in good financial condition (as shown by indicators such as increasing operating margins) are less diversified, but earn more revenue from diversification because they concentrate on programs in which they can gain market share. This contrasts with hospitals that are more diversified but have declining margins.[82] This suggests that successful hospital diversification strategies heed the warning that "A danger arises from diversification when the new products or markets differ radically from those the organization has previously known. Management may be unable to function effectively if it employs technology and expertise that is not appropriate for the new endeavor."[83]

As noted earlier, the potential for new sources of income is an overriding but not exclusive reason to diversify. Therefore, the best way to judge the success of diversification is whether the strategy contributes revenues that exceed the expense—the profitability—or whether it offers the promise of profits if it can be sustained through its developmental stages.

The data about hospital diversification for 1990 shown in Table 9.4 rank the degree to which diversification generates profits or breaks even. More than 60% of hospitals having freestanding outpatient surgery centers, freestanding outpatient diagnostic centers, inpatient physical rehabilitation units, or home health services generated profits from them in 1990. In all other categories (except wellness/health promotion) most hospitals at least broke even. This suggests that hospitals can continue these break-even activities until they do become profitable if they so choose. Yet, Table 9.4 shows quite clearly that not all diversifications meet the objective of profitability. Some may never do so.

Sometimes the decision to provide a new product/service or enter a new market is flawed. In other cases, other circumstances, including actions of competitors, may have changed during implementation. Diversification is successful because of careful screening and selection, good marketing, and effective implementation. Such programs contribute to an HSO's financial success. The economic dimensions of diversification are only one consideration, however. Hospitals, especially, must be careful in utilizing diversification strategies that may antagonize members of the clinical staff, typically physicians. Competition for outpatients is a significant source of con-

Table 9.4. Relative financial performance of hospital diversifications, 1990

Products/services	Percentage profitable	+	Percentage at break even	=	Success rate
Freestanding outpatient surgery center	76.4%		18.1%		94.5%
Freestanding outpatient diagnostic center	71.7		18.3		90.0
Physical rehabilitation	60.5		28.0		88.5
Home health service	60.4		27.2		87.6
Cardiac rehabilitation	42.2		38.5		80.7
Preferred provider organization	33.9		46.4		80.3
Industrial medicine	45.5		34.5		80.0
Women's medicine	39.3		38.5		77.8
Skilled nursing unit	39.7		32.9		72.6
Psychiatric service	49.0		22.5		71.5
Substance abuse treatment unit	39.2		30.9		70.1
Health maintenance organization	38.9		27.8		66.7
Intermediate care facility	34.2		32.5		66.7
Satellite urgent care facility	41.6		24.7		66.3
Retirement housing	29.4		35.3		64.7
Obstetrics	37.6		23.2		60.8
Pediatrics	24.7		34.3		59.0
Trauma center	26.1		31.8		57.9
Wellness/health promotion program	11.0		35.1		46.1

Reprinted from *Hospitals* 65, No. 1, by permission, January 5, 1991, Copyright © 1991, American Hospital Publishing, Inc.

flict between hospitals and physicians.[84] Diversifying in ways that minimize such economic competition is vital to good relations with practitioners, who, as noted in Chapter 7, are the engine that pulls the hospital train.

Only 11% of hospitals (see Table 9.4) that diversified into health promotion/wellness programs did so profitably; less than one half were profitable or breaking even. Despite this, by 1987 more than 70% of hospitals had diversified into health promotion/wellness programs, according to a survey that found that, while such services may not make money, "they can benefit a hospital by enhancing its reputation in the community and generating referrals."[85] Over time, these benefits translate into a stronger financial position just as surely as does a product/service that makes a more direct and immediate contribution to profitability.

To conclude, product/service diversification and market diversification were undertaken by hospital managers on a massive scale in the 1980s. Often, diversified activities have been profitable or have broken even, with the promise of future contributions to the financial health of the HSOs undertaking them. Indeed, against a background of declining revenue from traditional sources, diversifying has become a necessary and successful organization strategy that has enabled many HSOs to cope with their environments.

JOINT VENTURES

Joint ventures are a way HSOs can diversify. The joint venture is typically a limited partnership, which was described in Chapter 4. Joint ventures in health services commonly involve an acute care hospital as the general partner and physician members of its clinical staff as limited partners. The general partner usually invests the bulk of the capital and is the managing partner. Limited partners invest far less capital, sometimes insignificant amounts, a fact that has caused problems with the Internal Revenue Service for some not-for-profit HSOs. The primary reason to involve physicians in joint ventures, however, is not the capital they bring to the enterprise. It is because this ties them more closely to the hospital, and because they provide referrals to the health services delivery activity that is the purpose of the joint venture or, in the case of a medical office building (usually on the hospital campus), physicians rent space from the limited partnership and locate their practices there. Efforts to tie physicians who are independent contractors into the hospital are known as bonding. Various types of HSOs, even competitors, may engage in a joint venture to establish a shared service.

Well-conceived and well-executed joint ventures will help hospitals improve their profitability, market position, and physician relations. This explains why the level of joint venture activities has remained relatively stable in the 1980s.[86] In 1989, the various types of joint ventures with physicians in which hospitals engaged included outpatient diagnostic centers (23.2%), medical office buildings (17.0%), and surgery centers (5.9%).[87] Unsuccessful joint ventures, however, will split the medical communities, harm hospital occupancy, and create financial hardships for investors.[88] In 1984, only 12% of United States hospitals were involved in a joint venture.[89] In 1988, just 4 years later, 48% had at least one joint venture.[90]

HSOs should move cautiously in developing joint ventures. Hospitals with large clinical staffs that include physicians in competing medical groups must be especially wary, since inviting certain physicians will alienate those who do not share in the economic rewards or who do not have the competitive advantage gained by participating physicians. In addition to the economic and political risks (vis-à-vis clinical staff), the HSO must be aware that its community image may suffer should it be seen primarily as a business.

There are several reasons to organize a joint venture:

> Prevention of freestanding skimmers [HSOs that have lucrative niches] and competing ventures. Hospitals unwilling to divide the revenue pie with the [clinical] staff will find their physicians organizing a venture on their own or in cooperation with a provider of free-standing services.
> Creation of a "loss leader" to enhance overall revenue. To increase overall census, hospitals have joint ventured imaging centers, surgicenters, etc. This has increased the physician loyalty and overall utilization. (Joint ventures, however, have not generally achieved the objective of bonding physicians to the hospital.)[91]
> As a final strategy when conventional means of growing the business fail.
> To minimize the risk of specialty program start-up. Referring physician investment in a new specialty program such as lithotripsy, MRI [magnetic resonance imaging], and outpatient rehabilitation will increase the likelihood that referral patterns will shift toward that program.[92]

Problems with Joint Ventures

It is vital that the planning and implementation phases of a joint venture receive adequate attention. The literature stresses again and again that joint ventures are serious business activities that can, and often do, fail. An indicator of problems in joint ventures is the evolution of "salvage" firms whose modus operandi is to purchase failing joint-venture imaging and surgery centers.[93]

Joint ventures, especially those with physicians who are members of the clinical staff, raise potential legal problems under federal law. The two most significant are the Medicare and Medicaid fraud and abuse statute and challenges to the tax-exempt status of charitable HSOs resulting from issues of private benefit.

The Medicare and Medicaid Patient and Program Protection Act of 1987 (PL 100-93) addresses fraud and abuse in these programs and broadens earlier laws that dealt with kickbacks, bribes, and rebates. In mid-1991, the Health Care Financing Administration issued regulations that described "safe harbors."[94] Identifying safe harbors allows HSOs participating in Medicare and Medicaid to know what activities may be undertaken without penalty. Two examples of safe harbors related to joint ventures include detailed requirements about "small entities" and space and equipment. "Large entities" are defined as those HSOs that are publicly traded, with at least $50 million of net value in health care assets. The regulations for small entities focus on issues such as passive investors, marketing and furnishing of services to noninvestors, and proportional rate of return. Of great importance is that the percentage of gross revenue that may come from interested (physician) investors is limited to 40: "The 60/40 investment and revenue standards make it unlikely that typical physician joint ventures would fit within the small entities safe harbor."[95] The reason current joint ventures between hospitals and physicians will not fit into this safe harbor is because physicians who are also investors are usually the overwhelming source of referrals. A second safe harbor related to joint ventures is space and equipment. To qualify as a safe harbor the aggregate rental for space and equipment must be set in advance, consistent with fair market value, and not related to volume or referrals. "As a result, rental arrangements calculated on a per-use or percentage basis will not meet the safe harbor and will require case-by-case analysis to determine the risk of violating the illegal remuneration statute."[96] The limits established by these safe harbors suggest that the number of joint ventures is likely to decline in the future, or at the very least their structures will change significantly.

Issues of private benefit (inurement) have broad application to not-for-profit HSOs that are tax exempt under section 501(c)(3) of the Internal Revenue Code. These were discussed briefly in Chapter 4, but will be amplified here in the context of joint ventures. The law seeks to prevent private individuals from benefiting through misdirecting the tax advantages and special status of tax-exempt organizations. The Internal Revenue Service (IRS) has developed a three-part test for judging whether joint ventures further the charitable goals of the HSO and are not established for the benefit of limited partners. The joint venture:

> Must further the organization's exempt purposes;
> May not prevent the exempt organization from acting exclusively to further its exempt purposes (This may occur if the joint venture causes the organization's earnings to inure to private parties, or if the joint venture results in benefits to private parties other than as incidental to furthering public, exempt purposes.); and
> May not constitute the operation of an unrelated trade or business that becomes the exempt organization's primary purpose.[97]

Factors that the IRS considers in applying the three-part test include:

> Arm's length negotiations (negotiations by unrelated parties acting in their own self-interests);
> Parties to the transaction are not related (e.g., stockholders);
> Limits on hospital investment or loans;
> Adequate security;
> Reasonable return on investment;
> Indemnification or limited contractual liability of hospital;
> Hospital exercises control over joint venture;
> Limited rate of return to nonexempt limited partners; and
> Hospital has right of first refusal on sale of partnership assets or other events affecting the joint venture.[98]

This brief summary suggests that the issues of private benefit or inurement in joint ventures are complex and require specialized analysis and legal counsel. A tax-exempt HSO that violates prohibitions on private inurement risks its charitable status, a highly problematic situation.

Elements of Successful Joint Ventures

Several elements are important for successful joint ventures:

> *Joint ventures should possess an adequate number of referring physicians.* MRI [magnetic resonance imaging] ventures have a much easier time when key neurologists, neurosurgeons, and orthopedic surgeons are involved. Ventures should be inclusive versus exclusive, allowing for the addition of investors after the initial offering.
> *A strong source of financing should be available.* There is no guarantee that a joint venture will achieve its pro forma or even positive cash flow. Asking physician investors to cover a shortage in

operating funds can lead to a decline in investor confidence as well as significant political problems. So, in addition to a venture being adequately capitalized from the start, there should be a contingency plan for additional capital.

A successful venture must provide an attractive return to investors. Many ventures are structured so that all nonphysician investors defer their profits until the physician-investors receive distributions equal to their initial investment. Other ventures attempt to distribute profits at least quarterly as a timely reminder of venture participation. Recognizing Medicare fraud and abuse issues as a constraint, most physicians are looking for returns significantly above the prime rate.

The manager of the joint venture must be capable of producing a competitive product and willing to assume the risks associated with being a general partner. General partners ultimately assume the business risk of a venture, and that can result in personal financial hardship if the venture turns sour.[99]

In the 1990s, hospitals and physicians will become partners in delivering care, rather than just partners in facility investments. The real challenge and rewards will come from bringing physicians under the same umbrella as the hospital. This strategy includes purchasing group practices. "You gather the physicians together as a corporation under the umbrella of the hospital. Then the hospital and physician group can contract more effectively with managed care programs and employers."[100]

SUMMARY

Economic demands on HSOs during the 1990s will necessitate that they become more efficient if they are to retain their competitive position. Acute care hospitals have been and will be among the HSOs most significantly affected in this regard. Differentiation is part of this competitive strategy. A means of achieving these goals is innovative and judicious application of the information in this chapter. Interorganizational linkages, whether based on market transactions or voluntary or involuntary interorganizational linkages, will be increasingly important factors in the success of HSOs. While these linkages offer numerous potential advantages, there are significant risks associated with them.

Diversification is a means of offering new services, which may, in the process, create new interorganizational linkages. Joint ventures, too, are ways HSOs can cooperate with members of the clinical staff to enhance their activities and achieve mutual advantage. However, diversification and joint ventures sometimes fail, and the results of failure can be economically and politically disastrous for the HSO.

There is no one right way to structure an organization. It is important that senior managers first determine the HSO's objectives, assess the environment, and choose strategies. This assessment will determine whether the HSO must divest subsidiaries, diversify, downsize, consolidate GBs, centralize decision making, or restructure. Failure to organize the HSO in a manner to enable it to meet its objectives will lead to significant problems.

DISCUSSION QUESTIONS

1. Briefly distinguish among market transactions, voluntary interorganizational relationship transactions, and involuntary interorganizational relationship transactions as categories of linkage mechanisms in the health field.
2. Discuss the two types of negotiations that occur between interdependent organizations.
3. What four types of voluntary interorganizational relationship transactions are discussed? Describe them briefly.
4. Define and give an example of vertical integration in the health field.
5. List and briefly define the seven strategies that regulated organizations use to deal with their regulators.
6. What motives explain the extent of diversification in the health field in the 1980s?

7. Describe the two basic types of diversification discussed in this chapter.
8. Describe the relative degree of success hospitals have achieved through diversification strategies in the past decade.
9. Describe the risks and benefits of joint ventures. Outline an approach an acute care hospital could use in developing a joint venture with physician members of its clinical staff.
10. Identify the factors that inhibit HSOs from engaging in multiorganizational arrangements. What political and legal steps would you recommend to minimize them?

CASE STUDY 1: DOES IT MAKE SENSE?[101]

The following are comments from an executive in the medical equipment rental business:

"One particularly lucrative area for hospital diversification, designed to make it less dependent on inpatient revenues from third parties such as Blue Cross, has been the medical equipment rental market. Third parties, and particularly Medicare, have up until now focused on inpatient cost controls and have provided fairly comfortable ceilings in terms of payments. A crutch that costs $20, for example, can be rented to a discharged patient for $7 a month. Where else can the cost of a capital investment be recovered in less than 3 months?"

"This may seem like a nickel-and-dime candy store operation, and many administrators have ignored it because of this. On the average, a discharged hospital patient referred to one of these operations rents three to four different pieces of equipment (bed, respirator, and so on) in addition to consumables, such as oxygen, producing an average gross income per referral of as much as $2,000. These referrals have come often at the price of some holiday candy for the social workers."

"Many hospitals are now getting a bigger piece of the action, setting up their own subsidiaries to provide these supplies to patients or entering into joint ventures with particular suppliers, from which a moderate-sized hospital might expect to generate a million dollar surplus per year."

Questions

1. What type of diversification would this be for a hospital?
2. What interorganizational linkages might be needed to ensure success for a hospital entering the equipment rental field?

CASE STUDY 2: HOW TO TURN AN INTIMIDATING
GOVERNMENT BUREAUCRACY INTO A PARTNER AND ALLY[102]

John Henry, CEO of Crop Genetics International, had just left a boisterous hearing on Capitol Hill that had left him feeling as bleak as the late-winter Washington weather. The hearing had been called to investigate the questionable testing procedures of Advanced Genetic Sciences, Inc., which had apparently injected a test bacterium into 45 fruit trees at its corporate headquarters without Environmental Protection Agency (EPA) approval. Henry recognized that his own company's future could be gravely affected by the outcomes of that meeting. His company, only 5 years old, was embarking on genetic-engineering projects for plants that were every bit as significant as McCormick's reaper had been to the food industry. But the products of his company's research, and that of other companies like his, could potentially be so destructive if unanticipated consequences emerged, that government was understandably cautious, even antagonistic, about unprofessionally conducted activities.

Henry knew that his company's efforts would always be professional. But salable products were at least 5 years away for R&D currently ongoing, and he wanted to ensure that his firm's products had a chance to reach the marketplace.

It was then that Henry decided on an unusual strategy. He reasoned that it was not necessary that business and government be enemies. He asked himself, "Why not turn government into an ally and partner?" Further, he thought, "Why not consider environmental activists as a fourth branch of government?" He decided to make government relations the primary business of his firm for the immediate future.

Henry believed deeply in what he was doing, and so apparently did others. For example, one of his company's probable products could significantly reduce the level of chemical fertilizers used each year, thus helping reduce fish and bird kills and potential food-chain problems for human beings. He assembled a team of key former government officials to aid him in his quest. The team's members included:

William D. Ruckelshaus, twice former director of the EPA

Douglas M. Costle, head of the EPA during the Carter administration

Robert M. Teeter, a prominent Republican pollster who would eventually become co-chairman of the George Bush presidential transitional team

Elliot L. Richardson, former attorney general, who has held a number of other federal posts

The "team" met in brainstorming sessions for which participants received $1,000 per day plus certain stock options. These sessions produced a list of obstacles that Henry might face and strategies for overcoming them. The sessions also provided valuable insight into the workings of government and how a company could best work its way through the bureaucratic maze. The result? Crop Genetics became the first genetics firm to make it through the first round of regulator hoops without being delayed or stalled.

Questions

1. What is your assessment of the strategy Crop Genetics International used to manage its relationship with the Environmental Protection Agency (EPA)?
2. What other strategies might it have used?

CASE STUDY 3:   COMMUNITY HEALTH PLAN[103]

The CEO of Community Health Plan (CHP) had been approached by a community group from "north of the river." This area of the city was economically depressed and had lost many of its privately owned HSOs and physicians to the suburbs over the past several decades.

"North of the river" seemed to be in a downward vortex with no apparent bottom in sight. Increasing numbers of uninsured patients there meant that remaining HSOs were less able to continue serving the area. The large city-owned hospital had made several ill-fated attempts to serve "north of the river" with a clinic system, but its efforts had been scandal ridden. The system was a political football with little credibility.

The representatives from "north of the river" were community leaders, none of whom appeared to have any political ambitions. They seemed genuinely willing to do whatever they could to assist in delivering high-quality health services "north of the river." They proposed that CHP establish and staff three storefront clinics in the area. The community leaders stated they would organize volunteers to remodel the facilities and work in clerical capacities.

The CEO was describing the proposed activity to the CHP executive management committee, which included members of governance, managers, and physicians and others from clinical areas. In making the presentation, the CEO stressed the CHP's historical role in providing health services to those in need, its not-for-profit status, and its continuing modest surplus. The members listened patiently, but the minute the CEO was finished all of them seemed to speak at once.

Several were opposed and made the following points about the suggested venture:

1. "North of the river" was the city's responsibility. Providing care to the needy was not something a small, not-for-profit health plan should attempt.

2. CHP had a primary obligation to enhance benefits for its enrollees, rather than get involved in new schemes. There were numerous services that several of their physicians and many plan members had requested.

3. The modest surplus that the plan had accumulated over several years would quickly evaporate. The chief financial officer noted they were expecting an increase in reinsurance premiums in the next quarter.

4. If CHP pulled the city's political chestnuts out of the fire by providing even stop-gap assistance, the city would never get its house in order and develop the system needed "north of the river."

Several spoke in favor of working "north of the river":

1. Helping the "north of the river" community was the right thing to do. The people there deserved health services. It was noted that CHP's own start had come about when several physicians in the community had fought the prevailing attitude among their peers about prepaid practice.

2. Those opposed were putting dollars ahead of people's health. They must be willing to assist the less fortunate.

3. CHP's members would support such an initiative if it were properly explained to them.

4. The positive publicity would further CHP's interests by increasing the number of enrollees.

It seemed to the CEO this was a no-win situation. The organizational philosophy was not well developed, and the proposal was a major step, but it seemed that something should be done to assist the people "north of the river." The executive committee members were raising points that merited analysis.

Questions

1. Identify the management issues *and* the ethical issues in the case. Which are the most important? Why?

2. Outline three alternatives that could be used to assist the community "north of the river." Choose the one that you think is best and identify its negative and positive aspects.

3. What interorganizational linkages are used in each of the alternatives identified in question 2? Are these significant in choosing the "best" alternative?

4. Develop an implementation plan for the alternative you chose in question 2.

NOTES

1. Jaeger, B. Jon, Arnold D. Kaluzny, and Kathryn Magruder-Habib. *Multi-institutional systems management*, 16. Owings Mills, MD: AUPHA Press, 1987.

2. This section is adapted from Longest, Beaufort B., Jr. Interorganizational linkages in the health sector. *Health Care Management Review* 15 (Winter 1990): 17–28.

3. Freeman, R. Edward. *Strategic management: A stakeholder approach*. Boston: Pitman Publishing, Inc., 1984.

4. Starkweather, David B., and Karen S. Cook. Organization-environment relations. In *Health care management: A text in organization theory and behavior*, edited by Stephen M. Shortell and Arnold D. Kaluzny, 2d ed., 357. New York: John Wiley & Sons, 1988.

5. Rubin, Jeffrey Z., and Bert R. Brown. *The social psychology of bargaining and negotiation*, 2. New York: Academic Press, 1975.

6. Adapted from Greenberger, David, Stephen Strasser, Roy J. Lewicki, and Thomas S. Bateman. Perception, motivation, and negotiation. In *Health care management: A text in organization theory and behavior*, edited by Stephen M. Shortell and Arnold D. Kaluzny, 2d ed., 129. New York: John Wiley & Sons, 1988.

7. Adapted from Greenberger, Strasser, Lewicki, and Bateman, Perception, 131.

8. Thompson, James D. *Organizations in action*. New York: McGraw Hill, 1967.

9. Pointer, Dennis D., James W. Begun, and Roice D. Luke. Managing interorganizational dependencies in the new health care marketplace. *Hospital & Health Services Administration* 33 (Summer 1988): 167–177.

10. Eccles, Robert G. The quasi-firm in the construction industry. *Journal of Economic Behavior and Organization* 2 (December 1981): 335–357.

11. Starkweather, David B. *Hospital mergers in the making*. Ann Arbor, MI: Health Administration Press, 1981; Starkweather and Cook, Organization-environment.

12. Starkweather, *Hospital mergers*.

13. Souhrada, Laura. Hospitals' use of contract management approaches 50%. *Hospitals* 65 (February 5, 1991): 18.

14. Souhrada, Hospitals' use, 22.

15. Longest, Beaufort B., Jr., and James M. Klingensmith. Coordination and communication. In *Health care management: A text in organization theory and behavior,* edited by Stephen M. Shortell and Arnold D. Kaluzny, 2d ed., 234–264. New York: John Wiley & Sons, 1988.

16. Glassman, Roger. Persistence and loose coupling in living systems. *Behavioral Science* 18 (March 1973): 83–98.

17. Weick, Kenneth. Educational organizations as loosely coupled systems. *Administrative Science Quarterly* 21 (March 1976): 1–19.

18. Pointer, Begun, and Luke, Managing interorganizational, 170.

19. Luke, Roice D., and Bettina Kurowski. Strategic management. In *Health care management: A text in organization theory and behavior,* edited by Stephen M. Shortell and Arnold D. Kaluzny, 2d ed., 461–484. New York: John Wiley & Sons, 1983.

20. Shirely, R.C. Limiting the scope of strategy: A decision based approach. *Academy of Management Review* (April 7 1982): 262–268.

21. Astley, William, and Charles Fombrum. Collective strategy: Social ecology of organizational environments. *Academy of Management Review* 8 (October 1983): 576–587; Porter, Michael E. *Competitive advantage: Creating and sustaining superior performance.* New York: The Free Press, 1985; Pennings, Johannes M. Strategically interdependent organizations. In *Handbook of organizational design* edited by Paul C. Nystrom and William H. Starbuck, Vol. 1, 433–455. New York: Oxford University Press, 1981.

22. Pfeffer, Jeffrey and Gerald R. Salancik. *The external control of organizations: A resource dependence perspective,* 161. New York: Harper & Row, Publishers, 1978.

23. Shortell, Stephen M. Public policy and managerial implications. In *Hospital-physician joint ventures,* edited by Stephen M. Shortell, Thomas M. Wickizer, and J.R.C. Wheeler, 327. Ann Arbor, MI: Health Administration Press, 1984.

24. Blair, John D., Charles R. Slaton, and Grant T. Savage. Hospital-physician joint ventures: A strategic approach for both dimensions of success. *Hospital & Health Services Administration* 35 (Spring 1990): 4.

25. Luke, Roice D., James W. Begun, and Dennis D. Pointer. Quasi-firms: Strategic interorganizational forms in the health care industry. *The Academy of Management Review* 14 (January 1989): 13.

26. Pointer, Begun, and Luke, Managing interorganizational, 171.

27. Starkweather, *Hospital mergers,* 37–38.

28. Buzzell, Robert D. Is vertical integration profitable? *Harvard Business Review* 61 (Janaury–February 1983): 93.

29. Clement, Jan P. Vertical integration and diversification of acute care hospitals: Conceptual definitions. *Hospital & Health Services Administration* 33 (Spring 1988): 100.

30. Goldsmith, Jeff C. *Can hospitals survive? The new competitive health care market,* 136. Homewood, IL: Dow Jones-Irwin, 1981.

31. Conrad, Douglas A., and William L. Dowling. Vertical integration in health services: Theory and managerial implications. *Health Care Management Review* 15 (Fall 1990): 10.

32. Buzzell, Is vertical integration, 93–94.

33. Coddington, Dean C., and Keith D. Moore. *Market-driven strategies in health care,* 128. San Francisco: Jossey-Bass Publishers, 1987.

34. Porter, *Competitive advantage,* 394.

35. Luke, Roice D. Spatial competition and cooperation in local hospital markets. *Medical Care Review* 48 (Summer 1991): 219–220.

36. Kinzer, David M. Our realistic options in health regulation. *Frontiers of Health Services Management* 5 (Fall 1988): 3–43.

37. Altman, Drew, Robert Greene, and Harvey M. Sapolsky. *Health planning and regulation: The decision-making process,* 26–31. Ann Arbor, MI: AUPHA Press, 1981.

38. Luke, Begun, and Pointer, Quasi-firms, 12.

39. Thompson, *Organizations.*

40. Bolman, Larry G., and Terrence E. Deal. *Modern approaches to understanding and managing organizations.* San Francisco: Jossey-Bass Publishers, 1984.

41. Aldrich, Howard E., and David A. Whetton. Organization-sets, action-sets, and networking: Making the most of simplicity. In *Handbook of organizational design,* edited by Paul C. Nystrom and William H. Starbuck, Vol. 1, 385–408. New York: Oxford University Press, 1981.

42. Porter, *Competitive advantage,* 332–335.

43. Johnsson, Julie. Hospitals dismantle elaborate corporate restructurings. *Hospitals* 65 (July 5, 1991): 45.

44. Alexander, Jeffrey A. *The changing character of hospital governance,* 10. Chicago: The Hospital Research and Educational Trust, 1990.

45. Johnsson, Hospitals dismantle.

46. Johnsson, Hospitals dismantle, 41.

47. Coyne, Joseph S. Hospital performance in multihospital systems: A comparative study of system and independent hospitals. *Health Services Research* 17 (Winter 1982): 303.

48. Berman, Howard. Speech presented to the annual meeting of the Hospital Association of Pennsylvania, 1982.

49. Starkweather, David B. *Trends and types of multihospital arrangements, Part I.* Technical Assistance Memorandum No. 56. San Francisco: Western Center for Health Planning, 1980.

50. Starkweather, Trends and types.

51. Longest, Beaufort B., Jr. A conceptual framework for understanding the multi-hospital arrangement strategy. *Health Care Management Review* 5 (Winter 1980): 17.

52. Barrett, Diana. The trend line for multi-institutional systems can only be up. *Hospitals* 56 (April 1982): 81.

53. Brown, Montague, et al. Trends in multi-hospital systems: A multi-year comparison. *Health Care Management Review* 5 (Fall 1980): 9.

54. Longest, Conceptual framework, 17.

55. Longest, Conceptual framework, 17, 18.

56. Alexander, *Changing character,* 11.

57. Shortell, Stephen M. The evolution of hospital systems: Unfulfilled promises and self-fulfilling prophesies. *Medical Care Review* 45 (Fall 1988): 189.

58. Martinsons, Jane. Wade Mountz on the past, present, and future of hospital alliances. *Trustee* 41 (December 1988): 6, 7.

59. Larkin, Howard. Alliances: changing focus for changing times. *Hospitals* 63 (December 20, 1989): 34.

60. Larkin, Alliances, 36.
61. Larkin, Alliances.
62. Barrett, Trend line, 84.
63. Koska, Mary T. CEOs make the most of trustees' business acumen. *Hospitals* 64 (June 5, 1990): 29.
64. Alexander, *Changing character*, 11.
65. Koska, CEOs make, 30.
66. Robertson, E. Marie. Top hospital systems share a variety of characteristics. *Health Care Competition Week* 8 (April 29, 1991): 2.
67. Robertson, Top hospital, 1–2.
68. Zuckerman, Howard S. Multi-institutional systems: Promise and performance. *Inquiry* 16 (Winter 1979): 291.
69. This section is adapted from Longest, Beaufort B., Jr. In *Strategic issues in health care management: Point and counterpoint*, edited by W. Jack Duncan, Peter M. Ginter, and Linda E. Swayne, 14–33. Boston: PWS-Kent Publishing Company, 1992.
70. Shortell, Stephen M., Ellen M. Morrison, and Bernard Friedman. *Strategic choices for America's hospitals: Managing change in turbulent times,* 232. San Francisco: Jossey-Bass Publishers, 1990.
71. American Hospital Association. *Hospital statistics,* 7. Chicago, 1990.
72. American Hospital Association. *Hospital statistics,* xxxiv. Chicago, 1988.
73. Green, Jeffrey. 50 community hospitals closed, 43 opened in 1990. *AHA News* 27 (March 18, 1991): 1.
74. American Hospital Association, *Hospital statistics* (1988), 63.
75. Coddington and Moore, *Market-driven,* 114–115.
76. *AHA hospital statistics: 1991–1992 edition,* 7. Chicago, American Hospital Association, 1991.
77. Green, Jeffrey. Will claims of unfair competition hold up against subsidiaries? *AHA News* 27 (February 11, 1991): 1, 5.
78. Rue, Leslie W., and Phyllis G. Holland. *Strategic management: Concepts and experiences.* 2d ed., 57. New York: McGraw-Hill 1989.
79. Longest, Beaufort B., Jr. Interorganizational linkages in the health sector. *Health Care Management Review* 15 (Winter 1990): 17–28.
80. Luke, Begin, and Pointer, Quasi-firms.
81. Holt, David H. *Management: Principles and practices,* 2d ed., 198. Englewood Cliffs, NJ: Prentice Hall, 1990.
82. Moore, W. Barry. Hospitals win healthy margins by following business basics. *Hospitals* 64 (April 20, 1990): 56.
83. Kaluzny, Arnold D., and S. Robert Hernandez. Organizational change and innovation. In *Health care management: A text in organization theory and behavior,* edited by Stephen M. Shortell and Arnold D. Kaluzny, 2d ed., 400. New York: John Wiley & Sons, 1988.

84. Grayson, Mary, and Brian McCormick. Outpatients a source of M.D./hospital conflict. *Medical Staff Leader* 18 (March 1989): 1, 8.
85. American Hospital Association. *Vision, values, viability: Environmental assessment, 1989/1990,* 64. Chicago, 1988.
86. Hudson, Terese. Hospital-MD joint ventures move forward despite hurdles. *Hospitals* 65 (May 5, 1991): 22.
87. Hudson, Hospital-MD. 22.
88. Kaufman, Nathan. Joint ventures as competitive strategy. *Healthcare Executive* 3 (September/October 1988): 26.
89. Morrisey, Michael A., and Deal C. Brooks. Hospital-physician joint ventures: Who's doing what? *Hospitals* 59 (September 1, 1985): 86.
90. Jensen, J. Programs to support physician practices at 86% of hospitals. *Modern Healthcare* 19 (June 30, 1989): 36.
91. Grayson, Mary. Survey spots the tight turns in MD-CEO relations. *Hospitals* 62 (February 5, 1988): 53.
92. Kaufman, Joint ventures, 26.
93. Blair, Slaton, and Savage, Hospital-physician, 6. A useful discussion of planning and implementing a joint venture is found in Patton, James C., and Glenn T. Troyer. Planning and implementing the joint venture. *Topics in Health Care Financing* 13 (Fall 1986): 86–96.
94. Office of the Inspector General, U.S. Department of Health and Human Services. Medicare and state health care programs: Fraud and abuse; OIG anti-kickback provisions. Final rule. *Federal Register* 56 (July 29, 1991): 35952–35987.
95. Eiland, Gary W. Final safe harbors narrow and rarely navigable. *Health Care Financial Management* 45 (October 1991): 15–16.
96. Eiland, Final safe, 16.
97. Bromberg, Robert S. Current IRS audit issues. Paper presented at the 1991 Health Law Update of the National Health Lawyers Association, Chicago, Illinois, June 5–7, 1991, 17–18.
98. Bromberg, Current IRS, 21.
99. Kaufman, Joint ventures, 26–27.
100. Johnsson, Hospitals dismantle, 46.
101. Adapted from Smith, David B., and Arnold D. Kaluzny. *The white labyrinth: A guide to the health care system,* 2d ed., 172–173. Ann Arbor, MI: Health Administration Press, 1986.
102. Adapted from Higgins, James M. *The management challenge: An introduction to management,* 482–483. New York: Macmillan Publishing Company, 1991; based on Finnegan, Jay. All the president's men. *Inc.* (February 1989): 44–54; used by permission.
103. Adapted from Darr, Kurt. *Ethics in health services management* 2d ed., 88–89. Baltimore: Health Professions Press, 1991; used by permission.

BIBLIOGRAPHY

AHA hospital statistics: 1991–1992 edition. Chicago: American Hospital Association, 1991.

Alexander, Jeffrey A. *The changing character of hospital governance.* Chicago: The Hospital Research and Educational Trust, 1990.

Alexander, Jeffrey A. Diversification behavior of multihospital systems: Patterns of change, 1983–1985. *Hospital & Health Services Administration* (Spring 1990): 83–102.

American Hospital Association. *Vision, values, viability: Environmental assessment, 1989/1990.* Chicago, 1988.

Blair, John D., Charles R. Slaton, and Grant T. Savage. Hospital-physician joint ventures: A strategic approach for both dimensions of success. *Hospital & Health Services Administration* 35 (Spring 1990): 3–26.

Clement, Jan P. Vertical integration and diversification of acute care hospitals: Conceptual definitions. *Hospital & Health Services Administration* 33 (Spring 1988): 99–110.

Coddington, Dean C., and Keith D. Moore. *Market-driven strategies in health care.* San Francisco: Jossey-Bass Publishers, 1987.

Conrad, Douglas A., and William L. Dowling. Vertical integration in health services: Theory and managerial implications. *Health Care Management Review* 15 (Fall 1990): 9–22.

Eiland, Gary W. Final safe harbors narrow and rarely navigable. *Health Care Financial Management* 45 (October 1991): 15–16, 18.

Freeman, R.E. *Strategic management: A stakeholder approach.* Boston: Pitman Publishing, Inc., 1984.

Goldsmith, Jeff C. *Can hospitals survive? The new competitive health care market.* Homewood, IL: Dow Jones-Irwin, 1981.

Greenberger, David, Stephen Strasser, Roy J. Lewicki, and Thomas S. Bateman. Perception, motivation, and negotiation. In *Health care management: A text in organization theory and behavior,* edited by Stephen M. Shortell and Arnold D. Kaluzny, 2d ed., 129. New York: John Wiley & Sons, 1988.

Holt, David H. *Management: Principles and practices,* 2d ed. Englewood Cliffs, NJ: Prentice Hall, 1990.

Jaeger, B. Jon, Arnold D. Kaluzny, and Kathryn Magruder-Habib. *Multi-institutional systems management.* Owings Mills, MD: AUPHA Press, 1987.

Johnsson, Julie. Hospitals dismantle elaborate corporate restructurings. *Hospitals* 65 (July 5, 1991): 41–43, 45–46.

Kaluzny, Arnold D., and S. Robert Hernandez. Organizational change and innovation. In *Health care management: A text in organization theory and behavior,* edited by Stephen M. Shortell and Arnold D. Kaluzny, 2d ed., 379–417. New York: John Wiley & Sons, 1988.

Kaufman, Nathan. Joint ventures as competitive strategy. *Healthcare Executive* 3 (September/October 1988): 26–28.

Kinzer, David M. Our realistic options in health regulation. *Frontiers of Health Services Management* 5 (Fall 1988): 3–43.

Longest, Beaufort B., Jr. Interorganizational linkages in the health sector. *Health Care Management Review* 15 (Winter 1990): 17–28.

Longest, Beaufort B., Jr., and James M. Klingensmith. Coordination and communication. In *Health care management: A text in organization theory and behavior,* edited by Stephen M. Shortell and Arnold D. Kaluzny, 2d ed., 234–264. New York: John Wiley & Sons, 1988.

Luke, Roice D. Spatial competition and cooperation in local hospital markets. *Medical Care Review* 48 (Summer 1991): 207–237.

Luke, Roice D., James W. Begun, and Dennis D. Pointer. Quasi-firms: Strategic interorganizational forms in the health care industry. *The Academy of Management Review* 14 (January 1989): 9–19.

Luke, Roice D., and Bettina Kurowski. Strategic manage-ment. In *Health care management: A text in organization theory and behavior,* edited by Stephen M. Shortell and Arnold D. Kaluzny, 2d ed., 461–484. New York: John Wiley & Sons, 1983.

Morrisey, Michael A., and Deal C. Brooks. Hospital-physician joint ventures: Who's doing what? *Hospitals* 59 (September 1, 1985): 80–89.

Office of the Inspector General, U.S. Department of Health and Human Services. Medicare and state health care programs: Fraud and abuse; OIG anti-kickback provisions. Final rule. *Federal Register* 56 (July 29, 1991): 35952–35987.

Pennings, Johannes M. Strategically interdependent organizations. In *Handbook of organizational design* edited by Paul C. Nystrom and William H. Starbuck, Vol. 1, 433–455. New York: Oxford University Press, 1981.

Peters, Gerald R. Revamped, joint ventures make a comeback. *Healthcare Financial Management* 45 (August 1991): 62, 64, 66, 68, 70, 72, 74.

Pfeffer, Jeffrey, and Gerald R. Salancik. *The external control of organizations: A resource dependence perspective.* New York: Harper & Row, Publishers, 1978.

Pointer, Dennis D., James W. Begun, and Roice D. Luke. Managing interorganizational dependencies in the new health care marketplace. *Hospital & Health Services Administration* 33 (Summer 1988): 167–177.

Porter, Michael E. *Competitive advantage: Creating and sustaining superior performance.* New York: The Free Press, 1985.

Robertson, E. Marie. Top hospital systems share a variety of characteristics. *Health Care Competition Week* 8 (April 29, 1991): 1–2.

Rue, Leslie W., and Phyllis G. Holland. *Strategic management: Concepts and Experiences,* 2d ed. New York: McGraw-Hill, 1989.

Shortell, Stephen M. The evolution of hospital systems: Unfulfilled promises and self-fulfilling prophesies. *Medical Care Review* 45 (Fall 1988): 177–214.

Shortell, Stephen M. Public policy and managerial implications. In *Hospital-physician joint ventures,* edited by S.M. Shortell, T.M. Wickizer, and J.R.C. Wheeler, 327. Ann Arbor, MI: Health Administration Press, 1984.

Shortell, Stephen M., Ellen M. Morrison, and Bernard Friedman. *Strategic choices for America's hospitals: Managing change in turbulent times.* San Francisco: Jossey-Bass Publishers, 1990.

Sofaer, Shoshanna, and Robert C. Myrtle. Interorganizational theory and research: Implications for health care management, policy, and research. *Medical Care* 48 (Winter 1991): 371–409.

Starkweather, David B. *Hospital mergers in the making.* Ann Arbor, MI: Health Administration Press, 1981.

Starkweather, David B., and K.S. Cook. Organization-environment relations. In *Health care management: A text in organization theory and behavior,* edited by Stephen M. Shortell and Arnold D. Kaluzny, 2d ed., 357. New York: John Wiley & Sons, 1988.

Waterman, Robert H., Jr. *The renewal factor: How the best get and keep the competitive edge.* New York: Bantam Books, 1987.

V | Problem Solving, Quality Improvement, and Control in Health Services Organizations

10 / Managerial Problem Solving and Decision Making

We try to make management decisions that, if
everything goes right, will preclude future
problems. But everything does not always go
right, and managers therefore must be problem
solvers as well as decision makers.
James L. Hayes, President, American
Management Association[1]

Health services organizations (HSOs) are dynamic entities that exist in an ever-changing environment. The opening quote suggests the inevitability of change and that managers will always encounter problems. Figure 1.6 in Chapter 1, "The Management Process and Managerial Roles," conceptualized a management model in which HSOs were described as entities in a dynamic relationship with their broader environment. HSOs convert inputs (resources such as personnel, materials and supplies, technology, information, and capital) into outputs (individual and organizational work results) to achieve objectives such as patient care, education, or research. HSO managers cause that conversion when they integrate structure, tasks/technology, and people. Managers manage by engaging in functions, activities, and roles to accomplish organizational objectives. Managers are accountable for allocation and use of resources, as well as the results. Preventing problems by anticipating them or solving them when prevention fails are traditional management tasks; however, there must also be a focus on continuous improvement of quality. This proactive approach assumes that all processes can be improved and that managers must foster the appropriate environment and give employees the tools that enable them to make this improvement possible.

This chapter distinguishes problem solving from decision making. A problem-solving model is developed and the factors that influence managerial problem solving and decision making are discussed. The benefits of various group problem-solving strategies are discussed, and use of teams in quality improvement is emphasized. A model assists in determining when group versus individual problem solving is more effective.

DECISION MAKING

Much that a manager does involves either or both elements of problem solving—problem analysis and decision making. Problem analysis includes recognizing and defining a situation that requires a decision and implementing and evaluating alternatives chosen. Chapter 1 identified decision making as a managerial function that is defined as choosing among alternatives.[2] The key word is "choosing." Decision making occurs when managers choose. At its simplest, decision making has two steps: 1) identifying and evaluating alternatives, and 2) choosing an alternative.

Decision making is integral to all management functions, activities, and roles. For example, planning involves decisions (choosing), whether senior managers are formulating strategy or middle-level managers are selecting programs to implement. Decisions about organizing range from establishing authority–responsibility relationships to designing work systems, procedures and flows, and from structure–task–people relationships to making job assignments. In their staffing function, managers decide about numbers of staff, their pay and training, and appraisal of their performance. As managers lead, motivate, and communicate, they decide which motivational and leadership styles to use and how much information to impart, to whom, and when. When managers control, they compare individual and organizational work results with predetermined expectations and standards and decide whether results can be improved or standards increased. This means making decisions about what type of information to collect and report and which monitoring systems should be used to measure and compare HSO conversion activities and outputs with expectations and standards. Managers also decide which managerial roles to adopt, choosing among the interpersonal roles of figurehead, liaison, and influencer; the informational roles of monitor, disseminator, and spokesperson; and the decisional roles of change agent, disturbance handler, resource allocator, and negotiator. Figures 1.2 and 1.4 in Chapter 1 show interrelationship of decision making to other management functions and to managerial roles, respectively.

Types of Decisions

The types of decisions managers make can be classified in many ways. Three describe most decisions: 1) ends-means, 2) administrative-operational, and 3) programmed-nonprogrammed.

Ends-Means   Ends decisions determine which individual or organizational results are to be achieved (i.e., objectives). Means decisions choose the strategies or operational programs and activities that will accomplish desired results. For example, a decision to establish a quality and productivity improvement program in an HSO accomplishes the organizational objectives of enhanced quality of care and service, higher patient/customer satisfaction, and better resource use. In the management model shown in Figure 1.6, the output component represents ends—desired individual and organizational work results. Decisions about ends are inherent in strategic planning because such planning includes formulation of objectives and strategies. On a narrower plane, ends-means decision making occurs in departments and is reflected in departmental objectives and operational programs that contribute to overall HSO objectives.

Administrative-Operational   Many administrative decisions made by senior managers significantly affect the HSO and have major implications for resource allocation and utilization. Policy decisions are a synonym for administrative decisions. Examples include deciding how to finance facility construction or renovation, whether to recognize a union for collective bargaining without a certification election, whether to hire hospital-based physicians, whether to contract for laundry services, what pay increase to give employees, and the size of the capital equipment budget. In contrast, operational decisions are generally made by middle-level and first-line managers about day-to-day activities of a unit. Operational-level decisions include those about departmental equipment purchases, staff deployment, modification of work systems, and job assignments.

Programmable-Nonprogrammable   Programmed decisions are repetitive and routine. Because decisions can be programmed, procedures, rules, and manuals can be used to guide decisions.[3] Examples are patient admission, billing, scheduling, and inventory and supply ordering procedures.

Simon defines nonprogrammed decisions as "novel, unstructured, and consequential."[4] Examples of unique and nonroutine decisions that cannot be programmed are those to expand facilities; add, close, or share services; seek Medicare certification of skilled beds; restructure the organization into a corporate model; acquire a computer system; or add a residency program. Such decisions occur infrequently.

Overlap of Decision Types   Figure 10.1 shows that the three classes of decisions overlap, and decisions may include parts of each type. For example, merging with another HSO or establishing a satellite urgent care center or primary care preferred provider organization is a "means" decision because this achieves the organization's objectives or desired results. Furthermore, it is

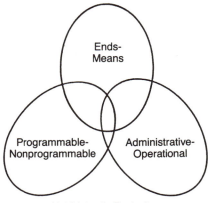

Figure 10.1. Types of decisions.

an administrative decision since it deals with major resource commitment, compared with a decision that carries out day-to-day activities and is primarily operational. Finally, the decision is nonprogrammable because it is unique and occurs infrequently.

MANAGERIAL PROBLEM SOLVING

All managers are problem solvers. Problems may be unstructured or structured, complex or simple, major or minor, urgent or nonurgent, and may involve varying degrees of cost, risk, and uncertainty. The problem-solving process includes a series of activities or steps by which managers cause change. It is "characterized by intentional reasoning about what the problem is and what the solution should be."[5] The purpose of problem solving, according to Vroom and Jago, is for the current state to more closely equal the desired state.[6] Consistent with terminology used in the management model, the purpose of problem solving is to introduce change so that actual HSO results or outputs more closely align with those desired. Briefly, the process by which managers solve problems consists of:

Identifying and analyzing a situation that requires a decision
Identifying and evaluating alternative solutions to address the situation
Choosing an alternative
Implementing the alternative
Evaluating the results after implementation

Figure 10.2 shows the relationships among problem solving, problem analysis, and decision making. Problem solving involves decision making; although the terms are often used interchangeably, they are not synonymous. All problem solving involves decision making (i.e., choosing from among alternatives), but not all decision making involves problem solving.[7] The distinction lies in the fact that problem solving includes problem analysis—predecision situation assessment and postdecision implementation and evaluation. The discussion here is relevant to both problem solving and decision making, and they are distinguished as necessary.

Managers perform a series of steps when undertaking either problem analysis or decision making. As with all processes, there are variables, conditions, and situations that influence the approach, manner, and style used. Problem solving skills are crucial to managerial success, and they are often more important than knowledge and skills in areas such as communication and

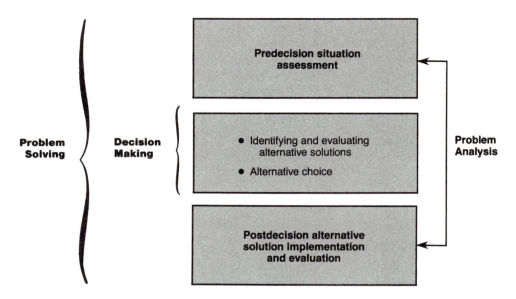

Figure 10.2.   Problem solving and decision making.

interpersonal relations. This does not mean that these skills and managerial functions, activities, and/or roles are unimportant. It does mean that problem solving is fundamental to everything a manager does and to effective managerial performance.

If one were required to describe a manager in five words or less, the description would be "problem solver and decision maker." The importance of problem solving to managerial effectiveness was shown by a major Canadian research study involving over 4,000 HSO (hospital, nursing facility, community health center, and medical clinic) managers, 2,500 of whom were chief executive officers (CEOs). Almost all of these managers identified problem solving, along with decision making, to be knowledge areas and skills that were among the most important.[8]

In a report by the American College of Hospital Administrators (now called the American College of Healthcare Executives) on the role of hospital CEOs in the United States, one major conclusion was that they had to improve the process of solving problems.[9] The 524 CEOs surveyed in hospitals of all types (investor owned, nonprofit, government, and those who were members of a multiorganizational system) indicated that the highest ranked problem areas were those dealing with community (i.e., stakeholder) relations, business and finance, medical care and medical staff, and personnel.[10]

PROBLEM-SOLVING PROCESS AND MODEL

Problem solving is a process in which managers analyze situations and make decisions to bring about change so that actual organization results (i.e., outputs) more closely approximate those that are desired. Problem solving may be classified as *prospective* if it is performed in anticipation of an event(s) that might cause organizational results to be inconsistent with those desired. It is *retrospective* when applied to deviations between actual and desired results that have already occurred. Retrospective problem solving identifies the cause of, and corrects the reason for, the deviation. Finally, problem solving is *concurrent* when the HSO is committed to a philosophy of continuously improving quality and productivity.

Conditions that Initiate Problem Solving

Another way to classify problem solving is by the conditions that initiate it.[11] Figure 10.3 shows the conditions and corresponding approaches to problem solving. The conditions are:

1. Opportunity/threat (prospective—might)
2. Crisis (immediate—will)
3. Deviation (retrospective—has/is)
4. Improvement (concurrent—seek)

Opportunity problem solving is prospective and anticipatory. It occurs when an event or situation is presented to the HSO that could be favorable to it and *might* enable it to more easily achieve or enhance desired organizational results.[12] The locus of opportunity may be internal or external. For example, fetal monitoring technology and changed consumer expectations enable a hospital to meet patient needs by offering a new service—a birth center—that takes advantage of this opportunity. Implementation involves problem analysis, consisting of predecision assessment and postdecision evaluation. The outcome is organizational results (new service) that align more closely with desired results, including improved patient service, higher patient satisfaction, and increased revenue.

The converse of opportunity problem solving is *threat problem solving*, which is also prospective and anticipatory. Threats are events or situations that, if not addressed, *might* cause future results to be less than desired. Their locus may be internal or external. For example, a competitor who initiates an aggressive marketing program to expand its service area presents a potential threat, and if no action is taken this might result in loss of market share.

Crisis problem solving is immediate.[13] It may be triggered by a threat that has been ignored or by an unanticipated but recognizable event, and it must be addressed immediately or organiza-

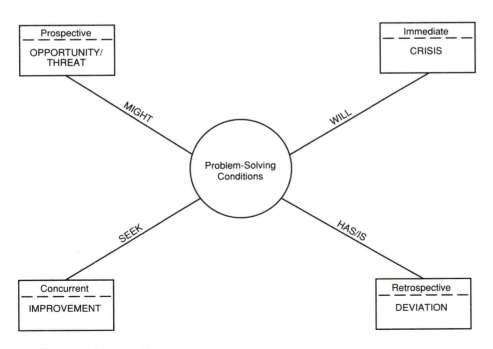

Figure 10.3. Problem-solving conditions.

tional results *will* be inconsistent with those desired. Examples of unanticipated crises are a local natural disaster, a strike by unionized employees, heart-lung bypass equipment malfunction during surgery, or a sudden reduction in Medicaid reimbursements that will severely affect the HSO's revenue. A crisis may also be something as simple as the loss of an employee with critical skills. Crises generally require a quick resolution of the problem.

Deviation problem solving is retrospective. It occurs after a difference between actual and desired organizational results *has* occurred and *is* detected. The deviation may be small, but it suggests the presence of a problem that, if left unsolved, could cause larger deviations.

Improvement problem solving is the opposite of deviation problem solving. It assumes all systems and processes can be improved, and initiates and supports activities to improve individual work and organizational results. Unlike deviation problem solving, improvement problem solving is not restricted or focused on the point suggested by the problem definition. The perspective, mind set, and process of achieving continuous improvement differ, particularly in problem analysis. First, the analysis is concurrent—one in which there is a continuous search for opportunities to improve results. The analysis is broad based and focuses on the whole organization. This includes all inputs and facets of the conversion process—the elements of structure, tasks/technology, and people, as well as the management process to integrate them—in order to generate *enhanced* outputs (see the management model, Figure 1.6). Second, there is a management philosophy that never-ending improvement is possible, leading to a cycle of continuously examining all systems, processes, and results and seeking ways to improve them. Another way of characterizing improvement problem solving is that managers (and employees) are *problem seekers* who systematically look for internal opportunities for improvement.[14]

The problem-solving process model that follows is described using the condition of deviation for several reasons. The primary purpose is to acquaint readers with the activities of problem solving—the steps in the process. The model is generic and is conceptually applicable for all types of problem solving except for that under the condition of improvement, where problem analysis differs. The reasons for this exception have been noted. Second, including all combinations of conditions would make the description overly complex and detract from the purpose of understanding the process. Third, research indicates that historically managers have engaged in problem solving most frequently under the condition of deviation[15] and infrequently under the condition of crisis.[16] Fourth, the strategic planning model (Figure 8.4) presented in Chapter 8, "Strategic Planning and Marketing," focuses on external opportunities and threats. Its salient elements (external and internal environment assessment, strategy choice, and implementation) are similar to those in problem solving (situation assessment, selection of an alternative, and implementation and evaluation), and this makes the skills readily transferrable. Finally, Chapter 11, "Quality and Productivity Improvement," focuses on continuous quality improvement, and problem solving is applied under the condition of improvement.

Problem-Solving Activities

The outcome of problem solving invariably affects allocation and utilization of resources and work results for which the manager is responsible. Much of a manager's time, particularly for senior and middle-level managers, is spent on problem solving. Managers continuously monitor resource use and work outcomes. Problem solving often is not easy and can be very time consuming. Frequently, situations are complex, unstructured, nonroutine, and sometimes beyond the manager's direct control. Yet, the process is essentially the same regardless of the type or scope of the problem or the conditions that initiate the need for problem solving. The time involved and intensity of analysis may vary, but not the process. Basic problem-solving includes:

> Problem analysis, specifically that part of problem recognition and definition (including gathering and evaluating information)

Making assumptions
Generation of tentative alternative solutions
Alternative solution evaluation and application of decision criteria
Selection of the alternative solution that most closely fits the criteria
Implementation
Evaluation of results

These steps are incorporated in the problem-solving process model shown in Figure 10.4. The remainder of this section describes them and references each by its number in Figure 10.4.

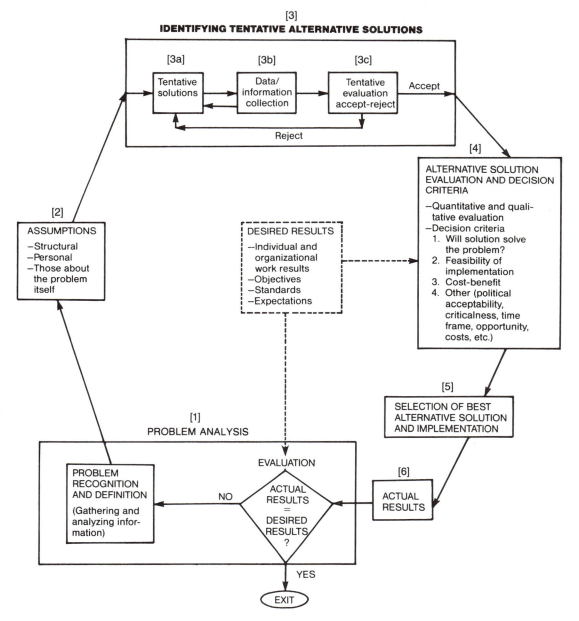

Figure 10.4. Problem-solving process model.

Problem Analysis (Recognition and Definition) [1]

The following discussion focuses on the typical type of problem solving, in which desired results are known by reference to objectives, standards, and similar measures and a deviation from these has occurred. Problem solving also occurs under conditions of change, as when opportunities or threats present managers with a new situation—one in which there are no previous data but analysis suggests a potential problem. For example, an HSO determines it must undertake a marketing program before service activity declines because of increased competition. Here, the HSO must solve the problem of responding to competition. The problem-solving process is the same, although there will be more unknowns, which adds complexity.

Problem solving under the condition of deviation begins when there are indications that actual results are, or will be, inconsistent with desired results. A problem is recognized because managers are monitoring their area of responsibility or the entire organization. "Desired results" in the middle of Figure 10.4 are the criterion or baseline against which actual results are compared. Desired results may be expressed in terms of: 1) overall organization objectives, such as quality of patient care, better client services, or financial solvency; 2) departmental objectives, such as reducing nursing service personnel turnover, surgical infection rates, ratio of inaccurate to accurate laboratory tests, radiograph retakes, magnetic resonance imager downtime, or budget variances; or 3) work results related to a particular individual's job. These expectations and desired results are standards against which monitoring and reporting systems compare actual results. Deviation may suggest that a problem exists.

One part of problem analysis is problem recognition and definition. As Cowan states:

> Problem recognition rarely occurs as a completely discrete event. In practice the process occurs through various time intervals (from seconds to years), amidst a variety of ongoing activities and in different ways depending on both situational and individual factors. At times, the process of problem recognition is automatic; at other times, it involves conscious effort. Often, it is a highly objective phenomenon resulting in problem descriptions that most anyone would agree on. At other times it is definitely a subjective process, where the nature of a problem description varies from individual to individual.[17]

Cowan suggests problem recognition has three stages. The first is gestation/latency, in which some cue or triggering event indicates a potential problem. Second is categorization, in which an individual is aware that a problem exists—that something is wrong—but cannot fully describe it. Third is diagnosis, in which there is the "attempt to achieve greater certainty about a problem description; it generally entails searching for additional information"[18] that will lead to problem definition.

Often, symptoms rather than causes clutter and confuse identification and definition of the problem's parameters. Some managers are better problem solvers partly because experience and knowledge allow superior problem recognition and definition. Sensitivity, the ability to identify and interpret information cues and perceive their meaning, ordered and systematic thinking about facts and their importance, knowing which questions to ask, and recognizing limits are skills that often only develop with experience.

In the recognition and definition stage of problem solving, information is gathered and systematically evaluated to determine the existence of a problem and its nature and extent. Sources of information may include routine reports and data sources, interviews and observation, information from work groups, and customer feedback.[19] In unstructured or complex situations, use of circumstantial evidence and deductive reasoning may be necessary. It may even be necessary to use exclusionary thinking to determine what the problem *is not*. Eventually, conclusions about the problem are reached, and it is classified by type, nature, and scope. Nutt labels this recognition-definition stage as formative "because it determines the nature of all subsequent action,"[20] especially generating alternatives. Furthermore, terminating the problem definition stage prematurely may also result in a low-quality solution or in solving the wrong problem.[21]

Making Assumptions [2]

The assumptions managers bring to problem solving affect the quality of the solution. Three categories encompass most assumptions: structural, personal, and those about the problem itself.[22]

Structural assumptions relate to the context of the problem. In a sense, they are boundary assumptions: the problem lies in (or out) of the manager's authority; additional resources are (or are not) available to solve the problem; other departments cause the problem; or the problem is caused by uncontrollable external factors such as a low patient census because of high local unemployment and fewer people having health insurance or lower levels of third-party reimbursement.

Personal assumptions are conclusions and biases that managers bring to the problem. They are often based on previous experience. Managers may have a high or low tolerance for the risk and uncertainty inherent in changes that invariably result from problem solving. A manager who has worked in an HSO where problem solving was equated with blame will have a low tolerance for risk and may make assumptions about the problem and/or alternatives that result in low-risk solutions. Also, assumptions may be made about the likely reaction of superiors, subordinates, or stakeholders to potential solutions. Personal biases, two of which are anchoring and escalating commitment, may also affect problem solving. Anchoring occurs when the individual "chooses a starting point (an 'anchor'), perhaps from past data, and then adjusts from the anchor based on new information."[23] If the anchor is incorrect, the resulting analysis based on that information will be flawed. The bias of escalating commitment is that of being unwilling to admit a previous mistake. Individuals who made earlier decisions about the situation that is now the problem "tend to be locked into a previously chosen course of action."[24]

Assumptions about the problem itself may cover a wide range, including perceived relative importance of the problem, the degree of risk, and how urgently a solution is needed. Other problem-centered assumptions include economic and political costs, the degree to which subordinates or superiors will accept solutions, and the likelihood of success of the solution that is implemented. Regardless, assumptions can limit the scope of problem solving, or even preclude identifying the best solution.[25]

Identifying Tentative Alternative Solutions [3]

Once the manager has recognized, defined, and analyzed the problem [1] and established its cause(s) and parameters and made assumptions [2], tentative alternative solutions are developed [3]. In Figure 10.4, this step includes considering tentative alternative solutions [3a]; collecting data/information [3b], if necessary; and evaluating the merits of each tentative alternative [3c] for an initial accept-reject decision. If tentative alternatives are unacceptable, the step is repeated. It is in the tentative alternative loop that imagination, creativity, and thoughts that occur "out of the blue" are identified. Unique, nontraditional, or innovative tentative solutions can be identified more readily if structural, personal, and problem assumptions are not overly restrictive.

Several factors influence the time and resources devoted to the tentative alternative solution loop. The two most important are the quality and precision of initial problem definition and the degree to which assumptions are not overly restrictive. Others are the sophistication of the HSO's information systems, availability of data, and degree to which the problem is structured. Unstructured problems are more complex, involve many variables, and take longer to solve. They require more attention than those that are simple, relatively obvious, or narrowly defined.

The tentative alternative solution loop has two hazards. Some managers spend excessive time and resources looking for the optimal solution when another solution is also acceptable. In addition, extensive attention to loop activities and reiteration may be an excuse for not taking action. "I need more information" may be an excuse for procrastinating and making no decision.[26]

Developing and Applying Decision Criteria [4]

The tentative alternative solution loop [3] produces a set of alternatives that are evaluated and compared. In evaluating alternatives [4], managers formally or informally develop decision criteria —the means by which alternative solutions are evaluated and compared. These include the criteria related to the "Desired Results" cell in the center of Figure 10.4. That is, will the alternative yield the desired results? In addition, at least three other types of decision criteria are usually applied: effectiveness of the alternative in solving the problem, feasibility of implementation, and acceptability of the alternative based on cost-to-benefit and advantage-to-disadvantage analysis.[27]

Some alternatives are unacceptable, such as those that do not solve the problem because they address only symptoms or are not permanent solutions. Exceptions as to absolute acceptability are made, for example, if taking action is critical, and it may be appropriate to select and implement a less than optimal solution because the consequences of doing nothing or waiting for a better solution are worse.

The feasibility of implementing an alternative is the second common criterion. Alternatives that are totally infeasible will be rejected in the tentative alternative solution loop. Those that survive may be implemented to varying degrees in terms of effort, structural boundaries and constraints, dependence on other people or departments or both, and costs. It may be appropriate that a manager not select an alternative that depends on people and departments beyond the manager's control. This is especially true if high political costs are associated with forcing implementation.

The third criterion concerns resource effectiveness, including cost-benefit analysis and assessment of qualitative advantages and disadvantages. Least cost should not be used as a sole criterion because both the costs and the benefits of an alternative must be considered. It is useful to perform both objective and subjective analysis of alternatives, including the opportunity costs associated with doing nothing. Objective evaluation means quantifying costs and benefits and should be attempted, despite the difficulty of quantifying some information. Subjective evaluation means being aware of considerations (advantages and disadvantages) that cannot be quantified. Information from both types of evaluation should be considered when evaluating alternatives and comparing them. If an alternative has high resource costs, but the problem solver concludes that subjective considerations are more important, a rational decision has been made.

Selecting and Implementing the Alternative Solution [5]

Almost always the manager selects an alternative (makes a decision) and implements it [5]. However, problem solving does not end. The results [6] of the intervention (change) must be monitored to determine if they are consistent with desired results [1]. If so, the problem is solved. If not, the problem-solving cycle begins anew, perhaps by fine-tuning an alternative previously identified or by developing new ones. Furthermore, intervening to solve one problem may create new problems. For example, decreasing an unusually high average length of stay will have revenue repercussions, creating another problem.

Implications for the Health Services Manager

Problem solving is not easy, but it is a major responsibility of health services managers. Done effectively, problem solving results in better allocation and utilization of resources, and individual and organizational work results are more consistent with what is desired. It may be, too, that results will improve. The level of management skill in problem solving, including decision making, will be directly reflected in the quality of solutions and interventions.

FACTORS INFLUENCING
PROBLEM SOLVING AND DECISION MAKING

Problem solving and its constituent, decision making, are dynamic activities that do not occur in a vacuum. Many factors shape how problem solving and decision making are performed, the style that is used, and the final outcome or quality of the alternative. Figure 10.5 presents three groups of factors: 1) attributes pertaining to the problem solver, 2) the nature of the situation, and 3) constraints in the environment.[28] To some degree, all of them can affect each problem-solving step (including decision making), beginning with problem definition and continuing through assumptions, identifying tentative alternative solutions, evaluating alternative solutions and choices, and implementation and evaluation.

Problem Solver Attributes

Knowledge, Experience, and Judgment   Among the most important attributes affecting problem solving are the experience, knowledge, and judgment of the problem solver—the one assessing the problem and making the decision. In health services, knowledge and experience are critical prerequisites for quality patient care, and this is recognized though licensing and certification. Physicians, dentists, nurses, pharmacists, and many types of technical specialists have years of formal education and clinical training. Nonmedical personnel such as HSO managers gain knowledge through education in graduate programs in health services administration or informally through continuing education and in-service programs. Their experience is enhanced by residencies and service in a variety of positions and organizations. Knowledge and experience are critical to good problem solving and decision making, and these are coupled with judgment. Sometimes, intuition and hunch are important.

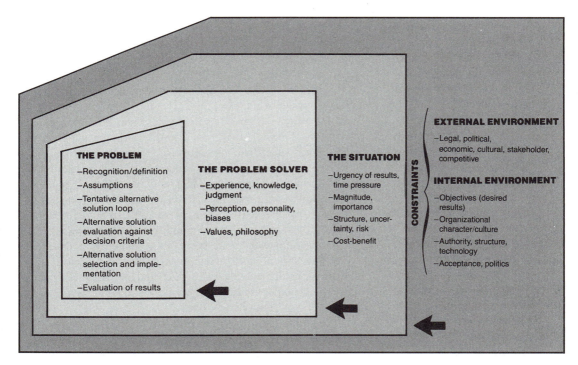

Figure 10.5.   Factors influencing problem solving and decision making.

Perception and Personality The problem solver's perceptions, personality, and biases influence problem solving and decision making. Perspective, one form of perception, is how the problem solver views a situation, problem, or environment. Those with a narrow perspective (tunnel vision) and who think vertically (and not horizontally) approach problems differently and will probably make lower quality decisions.[29] Traits such as temperament, aggressiveness, self-centeredness, self-assurance, and self-confidence, as well as demeanor (introvert-extrovert) and tolerance for risk, change, uncertainty, or instability, influence how managers solve problems and the quality of their decisions.

A nonaggressive, introverted, procrastinating person who is averse to risk and fears change (does not rock the boat) may make assumptions that limit the range of problem solving. Such a manager is likely to be less innovative in the tentative alternative solution loop. This person may hesitate to exit the loop because of a continuing search for the best solution (or an implicit hope that the problem will go away), and is more likely to make compromises or less bold decisions than a manager with other personality traits. Typically, such persons are reactive and must be forced to act. Proactive persons take the initiative, anticipate and manage events, and get the job done. The latter type of manager is usually more inclined to make difficult, bold, progressive, or nontraditional decisions.

Values and Philosophy Values and philosophy influence problem solving in two ways. Individual values, morals, and ethics affect assumptions and help define feasible alternatives. Those inconsistent with the problem solver's value system are excluded. Managers with a self-centered personal ethic may make decisions that provide positive, short-term, and self-serving benefit but are inconsistent with the long-term good of the HSO. A personal philosophy includes position on the political spectrum (liberal or conservative) as well as managerial leadership and motivational philosophy. The manager's personal philosophy can limit the alternatives that are considered and influence the approach to problem solving—whether it is unilateral or involves others, especially subordinates.

The Situation

Many facts about the situation within which a problem occurs and facts about the problem itself influence the problem-solving process and outcome. Those identified in Figure 10.5 are: how urgently a solution is needed and time pressure, magnitude and importance of the problem, degree of uncertainty and risk, and costs versus benefits.

Urgency of Solution and Time Pressures Sometimes immediate decisions are required because delay is too costly. Severe trauma or medical crises are examples. Similarly, problems such as impending work stoppage, major initiatives by competitors, or inadequate cash flow require action more quickly than other types of situations. The consequences of such problems are so significant that use of the tentative alternative solution loop will be quick and the evaluation process may be less thorough. In situations with little time pressure, such as under the conditions of opportunity, deviation, or improvement, the problem solver may use a different style, which involves consultation, collecting more information, and more thoroughly evaluating alternatives.

Magnitude and Importance The magnitude and importance of the problem directly affect the process—the time, energy, and resources spent in assessing the problem and making a decision. Ends-means and administrative decisions warrant greater attention and more intense evaluation than day-to-day operational decisions. Another measure of importance could be the cost implications of resource commitment and the opportunity cost of delay.

Problems with high cost or resource commitment, particularly under conditions of opportunity or improvement and when there is no urgency, justify devoting more time and collecting more information in the tentative alternative solution loop than do low-cost problems. The same is true for unstructured problems. A potential hazard for managers is that resources consumed (time and information collection) to find the best solution may begin to approach or exceed cost conse-quences of the problem. It is senseless to allocate $15,000 for resources such as management and staff time, feasibility studies, and special requests for nonroutine data to search for elaborate alternatives and the equipment to solve a medical records storage problem when space is available in the basement or old records can be moved off site. Managers must be mindful that the cost of searching for alternatives must not exceed the benefits of the one selected.

Structure, Uncertainty, and Risk   From a problem-solving perspective, structure refers to the degree to which the situation is clear: that is, the degree to which the scope and nature of problem and alternatives are precise.[30] Ends-means, administrative, and nonprogrammed deci-sion situations are inherently less structured than programmed or operational situations. Problems with equipment and material, job design, and process flow are more structured than those with behavioral dynamics or those involving external stakeholders and competitors. Risk is proportion-ate to certainty. The presence of certainty in a problem implies that the manager has complete information and can predict the outcomes of alternatives. Less information means greater risk because even carefully derived estimates contain a degree of uncertainty. For example, certainty of results is 100% if mismatched blood is transfused. Certainty is less than 100% when the problem-solving process determines that a free-standing family practice center should be estab-lished to provide inpatient referrals to a hospital. The more unstructured and uncertain the situa-tion, the greater the time spent and resources allocated and the more participative the problem-solving and decision-making processes are likely to be.

Cost-Benefit   Ultimately, problem solving results in selecting an alternative. Its selection will be based in part on quantitative cost-benefit and/or qualitative advantage-disadvantage crite-ria. Many problems are suited to cost-benefit analysis: which equipment will improve productiv-ity and decrease patient waiting time, or which new service will increase revenues. Another ex-ample is whether more nursing staff (cost) will decrease length of stay (benefit). Sometimes, however, measurable costs and benefits cannot be obtained or qualitative criteria may be more important. In fact, a choice among alternatives is appropriate only when all quantitative and qual-itative implications are considered. Exclusion of one detracts from the quality of the decision.

Environmental Constraints

The HSO's internal and external environments influence managerial problem solving by imposing variables management cannot control and constraints on the solution selected. This restricts the feasible alternatives.

External   Legal, political, economic, cultural, regulatory, stakeholder, competitive, and similar external forces are always present. The requirement to obtain a certificate of need for facility expansion or for adding new services constrains those alternatives; high local unemploy-ment with loss of employer-paid health insurance adversely affects revenues and increases bad debts. This may make capital expenditures infeasible. Changes in Medicare and Medicaid reim-bursement may limit the organization's ability to add new technology and equipment.

Internal   Internal environmental factors more directly affect problem solving. Organiza-tional objectives restrict alternatives that can be considered. Less precise, but influential nonethe-less, is organizational character and culture. All organizations have a unique character: it may be innovative or backward, aggressive or conservative, proactive or reactive, warm or cold. HSO characteristics such as these influence problem solving. Managers in an HSO with a reactive, slow-to-change character are unlikely to select bold, innovative, or nontraditional solutions. Sim-ilarly, managers of an HSO that moves quickly and with inadequate preparation are likely to be successful only by luck, not because of the quality of their decisions. Finally, any alternative considered or chosen must be consistent with the HSO's culture—the embedded and permeating values and beliefs. Those inconsistent with the culture should be rejected.

As managers apply decision criteria to the alternatives, they must consider implementation, which is affected by an array of factors ranging from resource availability to organizational commitment. Noteworthy factors are authority, structure, and technology. An alternative whose implementation is outside the scope of the manager's authority may not be feasible. The president of the professional staff has no authority to change the HSO's information system; the CEO has no authority to discharge a patient.

The existing organizational configuration may render implementation of one alternative infeasible, while absence of a technology base prohibits another. For example, physical plant layout may preclude changing patient and material flow patterns, union contracts may constrain how jobs are defined and designed, or the present computer system may be incapable of nursing station on-line terminal hookup.

Another influence is how decisions will be accepted by others in the organization. Acceptance by superiors and peers and/or subordinates is often critical to successfully implementing an alternative. A decision to decrease inpatient length of stay by decreasing turnaround time for diagnostic tests will be difficult to implement if those who read and interpret the tests are resistant. A decision to involve others in the problem-solving process will be partly influenced by the degree to which their acceptance is critical to implementation. Finally, the nature of organizational politics influences both the problem-solving process and the outcome. The degree of informal influence, conflict, and competition among power factions such as professional staff and nursing service may cause a manager to negotiate, collaborate, compromise, or "satisfice" (find a workable, if imperfect, solution) when solving problems.

Implications for the Health Services Manager

The attributes of the problem solver, the nature of the situation, and the environmental constraints presented in Figure 10.5 influence problem solving—how it is done, time and resources spent performing it, and the quality of the ultimate decision. However, these influences are not mutually exclusive. Some persons with a given perception, personality, and value set function better in a highly politicized environment and cope better with unstructured and risk-laden situations than others. Also, one variable may supersede or preempt others: an urgent situation that requires immediate solution can force the manager who usually seeks input, develops wide-ranging alternatives, and does extensive evaluation to act quickly and unilaterally.

These attributes have several implications for health services managers. Managers should recognize and be sensitive to the factors that affect problem solving, change their methods as appropriate, modify and mitigate detrimental influences when possible, and cope with those that cannot be changed. In this way, they will improve the quality of problem solving.

GROUP PROBLEM SOLVING

Managers solve problems and make decisions in their areas of responsibility. They are accountable for results as well as resource allocation and utilization. Managers may choose to solve problems and make decisions on their own (unilateral problem solving), or they may choose to involve superiors, peers, or subordinates to a degree that can range from some involvement and participation, perhaps in a consultative information-gathering capacity, to group involvement in which participants share equally in problem solving.

Each approach has advantages and disadvantages. Unilateral problem solving has the advantage of being time efficient. Involving others is time consuming, particularly in group forums, and there are overhead costs such as staff time in group problem solving, especially if the number of people involved is large.[31] Another disadvantage of group problem solving is that there may be social pressure to conform and concur with a decision, the extreme of which is groupthink. Groupthink occurs when the group ignores important clues and cues about the problem, others outside of the group are stereotyped (usually as being hostile to the group), there is pressure on dissenters to conform, group censorship and the illusion of unanimity are present, and information contrary to the group's position is discounted.[32] In the political arena, Watergate is the classic example of groupthink.[33]* An example in the health services area would be a conscious group decision on the part of a hospital's senior management and/or governing body not to inform former patients who received invasive treatment from a staff member who died from acquired immunodeficiency syndrome (AIDS). Simply put, remaining silent in such a situation is unethical. Finally, in group problem solving the phenomenon of "risky shift" can occur. Diffused responsibility encourages more risky decisions than when one person is responsible for a decision.[34]

As a rule, however, group problem solving generally results in better quality solutions because multiple perspectives and more information and experience are brought to bear. Other people, especially subordinates, may be able to help define a problem and its parameters and assist in identifying tentative alternative solutions because they have more knowledge about the problem. Involving persons knowledgeable about a problem or process is critical to successful quality improvement activities. A greater variety of alternatives may be considered because restrictive problem assumptions are likely to be challenged. Furthermore, involving others enhances acceptance and facilitates implementation. Those involved take greater pride of ownership and usually are more committed to implementing the selected alternative. Finally, group problem solving enhances communication and coordination because those implementing the decision have greater knowledge about the solution and the process by which it was obtained.

The benefits of employee participation in problem solving and decision making are well documented in the behavioral science literature. Involved employees have greater identification with the HSO and what it does. Kaluzny advocates a new focus on group problem solving in HSOs, particularly as related to quality improvement. He calls it a model of involvement and commitment,[35] and it includes two thrusts. The first is that senior management rethink the problem-solving role and responsibility of middle-level managers. The aim is to enlarge their role and increase their authority and responsibility. The second is that middle-level managers rethink the superior-subordinate relationship with the aim of involving their subordinates more in problem solving in order to achieve greater commitment to the HSO's objectives. In doing so, Kaluzny concludes, the advantage of group problem solving or

> a team approach to department or unit management is that each individual is able to participate in complex decisions and to add relevant expertise. This level of commitment not only facilitates the performance of the group/unit, but enhances the overall level of commitment within the organization.[36]

Quality Circles as a Problem-Solving and Quality Improvement Technique

Certain conditions must exist if group problem solving is to be effective. First, there must be a climate of openness that permits free expression of ideas, and the focus must be on solutions rather than fault finding.[37] Second, participation in problem solving must be legitimate in that those involved, usually subordinates, know that managers are truly interested in the group's reasonable recommendations. Crosby calls this situation "empowering," because subordinates actually influence decisions.[38] One group problem-solving method linked to productivity and quality improvement is quality circles. Lawler and Mohrman state that:

---

*Watergate is the apartment complex in Washington, D.C., that housed the headquarters of the Democratic National Committee during the 1972 presidential election campaign. Operatives of the (Republican) Committee to Re-elect the President (Richard M. Nixon) broke into these headquarters and were apprehended. The subsequent political stonewalling by President Nixon, the resulting scandal, and the eventual resignation of the president are collectively called "Watergate." The decision-making process and mindset of those involved in the break-in exemplify groupthink.

Quality circles are a parallel-structure approach to involving employees in problem solving. A parallel structure is one that is separate and distinct from the regular, ongoing activities of an organization and, as such, operates in a special way. In quality circle programs, groups are composed of volunteers from a work area who meet with a special type of leader and/or facilitator for the purpose of examining productivity and quality problems.[39]

To be effective, quality circle programs must have commitment from senior management in terms of both process and outcomes. Resources that include member meeting time and employee training in problem solving may be substantial. Furthermore, there must be management commitment to acting on appropriate recommendations made by the group. Failure to do so will cause quality circle members to conclude that their participation is not legitimate or cause them to perceive that their efforts are unimportant. Benefits include better problem solving, because it is based on employee knowledge and expertise about the work they perform, and greater employee involvement with and commitment to the HSO, leading to higher motivation, morale, and job satisfaction.[40] Given the opportunity, employees can contribute significantly to solving problems.

Other Group Formats

Group problem solving need not be restricted to an institutionalized format such as quality circles. Ad hoc task forces, particularly for solving major organization-wide problems or for addressing unstructured and major problems under the conditions of opportunity or threat, may be formed. Focus group teams[41] or quality improvement teams (similar to quality circles) may be used. They may be interdepartmental and may focus on quality improvement initiatives that span the organization and levels in the hierarchy.[42] Finally, managers may encourage problem-solving participation from their subordinates. Such participation may be frequent or infrequent and may involve few or many subordinates separately or in groups, and it need not be formalized or institutionalized, as are quality circles and quality improvement teams.

PROBLEM-SOLVING AND DECISION-MAKING STYLES

The manager's style of problem solving and decision making may involve subordinates individually or in groups. The style is influenced by the nature and importance of the problem, the extent to which the manager has sufficient information to define it, and the degree to which solution acceptance by other organization members is critical to implementing the alternative chosen. This section presents a conceptual model of problem-solving/decision-making styles useful to managers in determining whether and to what degree others should be involved and under what conditions their participation should occur. The model focuses on subordinate involvement, but it can be applied to peers or superiors.

Table 10.1 shows five problem-solving and decision-making styles that are based on research by Victor Vroom.[43] Each represents a different degree of subordinate involvement.[44] Vroom's AI style is unilateral (autocratic), with no subordinate involvement either in predecision assessment or choice of alternative. The AII style is a variant of AI in which subordinates are involved only to provide information. The CI (consultative) and CII styles represent degrees to which subordinates' opinions are elicited and considered by the manager. The GII (group) style represents full subordinate involvement, including the manager's acceptance of the group decision. These styles and the model presented in Figure 10.6 are also discussed in Chapter 14, which focuses on leadership.

If it is presumed that effective problem solving is a function of: 1) the quality of the decision and 2) its acceptance, there are situations in which involving others may contribute to problem-solving effectiveness, thus both improving the decision's quality and enhancing its acceptance. Figure 10.6 presents a problem-solving/decision-making style model identifying appropriate styles (AI through GII) under different situations.

Table 10.1. Management problem-solving and decision-making styles

AI	The manager solves the problem or makes the decision unilaterally, using information available at that time.
AII	The manager obtains necessary information from subordinate(s), then develops and selects the solution unilaterally. Subordinates may or may not be told what the problem is when the manager gets information from them. Subordinates provide necessary information rather than generating or evaluating alternative solutions.
CI	The manager shares the problem with relevant subordinates individually, getting their ideas and suggestions without bringing them together. The manager's decision may or may not reflect the subordinates' contribution.
CII	The manager shares the problem with subordinates as a group, obtains their ideas and suggestions, and then makes the decision that may or may not reflect the subordinates' contribution.
GII	The manager shares the problem with subordinates as a group. Together they generate and evaluate alternatives and attempt to reach agreement (consensus) on a solution. The manager's role is much like that of chairperson—not trying to influence the group to adopt a particular solution. The manager is willing to accept and implement any solution supported by the group.

Adapted from Vroom, Victor H. A new look at managerial decision making. *Organizational Dynamics* 1 (Spring 1973): 66–80; reprinted by permission. © 1973. American Management Association, New York. All rights reserved.

Situational Variables (Problem Attributes)

The situational variables influencing style are characterized by seven different problem attributes. In Figure 10.6 these problem attributes are identified at the top of the model by the lower case notations *a* through *g*. The problem-solving style outcomes in Figure 10.6 have capital letter notation AI to GII. The first four problem attributes, *a* through *d*, denote the importance of decision quality and acceptance by others. The last three problem attributes, *e* through *g*, moderate the effects of subordinate participation on quality and acceptance (*a* through *d*). The seven problem attributes in the model (Figure 10.6) are replicated in Table 10.2, along with diagnostic questions that yield yes-or-no results.

Situations and Styles

On the basis of answers to the diagnostic questions for the seven problem attributes in Table 10.2, there are 14 different possible situations. They are identified by the numbers 1–14 in the model in Figure 10.6. Associated with each is the most appropriate problem-solving/decision-making style (AI through GII). It should be noted that each result and each style shown is the *most restrictive* for that set of problem attributes (note that, among Vroom's styles, AI is the most restrictive and GII the least), based on the assumption that the manager wishes to minimize time taken to solve the problem. For example, for situation 1 in Figure 10.6, the manager could use an AII, CI, CII, or GII style; however, more time would be needed to solve the problem using any of these. Therefore, given the problem attributes, the AI style is both appropriate for the circumstances and less time consuming than less restrictive styles.

Use of the Model

As the manager assesses the situation by examining problem attributes *a* through *g* and drawing yes-or-no conclusions, the model in Figure 10.6 will indicate the style (AI through GII) most appropriate for the particular situation. To demonstrate how the problem-solving and decision-making style model in Figure 10.6 can be used by managers, the logic flow is traced for situations 1, 2, 3, 11, 12, 13, and 14. The reader is invited to independently follow the logic of the other situations.

Situations 1, 2, and 3 If there is no decision quality requirement [a] and there are a number of obvious alternatives, all relatively meritorious, it is implied that the decision maker has sufficient information [b] to solve the problem unilaterally; the problem therefore must be relatively structured [c]. The next attribute or situational variable of consequence is whether subordi-

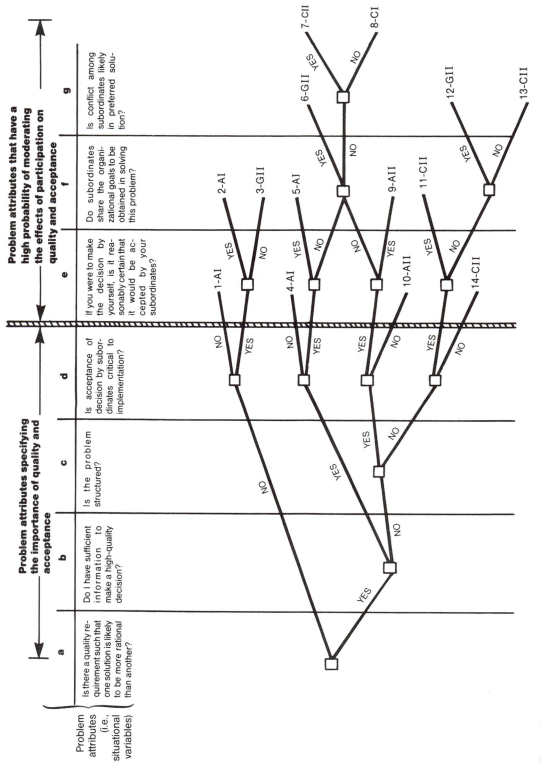

Figure 10.6. Problem-solving and decision-making style model. (Adapted from Vroom, Victor H. A new look at managerial decision making. *Organizational Dynamics* 1 [Spring 1973]: 66–80; reprinted by permission. © 1973. American Management Association, New York. All rights reserved.)

Table 10.2. Problem attributes used in the problem-solving and decision-making style model (Figure 10.6)

Problem attributes	Diagnostic questions
a. Importance of the quality of the decision	Is quality requirement such that one solution is likely to be more rational (better) than another? (Another way of discerning the quality is: If the alternatives are *not* equally meritorious—some are or can be much better than others—there is a quality requirement.)
b. Extent to which the decision maker possesses sufficient information/expertise to make a high-quality decision unilaterally	Do I have sufficient information to make a high-quality decision?
c. Extent to which problem is structured	Is problem structured? (Does decision maker know what information is needed and where to find it?)
d. Extent to which acceptance or commitment of subordinates is critical to effective implementation	Is acceptance of decision by subordinates critical to effective implementation?
e. Prior probability that a unilateral decision will receive acceptance by subordinates	If decision is made unilaterally, will it probably be accepted by subordinates?
f. Extent to which subordinates are motivated to attain organizational goals as represented in objectives explicit in statement of problem	Do subordinates share organizational goals to be obtained in solving problems?
g. Extent to which subordinates are likely to be in conflict over preferred solutions	Is conflict among subordinates likely to occur in preferred solutions?

Adapted from Vroom, Victor H. A new look at managerial decision making. *Organizational Dynamics* 1 (Spring 1973): 66–80; reprinted by permission. © 1973. American Management Association, New York. All rights reserved.

nate acceptance of the decision is critical to implementation [d]. If not, the manager can quite appropriately use unilateral style AI for situation 1 (1-AI in Figure 10.6). (The reader should note that each style presented is the most restrictive. Other, less restrictive styles, such as AII, CII, or GII, could be used in situation 1, if time to solve the problem were not a concern.)

If subordinate acceptance is critical to implementation, attribute *e* is evaluated. If it is likely that subordinates would accept the unilateral decision, the manager can appropriately use style AI for situation 2 (2-AI in Figure 10.6).

If subordinates probably would not accept the manager's decision, then style GII would be appropriate for situation 3 (3-GII in Figure 10.6). Group involvement (style GII) is appropriate because subordinate participation in solving the problem increases acceptance. Also, the manager is indifferent as to which alternative is chosen because all are relatively meritorious and there is no quality requirement [a].

Situations 11, 12, 13, and 14   Existence of a quality requirement [a] means that not all alternatives are equally good or others that may be possible are not clear. If this is the case and the manager does not have sufficient information to make high-quality decisions [b], and if the problem is not structured [c], the attribute of subordinate acceptance [d] is important in determining the appropriate problem-solving and decision-making style.

If subordinate acceptance is not critical to implementation [d], the consultative style CII is appropriate for situation 14 (14-CII in Figure 10.6). In this situation, sharing the problem with subordinates and obtaining their ideas and suggestions provides information the manager needs, yet the decision made need not necessarily reflect subordinates' influence.

If subordinate acceptance is critical to implementation [d], the manager determines whether they would be likely to accept the decision [e]. If so, style CII is appropriate for situation 11 (11-CII in Figure 10.6).

If the conclusion reached for attribute *e* is "no" (i.e., subordinates probably would not accept the manager's unilateral decision), the manager assesses attribute *f* to determine if subordinates share the organizational goals to be achieved in solving the problem. If the answer is no, style CII is appropriate for situation 13 (13-CII in Figure 10.6). If the answer is "yes," group style GII is appropriate (12-GII in Figure 10.6). Group involvement is appropriate because acceptance, which is critical to implementation of the alternative, will be enhanced. Since all participants have the same goals, there is no concern that the group will make a decision incompatible with the decision that the manager would have made.

Implications for the Health Services Manager

The problem-solving and decision-making style model presented in Figure 10.6 sets forth a logical sequence to suggest styles appropriate under different conditions (i.e., problem attributes). Although it is designed as a function of the degree of subordinate involvement in problem solving, similar analyses could be made for peer or superior involvement using the same model.

The importance of this model is not necessarily the style outcome, since other individual, situation, and environmental variables (see Figure 10.5) can influence style. What is important is that the model is a systematic way for the manager to think about whether others should be involved and to what degree, as well as how involvement of others can affect the quality of the problem solution and the success of implementation.

SUMMARY

This chapter focuses on managerial problem solving and decision making in HSOs. Problem solving is an activity that managers continuously perform to bring about change so that actual work and organization results are consistent with those that are desired. A distinction between problem solving and decision making is made, and types of managerial decisions are described. The conditions that initiate problem solving are presented in Figure 10.3. Those conditions are opportunity/threat, crisis, deviation, and improvement. The problem-solving activities or steps presented in the model (Figure 10.4) include the following: problem analysis (including problem recognition and definition), assumptions, identification of alternative solutions, alternative solution evaluation relative to decision criteria, selection of an alternative, and implementation and evaluation of results. Attributes of each step and implications for the manager are discussed.

A number of factors influence the problem-solving process and the quality of the outcome. They are characteristics of the problem solver, such as experience and values; factors related to the situation, such as the urgency of taking action and costs-benefits; factors related to the external HSO environment, such as legal constraints and competition; and factors internal to the HSO, including objectives and culture.

The advantages of group problem solving are presented, and quality circles are described as one formalized technique for problem solving, particularly under the condition of improvement. Employee participation not only enhances the quality of problem definition and solution, but also increases the commitment of the participants to the HSO.

The concluding section presents a problem-solving and decision-making style model (Figure 10.6) that suggests the extent to which subordinates may be involved. It describes a set of logic criteria that yield a managerial problem-solving and decision-making style ranging from unilateral to group involvement that is appropriate for a particular situation having certain attributes.

Skill in problem solving and as a decision maker is critical for health services managers. If they understand the process, are aware of factors that influence it, and assess appropriateness of subordinate (or superior or peer) involvement, the quality of their decisions will be enhanced.

DISCUSSION QUESTIONS

1. Explain why decision making is considered a distinct management function and why it is linked to all other management functions. Identify the three managerial decision classifications and give examples of each.

2. What conditions initiate problem solving? Discuss how problem solving under the condition of improvement can (conceptually) be related to problem solving under the condition of opportunity.

3. How are problem solving and decision making related? What predecision and postdecision activities are inherent in problem solving? What are the steps of problem solving?

4. Using the problem-solving process model in Figure 10.4, discuss and give examples of:
   1. How assumptions affect problem solving
   2. Positive and negative results that can occur in the tentative alternative solution loop
   3. Why both qualitative and quantitative considerations are important when evaluating and choosing an alternative

5. Identify the factors that influence problem solving. Describe several situations and indicate which factors were influential in shaping the outcome.

6. What are the advantages of group problem solving? List reasons why you think it is critical to the success of an organization-wide quality improvement program. Think of a situation that you have experienced in which the phenomenon of groupthink occurred and be prepared to describe that situation.

7. Identify the types of problem-solving and decision-making styles (see Table 10.1). Use the model in Figure 10.6 and problem attribute descriptions in Table 10.2 to describe a situation that shows each of the following styles: AI, CI, and GII.

CASE STUDY 1:   THE NEW CHARGE NURSE

You are a third shift (11:00 P.M.–7:00 A.M.) nurse supervisor to whom a number of charge nurses report. Six months ago you promoted Sally Besnick to charge nurse on that shift. One year ago she graduated with a bachelor of science in nursing (B.S.N.) from an out-of-state university that trains its students in a primary nursing philosophy. She is the same age as the five registered nurses (RNs) she supervises, who graduated from a diploma program at a local hospital. She is the only nurse with a B.S.N. who reports to you.

Besnick received the same in-service training that all other charge nurses receive, but she is failing on the job. Morale among her subordinates is low, absenteeism is high, and not all the work on her unit is getting done. You think her main difficulty is that she does not seem able to control, lead, discipline, or correct her subordinates. She seems very easygoing. Her subordinates refer to her as "Soft Sally" and feel that they know how to deliver technically better patient care than she does. However, you have no indication that the quality of care is any different on her unit than on the others.

Besnick is personable and well liked by all the other charge nurses and by you. She socializes with them after hours and has made it a point to participate in American Nurses Association professional activities, just like the other charge nurses. She and her husband just bought a new house in the community after renting for the year she has worked at your hospital. They adopted a baby 2 months ago.

You are concerned that if you demote Besnick, her pride will be hurt and she will quit. You do not want to lose a good RN.

Questions

1. What should you do in this situation? Why?
2. Evaluate this situation using each step in the problem-solving process model in Figure 10.4.

CASE STUDY 2:   THE NURSE AIDE

You are the supervisor on the day shift at a 100-bed nursing facility. In one 20-bed unit the work load relative to other units has been extremely heavy for the past month. In that unit you observed family members of a bedridden patient turning the patient. When you asked why they were doing that the family members said: "Nurse aide Johnson told us that the staff was too busy. If we want our father turned we would have to do it ourselves, or wait 3–4 hours before the staff could do it." On several occasions during the past week you noticed Johnson sitting in the utility room for long periods of time.

Questions

1. What is the problem? What results are inconsistent with desired results?
2. Identify several alternatives that could potentially solve the problem.
3. Choose an alternative.
4. Compare the alternative you chose to those chosen by other class members. What assumptions about the problem, personal assumptions, and structural assumptions have you made that are different from class members who chose a different alternative?

CASE STUDY 3: PREFERRED PROVIDER ORGANIZATION

You are the senior vice president and chief operating officer of a 400-bed acute care hospital and medical center. The president of your hospital asked you to investigate what he thinks is a problem and to identify alternatives to solve it. The hospital's inpatient days, occupancy rate, ancillary service units, and outpatient visits have been declining for a year; the president's estimate is at least 10% in each category. The president thinks this is caused by competition from a local health maintenance organization (HMO) established a year ago and from two investor-owned free-standing emergency centers that opened 6 months ago. The other two hospitals in your city of 300,000 have not done anything different this year compared to the past. The only exception is that uncollectible accounts have increased for all.

You know that the professional staff organization membership has not changed over the period, your hospital enjoys good press and has good stakeholder relations, there have been no quality problems, and your hospital's inpatient and outpatient charges are about 5% less than those of the other two hospitals. It seems that inpatient days and outpatient visits should have increased since your hospital completed a new building expansion 6 months ago, especially because it added space to the outpatient department. In fact, it was completed ahead of schedule and under budget. The area's 13% unemployment allowed contractors to accelerate construction because skilled workers were readily available.

You are perplexed as to why this supposed problem exists. To your knowledge, the HMO has an enrolled population from only one of the many local major manufacturing firms and, as far as you know, that firm's employees and dependents never represented more than 4% of your hospital's business.

You must submit your recommendation to the president in 2 weeks. Your are considering calling a meeting of your subordinates, who include the vice president of nursing service, two operations vice presidents, and the vice president of human resources. Two other individuals who report directly to the president have been invited by you to attend the meeting. They are the vice president for professional staff liaison and the chief financial officer. Your subordinates are united in purpose and easy to work with. The other two individuals who report to the president see the world differently than you do. They always look at problems from the viewpoint of their area of responsibility versus the hospital as a whole, and they do not always agree and cooperate with you.

You have been thinking about forming a preferred provider organization (PPO) in which your hospital would contract with solo and group practice fee-for-service physicians to provide inpatient and outpatient services at a contracted discounted rate. This program would be marketed to local businesses. You believe this arrangement will solve the problem by increasing patient volume. In fact, the more you think about it, the more you wonder if you need to hold that meeting.

Questions

1. Use the information in Figure 10.6 and Tables 10.1 and 10.2 to identify the appropriate problem-solving and decision-making style you should use in solving the problem. Should the meeting be held? Why? Be prepared to discuss why you selected a particular style.
2. Assume you unilaterally made a decision and recommended the PPO alternative to the president. Use the problem-solving model (Figure 10.4) to identify the activities that were not done or were not done well, and why.

NOTES

1. Hayes, James L. Quotation. Cited in *The manager's book of quotations,* edited by Lewis D. Eigen and Jonathan P. Siegel, 107. New York: American Management Association, 1989.
2. Drucker, Peter F. *An introductory view of management,* 396. New York: Harper's College Press, 1977; Pearce, John A. III, and Richard B. Robinson, Jr. *Management,* 62. New York: Random House, 1989.
3. Pearce and Robinson, *Management,* 63–64.
4. Simon, Herbert A. *The new science of management decision,* 6. New York: Harper and Brothers, Publishers, 1960.
5. Gallagher, Thomas J. *Problem solving with people: The cycle Process,* 9. New York: University of America Press, 1987.
6. Vroom, Victor H., and Arthur G. Jago. *The new leadership: Managing participation in organizations,* 56. Englewood Cliffs, N.J: Prentice Hall, Inc., 1988.
7. Higgins, James M. *The management challenge: An introduction to management,* 70–71. New York: Macmillan Publishing Company, 1991.
8. Hastings, John E.F., William R. Mindell, John W. Browne, and Janet M. Barnsley. Canadian health administrator study. *Canadian Journal of Public Health* 72, suppl. 1 (March/April 1981): 46–47.
9. American College of Hospital Administrators. *The evolving role of the hospital chief executive officer,* 90. Chicago: The Foundation of the American College of Hospital Administrators, 1984.
10. American College of Hospital Administrators, *Evolving role,* 59.
11. Cowan, David A. Developing a process model of problem recognition. *Academy of Management Review* 11 (Spring 1986): 763–764.
12. Gallagher, *Problem solving,* 77; Pearce and Robinson, *Management,* 65.
13. Brightman, Harvey J. *Problem solving: A logical and creative approach,* 7. Atlanta: Business Publication Division, College of Business Administration, Georgia State University, 1980.
14. Postal, Susan Nelson. Using the Deming quality improvement method to manage medical record department product lines. *Topics in Health Record Management* 10 (June 1990): 36.
15. Cowan, Developing a process, 764.
16. Nutt, Paul C. How top managers in health organizations set directions that guide decision making. *Hospital & Health Services Administration* 36 (Spring 1991): 67.
17. Cowan, Developing a process, 764.
18. Cowan, Developing a process, 766.
19. Andriole, Stephen J. *Handbook of problem solving: An analytical methodology,* 25. New York: Petrocelli Books, Inc., 1983.
20. Nutt, How top managers, 59.
21. For a discussion on problem definition, see Chow, Chee W., Kamal M. Haddad, and Adrian Wong-Boren. Improving subjective decision making in health care administration. *Hospital & Health Services Administration* 36 (Summer 1991): 192–193.
22. For a good presentation of problem-solving constraints, including assumptions, see Brightman, *Problem solving,* chpt. 3.
23. Chow, Haddad, and Wong-Boren, Improving subjective, 194.
24. Chow, Haddad, and Wong-Boren, Improving subjective, 202.
25. Chow, Haddad, and Wong-Boren, Improving subjective, 192.
26. Etzioni, Amitai. Humble decision making. *Harvard Business Review* 89 (July-August 1989): 125.
27. Pearce and Robinson (*Management,* 75) describe these criteria as: Will the alternative be effective?, Can the alternative be implemented?, and What are the organization consequences?, respectively.
28. For good presentations of problem solving in general and factors influencing the problem-solving process, see: Ackoff, Russell L. *The art of problem solving.* New York: John Wiley & Sons, 1978; Brightman, *Management;* Ivancevich, John M., James H. Donnelly, Jr., and James L. Gibson. *Management principles and functions,* 4th ed. Homewood, IL: Irwin, 1989; Kepner, Charles H., and Benjamin B. Tregoe. *The rational manager: A systematic approach to problem solving and decision making.* New York: McGraw-Hill Book Company, 1965; Nutt, How top managers.
29. Brightman, *Problem solving,* 83–84.
30. Vroom and Jago, *New leadership,* 56.
31. Vroom and Jago, *New leadership,* 28.
32. Brightman, Harvey J. *Group problem solving: An improved managerial approach,* 51. Atlanta: Business Publication Division, College of Business Administration, Georgia State University, 1988.
33. Ways, Max. Watergate as a case study in management. *Fortune* 88 (November 1973): 196–201.
34. Higgins, *Management challenge,* 87.
35. Kaluzny, Arnold D. Revitalizing decision making at the middle management level. *Hospital & Health Services Administration* 34 (Spring 1989): 42.
36. Kaluzny, Revitalizing decision making, 45.
37. Crosby, Bob. Why employee involvement often fails and what it takes to succeed. In *The 1987 annual: Developing human resources,* edited by J. William Pfeiffer, 179. San Diego, CA: University Associates, Inc., 1987.
38. Crosby, Why employee involvement, 181.
39. Lawler, Edward E., III, and Susan A. Mohrman. Quality circles: After the honeymoon. In *The 1988 annual: Developing human resources,* edited by J. William Pfeiffer, 201. San Diego, CA: University Associates, Inc., 1988.

40. Kahn, Susan. Creating opportunities for employee participation in problem solving. *Health Care Supervisor* 7 (October 1988): 39.
41. Dailey, Robert, Frederick Young, and Cameron Barr. Empowering middle managers in hospitals with team-based problem solving. *Health Care Management Review* 16 (Spring 1991): 55.
42. Barger, Gene, Paul Hofmann, James Shumake, and Walter Daves. Improved patient care through problem-solving groups. *Health Progress* 68 (September 1987): 43.
43. Vroom, Victor H. A new look at managerial decision-making. *Organizational Dynamics* 1 (Spring 1973): 66–80.
44. See also Vroom, Victor, H., and Philip W. Yetton. *Leadership and decision-making*. Pittsburgh: University of Pittsburgh Press, 1973; Vroom and Jago, *New leadership*.

BIBLIOGRAPHY

Ackoff, Russell L. *The Art of Problem Solving*. New York: John Wiley & Sons, 1978.

American College of Hospital Administrators. *The Evolving Role of the Hospital Chief Executive Officer*. Chicago: The Foundation of the American College of Hospital Administrators, 1984.

Andriole, Stephen J. *Handbook of Problem Solving: An Analytical Methodology*. New York: Petrocelli Books, Inc., 1983.

Brightman, Harvey J. *Problem Solving: A Logical and Creative Approach*. Atlanta: Business Publication Division, College of Business Administration, Georgia State University, 1980.

Brightman, Harvey J. *Group Problem Solving: An Improved Managerial Approach*. Atlanta: Business Publication Division, College of Business Administration, Georgia State University, 1988.

Chow, Chee W., Kamal M. Haddad, and Adrian Wong-Boren. Improving subjective decision making in health care administration. *Hospital & Health Services Administration* 36 (Summer 1991): 191–210.

Cowan, David A. Developing a process model of problem recognition. *Academy of Management Review* 11 (Spring 1986): 763–776.

Crosby, Bob. Why employee involvement often fails and what it takes to succeed. In *The 1987 Annual: Developing Human Resources,* edited by J. William Pfeiffer. San Diego, CA: University Associates, Inc., 1987.

Dailey, Robert, Frederick Young, and Cameron Barr. Empowering middle managers in hospitals with team-based problem solving. *Health Care Management Review* 16 (Spring 1991): 55–63.

Drucker, Peter F. *An Introductory View of Management*. New York: Harper's College Press, 1977.

Etzioni, Amitai. Humble decision making. *Harvard Business Review* 89 (July–August 1989): 122–126.

Gallagher, Thomas J. *Problem Solving with People: The Cycle Process*. New York: University of America Press, 1987.

Hastings, John E.F., William R. Mindell, John W. Browne, and Janet M. Barnsley. Canadian health administrator study. *Canadian Journal of Public Health* 72, suppl. 1 (March/April 1981): 1–60.

Higgins, James M. *The Management Challenge: An Introduction to Management*. New York: Macmillan Publishing Company, 1991.

Ivancevich, John M., James H. Donnelly, Jr., and James L. Gibson. *Management Principles and Functions,* 4th ed. Homewood, IL: Irwin, 1989.

Kaluzny, Arnold D. Revitalizing decision making at the middle management level. *Hospital & Health Services Administration* 34 (Spring 1989): 39–51.

Kepner, Charles H., and Benjamin B. Tregoe. *The Rational Manager: A Systematic Approach to Problem Solving and Decision Making*. New York: McGraw-Hill Book Company, 1965.

Lawler, Edward E., III, and Susan A. Mohrman. Quality circles: After the honeymoon. In *The 1988 Annual: Developing Human Resources,* edited by J. William Pfeiffer. San Diego, CA: University Associates, Inc., 1988

Nutt, Paul C. How top managers in health organizations set directions that guide decision making. *Hospital & Health Services Administration* 36 (Spring 1991): 57–75.

Pearce, John A. III, and Richard B. Robinson, Jr. *Management*. New York: Random House, 1989.

Simon, Herbert A. *The New Science of Management Decision*. New York: Harper and Brothers, Publishers, 1960.

Vroom, Victor H. A new look at managerial decision-making. *Organizational Dynamics* 1 (Spring 1973): 66–80.

Vroom, Victor H., and Arthur G. Jago. *The New Leadership: Managing Participation in Organizations*. Englewood Cliffs, NJ: Prentice Hall, Inc., 1988.

Vroom, Victor, H., and Philip W. Yetton. *Leadership and Decision-Making*. Pittsburgh: University of Pittsburgh Press, 1973.

Ways, Max. Watergate as a case study in management. *Fortune* 88 (November 1973): 109–112, 196–201.

11 / Quality and Productivity Improvement

The CQI Challenge: Continuous Quality Improvement demands that health care providers answer three questions. Are we doing the right things? Are we doing things right? How can we be certain that we do things right the first time, every time?
Brent C. James, The Hospital Research and Educational Trust, Quality Measurement and Management Project[1]

The management model in Chapter 1 (see Figure 1.6) shows how HSOs convert input resources into outputs. Individual and organizational work results (i.e., outputs) are achieved only when structure, tasks/technology, and people elements are integrated. The quality of output is affected by this conversion process and by the types and nature of inputs.

This chapter presents two dimensions of the quality of output. The philosophy of continuous quality improvement (CQI) is defined and the importance of improving the processes used to generate output is discussed. The relationships among CQI, productivity, and cost effectiveness are analyzed. The work of quality experts W. Edwards Deming, Joseph M. Juran, and Philip B. Crosby is profiled. The chapter introduces two CQI process improvement models, and the relationship between problem solving and the team approach to process improvement is discussed. The potential conflict between CQI and professional autonomy in health services organizations (HSOs) is explored. Productivity and productivity improvement (PI) are defined, and various PI methods to improve work systems and job design, capacity and facilities layout, and production control, scheduling, and materials handling are presented. Finally, the link between CQI and PI is described.

There has been a shift in the health services paradigm (model) with respect to quality.[2] It occurred at two levels: the definition of quality output, and the focus, or how to achieve it. First, the traditional definition of quality of care and service (i.e., output) has been expanded beyond meeting specifications or standards to that of conformance to requirements and fitness for use that includes patient/customer satisfaction and meeting customer expectations. Second, there is recognition of the importance of focusing on improving the inputs and processes that generate outputs (product and service outcomes).[3] This expanded definition of quality output and the focus on improving inputs and processes are the twin pillars of CQI. Adopting the philosophy and methods of CQI will positively affect HSO management and organizational arrangements; resource allocation, utilization, cost effectiveness, and PI; the quality of services provided; and the HSO's competitive position.

Intense international competition and increased consumer demands and expectations for quality products *and* services profoundly affected the American industrial sector in the 1970s and 1980s, and industry was found wanting. The result has been an increased awareness by business of the importance of quality, the implementation of initiatives to improve the quality of outputs to be more effective in the face of global competition, and, as described by Deming, the beginning of the transformation of American business.[4]

Like industry, the health services system in the United States is undergoing profound change. The 1980s were years of turmoil for HSOs, especially hospitals. Environmental changes in the 1980s—revenue and cost pressures; increased competition from alternate forms of delivery, such as managed care organizations and freestanding or satellite ambulatory surgery centers; and health services system restructuring, with formation of multiorganizational systems, closures, mergers, and consolidations[5]—will continue into the 1990s and create a hostile environment for HSOs. Additionally, there have been demands from customers for lower cost care with improved quality. These customers include patients as well as major payors such as government and self-insured businesses.[6] HSOs must respond to all these customer and stakeholder expectations.

QUALITY—TWO DIMENSIONS

Traditionally, quality in HSOs focused on product or service content[7] and meeting specifications or standards. Evaluation of quality tended to be retrospective and assessed the product or service using predetermined criteria. HSO examples are accuracy of diagnosis, physiological change and improvement in patients at discharge, mortality rates, and the efficacy of medical procedures and drugs. Methods of quality evaluation include inspection, peer review, and quality assurance, as well as tracking indicators such as infection rates, unanticipated readmissions after discharge, and accuracy and timeliness of diagnostic tests.

The contemporary view of quality* in HSOs includes two dimensions: conformance to requirements and fitness for use—both of which incorporate satisfying customer needs and meeting customer expectations.[9] "When an organization or individual generates outputs, either as products or services, and delivers these outputs to other organizations or individuals, then a quality judgment can occur."[10] Quality considerations include questions such as: Are there defects? Does the product work? Was the service appropriate? Is treatment reliable? Was the service on time? Was it delivered in a friendly manner? Was it the right service? Did it meet the customer's needs? The answers to such questions about expectations by customers are influenced by their experiences, perceptions, and values. The Hospital Research and Educational Trust Quality Measurement and Management Project (QMMP) terms this "delivery quality," and it "refers to all aspects of the organization's interaction with the customer in delivery of output."[11] In a general way, delivery quality describes the patients' satisfaction with their experiences based on interacting with the HSO.

In HSOs, conformance and expectation quality monitoring and improvement must be directed at every level and at every process.[12] Customers are not just patients and external stakeholders;[13] customers are also any internal downstream user of a unit's output.[14] For example, nursing service is a customer of pharmacy with regard to medications and of dietary services with regard to food service for patients; physicians are customers of diagnostic testing; the intensive care unit is a customer of the emergency department with respect to trauma patients being admitted; third-party payors are customers of patient billing; and all HSO departments and units, to some degree, are customers of administration. Depending on the transaction, any HSO process, department, unit, or person may switch from supplier to customer.[15] Figure 11.1 shows how a hospital's functional departments have internal and external customers.

---

*The American Production and Inventory Control Society defines quality as: "Conformance to requirements, or fitness for use. Quality can be defined through five principal approaches: (1) Transcendent quality is an ideal, a condition of excellence. (2) Product-based quality is based on a product attribute. (3) User-based quality is fitness for use. (4) Manufacturing based quality is the conformance to requirements. (5) Value-based quality is the degree of excellence at an acceptable price. Also, quality has two major components: (1) quality of conformance—quality is defined by the absence of defects, and (2) quality of design—quality is measured by the degree of customer satisfaction with a product's characteristics and features."[8] For ease of reading, these two components of quality will be referred to as conformance/expectation quality.

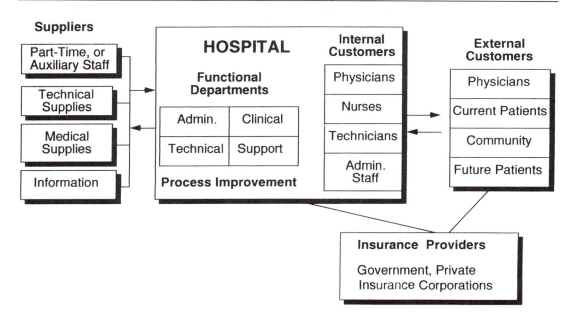

Figure 11.1. Internal and external customers of hospital functional departments. (Reprinted with permission from Carol Greebler, TQM Plus. San Diego, CA [1989].)

CONTINUOUS QUALITY IMPROVEMENT

A new philosophy about quality is emerging in health services. Largely based on the work of the industrial quality experts W. Edwards Deming,[16] Joseph M. Juran,[17] and Philip B. Crosby,[18] this philosophy has four attributes. First, output quality includes meeting customer expectations. Second, monitoring and evaluating the quality of outputs is both retrospective (after the fact) *and* prospective (before the fact); poor quality can be prevented. Third, "quality is not the responsibility of just one department or individual;"[19] it is organization-wide and involves all HSO staff. Fourth, quality and quality improvement focus on both process (and inputs) *and* outcomes, not just outcomes. (For ease of reading, when reference is made to process improvement, it also includes input improvement.) The Joint Commission on Accreditation of Healthcare Organizations's (Joint Commission's) *Agenda for Change* recognizes the need for outcome and process quality.[20] The philosophical context of the agenda for change is based on quality improvement that *emphasizes* the following:

> Quality as a central priority: organization-wide devotion to quality, leadership involvement in promoting and improving quality.
> Customers: attention to customer needs, feedback from internal and external customers, customer-supplier dialogue.
> Work processes: describing key clinical and managerial processes, systems approach, and cross-disciplinary teams.
> Measurement: use of data, understanding of variation, search for underlying causes.
> Improvement: never-ending commitment to improving performance.[21]

Continuous quality improvement is sometimes called quality management,[22] total quality management (TQM),[23] total quality care,[24] or quality improvement.[25] CQI is used here rather than TQM. CQI suggests the major break with previous efforts to achieve quality, it is the most positive way to state the concept, and it eliminates the suggestion that quality is only the job of managers.

CQI is defined as *an ongoing, organization-wide framework in which HSOs and their employees are committed to and involved in monitoring and evaluating all aspects of the HSO's activities (inputs and processes) and outputs in order to continuously improve them.*[26] The essential elements of this definition are:

CQI is organization wide. CQI can only be successful if the organization is transformed to seek quality in all that it does. It requires a total commitment to quality—a philosophical transformation—by the governing body and senior management and involves all HSO employees.

CQI is process focused. CQI seeks to understand processes, identify process characteristics that should be measured, and monitor processes as changes are made to determine the effect of changes. The result is more efficient and effective processes that improve productivity through better use of resources. In sum, CQI improves conversion processes, thereby generating higher quality products and service (outputs).

CQI uses output or inspection measures. Outcomes of care (indicators) provide macro-level measures to determine how well groups of processes and the HSO as a whole are performing. Indicators allow an HSO to perform time series comparisons and do inter-HSO comparisons, for example. They are crude arrows that point the HSO toward needs for process analysis and improvement.

CQI is customer driven. The goal is to meet or exceed customer expectations. "Customer" is defined in its broadest possible sense, both internally and externally.

The literature is replete with CQI applications in HSOs. Selected examples are individual hospitals,[27] multiorganizational systems,[28] and medical speciality clinics.[29] Success stories in specific departments abound—clinical medicine,[30] laboratory,[31] diagnostic radiology,[32] medical records,[33] and pharmacy.[34]

CQI Model

The chapter's opening quote stated the CQI challenge as expressed by the Hospital Research and Educational Trust QMMP. It poses three questions: Are we doing the right things? Are we doing things right? How can we be certain that we do things right the first time, every time? Figure 11.2 answers these questions in the context of a CQI model. The discussion in this section references components of the model by number.

Are We Doing the Right Things? Output quality [3] is the first pillar of CQI and determines if the HSO is doing the right things. Products and services that meet customer expectations result in the HSO doing the right things. From the CQI perspective, customers are not only patients and external stakeholders, but also internal users of a department, unit, or individual's outputs. Customers are the next downstream process that relies on an upstream process for inputs.[35] Output that is in conformance/meets customers' expectations is a quality product or service and means that the HSO is doing the right things.

Are We Doing Things Right? Process improvement [2] is the second pillar of CQI for three reasons. First, output quality can be improved only by improving the processes that produce it (and/or the inputs used in the process). Second, all processes can be improved. As observed by the president of the Joint Commission, "patient care systems, particularly because of their high degree of human dependency, can always be improved."[36] He states further, "quality improvement turns us 180 degrees from where we have been. It means if it ain't broke, it can still be improved."[37]

Third, monitoring, evaluating, and intervening to improve processes is continuous. A prerequisite is systematic understanding and documentation of processes. In addition, all employees must seek opportunities to improve work results and the way they produce them. The outcome is

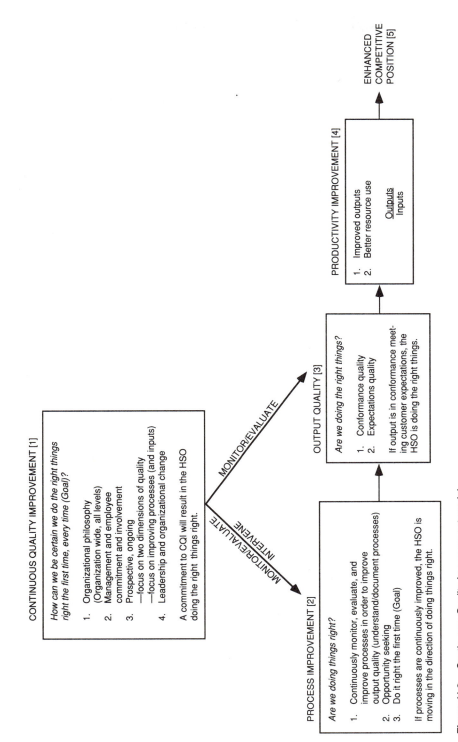

CONTINUOUS QUALITY IMPROVEMENT [1]

How can we be certain we do the right things right the first time, every time (Goal)?

1. Organizational philosophy
   (Organization wide, all levels)
2. Management and employee
   commitment and involvement
3. Prospective, ongoing
   —focus on two dimensions of quality
   —focus on improving processes (and inputs)
4. Leadership and organizational change

A commitment to CQI will result in the HSO doing the right things right.

MONITOR/EVALUATE
INTERVENE

MONITOR/EVALUATE

PROCESS IMPROVEMENT [2]

Are we doing things right?

1. Continuously monitor, evaluate, and
   improve processes in order to improve
   output quality (understand/document processes)
2. Opportunity seeking
3. Do it right the first time (Goal)

If processes are continuously improved, the HSO is moving in the direction of doing things right.

OUTPUT QUALITY [3]

Are we doing the right things?

1. Conformance quality
2. Expectations quality

If output is in conformance meeting customer expectations, the HSO is doing the right things.

PRODUCTIVITY IMPROVEMENT [4]

1. Improved outputs
2. Better resource use

Outputs
Inputs

ENHANCED
COMPETITIVE
POSITION [5]

Figure 11.2. Continuous Quality Improvement model.

411

not only improved output quality [3], but also PI in which there is more effective resource use [4]. The goal of process improvement, as expressed by Crosby, is to do it right the first time.[38] Although this ultimately may never be attained, if an HSO continuously improves processes, it is moving in the direction of "do it right the first time," and doing things right.

How Can We Be Certain We Do the Right Things Right the First Time, Every Time? The goal of CQI is doing the right things right the first time, every time. If there is quality output (the right things) and process improvement (doing things right) with CQI, the HSO will move in the direction of doing things right the first time, every time (goal).[39] The essential attributes of CQI [1] are (see Figure 11.2):

> CQI is a philosophy that becomes part of the culture—the ingrained beliefs and values of the HSO. It is pervasive throughout the organization. This requires transformation of the existing beliefs and values regarding quality and is customer driven.

> CQI requires total commitment and involvement of everyone in the HSO. Management must commit resources and create an atmosphere conducive to continuous improvement in which quality is integral to the work of all employees.[40] Employees must participate and be committed to continuously improving their work results and the way those results are achieved. This requires extensive collaboration and cross-functional coordination among work units and departments.[41] Employees must be involved in problem solving—particularly as it relates to seeking and identifying opportunities for improvement.

> CQI is prospective and ongoing. The focus on output quality must be prospective, not just retrospective. The aim is to prevent poor quality before it happens and to seek opportunities to improve processes in an organized fashion.

> CQI requires management to meet its leadership responsibility to train employees; to encourage innovation, worker participation, and team building so employees can contribute to process improvement problem solving; and to facilitate organizational change that leads to improvement.

CQI, Productivity Improvement, and Cost Effectiveness

The result of the CQI paradigm is the reciprocal of the traditional PI and cost-containment initiatives prevalent during the 1970s and 1980s. In the context of the management model in Figure 1.6, PI focused on increasing the ratios of outputs to inputs. Such initiatives were narrowly applied, episodic, and short term. They often had low worker involvement and commitment, and primarily focused on reducing input costs rather than enhancing output quality. In the CQI model, improvement initiatives are broad based, long term, and ongoing, have high management and employee involvement and commitment, are customer driven, and focus on improving both process and output quality versus simply reducing costs.

Figure 11.2 depicts how CQI achieves improved quality and PI [4]. Deming asserts that PI does not necessarily result in improved output quality, but that improved quality does result in PI. Consequently, the HSO's competitive position is enhanced [5]. According to Deming, the CQI philosophy causes a chain reaction: improved quality results in better resource use (lower costs) because improved processes result in less rework (readmissions), fewer mistakes (repeats of tests), fewer delays (waiting for service), and better use of resources. These results occur because the prospective and continuous assessment of and changes made to work processes and inputs yield both improved quality *and* productivity.[42]

APPROACHES TO QUALITY IMPROVEMENT

Three recognized leaders on achieving quality—W. Edwards Deming, Joseph M. Juran, and Philip B. Crosby—have greatly influenced the philosophy and practice of CQI, and their principles are being adopted in HSOs.[43] These experts provide philosophies and methodologies for organizations seeking to establish a quality culture. They are not of like mind on many of the specifics of how to achieve quality improvement: Deming is the philosopher and statistician; Juran uses a more managerial approach; and Crosby is the organizational behavioralist and motivator. Although the routes differ somewhat, their destination is the same. They are three different preachers with the same religion—quality.[44]

W. Edwards Deming

Deming was most influential in assisting post–World War II Japan in transforming its industry into the economic power it became. His underlying premise, like that of Juran, is that poor quality is due to badly designed or malfunctioning processes—not to worker behavior—and that poor quality can be prevented. Therefore, his approach emphasizes monitoring and evaluating processes through statistical quality control and searching for ways to improve processes. Like Crosby and Juran, Deming incorporates the essential characteristics of CQI: total organization commitment and worker involvement and education in the improvement of processes. The following profile of Deming is insightful:

> Quality must become a central focus of the corporation. The emphasis must shift from inspection to prevention. Preventing defects before they occur and improving the process so that defects do not occur, are goals for which a company should strive.
>
> Training and retraining of employees is critical to the success of the corporation. Deming believes that it is management's job to coach employees. Education and training are investments in people. They help to avoid employee burnout, reenergizing employees, and give a clear message to employees that management considers employees to be a valuable resource. Finally, Deming also believes that management must pay attention to variability within processes. He advocates systematic understanding of variation and reduction of variations as a strategy to improve processes.
>
> Deming believes that the road to enhanced productivity is through continuous quality improvement called the Deming Chain Reaction. Improving quality through improving processes leads to a reduction of waste, rework, delays, and scrap. This reduction causes productivity as well as quality to improve.[45]

The Deming chain reaction is presented in Figure 11.3. It indicates that improving quality and eliminating variability in processes decreases costs, increases productivity, and enhances the organization's competitive position. This sequence is incorporated in the CQI model in Figure 11.2.

The Deming method has two distinct components. The first step is critical: Managers must establish and perpetuate an environment in which quality improvement is integral to the work of all employees. For most HSOs this means a transformation—a major philosophical shift and commitment to quality. The second, and concurrent, component is that efforts to improve quality are supported by statistical analysis of activities—management must understand what the organization is doing and how well it is being done. These data and their analyses allow managers to identify and correct problems.

Deming's 14 points for quality[46] have been discussed extensively by other writers.[47] The 14 points have been applied to HSOs by Bataldan and Vorlicky, as cited in Deming[48] and Darr.[49]

1. *Create constancy of purpose toward improvement of product and service with the aim to become competitive, to stay in business, and to provide jobs.*[50] This means identifying customers, giving good quality service to them, and ensuring organization survival through innovation and constant improvement.
2. *Adopt the new philosophy.* Commonly accepted levels of nonquality are unacceptable.
3. *Cease dependence on inspection to achieve quality.* Health services should

   require statistical evidence of quality of incoming materials, such as pharmaceuticals, serums, and equipment. Inspection is not the answer. Inspection is too late and is unreliable. Inspection does not produce quality. . . . Require corrective action, where needed, for all tasks that are performed in the

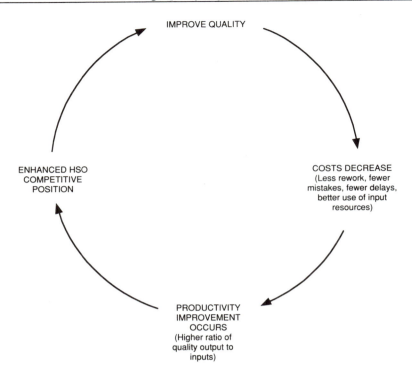

IMPROVE QUALITY

COSTS DECREASE
(Less rework, fewer
mistakes, fewer delays,
better use of input
resources)

PRODUCTIVITY
IMPROVEMENT
OCCURS
(Higher ratio of
quality output to
inputs)

ENHANCED HSO
COMPETITIVE
POSITION

Figure 11.3.   Deming chain reaction (quality, cost, PI, competitive position). (Modified from Deming, W. Edwards. *Out of the crisis.* Boston: Massachusetts Institute of Technology, 1986; and James, Brent C. *Quality management for health care delivery—Quality Measurement and Management Project.* Chicago: The Hospital Research and Educational Trust, 1989.)

hospital or other facility, ranging all the way from bills that are produced to processes of registration. Institute a rigid program of feedback from patients in regard to their satisfaction with services.[51]

4. *End the practice of awarding business on the basis of price tag.* The intent is to develop long-term relations with suppliers so that they can improve the quality of the products (and services) they provide as an input to the HSO.

5. *Improve constantly and forever the system of production and service, to improve quality and productivity, and thus constantly decrease costs.* Improvement is not a one-time effort. Management is obligated to continually look for ways to reduce waste and improve quality.

6. *Institute training on the job.* Too often, workers learn their jobs from other workers who were never trained properly. They cannot do their jobs well because no one tells them how.

7. *Institute leadership.* A supervisor's job is not to tell people what to do or to punish them, but to lead.

Supervisors need time to help people on the job. Supervisors need to find ways to translate the constancy of purpose to the individual employee. Supervisors must be trained in simple statistical methods for aid to employees, with the aim to detect and eliminate special causes of mistakes and rework.[52]

8. *Drive out fear, so that everyone may work effectively for the company.* Many workers are afraid to take a position or ask questions even when they do not understand the job, or what is right or wrong.

We must break down the class distinctions between types of workers within the organization—physicians, nonphysicians, clinical providers versus nonclinical providers, physician to physician. . . . Cease to blame employees for problems of the system. Management should be held responsible for faults of the system. People need to feel secure to make suggestions.[53]

9. *Break down barriers between departments.* Often areas compete with one another or have conflicting goals. They do not work as a team to solve or foresee problems. Worse, one department's goals may cause trouble for another department.

10. *Eliminate slogans, exhortations, and targets for the workforce asking for zero defects and new levels of productivity.* "Instead, display accomplishments of the management in respect to assistance to employees to improve their performance."[54]

11. *Eliminate work standards (quotas) on the factory floor.* Quotas that represent measured day work or output alone without regard to quality should be eliminated. "It is better to take aim at rework, error, and defects [all measures of quality], and to focus on help to people to do a better job."[55]

12. *Remove barriers that rob the hourly worker of the right to pride of workmanship.* People are eager to do a good job and distressed when they cannot. Too often, misguided supervisors, faulty equipment, and defective materials stand in the way. These barriers must be removed.

13. *Institute a vigorous program of education and self-improvement.* "Institute a massive training program in statistical techniques. Bring statistical techniques down to the level of the individual employee's job, and help him to gather information in a systematic way about the nature of his job."[56] Also, the training "program should keep up with changes in model, style, materials, methods, and if advantageous, new machinery."[57]

14. *Put everyone in the company to work to accomplish the transformation.* As observed by Darr, "taking action to accomplish the transformation . . . will take a special top management team with a plan of action to carry out the quality mission. Workers can't do it on their own, nor can managers."[58]

Joseph M. Juran

Joseph M. Juran, consultant and head of the Juran Institute, is a leading advocate of total quality management (TQM). He defines quality as fitness for use, which includes freedom from deficiencies and meeting customer needs.[59] "Juran has developed the 'Quality Trilogy' as a universal way of thinking about quality that fits all functions, levels, and product lines."[60] The quality trilogy involves three activities: quality planning, quality control, and quality improvement.

Quality Planning. This is the activity of developing the products and services required to meet customers' needs. It involves a series of universal steps essentially as follows:

1. Determine who the customers are.
2. Determine the needs of customers.
3. Develop product features that respond to customers' needs.
4. Develop the processes that are able to produce those product features.
5. Transfer the resulting plans to the operating forces.

Quality Control. This process consists of the following steps:

1. Evaluate actual quality performance.
2. Compare actual performance to quality goals.
3. Act on the differences.

Quality Improvement. This process is a means of raising quality performance to unprecedented levels ("breakthrough"). The methodology consists of a series of universal steps:

1. Establish the infrastructure needed to secure annual quality improvement.
2. Identify the specific needs for improvement—the improvement *projects.*
3. For each project, establish a project team with clear responsibility for bringing the project to a successful conclusion.
4. Provide the resources, motivation, and training needed by teams to—diagnose the causes, stimulate establishment of a remedy, (and) establish controls to hold the gains.[61]

Juran, like Crosby, argues that there is a cost to nonquality, including reworking of defective products, scrap, liability from lawsuits, and lost sales from previously dissatisfied customers or customers who purchase competitors' products or services because of their better quality.[62]

The relationship of the parts of the trilogy is presented in Figure 11.4. Juran describes it as follows:

> The Juran Trilogy diagram is a graph with time on the horizontal axis and cost of poor quality (quality deficiencies) on the vertical axis. The initial activity is quality planning. The planners determine who are the customers and what are their needs. The planners then develop product and process designs that are able to respond to those needs. Finally, the planners turn the plans over to the operating forces.
>
> The job of the operating forces is to run the processes and produce the products. As operations proceed it soon emerges that the process is unable to produce 100 percent good work. [Figure 11.4] shows that 20 percent of the work must be redone as a result of quality deficiencies. This waste then becomes chronic because *the operating process was designed that way.*
>
> Under conventional responsibility patterns, operating forces are unable to get rid of that planned chronic waste. What they do instead is carry out *quality control*—to prevent things from getting worse. Control includes putting out the fires, such as that sporadic spike.
>
> The chart also shows that in due course the chronic waste is driven down to a level far below the level that was planned originally. That gain is achieved by the third process of the trilogy: quality improvement. In effect, it is realized that chronic waste is also an opportunity for improvement. So steps are taken to seize that opportunity.[63]

Juran advocates quality improvement (QI), the third step in the trilogy, as a way to improve an existing process (redesigned, if necessary) so that the "original zone" of quality control and the chronic waste associated with it can be reduced below the (original) existing level. This is represented in Figure 11.4 by the "new zone" of quality control. Juran views QI as seeking and finding opportunities for improvement that result in achieving the new zone. In his earlier writings, Juran called this the "breakthrough" zone consisting of a new and better level of performance and qual-

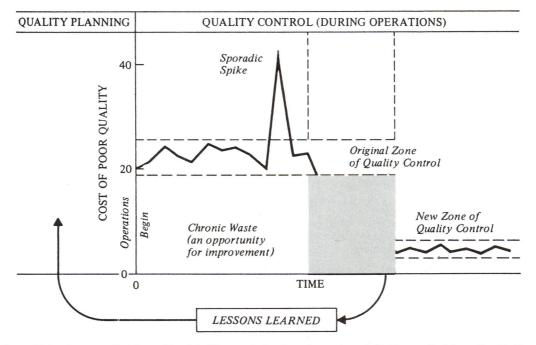

Figure 11.4. Juran quality trilogy. (Reprinted by permission from Juran, Joseph M. The quality trilogy. *Quality Progress*, 19:8, August 1986, p. 20.)

ity. A breakthrough necessitates accepting the premise that current performance is not good enough and can be improved, as well as a change in attitude about quality that becomes part of the organizational culture.[64] In Crosby's terms it involves attaining and surpassing the enlightenment stage of organization maturity and moving to the certainty stage.

Philip B. Crosby

Crosby, a former vice president of ITT and consultant to many industrial organizations, states that "Quality is free. It's not a gift, but it is free. What costs money are the unquality things—all the actions that involve not doing jobs right the first time."[65] Crosby views quality as "conformance to requirements," and he states to "satisfy the customer first, last, and always."[66] Sahney and Warden profile Crosby and his basic principles as follows:

> Crosby strongly advocates a system of quality improvement that focuses on prevention rather than appraisal. Prevention involves careful understanding of the process and identification of problem areas, followed by improvement of the process.
>
> Crosby strongly advocates the ultimate goal of quality as "Zero Defects" and that a company should constantly strive to achieve this goal. He believes that the best measure of quality is "cost of quality" and that this cost can be divided into two components: the price of nonconformance, and the price of conformance. The price of nonconformance includes the cost of internal failures (i.e., the cost of reinspection, retesting, scrap, rework, repairs, and lost production) and external failures (i.e., legal services, liability, damage claims, replacement, and lost customers). Crosby estimates that an organization's cost of nonconformance can be as high as 25 to 30 percent of operating costs. The price of conformance, on the other hand, includes the cost of education, training, and prevention as well as costs of inspection and testing. An organization must minimize the sum of both costs. The focus on process improvement, error-cause removal, employee training, management leadership, and worker awareness of quality problems are all important tenets.[67]

Crosby also emphasizes that organizations should recognize the hidden costs of poor quality. In health services, malpractice is one such cost. Figure 11.5 uses an iceberg model to present examples of the visible and hidden costs of poor quality for an HSO. Crosby's ultimate goal of "do it right the first time" and the derivative concept of "zero defects"* are just that—ultimate goals, which may never be attained but which give direction for the organization with regard to quality.[68] To move in this direction the HSO must go through a maturing process with respect to a philosophy about quality and then use Crosby's 14 steps of QI.

Crosby's organization maturity model includes the stages of uncertainty, awakening, enlightenment, wisdom, and certainty.[69] Enlightenment is the stage in which management's understanding and attitude about QI are heightened and management is supportive of and accepts QI; problems are faced openly and resolved in an orderly manner; and there is implementation of the 14-step approach to quality. Crosby states that in the last stage, certainty, CQI is ingrained in the organization's culture.

Crosby's 14 steps of QI are not necessarily consecutive; in fact, many are parallel:[70]

1. Management commitment to and involvement in quality
2. Use of QI teams composed of persons with process knowledge and a commitment to action
3. Quality measurement so that areas for improvement can be identified and action taken
4. Measuring the cost of quality—meaning the cost of nonquality
5. Quality awareness by all organization members

---

*The industrial concept of zero defects means conformance to standards or specifications. For example, size is allowed to vary by plus or minus 3 millimeters. "Zero defects" does not mean the product is perfect, although "zero defects" has been used in industry as a slogan—an exhortation directed at workers. Deming opposes setting specifications except as general guides. He argues that efforts to seek perfection are thwarted if the goal is only to meet specifications. Deming's point 10 expresses his opposition to slogans. In his judgment, management has been unwilling to accept blame for poor processes and, instead, blamed the workers, an attitude that caused management to substitute slogans for process improvement. Deming believes slogans alone only cause worker anger and frustration.

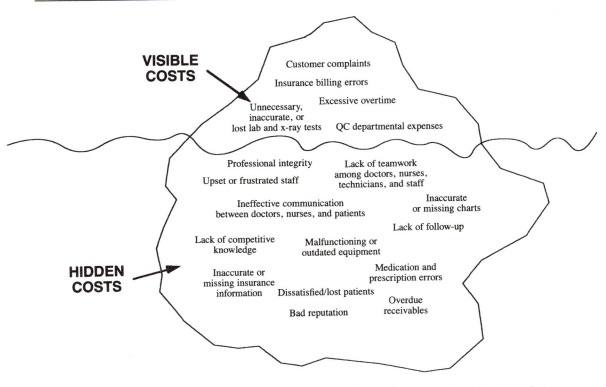

Figure 11.5. Visible and hidden costs of poor quality. (Reprinted with permission from Carol Greebler, TQM Plus. San Diego, CA [1989].)

6. Corrective actions—seek opportunities for improvement
7. Zero defects planning—striving to "do it right the first time"
8. Employee education with formal orientation at all levels of management (and employees) about the 14 steps
9. Zero Defect Day, which is management's demonstration of its commitment to quality
10. Goal setting—the ultimate is zero defects, but "intermediate goals move in that direction"
11. Error-causal removal, in which persons describe problems that prevent error-free work
12. Recognition of those who meet their goals
13. Quality councils composed of quality professionals assisting others in QI
14. Do it all (steps 1 through 13) over again

Crosby states that his 14-step program is "a systematic way of guaranteeing that organized activities happen the way they are planned."[71] It results in doing the right things the right way and doing them right the first time.

STATISTICAL CONTROL

Deming and Juran believe that poor quality is overwhelmingly caused by processes rather than by workers. They emphasize the use of statistical methods for quality control and to identify process variation.[72] Deming is especially vocal in support of his contention that most poor quality results from variation. He defines variation "in statistical control as performance within three standard deviations of the mean—a generous amount of variation, although management can set more stringent limits."[73] Variation within these limits is common variation and results from the process itself. "Variation beyond these limits is called special variation and can be either positive or negative. Causes of negative special variation must be identified and corrected immediately."[74] Examples are staffing shortages in nursing service, malfunctioning or broken equipment, or delays in service due to an unanticipated surge in arrivals in the emergency department—which may indicate a capacity problem. Special variation for Juran is the "sporadic spike" where a process is not "in control." Deming and Juran believe that once processes are in control they can be improved. In Juran's terminology, this is moving to the "new zone of quality control." In Deming's, it is improving the process by decreasing common variation around the mean. For Crosby, it is moving through the organizational maturity stages toward certainty and striving for the goal of "do it right the first time."

Deming uses control charts to determine if a process is in control. The applications of such charts are numerous and can range from analyzing customer waiting time in the admitting office or units of output from a laboratory to monitoring equipment and capacity utilization. Figure 11.6 is a control chart of average patient waiting time from arrival to the start of service in the admitting office. The mean waiting time is four minutes with an upper control limit (UCL) of eight minutes. The lower control limit (LCL) is zero—no patient on a given day waited for service. Common variation is between the UCL and LCL. Average patient waiting time for this set of observations exceeded the UCL on days 5 and 10. Deming advocates finding the reason for this special cause variation. Perhaps a computer was down or a new, untrained employee was on duty. Once found, the special cause variation is corrected.

Because it will do most to improve quality, the more important focus must be reducing common variation in a process that is in statistical control. Deming avers that all processes can be improved and that initiatives to lower the UCL to UCL' (prime) (see Figure 11.6) will result in higher quality (greater customer satisfaction) as well as PI. In Juran's terminology this is moving to the new zone of quality control. In Crosby's terminology this is moving toward the goal of zero defects.

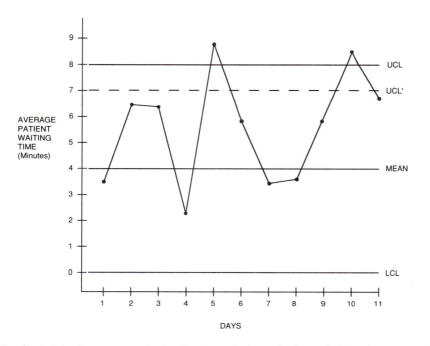

Figure 11.6.   Control chart—average patient waiting time prior to service in an admitting department. UCL and LCL are ±3 standard deviations from the mean.

PROCESS IMPROVEMENT—TWO MODELS, SAME RESULTS

CQI uses statistical techniques such as control charts to understand a process. As monitoring continues, changes are made to proactively improve the process. Two similar CQI process improvement models are presented. The first was developed by the Hospital Corporation of America. The second resulted from the Hospital Research and Educational Trust Quality Measurement and Management Project (QMMP) as part of a 3-year undertaking supported by 15 hospital systems and alliances.[75]

The Hospital Corporation of America's FOCUS-PDCA process improvement model is shown in Figure 11.7. Table 11.1 is a detailed description of the FOCUS and the Plan-Do-Check-Act (PDCA) cycle.* Data collection is important throughout to monitor and evaluate, to determine if an opportunity for improvement is present, to clarify the current understanding of and knowledge about the process under investigation, and to uncover causes of variation.

The Hospital Research and Educational Trust QMMP model for process improvement has steps like those in Figure 11.7. They are:

1. Find a process that needs improvement.
2. Assemble a team that knows the process. Generally those who understand it best are the employees involved in it. "Through its members, the team must also have an understanding of continuous quality improvement principles, statistical quality control, the use of data management systems, and access to management so that organizational roadblocks to improvement can be overcome."[76]
3. Identify customers and process outputs and measure customer expectations regarding outputs. Different processes have different outputs and "the team's first task is therefore to list the outputs of the process, identify its customers, and measure expectations of outputs."[77] Customers may be patients, external stakeholders, or an internal downstream process.
4. Document the process.

   A process consists of a series of steps that convert inputs to outputs. They are usually hierarchical; that is, the main process may be broken down into subprocesses, each with subinputs and suboutputs. The hierarchical chain may be followed to that level of detail necessary to understand the process.[78]

5. Generate output and process specifications. "A specification is an explicit, measurable, statement regarding an important attribute of an output (a customer expectation) or the (sub)process that produces it."[79]
6. Eliminate inappropriate variation (Implement).
7. Document continuous improvement (Innovate).

   The team can select those ideas that seem most promising and then apply them on a test basis within their process. . . . The proposed change can then be discarded, implemented, or modified and tried again, based on the results of the test.[80]

Understanding and Measuring a Process

The first step in process improvement in both the FOCUS-PDCA and the QMMP models is to select a process to improve. People with process knowledge are critical to understanding and documenting the process. Flowcharts are used to describe it. It is only after the process is understood that data about process variables can be collected to determine if the process is in control. If the process is not in control, it must be brought into control, which means eliminating special cause variation. Once a process is in control, process variables can be measured and decisions can be made as to where changes should be made. Data collection is continued so the effects of changes can be measured.

---

*The technical name is the Shewhart cycle, for Walter Shewhart, who developed it. Because of Dr. Deming's work it is known as the Deming cycle in Japan.

Table 11.1. What to look for on a FOCUS-PDCA storyboard

F(ind)
- Who is the customer?
- What is the name of the process?
- What are the process boundaries?
- Is the opportunity statement there? Is it clear?
- Who will benefit from the improvement?
- How is the process tied to the hospital as a system and its priorities?

O(rganize)
- How big is the team?
- Do the members represent people who work in the process or did the "organizational chart" show up?
- Does the team's knowledge of the process align with the boundaries in the opportunity statement?

C(larify)
- Is the process presented at a level of detail that identifies possible causes of variation?
- Is there evidence of agreement on a best method as represented by a single flow diagram?
- Do the boundaries of the flow diagram align with the opportunity statement and the team?
- Were there quick and easy improvements made in the "C" phase using PDCA? Did the team defer any improvements to the "S" phase?
- Is there evidence that the "actual" flow of the process was documented rather than some perceived flow?

U(nderstand)
- How did the team identify the key quality characteristic (KQC) and potential key process variables (KPVs)?
- Is there an operational definition for the KQC and the potential KPV?
- Is there a data collection plan? Is it clear how the data will be collected? Who will collect them?
- Does the team understand how long it will take to collect enough data to make a decision?
- How does the performance of the process vary over time?
- Can the team show a relationship between the KQC and the KPV?

S(elect)
- How did the team select the opportunity for improvement?
- Are there any data or other evidence to support the selection?
- What were the criteria for making the decision?

Roadmap
- Does the roadmap indicate key actions that the team is likely to take?
- What is the time frame?
- Is the team on track?
- Is there evidence of updating or reviewing the roadmap?
- Where is the team on the roadmap?

P(lan)
- Does the team have a plan for piloting the improvement and collecting data?
- Does the pilot plan indicate dates, communications, and ownership of specific steps?
- What training was necessary?

D(o)
- How was the plan executed?
- Did any contingencies arise?
- Were dates on the data collection plan met?

C(heck)
- Do the data on the run chart suggest that the process changed?
- How did the data change?
- Does the team know anything that helps explain any evident change?
- Is the team comfortable that enough data are present to support an action?
- If the team is not comfortable with the amount of data or the knowledge provided by the data, what is the plan for obtaining more?

A(ct)
- Did the team act to implement the process gain beyond the pilot?
- Did the team act to generalize the lessons learned from the pilot? Or did the team act to discard the planned improvement?
- Can the team find another opportunity for improvement within this process?
- What did the team learn from the effort?

Figure 11.2 shows that monitoring and evaluation are crucial elements of process improvement. There are many formal sources, such as reports, data from control charts, and customer questionnaires, as well as informal sources (i.e., complaints) from which information can be obtained. These data must be organized so they become information usable for decision making. Two examples of such organization are helpful.

Pareto analysis is a way to prioritize—to separate the "important few" from the "trivial many."[81] The principle is that 80% of defects, errors, volume, or whatever is being measured are caused by 20% of the variables or process factors. The 80/20 rule in marketing is an application of the Pareto principle. That is, 80% of sales are derived from 20% of a firm's products. In a hospi-

FOCUS-PDCA

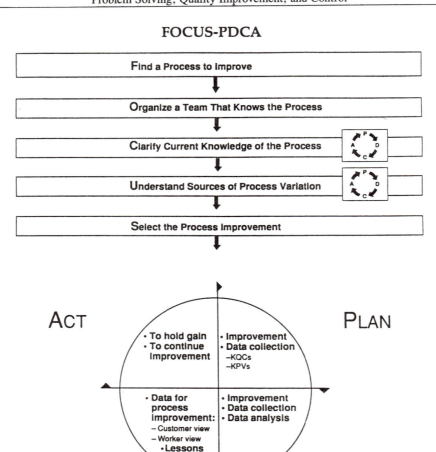

Figure 11.7. Process improvement model. *KQCs,* key quality characteristics; *KPVs,* key process variables. (From Hospital Corporation of America, Nashville, TN; reprinted by permission. FOCUS-PDCA is a registered servicemark of Hospital Corporation of America.)

tal, Pareto analysis would indicate that 80% of operative case delays are caused by 20% of surgeons.[82] The 80/20 ratio is not fixed or magical; instead, it is the notion of understanding relationships that is important. A Pareto diagram is a useful tool in understanding what is happening in a process and for prioritizing, because it shows the relative importance of elements in a process that contribute to a result. Figure 11.8 is an example of a Pareto diagram. It shows that physicians' untimed routine orders and discharge orders are the two areas in which greatest improvement can occur, and attention should be focused there.

Figure 11.9 is a second way to display data. Scatter diagrams depict the relationship between two variables. Here, the relationship is that between number of operations per year (x axis) and percentage mortality (quality) for coronary artery bypass graft operations (y axis). The data suggest a decline in mortality as the number of operations increases, perhaps as a result of a learning or experience curve.

The statistical technique of least squares linear regression can be applied to scatter diagram plots to show a "best fit line" as well as UCLs and LCLs, which are set by some number of positive and negative standard deviations, respectively, from the best fit line. If three standard deviations

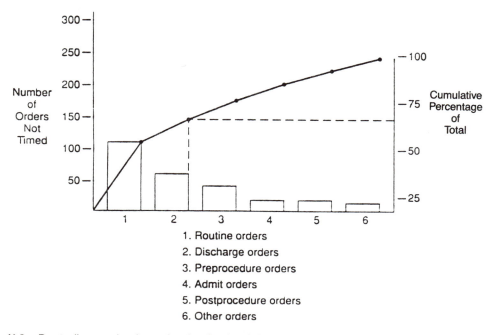

Figure 11.8. Pareto diagram showing rank order of untimed physicians' orders in a major hospital. This diagram ranks classes of orders that failed to be timed with a plot line showing that the correction of the first two classes of orders would lead to a greater than 50% improvement in all untimed orders. (From Re, Richard N., and Marie A. Krousel-Wood. How to use continuous quality improvement theory and statistical quality control tools in a multispecialty clinic. *Quality Review Bulletin* 16 [November 1990]: 394. Copyright 1990 by the Joint Commission on Accreditation of Healthcare Organizations, Oakbrook Terrace, IL; reprinted by permission.)

are used, there is 99.74% confidence that an outlying plot is not due to chance. Figure 11.9 indicates that the single outlying plot above the UCL and the two below the LCL would be, in Deming's terms, special variation, and in Juran's terms, a sporadic spike. All three outliers are of interest. The one above the UCL would be investigated to determine why the undesirable result occurred so it might be prevented in the future. Those below the LCL would be investigated to understand the reasons for the good results and to learn, for example, whether a surgical team was doing something that could be replicated by other teams. Deviation of the outliers may result from input differences such as the skill and training of surgical teams or the acuity of the patient, or from the process—the way the surgery was performed and techniques used.

At a macro level, systematic data collection provides information that allows priorities to be set about which processes to improve. At a process improvement level—a more micro level—data enable the quality improvement team to understand variables in a process, a requisite to improvement.

Improvement and Problem Solving

Process improvement requires problem solving[83] and uses the steps in the problem-solving model presented in Chapter 10 (see Figure 10.4). Conditions that initiate problem solving are deviation (actual results are inconsistent with desired results), crisis, opportunity or threat, and improvement (see Figure 10.3 in Chapter 10). Problem solving under the condition of improvement, as under the other conditions, involves: 1) problem analysis, 2) making assumptions, 3) identifying tentative alternatives, 4) evaluating alternatives by comparing them to decision criteria, 5) selecting the alternative that best fits the criteria, and 6) implementation. Results of the change are compared with desired results.

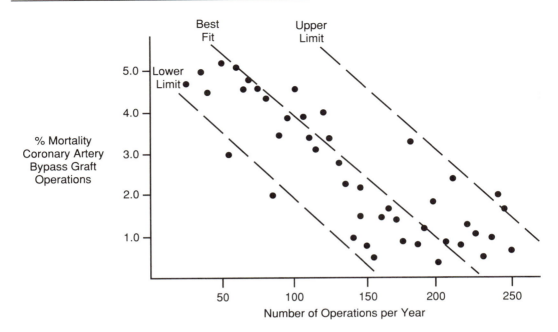

Figure 11.9. Scatter diagram used to determine a possible relationship between two variables: the mortality rate for a surgical procedure and the number of times the procedure is performed during a 12-month period. Each dot represents one surgical team. (From Merry, Martin D. Total quality management for physicians: Translating the new paradigm. *Quality Review Bulletin* 16 [March 1990]: 103. Copyright 1990 by the Joint Commission on Accreditation of Healthcare Organizations, Oakbrook Terrace, IL, reprinted by permission.)

The steps of process improvement in Figure 11.7 and the PDCA cycle are similar to problem solving. CQI also involves problem solving under the condition of deviation when outliers are investigated, for example. However, CQI is primarily concerned with improving processes—proactively seeking opportunities for improvement. In applying the problem-solving model to seeking opportunities for improvement, the situation analysis step is different. It involves collecting and evaluating information not in terms of recognizing or defining a problem (as under the condition of deviation), but in terms of recognizing and defining opportunities to improve a process that is in control—that is, to make the acceptable better. Improvement problem solving for Deming is reducing common variation; for Juran, it is moving a process to the new zone of quality control; and for Crosby, it is moving toward the goal of doing it right the first time.

The Improvement Team

The discussion of the "assumptions step" in problem solving in Chapter 10 states that narrow, restrictive structural and personal assumptions and assumptions about the problem itself result in lower quality solutions. This occurs because assumptions narrow the range of alternatives that is considered. The same issue arises in process improvement. Organizing for improvement means assembling persons with process knowledge. This necessitates large-scale worker involvement because workers are most knowledgeable about the process.[84] The advantages of group problem solving and quality circles presented in Chapter 10 apply to process improvement. Beyond these advantages, a quality improvement team's (QIT's) members will learn new tasks and become aware of each other's problems. They will be more eager to assist one another in solving problems, team spirit will develop, and motivation and sense of worth will be enhanced.[85]

Commitment by management to provide resources, a participative philosophy, and employee team building[86] are essential. Deming, Juran, and Crosby advocate giving employees authority to act. Others call it empowerment.[87] QITs, sometimes called process improvement teams, permit a systematic dissection of the process being investigated and greater understanding of it. The cause-and-effect diagram presented in Figure 11.10 assists a team in brainstorming and identifying the problems in a process, as well as ways to solve them.

Walton indicates that the cause-and-effect diagram is "also known as the 'fishbone' diagram because of its shape, or the Ishikawa diagram, after its originator Kaoru Ishikawa." These diagrams "are used in brainstorming sessions to examine factors that may influence a given situation. An 'effect' is a desirable or undesirable situation, condition, or event produced by a system of 'causes'."[88] The cause-and-effect diagram in Figure 11.10 shows reasons for laboratory test delays for patients in an emergency department. Primary process variables are represented by the long arrows, and minor process variables relate to each of the primary variables.

A cause-and-effect diagram is a systematic way to identify key process variables. This is critical to a QIT's understanding of a process in which it is believed an opportunity for improvement exists. The QMMP step of "document the process" requires that "fundamental knowledge about it" be gathered. This knowledge "usually resides in front-line workers who deal with the process in a detailed manner on a daily basis."[89] Understanding the process leads to ideas about how it can be improved.

CQI AND PROFESSIONAL AUTONOMY

If CQI is to work, barriers inherent in how HSOs are organized must be overcome. HSOs are unique and differ from industrial organizations because they are a structural blend of administrative and patient care activities in which clinical personnel are accorded significant individual autonomy. Historically, the blended structure created conflict between the two and this conflict can be heightened by moving toward CQI.

McLaughlin and Kaluzny identify sources of conflict that may occur when the traditional autonomy relationship is changed. They use the term "clinical professional model" to describe the traditional HSO and the term "TQM model" to denote an HSO that is implementing CQI. (As used here, TQM is synonymous with CQI and therefore is used in the following discussion.) Potential areas of conflict include:

1. *Responsibility* The clinical professional model places responsibility for performance on the individual; the TQM model puts it on the process.
2. *Leadership* The clinical professional model puts leadership in patient care activities on the professional; the TQM model puts it on management. TQM

   demands that management take a more participative approach. Managers are required to involve clinical professionals in the decision making process, leaving it up to them to solve quality problems as they arise. Yet, while this is a participative program, it is clearly a management initiative.[90]

3. *Autonomy and accountability* The clinical professional model is predicated on the autonomy and accountability of professionals for their own work results. The TQM model "does not, however, respect professional autonomy as much as it respects personal autonomy. At the same time it demands that clinical professionals hold themselves accountable for both outcomes and process performance on a continuing basis."[91]

Other potential conflicts between the clinical professional and TQM (i.e., CQI) models include goal versus performance and process expectations; retrospective versus concurrent performance appraisal; and traditional quality assurance versus continuous improvement. The writers' point relative to the clinical professional is that "this [TQM] approach represents a paradigm shift in health care management and presents a series of potential conflict areas in the way health care organizations are organized."[92]

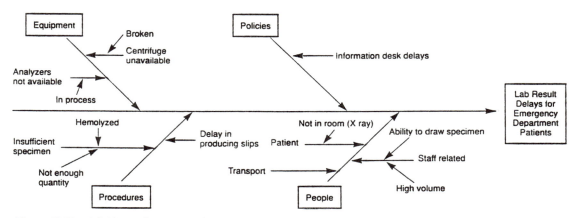

Figure 11.10.   A fishbone diagram examining reasons for delays in laboratory test results for emergency department patients. The fishbone, or cause-and-effect, diagram is drawn after a brainstorming session. The central problem is visualized as the head of the fish, with the skeleton divided into branches showing contributing causes of different parts of the problem. (From Merry, Martin D. Total quality management for physicians: Translating the new paradigm. *Quality Review Bulletin* 16 [March 1990]: 102. Copyright 1990 by the Joint Commission on Accreditation of Healthcare Organizations, Oakbrook Terrace, IL; reprinted by permission.)

As a final point, McLaughlin and Kaluzny make the salient observation that TQM "is a fundamental challenge to the way all professionals think about quality, evaluate and regulate themselves, and protect their professional autonomy."[93] This is especially true for physicians. Physician-writers, however, are enthusiastic about TQM, and it is likely that physicians who understand TQM will embrace it. First, TQM is process oriented rather than person oriented.[94] Second, it seeks to improve the quality of medical outcomes, which is also the objective of medical care.[95] It results in better mobilization of HSO resources to meet the needs of physicians' patients.[96] Third, QITs study processes and outcomes using a scientific method,[97] and physicians should be comfortable with this data-driven, systematic-scientific approach. In his experience, James, a physician and author of the QMMP report, concludes that when TQM (i.e., CQI) "methods and ideas are advanced within the established professional framework for quality improvement, when the hospital supplies the necessary data management and analysis infrastructure, and when physicians are asked to concentrate on clinical products, then physicians adopt TQM easily."[98]

PRODUCTIVITY IMPROVEMENT

Cost (resource use) effectiveness and productivity improvement (PI) result from CQI. Figure 11.2 indicates that process improvement [2] leads to higher quality outputs [3], which leads to PI and better resource use [4], and, thus, enhanced competitive position [5]. The Deming chain reaction in Figure 11.3 shows that improved quality decreases costs, and this results in PI and an enhanced competitive position. CQI and PI are integral. They cannot be separated, nor can input resource costs be separated from output quality. They must be evaluated simultaneously.

Productivity and Productivity Improvement

Productivity is the index of outputs relative to inputs.[99] Alternately, productivity is results achieved relative to resources consumed:[100]

$$\text{Productivity} = \frac{\text{Outputs}}{\text{Inputs}} = \frac{\text{Results achieved}}{\text{Resources consumed}}$$

Productivity is increased by any change that increases the ratio of outputs to inputs, which is achieved by altering either the conversion process (structure, tasks/technology, people) or the inputs. For example, fewer nurses caring for the same number of patients increases productivity: same output, fewer inputs. More radiographic procedures per day with the same personnel and equipment has the same result. However, increasing productivity (output) without maintaining the level of quality *does not* lead to PI. Producing poor-quality radiographs or performing unnecessary radiographic procedures is not PI. PI occurs *only* when the index ratio of outputs to inputs increases and conformance/expectation quality is maintained or enhanced. This is denoted in the following formula:[101]

$$PI = \frac{Outputs}{Inputs} = \frac{Quantity + Quality}{Inputs} = \frac{Results\ achieved}{Resources\ consumed}$$

CQI and Productivity Improvement

Figure 11.11 shows the relationship of the PI triangle to CQI. PI occurs only when lowest reasonable costs (inputs) are consistent with highest possible quality (outputs). The QMMP calls this the "value of health care."[102] Since PI focuses on the relationship of outputs and quality to inputs and costs, both inputs and processes are investigated in PI, as they are in CQI.

HSOs are service organizations with high levels of customer interaction. Most HSOs, but especially hospitals, must have flexible capacity to meet surges in demand.[103] For others, such as nursing facilities, there is little need for flexible capacity, particularly when occupancy is 100%.

CQI focuses on improving processes (see Figure 11.7), which commonly necessitates evaluating inputs. For example, a QIT may determine that a process will be more efficient if better skilled employees are recruited, or if employees are cross-trained so reassignment is more flexible when workloads change. Enhancing technology inputs can improve work systems and substitute equipment for people. Magnetic resonance imaging improves clinical diagnosis, and microcomputers enhance accuracy and productivity in billing and admitting. Other techniques may be used to add efficiency to inputs: increasing the quality of materials and supplies by working closely with suppliers (Deming advocates sole-source suppliers); using a just-in-time inventory system to

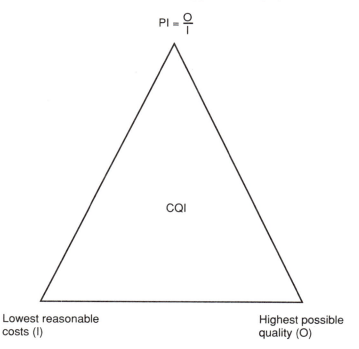

Figure 11.11. Productivity Improvement triangle.

eliminate inventory beyond that needed for safety stock; and using ABC inventory analysis* (similar to Pareto analysis) to indicate which supplies are most expensive and require special attention. Management information systems provide data for control and utilization evaluation, and forecasting enables managers to anticipate demand and alter capacity. Use of work measurement to monitor employee utilization and work loads and information from a patient acuity classification system permit efficient nurse staffing patterns.

Productivity may be improved in numerous ways other than by analyzing inputs. Examination of a process or work system in a CQI framework should ask questions such as: Is what we do really necessary? Are we doing the right things? Can the work be done in another way with the same or improved quality? How are the work results of one job interdependent with other jobs, materials, or processes? Can we improve the process with a different mix of resources that will improve quality, decrease costs, or both? The following sections describe methods to answer these questions: 1) analysis and improvement of work systems and job design, 2) capacity planning and facilities layout, and 3) scheduling and materials handling. Inputs are integral to each of them.

Analysis and Improvement of Work Systems and Job Design

Analysis and improvement of work systems and job design is integral to CQI process improvement and leads to PI. The basic objectives are to find better ways to work in general, improve specific jobs in particular, and increase the ratio of quality relative to costs—with the same, fewer, or a different mix of inputs.

Work systems (i.e., processes) are interrelated and connected jobs that form an integrated whole. Hospitals, for example, have many systems and subsystems: non–patient care systems, such as admitting, discharge, accounts payable, transportation, central services, material distribution, patient food delivery, medication order fulfillment; direct patient care, including nursing service; ancillary services such as laboratory, radiology, and respiratory therapy; and administration. Analysis of a system can be exclusive (how it functions) or inclusive (how it interrelates with other systems); the purpose is to identify ways to improve systems so output quality and productivity are enhanced.

Process and methods analysis are techniques used to evaluate systems.[104] In health services, processes are the series of operations, steps, or activities through which patients, material, or information flow. Documenting flow permits evaluation of the sequence of events[105] and whether altering the flow, combining or eliminating operations, or methods redesign will result in higher quality outputs and PI.[106] One of the first activities of a QIT is to flow diagram the process.

Figure 11.12 is an example of a flow diagram of a process. Understanding the sequence of events in a physician's order will show how the process can be improved—the bottlenecks, delays, or steps that can be eliminated. In processes with high customer interaction, flow analysis will indicate where interactions may be enhanced or lessened, if either results in higher patient satisfaction.

Because HSO work systems are interdependent, multisystem process flow analysis is necessary to identify areas for improvement. For example, timely reading and reporting of test results (radiology, electrocardiogram, electroencephalogram, and laboratory) positively affects patient care and shortens length of stay; delayed reading or reporting negatively affects patient care and increases length of stay. Knowledge about and improvement of system or process output that becomes a downstream customer's input positively affects productivity elsewhere.

Methods analysis involves evaluating how work is done—the specific operations, steps, or activities performed. Such analyses include evaluating the appropriateness of the operations,

---

*In ABC inventory analysis, items are classified into A, B, or C groups based on volume or dollar value. A is high; C is low. The A group should have highest priority.

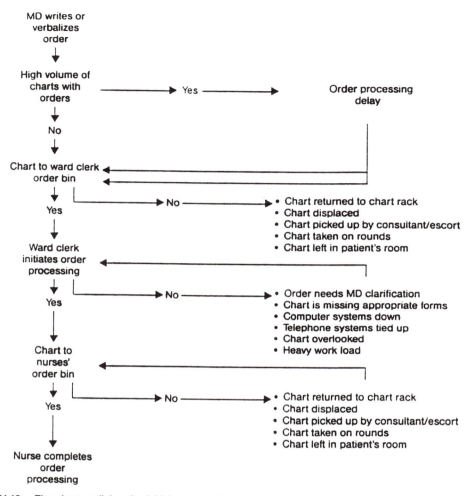

Figure 11.12. Flowchart outlining the initial steps in implementing physicians' orders, clearly identifying points of consumer-producer interchange (e.g., the interaction of physician and ward clerk) and sites of possible system failure or delay. (From Re, Richard N., and Marie A. Krousel-Wood. How to use continuous quality improvement theory and statistical quality control tools in a multispecialty clinic. *Quality Review Bulletin* 16 [November 1990]: 393. Copyright 1990 by the Joint Commission on Accreditation of Healthcare Organizations, Oakbrook Terrace, IL; reprinted by permission.)

steps, or activities; considering alternative inputs, such as personnel and equipment substitution, redesigning jobs; or evaluating information flow and the media used. For example, evaluating how patient orders are processed may show that redesigned, multipart forms with copies for ancillary services, patient accounts, and medical records will decrease the time spent on paperwork (PI) and reduce transcription errors (QI).

At a micro level, job design improvement evaluates the tasks in a job or a cluster of jobs that constitute an operation or activity in a process. Included are the sequence of job tasks, design of physical layout, and people-machine relationships, including equipment, material, and supplies used. Job design improvement or a variant, work simplification, is used to eliminate unnecessary tasks, reduce time between tasks, reallocate tasks among different jobs, combine jobs, or centralize common tasks in one job (i.e., specialization).

Finally, work simplification, which involves dividing work into specific tasks and making it easier, is a way to evaluate and improve jobs and enhance work results. User-friendly, menu-driven microcomputers in the admissions department enable employees to admit patients faster, with greater accuracy—both of which improve quality as well as productivity.

Capacity Planning and Facilities Layout

Facilities analysis is an important dimension of process improvement. It focuses on the physical aspects of a process, the need for flexibility in meeting variable demand, and balancing timeliness of service and idle resources. Facility layout is the arrangement of equipment and work areas. Facilities, process flow, equipment, and work stations may be rearranged to improve sequence and flow, decrease unnecessary worker movement and material transportation, eliminate bottlenecks and congestion, and yield faster patient throughput. Layout analysis can be done by using drawings, proximity charts, templates, or three-dimensional models. Computer simulation can be used to design physical layout of a facility within predetermined constraints and assumptions.

Analysis of traffic patterns and material flows consists of observing and recording movement to decrease travel, eliminate or reduce delays, or substitute alternate material handling or delivery methods. For example, analysis of traffic patterns may reveal that restricting use of certain elevators to patients and employees reduces delays in transporting patients and equipment. Similarly, materials and supplies flow analyses may justify an exchange cart system to improve logistical movement, decrease inventory and staffing, and have patient care supplies and medications at units when needed.

Production Control, Scheduling, and Materials Distribution

Production control in HSOs involves matching workload with capacity through work scheduling, and is applicable to many areas: admitting, operating rooms, diagnostic testing, clinics, physician offices, and outpatient services. Often, production-smoothing techniques are used to spread workload throughout a shift. For example, if all patients were brought to radiology or all outpatients arrived at 9:00 A.M., waiting lines build, staff are overworked, and quality—patient satisfaction—is reduced because of increased waiting time. In the afternoon staff are underutilized. If workload can be spread throughout the day, patient waiting time is minimized and staff are productive during the entire shift. If demand cannot be controlled through scheduling, part-time staff may be used or other adjustments made to meet peak load demands.

Another PI technique is lot sizing, or batching work. Because jobs such as preparing intravenous fluid solutions, sterilizing equipment, preparing meals, and washing laundry require a setup procedure, the economic lot size must be determined. This improves use of people and equipment and decreases setup and down time for workers and equipment. For example, when preparing intravenous solutions, it may be better to prepare many at one time and refrigerate them rather than prepare each one as an order is received. This also smooths workload, since these can be prepared when other work is slack.

Workload balancing through proper scheduling of demand or capacity ensures that staff, equipment, and facilities are used efficiently and customer waiting time is lessened. Many manual and computerized scheduling techniques are available, including short-interval scheduling, multiple activity charts, and work distribution analysis. Another is simulation, which is discussed in Chapter 12.

Timely distribution of materials and supplies is important to downstream processes. Improvement techniques are as simple as using general stores exchange carts to deliver supplies to nursing units. Each day one is filled and the other is used. Once a day they are exchanged. In the operating room, a case cart system may be used. Each surgeon has a list of supplies and equipment needed for each procedure, and, before the start of surgery, the case cart for that procedure is packed and delivered to the operating room. The unit dose distribution system is used to distribute drugs. Medications are purchased individually prepackaged or are packaged in the pharmacy and distributed to nursing units. Each dose of medication is available, as needed by the patient, and the risk of error is reduced.

SUMMARY

This chapter examines the health services paradigm shift with respect to quality. Quality must incorporate the dimension of how well patient and customer expectations are met. The philosophy of continuous quality improvement (CQI) is described and modeled. CQI is defined as an ongoing, organization-wide framework that commits managers and employees to improving quality and involves them in monitoring and evaluating all HSO activities (inputs and processes) and outputs to improve them.

The CQI model presented in Figure 11.2 rests on two pillars: improving output quality and improving processes. Through both, productivity improvement (PI) occurs and the HSO's competitive position is enhanced.

Profiles of three quality experts—W. Edwards Deming, Joseph M. Juran, and Philip B. Crosby—are presented. Included are Deming's 14 points for improved quality and organization transformation, Juran's quality trilogy, and Crosby's 14 steps for quality improvement. The role of statistical quality control is emphasized.

Two process improvement models are presented: the FOCUS-PDCA and the QMMP models. Both are similar and suggest steps to improve processes. CQI and problem solving, the role of quality improvement teams (QITs), and methods that can assist QITs in analyzing processes are discussed. For CQI to be effective, there must be commitment to it by all HSO members. Potential areas of conflict between traditional professional autonomy and CQI are raised.

The subjects of productivity and PI are presented. Productivity is the index of outputs to inputs. PI is a function of the index of results achieved—which includes quantity and quality—relative to resources consumed. The PI triangle (Figure 11.12) presents the relationship between CQI and PI, and indicates that PI occurs only when the highest quality possible (outputs) is attained for the lowest reasonable costs (inputs). Various approaches to PI are presented: analysis and improvement of work systems and job design; capacity planning and facilities layout; and production control, scheduling, and materials distribution.

DISCUSSION QUESTIONS

1. What are some of the important changes that occurred in health services delivery in the 1980s that induced HSOs to adopt the philosophy of CQI in the 1990s?
2. Define CQI. Why is it an organizational philosophy? What are its attributes? How can CQI lead to an enhanced HSO competitive position?
3. Think about nursing service in a hospital. Who or what are its customers? If nursing service is the customer, who or what provides inputs (is the supplier)?
4. Based on the profiles of Deming, Juran, and Crosby, identify the similarities and differences in their approaches to quality.
5. Compare the FOCUS-PDCA and QMMP process improvement models. What are the similarities and differences? How do they relate to the problem solving model in Chapter 10 (Figure 10.4)?
6. Explain how the elements in the PI triangle are related (see Figure 11.11).

CASE STUDY 1:   FED UP IN DALLAS[107]

Dear Ann Landers:

I've done at least $20,000 worth of business with a local printer. I've always paid my bills in installments, some as large as $1,000 a month.

My printer told me my payments were too small and she had to have all her money in one lump from then on. I paid her off and took my printing elsewhere.

I've patronized the same dry cleaner for five years. They know me on sight and have never asked for identification when they cash my checks. Suddenly, they are losing and damaging my clothes and acting as if it's not their fault.

This morning I drove into the service station where I've been a customer for three years. I asked the man to please check the pressure in a low tire. I was told that I'd have to buy gas in order to get full service. When I said, "OK," the attendant continued to gripe and then the owner got into the act. I told them to forget it, that I'd go elsewhere. The attendant replied, "You want me to take the air back out of your tire?" Needless to say, they won't see me again.

I've even had a run-in with a doctor I've been seeing for six years. I walked out of his office after being kept waiting for an hour and a half.

Ann, what's wrong with these people? Why don't they value those of us who keep them in business? In these times of economic hardship, you'd think they would do everything possible to please their customers. Am I wrong to expect a little service and courtesy in exchange for my business?

—Fed Up in Dallas

Questions

1. CQI focuses on improving processes and quality. It is customer oriented. In the letter to Ann Landers, it is evident that "Fed Up in Dallas" is not a satisfied customer. In our society in general, why do you think there is indifference to customers by organizations (and their employees) that provide products and services?
2. Describe instances where you or acquaintances encountered a negative customer orientation by an HSO. What was your (their) reaction?

CASE STUDY 2: THE CARBONDALE CLINIC[108]

The Carbondale Clinic, located in Carbondale, Illinois, is a large group practice of about 30 physicians. The clinic employs about 100 people and serves a regional population of about 100,000. Specialties ranging from pediatrics to psychiatry are offered by the clinic, which also operates its own lab, x-ray room, and outpatient surgical center.

For some years, the clinic has been receiving complaints from its patients that appointment times are not being met. For instance, a patient with an appointment for two o'clock might not get in to see the physician until four o'clock. However, the clinic has felt that such delays are unavoidable due to the uncertainty involved in the time it takes to adequately examine each patient and the possibility of emergency cases that must be inserted into the schedule.

Several criteria are used for scheduling. For instance, many patients are scheduled for annual physical exams. These are usually scheduled at least several weeks in advance because they require coordination of lab facilities and the physician's time. However, some physicians will begin examining a patient and decide that the patient needs a physical immediately. The physicians feel this does not really cause problems because they can send the patient down to the lab while they continue to see other patients.

Some patients also phone the clinic for an appointment when they have nonemergency, routine problems such as a mild fever or sore throat. Such patients are scheduled into available time slots as soon as possible—usually a day or two from the time they call. The objective here is to fit such patients in as quickly as possible without overloading the schedule with more patients than can reasonably be examined in a time period. Usually the plan is to schedule four patients per hour.

However, each day various emergencies occur. These can range from a splinter in the eye to a heart attack, and these cases cannot wait. For an emergency that is not life threatening, the approach is to try to squeeze the person into a time slot that is not too heavily scheduled. However, a case of life or death—such as a heart attack—means that the schedule must be disrupted and the patient treated immediately.

Currently, all scheduling of appointments is done centrally. However, this frequently causes problems because the people making appointments often do not know how long it should take to examine a patient with a particular complaint. On the other hand, the nurses in each department are usually too busy to do the scheduling themselves. Generally, if there is a doubt about whether a patient can be fitted into a time slot, the preference is to go ahead and schedule the patient. This is because the physicians prefer not to have any empty times in their schedules. At times, if it looks as if there might be an available opening, the clinic even calls patients who were originally scheduled for a later time and asks them to come in early.

Questions

1. "For some years, the clinic has been receiving complaints from its patients that appointment times are not being met." Why do you suppose that no action to correct the situation has been taken?
2. As a member of a QIT, you are charged with evaluating the appointment/scheduling process. Are there some "assumptions" in the narrative that you question? If there were sufficient data to prepare a Pareto diagram, what do you think the items would be? Please list them.
3. Draw a cause-and-effect diagram (fishbone chart) of this situation.
4. What recommendations would you make to improve the situation and decrease patient waiting time?

CASE STUDY 3: TOTAL QUALITY MANAGEMENT (TQM) INVENTORY[109]

Continuous Quality Improvement (CQI) and Total Quality Management (TQM) are used interchangeably in the literature. This TQM inventory is an instrument to measure an organization's TQM (or CQI) orientation. It contains three parts, eight criteria questions, a scoring sheet, and an interpretation sheet.

Part 1: TQM Inventory

Instructions: For each of the eight total quality management criteria listed below, circle the statement that best describes the present situation in your organization.

Criterion 1: Top Management Leadership and Support

A. Top managers are directly and actively involved in activities that foster quality.
B. Top managers participate in quality leadership activities.
C. Most top managers support activities that foster quality.
D. Many top managers are supportive of and interested in quality improvement.
E. Some top managers are beginning to tentatively support activities that foster quality.
F. No top management support exists for activities involving quality.

Criterion 2: Strategic Planning

A. Long-term goals for quality improvement have been established across the organization as part of the overall strategic planning process.
B. Long-term goals for quality improvement have been established across most of the organization.
C. Long-term goals for quality improvement have been established in key parts of the organization.
D. Short-term goals for quality improvement have been established in parts of the organization.

   E.   The general goals of the organization contain elements of quality improvement.

   F.   No quality improvement goals have been established anywhere in the organization.

Criterion 3: Focus on the Customer

   A.   A variety of effective and innovative methods is used to obtain customer feedback on all organizational functions.

   B.   Effective systems are used to obtain feedback from all customers of major functions.

   C.   Systems are in place to solicit customer feedback on a regular basis.

   D.   Customer needs are determined through random processes rather than by using systematic methods.

   E.   Complaints are the major methods used to obtain customer feedback.

   F.   No customer focus is evident.

Criterion 4: Employee Training and Recognition

   A.   The organization is implementing a systematic employee training and recognition plan that is fully integrated into the overall strategic quality planning process.

   B.   The organization is assessing the employee training and recognition needed, and the results of that assessment are being evaluated periodically.

   C.   An employee training and recognition plan is beginning to be implemented.

   D.   An employee training and recognition plan is under active development.

   E.   The organization has plans to increase employee training and recognition.

   F.   There is no employee training, and there are no systems for recognizing employees.

Criterion 5: Employee Empowerment and Teamwork

   A.   Innovative, effective employee empowerment and teamwork approaches are used.

   B.   Many natural work groups are empowered to constitute quality improvement teams.

   C.   A majority of managers support employee empowerment and teamwork.

   D.   Many managers support employee empowerment and teamwork.

   E.   Some managers support employee empowerment and teamwork.

   F.   There is no support for employee empowerment and teamwork.

Criterion 6: Quality Measurement and Analysis

   A.   Information about quality and timeliness of all products and services is collected from internal and external customers and from suppliers.

   B.   Information about quality and timeliness is collected from most internal and external customers and from most suppliers.

   C.   Information about quality and timeliness is collected from major internal and external customers and from major suppliers.

   D.   Information about quality and timeliness is collected from some internal and external customers.

   E.   Information about quality and timeliness is collected from one or two external customers.

   F.   There is no system for measuring and analyzing quality.

Criterion 7: Quality Assurance

   A.   All products, services, and processes are designed, reviewed, verified, and controlled to meet the needs and expectations of internal and external customers.

   B.   A majority of products, services, and processes are designed, reviewed, verified, and controlled to meet the needs and expectations of internal and external customers.

C. Key products, services, and processes are designed, reviewed, verified, and controlled to meet the needs and expectations of internal and external customers.

D. A few products and services are designed, reviewed, and controlled to meet the needs of internal and external customers.

E. Products and services are controlled to meet internally developed specifications that may or may not include customer input.

F. There is no quality assurance in this organization.

Criterion 8: Quality and Productivity Improvement Results

A. Most significant performance indicators demonstrate exceptional improvement in quality and productivity over the past 5 years.

B. Most significant performance indicators demonstrate excellent improvement in quality and productivity over the past 5 years.

C. Most significant performance indicators demonstrate good improvement in quality and productivity.

D. Most significant performance indicators demonstrate improving quality and productivity in several areas.

E. There is evidence of some quality and productivity improvement in one or more areas.

F. There is no evidence of quality and productivity improvement in any area.

Part 2: Total Quality Management (TQM) Inventory Scoring Sheet

To determine your scores on the inventory, complete the following three steps:

1. For each of the *Total Quality Management Criteria* listed in the left column, find the letter under the heading labeled *Response Categories/Points* that corresponds to the one you chose on the questionnaire.

2. Then circle the one- or two-digit *Point* number that corresponds to the letter you chose.

3. Finally, add up the points circled for all eight criteria to determine your *Overall Score*.

Note: The numbers you are about to circle correspond to the relative weights attached to individual Quality/Productivity Criteria in the President's Award.* Therefore, in addition to helping to score your responses, the points also identify the categories that are more significant than others. For example, scores on Criterion 8 (Quality and Productivity Improvement Results) are better indicators of an organization's orientation toward quality and productivity than are its scores on Criterion 4 (Employee Training and Recognition).

Total Quality Management Criteria	Response Categories/Points					
	A	B	C	D	E	F
1. Top Management Leadership and Support	20	16	12	8	4	0
2. Strategic Planning	15	12	9	6	3	0
3. Focus on the Customer	40	32	24	16	8	0
4. Employee Training and Recognition	15	12	9	6	3	0
5. Employee Empowerment and Teamwork	15	12	9	6	3	0
6. Quality Measurement and Analysis	15	12	9	6	3	0
7. Quality Assurance	30	24	18	12	6	0
8. Quality and Productivity Improvement Results	50	40	30	20	10	0
Scores for Choice Categories:	___	___	___	___	___	___
Overall Score:	___ (Range: 0–200)					

*This instrument is based on the Federal Quality Institute's *Federal Total Quality Management Handbook 2: Criteria and Scoring Guidelines for the President's Award for Quality and Productivity Improvement,* Washington D.C.: Office of Personnel Management, 1990.

Part 3: Total Quality Management (TQM) Inventory Interpretation Sheet

160–200 points: An overall score in this range indicates a "world-class" organization with a deep long-term and active commitment to improving quality and productivity. At this level, goals should focus on the challenge of maintaining gains as well as seeking ways to attain even higher levels of quality and productivity.

120–159 points: An overall score in this range indicates that an organization with a sound, well-organized philosophy of quality and productivity improvement is beginning to emerge. At this level, goals should focus on fully implementing a sound TQM effort while continuing to build on current levels of excellence.

80–119 points: An overall score in this range indicates an organization that is starting to learn about and plan quality and productivity improvements. At this level, goals should focus on moving from the planning stages to actually implementing a TQM effort in order to gain the necessary hands-on experience.

40–79 points: An overall score in this range indicates an organization that is vaguely aware of quality and productivity improvement but has no plans to learn about or implement such activity. Scores at this level approach the danger point; if long-term organizational viability is sought, progress must be made quickly. Goals should focus on strongly encouraging top managers to learn more about TQM while re-examining their assumptions about possible contributions that the process can make to the health of their organization.

0–39 points: An overall score in this range indicates an organization that currently has neither an awareness of nor an involvement with quality- and productivity-improvement programs. Unless an organization has an absolute, invulnerable monopoly on extremely valuable products or services, this level represents a de facto decision to go out of business. Goals should focus on an emergency turnaround. Learning about total quality management must occur at an accelerated rate, and plans to bring quality and productivity consciousness to the organization must be implemented immediately.

CASE STUDY 4: NONINVASIVE CARDIOVASCULAR LABORATORY (REVISED)

The associate vice president for operations at Barbarosa Hospital had a problem concerning the noninvasive cardiovascular laboratory (NCVL). First, patients were complaining to their physicians about long waits and interruptions during tests. Second, the NCVL technician was complaining about being overworked. After observing the technician and talking with him and his supervisor, the following information was obtained.

The NCVL is located on the third floor of the hospital. It is adjacent to the stress test laboratory, which has twice the space of the noninvasive lab but uses only half of it. Also, the stress technician is productive only 60% of the time. Loren Findley is the only technician assigned to the NCVL. Findley's work space is cramped and crowded with two patient beds, a very large desk, and supplies in stacked boxes. The equipment layout in the room does not permit easy movement and some of it must be placed in the hall. Consequently, Findley spends an average of 10 minutes moving equipment in or out of the room when setting up for a test different from the preceding one.

Findley is qualified to administer the following three tests:

1. ECHOs. An echocardiogram (ECHO) is a graphic recording generated by ultrasound that is used for studying the structures and motions of the heart.
2. OPGs. An ocular plethysmograph (OPG) is a test that measures the change in size and volume of the eye.
3. PVRs. A pulse volume recording (PVR) plethysmograph is a test to measure changes in volume of a cross section of a blood vessel over several heartbeats.

Findley schedules the inpatient and outpatient tests ordered by house staff and attending physicians. Frequent phone calls to schedule tests are received throughout the day. On average, three of four tests Findley administers are interrupted by phone calls. It takes 10 minutes to return to the point before the interruption (2 minutes talking on the phone, and 8 minutes to restart the test).

From extensive observation, the following standard times for each of these tests were determined (assume there is no standard time difference for inpatients and outpatients):

Test	Standard time
ECHO	1 hour
OPG	½ hour
PVR	½ hour

With the expansion of the professional staff organization at the beginning of the year the number of tests ordered increased. Findley complained to his supervisor about being overworked and being unable to keep up with the workload. He stated that he wanted a full-time assistant or he might quit. The hospital has no other employees who could perform the tests even though they are not difficult to learn. Findley could train someone to perform the tests in about 2 months.

Hospital records were used to determine the number of tests performed during the previous year, and these data were compared with the number of tests performed in the first 3 months of this year:

	Number performed		
		This year	
Test	Previous year	First 3 months	Annualized
ECHO	800	300	1,200
OPG	200	75	300
PVR	200	75	300

The typical pattern for scheduled tests on any given day is: ECHO, ECHO, OPG, ECHO, ECHO, PVR, ECHO, ECHO, OPG, ECHO, ECHO, PVR.

Questions

1. Is Findley overworked? Why or why not? Should another technician be hired?
2. Assume that the addition of a new technician is not considered a viable alternative. How can the present NCVL process be changed to improve quality and productivity?

CASE STUDY 5: THE CLINIC LAYOUT

A physician group practice is planning to open a free-standing ambulatory center to treat minor emergencies. They developed two facility layout plans. It is expected that two physicians will be on duty at a time.

Plan A calls for fully equipped patient care areas; therefore, the patient is kept in one location for the entire visit. This necessitates a team approach to treating the patient.

Plan A Layout

Six examination rooms with supplies stocked totally in the rooms (three rooms assigned to each physician)

Two portable X-ray machines (one for each physician)
One laboratory
One storage room
Two nurses (one works with each physician)

Plan B takes a different approach. In it, work stations (e.g., X-ray and holding room) are used to process patients. The jobs are more specialized; it was thought that this arrangement might be more efficient.

Plan B Layout

Four examination rooms
One X-ray room
One recovery (holding) room
One laboratory
One central supply room
Two float nurses

You have been asked to recommend Plan A or Plan B.

Questions

1. What criteria—primary considerations—should be used when evaluating the layout plans?
2. Which plan do you recommend? Why?
3. Should other information be available? If so, what?

NOTES

1. James, Brent C. *Quality management for health care delivery—Quality Measurement and Management Project*, 7. Chicago: The Hospital Research and Educational Trust, 1989.
2. Laffel, Glenn, and David Blumenthal. The case for using industrial management science in health care organizations. *Journal of the American Medical Association* 262 (November 24,1989): 2870; Merry, Martin D. Total quality management for physicians: Translating the new paradigm. *Quality Review Bulletin* 16 (March 1990): 104; McLaughlin, Curtis P., and Arnold D. Kaluzny. Total quality management in health: Making it work. *Health Care Management Review* 15 (Summer 1990): 7.
3. American Hospital Association. *Quality Management: A management advisory*, 1. Chicago: American Management Association, 1990; James, *Quality management*, 10; Laffel and Blumenthal, Case for using, 2870; O'Connor, Stephen J. Service quality: Understanding and implementing the concept in the clinical laboratory. *Clinical Laboratory Management Review* 3 (November/ December 1989): 330; Schumacher, Dale N. Organizing for quality competition: The coming paradigm shift. *Frontiers of Health Services Management* 5 (Summer 1989): 113. For a useful model of quality, see Lanning, Joyce A., and Stephen J. O'Connor. The health care quality quagmire: Some signposts. *Hospital & Health Services Administration* 35 (Spring 1990): 42.
4. Deming, W. Edwards. *Out of the Crisis*, 18. Boston: Massachusetts Institute of Technology, 1986.
5. Milakovich, Michael E. Creating a total quality health care environment. *Health Care Management Review* 16 (Spring 1991): 9.
6. Casurella, Joe. Managing a "total quality" program.

Federation of American Health Systems Review 22 (July/ August 1989): 31.
7. James, *Quality Management*, 11.
8. American Production and Inventory Control Society. *APICS dictionary*, 7th ed. 41. Falls Church, VA: American Production and Inventory Control Society, Inc., 1992.
9. For further discussion of quality, see: Casalou, Robert F. Total quality management in health care. *Hospital & Health Services Administration* 36 (Spring 1991): 135; James, Brent C. Implementing continuous quality improvement. *Trustee* 43 (April 1990): 16; Juran, Joseph M. *Juran on planning for quality*, 4. New York: The Free Press, 1988; Re, Richard N., and Marie A. Krousel-Wood. How to use continuous quality improvement theory and statistical quality control tools in a multi-specialty clinic. *Quality Review Bulletin* 16 (November 1990): 392.
10. James, *Quality management*, 10.
11. James, *Quality management*, 11.
12. Re and Krousel-Wood, How to use, 392.
13. Milakovich, Creating a total, 11.
14. McLaughlin and Kaluzny, Total quality management, 8.
15. Marszalek-Gaucher, Ellen, and Richard J. Coffey. *Transforming healthcare organizations: How to achieve and sustain organizational excellence*, 85. San Francisco: Jossey-Bass Publishers, 1990.
16. Deming, W. Edwards. Improvement of quality and productivity through action by management. *National Productivity Review* 1 (Winter 1981–82): 12–22; Deming, W. Edwards. *Quality, productivity, and competitive position*. Boston: Massachusetts Institute of Technology, 1982; Deming, W. Edwards. Transformation of Western

style management. *Interfaces* 15 (May/June 1985): 6–11; Deming, *Out of the crisis.*

17. Juran, Joseph M. *Managerial breakthrough: A new concept of the manager's job.* New York: McGraw-Hill Book Company, 1964; Juran, Joseph M. The quality trilogy. *Quality Progress* 19 (August 1986): 19–24; Juran, Joseph M. *Juran on leadership for quality.* New York: The Free Press, 1989; Juran, *Juran on planning.*

18. Crosby, Philip B. *Quality is free.* New York: McGraw-Hill Book Company, 1979; Crosby, Philip B. *Let's talk quality.* New York: McGraw-Hill Publishing Company, 1989; Crosby, Philip B. *Quality without tears.* New York: McGraw-Hill Book Company, 1984.

19. American Hospital Association, *Quality management,* 2.

20. Joint Commission on Accreditation of Healthcare Organizations. *The Joint Commission's agenda for change: Stimulating continual improvement in the quality of care,* 1–4. Oakbrook Terrace, IL, 1990; Joint Commission on Accreditation of Healthcare Organizations. *Transitions: From QA to CQI—using CQI approaches to monitor, evaluate, and improve quality,* 6–7. Oakbrook Terrace, IL, 1991.

21. Joint Commission on Accreditation of Healthcare Organizations. Brief overview of *Joint Commission's agenda for change.* (internal working document), 1. Oakbrook Terrace, IL, 1990.

22. James, *Quality management,* 1.

23. Anderson, Craig A., and Robin D. Daigh. Quality mindset overcomes barriers to success. *Healthcare Financial Management* 45 (February 1991): 21; Kronenberg, Philip S., and Renee G. Loeffler. Quality management theory: Historical context and future prospect. *Journal of Management Science & Policy Analysis* 8 (Spring/Summer 1991): 204; McLaughlin and Kaluzny, Total quality management, 7; Sahney, Vinod K., and Gail L. Warden. The quest for quality and productivity in health services. *Frontiers of Health Services Management* 7 (Summer 1991): 2.

24. Milakovich, Creating a total, 9.

25. McEachern, J. Edward, and Duncan Neuhauser. The continuous improvement of quality at the Hospital Corporation of American. *Health Matrix* 7 (Fall 1989): 7; Postal, Susan Nelson. Using the Deming quality improvement method to manage medical records department product lines. *Topics in Health Records Management* 10 (June 1990): 34.

26. American Hospital Association, *Quality management,* 2; James, *Quality management,* 1; Lynn, Monty L., and David P. Osborn. Deming's quality principles: A health care application. *Hospital & Health Services Administration* 36 (Spring 1991): 113.

27. Lynn and Osborn, Deming's quality principles.

28. Green, Deborah K. Implementing a corporate quality management program: The AMI experience. *Topics in Health Records Management* 10 (March 1990): 23–31; Postal, Using the Deming; McEachern and Neuhauser, Continuous improvement of quality; Sahney and Warden, Quest for quality; Walton, Mary. *Deming management at work.* New York: G.P. Putnam's Sons, 1990.

29. Re and Krousel-Wood, How to use.

30. James, Brent C. TQM and clinical medicine. *Frontiers of Health Services Management* 7 (Summer 1991): 42–46.

31. Laffel and Blumenthal, Case for using.

32. Cascade, Philip N. Quality improvement in diagnostic

radiology. *American Journal of Radiology* 154 (May 1990): 1117–1120.

33. Postal, Using the Deming.

34. Peterson, Charles D. Quality improvement in pharmacy: A prescription for change. *Quality Review Bulletin* 16 (March 1990): 106–108.

35. Casalou, Total quality management, 138.

36. O'Leary, Dennis S. CQI—a step beyond QA. *Joint Commission Perspectives* 10 (March/April 1990): 2.

37. President of the Joint Commission, cited in Patterson, Pat. JCAHO shifts its emphasis to QI—quality improvement. *OR Manager* 6 (May 1990): 1.

38. Crosby, *Let's talk quality,* 63.

39. See also Berwick, Donald M., A. Blanton Godfrey, and Jane Roessner. *Curing health care: New strategies for quality improvement,* 32–43. San Francisco: Jossey-Bass Publishers, 1990.

40. Darr, Kurt. Applying the Deming method in hospitals: Part 1. *Hospital Topics* 67 (November/December 1989): 4.

41. Milakovich, Creating a total, 12.

42. Deming, *Out of the crisis,* 3; Walton, Mary. *The Deming management method,* 25. New York: Perigee Books (Putnam Publishing Group), 1986.

43. Lowe, Ted A., and Joseph M. Mazzeo. Crosby, Deming, Juran: Three preachers, one religion. *Quality* 25 (September 1986): 22–25; Sahney and Warden, Quest for quality, 4–7.

44. Lowe and Mazzeo, Crosby, Deming, Juran, 22.

45. Sahney and Warden, Quest for quality, 4–5.

46. Deming, Improvement of quality; Deming, *Quality, productivity;* Deming, *Transformation of Western;* Deming, *Out of the crisis.*

47. Darr, Applying the Deming method (Part 1); Darr, Kurt. Applying the Deming method in hospitals: Part 2. *Hospital Topics* 68 (Winter 1990): 4–6; Gabor, Andrea. *The man who discovered quality: How W. Edwards Deming brought the quality revolution to America—the stories of Ford, Xerox, and GM.* New York: Random House, 1990; Gitlow, Howard S., and Shelly J. Gitlow. *The Deming guide to quality and competitive position.* Englewood Cliffs, NJ: Prentice Hall, Inc., 1987; Neuhauser, Duncan. The quality of medical care and the 14 points of Edwards Deming. *Health Matrix* 6 (Summer 1986): 7–10; Scherkenbach, William W. *The Deming route to quality and productivity.* Washington, DC: Ceep Press Books, 1986; Walton, *Deming management method.*

48. Deming, *Out of the crisis,* 199–203.

49. Darr, Applying the Deming method (Part 1), 4.

50. Deming's 14 points (in italics) are drawn from Deming, *Out of the crisis,* 22–24.

51. Deming, *Out of the crisis,* 200.

52. Deming, *Out of the crisis,* 201.

53. Deming, *Out of the crisis,* 202.

54. Deming, *Out of the crisis,* 202.

55. Deming, *Out of the crisis,* 202.

56. Deming, *Out of the crisis,* 203.

57. Deming, Improvement of quality, 22.

58. Darr, Applying the Deming method (Part 1), 5.

59. Juran, *Managerial breakthrough;* Juran, Quality trilogy; Juran, *Juran on planning;* Juran, *Juran on leadership,* 361.

60. Sahney and Warden, Quest for quality, 6–7.

61. Juran, *Juran on leadership,* 20–21.

62. Juran, *Juran on planning,* 1.

63. Juran, *Juran on leadership,* 21–22.
64. Juran, *Managerial breakthrough,* 7.
65. Crosby, *Quality is free,* 1.
66. Crosby, *Let's talk quality,* 104.
67. Sahney and Warden, Quest for quality, 6.
68. Crosby, *Let's talk quality,* 9.
69. Crosby, *Quality is free,* 38–39.
70. Crosby, *Quality is free,* 132–138; Crosby, *Quality without tears,* 101–124; Crosby, *Let's talk quality,* 106–107. The quotation in point 10 is from Crosby, *Quality without tears,* 117.
71. Crosby, *Quality is free,* 22.
72. Lowe and Mazzeo, Crosby, Deming, Juran, 23.
73. Darr, Applying the Deming method (Part 2), 4.
74. Darr, Applying the Deming method (Part 2), 4.
75. James, *Quality management,* iii.
76. James, *Quality management,* 26.
77. James, *Quality management,* 26.
78. James, *Quality management,* 27.
79. James, *Quality management,* 27–28.
80. James, *Quality management,* 32.
81. Vonderembse, Mark A., and Gregory P. White. *Operations management: Concepts, methods, and strategies,* 2d ed., 723. St. Paul, MN: West Publishing Co., 1991.
82. Werner, John P. Productivity and quality management. In *Productivity and performance management in health care institutions,* edited by Mark D. McDougall, Richard P. Covert, and V. Brandon Melton, 110. Chicago: American Hospital Publishing, Inc., 1989.
83. Mosard, Gil R. A TQM technical skills framework. *Journal of Management Science & Policy Analysis* 8 (Spring/Summer 1991): 242-244.
84. James, Implementing continuous quality, 16.
85. Goldense, Robert A. Attaining TQM through employee involvement: Imperatives for implementation. *Journal of Management Science & Policy Analysis* 8 (Spring/Summer 1991): 268.
86. Schermerhorn, John R., Jr. Improving health care productivity through high-performance managerial development. *Health Care Management Review* 12 (Fall 1987): 51.
87. Kazemek, Edward A., and Rosemary M. Charny. Quality enhancement means total organizational involvement. *Healthcare Financial Management* 45 (February 1991): 15; Kronenberg and Loeffler, Quality management theory, 211–212.
88. Walton, *Deming management method,* 99.
89. James, *Quality management,* 27.
90. McLaughlin and Kaluzny, Total quality management, 10.
91. McLaughlin and Kaluzny, Total quality management, 10.
92. McLaughlin and Kaluzny, Total quality management, 7.
93. McLaughlin and Kaluzny, Total quality management, 8.
94. Re and Krousel-Wood, How to use, 392.
95. Schumacher, Organizing for quality, 11.
96. Laffel and Blumenthal, Case for using, 2870.
97. James, TQM and clinical medicine, 43.
98. James, TQM and clinical medicine, 43.
99. Eastaugh, Steven R. *Financing health care: Economic, efficiency, and equity,* 258. Dover, MA: Auburn House Publishing Co., 1987.
100. Fogarty, Donald W., Thomas R. Hoffmann, and Peter W. Stonebraker. *Production and operations management,* 18. Cincinnati, OH: South-Western Publishing Co., 1989.
101. Selbst, Paul L. A more total approach to productivity improvement. *Hospital & Health Services Administration* 30 (July/August 1985): 86.
102. James, *Quality management,* 7.
103. Shukla, Ramesh K. Effect of an admission monitoring and scheduling system on productivity and employee satisfaction. *Hospital & Health Services Administration* 35 (Fall 1990): 430.
104. Laliberty, Rene, and W. I. Christopher. *Enhancing Productivity in Health Care Facilities,* Chpt. 5. Owings Mills, MD: National Health Publishing, 1984.
105. Mosard, TQM technical skills, 237.
106. Anderson and Daigh, Quality mind-set, 26.
107. From *Akron Beacon Journal* (July 12, 1991): C14; reprinted by permission of Ann Landers and Creators Syndicate, *The Chicago Tribune,* Chicago, IL.
108. From Vonderembse, Mark, and Gregory White. *Operations management: Concepts, methods, and strategies,* 2d ed., 549–550. St. Paul, MN: West Publishing Company, 1991; reprinted by permission. (Copyright © 1991 by West Publishing Company. All rights reserved.)
109. Gaylord Reagan, "Total Quality Management (TQM) Inventory." Reprinted from J. William Pfeiffer (Ed.), *The 1992 Annual: Developing Human Resources,* San Diego, CA: Pfeiffer & Company, 1992. Used with permission. This instrument is based on the Federal Quality Institute's *Federal Total Quality Management Handbook 2: Criteria and Scoring Guidelines for the President's Award for Quality and Productivity Improvement,* Washington, DC: Office of Personnel Management, 1990.

BIBLIOGRAPHY

American Hospital Association. *Quality management: A management advisory,* 1–3. Chicago: American Management Association, 1990.

Anderson, Craig A., and Robin D. Daigh. Quality mind-set overcomes barriers to success. *Healthcare Financial Management* 45 (February 1991): 21–22, 26–32.

Berwick, Donald M., A. Blanton Godfrey, and Jane Roessner. *Curing health care: New strategies for quality improvement,* San Francisco: Jossey-Bass Publishers, 1990.

Casalou, Robert F. Total quality management in health care. *Hospital & Health Services Administration* 36 (Spring 1991): 134–146.

Cascade, Philip N. Quality improvement in diagnostic radiology. *American Journal of Radiology* 154 (May 1990): 1117–1120.

Casurella, Joe. Managing a "total quality" program. *Federation of American Health Systems Review* 22 (July/August 1989): 31–33.

Crosby, Philip B. *Quality is free.* New York: McGraw-Hill Book Company, 1979.

Crosby, Philip B. *Quality without tears.* New York: McGraw-Hill Book Company, 1984.

Crosby, Philip B. *Let's talk quality.* New York: McGraw-Hill Book Company, 1989.

Darr, Kurt. Applying the Deming method in hospitals: Part 1. *Hospital Topics* 67 (November/December 1989): 4–5.

Darr, Kurt. Applying the Deming method in hospitals: Part 2. *Hospital Topics* 68 (Winter 1990): 4–6.

Deming, W. Edwards. Improvement of quality and productivity through action by management. *National Productivity Review* 1 (Winter 1981–82): 12–22.

Deming, W. Edwards. *Quality, productivity, and competitive position.* Boston: Massachusetts Institute of Technology, 1982.

Deming, W. Edwards. Transformation of Western style management. *Interfaces* 15 (May/June 1985): 6–11.

Deming, W. Edwards. *Out of the crisis.* Boston: Massachusetts Institute of Technology, 1986.

Eastaugh, Steven R. *Financing health care: Economic, efficiency, and equity.* Dover, MA: Auburn House Publishing Co., 1987.

Fogarty, Donald W., Thomas R. Hoffmann, and Peter W. Stonebraker. *Production and operations management.* Cincinnati, OH: South-Western Publishing Co., 1989.

Gabor, Andrea. *The man who discovered quality: How W. Edwards Deming brought the quality revolution to America—the stories of Ford, Xerox, and GM.* New York: Random House, 1990.

Gitlow, Howard S., and Shelly J. Gitlow. *The Deming guide to quality and competitive position.* Englewood Cliffs, NJ: Prentice Hall, Inc., 1987.

Goldense, Robert A. Attaining TQM through employee involvement: Imperatives for implementation. *Journal of Management Science & Policy Analysis* 8 (Spring/Summer 1991): 263–274.

Green, Deborah K. Implementing a corporate quality management program: The AMI experience. *Topics in Health Records Management* 10 (March 1990): 23–31.

James, Brent C. *Quality management for health care delivery—Quality Measurement and Management Project.* Chicago: The Hospital Research and Educational Trust, 1989.

James, Brent C. Implementing continuous quality improvement. *Trustee* 43 (April 1990): 16–17.

James, Brent C. TQM and clinical medicine. *Frontiers of Health Services Management* 7 (Summer 1991): 42–46.

Joint Commission on Accreditation of Healthcare Organizations. Brief overview of *Joint Commission's agenda for change.* (internal working document), 1–4. Oakbrook Terrace, IL, 1990.

Joint Commission on Accreditation of Healthcare Organizations. *Transitions: From QA to CQI—using CQI approaches to monitor, evaluate, and improve quality.* Oakbrook Terrace, IL, 1991.

Juran, Joseph M. *Managerial breakthrough: A new concept of the manager's job.* New York: McGraw-Hill Book Company, 1964.

Juran, Joseph M. The quality trilogy. *Quality Progress* 19 (August 1986): 19–24.

Juran, Joseph M. *Juran on planning for quality.* New York: The Free Press, 1988.

Juran, Joseph M. *Juran on leadership for quality.* New York: The Free Press, 1989.

Kronenberg, Philip S., and Renee G. Loeffler. Quality management theory: Historical context and future prospect. *Journal of Management Science & Policy Analysis* 8 (Spring/Summer 1991): 203–221.

Laffel, Glenn, and David Blumenthal. The case for using industrial management science in health care organizations. *Journal of the American Medical Association* 262 (November 24, 1989): 2869–2873.

Laliberty, Rene, and W. I. Christopher. *Enhancing Productivity in Health Care Facilities,* Chpt. 5. Owings Mills, MD: National Health Publishing, 1984.

Lanning, Joyce A., and Stephen J. O'Connor. The health care quality quagmire: Some signposts. *Hospital & Health Services Administration* 35 (Spring 1990): 39–54.

Lowe, Ted A., and Joseph M. Mazzeo. Crosby, Deming, Juran: Three preachers, one religion. *Quality* 25 (September 1986): 22–25.

Lynn, Monty L., and David P. Osborn. Deming's quality principles: A health care application. *Hospital & Health Services Administration* 36 (Spring 1991): 111–120.

Marszalek-Gaucher, Ellen, and Richard J. Coffey. *Transforming healthcare organizations: How to achieve and sustain organizational excellence.* San Francisco: Jossey-Bass Publishers, 1990.

McEachern, J. Edward, and Duncan Neuhauser. The continuous improvement of quality at the Hospital Corporation of American. *Health Matrix* 7 (Fall 1989): 5–10.

McLaughlin, Curtis P., and Arnold D. Kaluzny. Total quality management in health: Making it work. *Health Care Management Review* 15 (Summer 1990): 7–14.

Merry, Martin D. Total quality management for physicians: Translating the new paradigm. *Quality Review Bulletin* 16 (March 1990): 101–105.

Milakovich, Michael E. Creating a total quality health care environment. *Health Care Management Review* 16 (Spring 1991): 9–20.

Mosard, Gil R. A TQM technical skills framework. *Journal of Management Science & Policy Analysis* 8 (Spring/Summer 1991): 223–245.

Neuhauser, Duncan. The quality of medical care and the 14 points of Edwards Deming. *Health Matrix* 6 (Summer 1988): 7–10.

O'Connor, Stephen J. Service quality: Understanding and implementing the concept in the clinical laboratory. *Clinical Laboratory Management Review* 3 (November/December 1989): 329–335.

O'Leary, Dennis S. CQI—a step beyond QA. *Joint Commission Perspectives* 10 (March/April 1990): 2–3.

Peterson, Charles D. Quality improvement in pharmacy: A prescription for change. *Quality Review Bulletin* 16 (March 1990): 106–108.

Postal, Susan Nelson. Using the Deming quality improvement method to manage medical records department product lines. *Topics in Health Records Management* 10 (June 1990): 34–40.

Re, Richard N., and Marie A. Krousel-Wood. How to use continuous quality improvement theory and statistical quality control tools in a multispecialty clinic. *Quality Review Bulletin* 16 (November 1990): 391–397.

Sahney, Vinod K., and Gail L. Warden. The quest for quality and productivity in health services. *Frontiers of Health Services Management* 7 (Summer 1991): 2–41.

Scherkenbach, William W. *The Deming route to quality and productivity.* Washington, DC: Ceep Press Books, 1986.

Schermerhorn, John R., Jr. Improving health care productivity through high-performance managerial development. *Health Care Management Review* 12 (Fall 1987): 49–55.

Schumacher, Dale N. Organizing for quality competition: The coming paradigm shift. *Frontiers of Health Services Management* 5 (Summer 1989): 4–30.

Selbst, Paul L. A more total approach to productivity improvement. *Hospital & Health Services Administration* 30 (July/August 1985): 85–96.

Shukla, Ramesh K. Effect of an admission monitoring and scheduling system on productivity and employee satisfaction. *Hospital & Health Services Administration* 35 (Fall 1990): 429–441.

Vonderembse, Mark A., and Gregory P. White. *Operations management: Concepts, methods, and strategies,* 2d ed. St. Paul, MN: West Publishing Co., 1991.

Walton, Mary. *The Deming management method.* New York: Perigee Books (Putnam Publishing Group), 1986.

Walton, Mary. *Deming management at work.* New York: G.P. Putnam's Sons, 1990.

Werner, John P. Productivity and quality management. In *Productivity and performance management in health care institutions,* edited by Mark D. McDougall, Richard P. Covert, and V. Brandon Melton, 83–118. Chicago: American Hospital Publishing, Inc., 1989.

Control, Risk Management, Quality Assessment/ Improvement, and Resource Allocation

Control in HSOs requires a sensor component that gathers data on the quantity of services rendered, the quality and other characteristics of these services, and the resources consumed in their provision. Data from the sensor are monitored against preestablished standards of quantity (production and service goals), quality of care, and the efficiency of the service process. When standards are not met, a control process is activated to initiate necessary changes and improvement.

Charles J. Austin[1]

Chapter 11 focuses on quality—doing the right things right—and productivity improvement—providing the highest quality products and services at the lowest reasonable cost. This chapter focuses on control and resource allocation. How do we know if a health services organization's (HSO's) products and services are high quality? How do we determine if processes that generate output are functioning effectively? How do we know if input resources are high quality, if they are properly allocated, and if the amount used is appropriate? One word answers these questions—control. Those who understand HSOs know about quality control, infection control, quality assessment and improvement, risk management, cost control, utilization review, narcotics control, and credentials review. All are control or control-like activities.

In this chapter, a control model that integrates continuous quality improvement (CQI) is presented. It compares actual results to standards and expectations and suggests appropriate action when deviation occurs. Control is information dependent, and management information systems and their applications are discussed.

A special section addresses risk management and quality assessment and improvement, which are critical to control in HSOs. Other methods of control examined are budgeting, case-mix accounting, ratio analysis, and network programming. The final section discusses analytical techniques relevant to resource allocation and use, such as volume analysis, capital budgeting, cost-benefit analysis, and simulation.

CONTROL AND PLANNING

Managers control to ensure that what is planned and expected actually occurs. Organization results occur when HSO managers integrate structure-tasks/technology-people components and allocate and use input resources. As the opening quote suggests, to ensure that individual work results are desirable and organization objectives are accomplished, managers consciously and continuously monitor, evaluate, and, if warranted, intervene. As indicated by the management process model in Chapter 1 (see Figure 1.6), managers use control to ensure that actual and desired output are consistent, work and conversion processes are effective, and resource consumption is appropriate.

Chapter 1 described the controlling function as being technical and focusing on monitoring the organization's activities. Control is defined here *as gathering information about and monitoring the HSO's activities, comparing actual results with expected results, and, when appropriate, intervening to take corrective action by changing inputs or processes.* Control is also the means "by which managers assure that the organization is reaching its objectives and carrying out associated plans in an effective and efficient manner."[2] Control and planning are the Siamese twins of management—the standards and desired results used in control are derived from the HSO's strategic and operational plans.[3]

MONITORING (CONTROL) AND INTERVENTION POINTS

Control systems are information based. Figure 12.1 shows a generic control system that identifies monitoring (control) and intervention points. In the process of control, information is collected at three monitoring points: input utilization, functioning of conversion processes, and outputs. If results at these three monitoring points are inconsistent with expectations or standards, intervention can occur at the input [A] or process [B] points or both.

Output Control

The best known type of control is exercised over output. It is often called feedback control[4] and is retrospective—after the fact. Feedback in HSOs focuses on all levels of quantitative and qualitative output and ranges from individual and departmental to overall organization results. Throughout, standards and expectations denote desired results, which are usually expressed numerically. Examples at the individual and departmental levels include individual job performance and departmental measures such as number or units of output (e.g., laboratory tests, radiographs, surgical procedures, meals served, patients admitted, drug orders filled, and pounds of laundry processed), as well as quality dimensions of outputs such as accuracy, timeliness, and customer satisfaction. At the organization level, examples are outpatient visits, average length of stay, occupancy rate, quality of care, range of services, stakeholder satisfaction, financial integrity, and market share. Output standards and expectations are derived from and reflect departmental and organizational objectives.

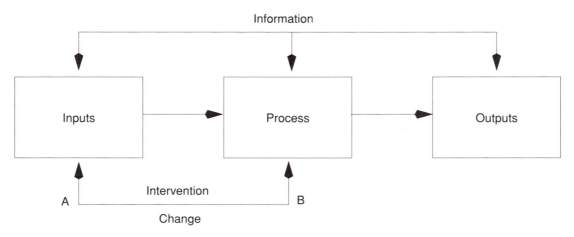

Figure 12.1. Generic control system.

Process Control

Converting inputs to outputs requires processes. The quality of outputs is determined by efficacy and efficiency of process, amount and appropriateness of inputs, or both. In controlling, attention is usually directed at outputs (quantity and quality of care), but it is equally important to monitor the myriad integrative conversion processes whose total effort generates outputs. The principle of continuous quality improvement (CQI) is that processes can be improved. For this to occur there must be a monitoring system to identify how well they are functioning. Examples of integrative conversion processes in HSOs include:

> Work systems such as patient admitting and discharge, transportation, materials handling and distribution, direct patient care, and ancillary services
>
> Specific job design and staff, and machine, technology, and facility interrelationships
>
> Financial record keeping and information collection, storage, retrieval, and dissemination systems
>
> Decision and resource allocation and planning processes
>
> Managerial methods, practices, and styles along with organizational structuring, coordination, and communication methods and flows

Since process (in combination with inputs) yields outputs, concurrent process control is important. Also referred to as screening control, it "focuses on activities that occur as inputs are being transformed to outputs."[5] Furthermore, process is one of two points at which intervention can occur if outputs are inconsistent with expectations (see point B in Figure 12.1). Standards and expectations are easier to develop for processes that deal with things, are consistent, and are simple to document and understand. It is more difficult when a process is less tangible. For example, what are the effects on conversion (and ultimately on output) of different managerial methods of problem solving and decision making, leadership and supervisory styles, approach to motivation, or methods of communication? Perhaps this is one reason why control has historically focused more on outputs generated and inputs consumed and less on process. One inherent element of CQI is that control is directed at process.

Input Control

As stated in the opening quotation, control must focus on "resources consumed" in creating outputs. Virtually all HSOs exercise control over input by developing standards and expectations about resource consumption. Examples include nursing hours per patient day, materials and supplies consumed, and the ratio of personnel to beds. Often called "feedforward" control, "it is an approach to control that uses inputs to a system of organizational activities as a means of controlling the accomplishment of organizational objectives [outputs]."[6] The philosophy of CQI suggests choosing the best inputs before conversion to avoid problems. In HSOs, one way to control the quality of human resource inputs is credentialing and licensure, which help ensure HSOs that clinical staff possess certain levels of training and skills. Input control alone, however, is no substitute for process and output control.

CONTROL MODEL

Thus far, control has been described as a process by which information is gathered about results and performance at the monitoring (control) points of inputs, process, and outputs. Comparing actual results with preestablished standards and expectations, appraising comparisons, and making interventions and changes at the inputs and/or process points as needed are the remaining components of control. Figure 12.2 incorporates these components in a control process model and shows that actual results are measured and compared with standards and expectations. Depending on results, the control process follows one of four loops, each of which indicates whether intervention and change are necessary.

In Control Loop

In Figure 12.2, the "in control loop" is the simplest. When appraisal of results indicates that they meet standards and expectations, no change is required. Whatever is being monitored is judged to be in control; activity continues.

Acceptance Control Loop

When appraisal indicates that actual results and performance do not meet standards and expectations, managers investigate to determine the cause of the deviation. If the deviation is desirable or acceptable, or its cause is uncontrollable, activities continue with no intervention or change. For example, higher (actual results) than budgeted (standard) overtime may be acceptable if the census is higher than expected.

Deviation is undesirable; if the cause is uncontrollable, however, actual results and performance must be accepted. For example, a decrease in the ratio of registered nurse hours per patient, to below the desired standard but above the minimum needed for good patient care, may be due to a shortage of registered nurses—an inadequate pool of this resource in the service area.

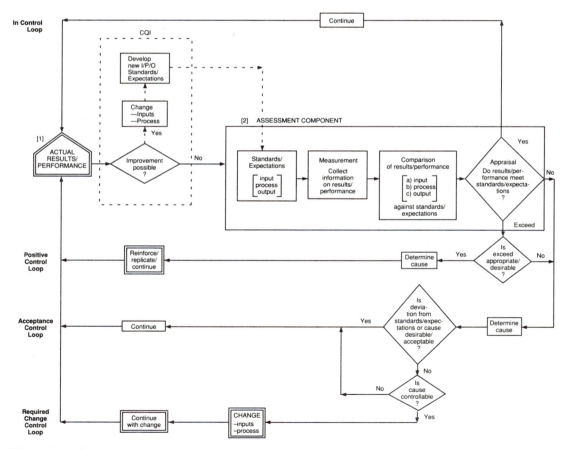

Figure 12.2. Control model.

Required Change Control Loop

When deviation is unacceptable and the cause is controllable, intervention should occur. For example, if average length of stay is substantially above standard, intervention and change are required. This may occur if physicians (input point) do not discharge patients in a timely manner or if work systems (process point) are ineffective and there are delays in administering and reporting tests. Another example is higher than normal personnel turnover, which may result from a poor organizational climate, inadequacy of the compensation system, or poor supervision. Here, too, intervention and change are required.

Positive Control Loop

There is a general perception that control has a negative focus; however, this is not always the case. For example, if performance is better than standards, the cause should be identified, reinforced, frozen in place, and replicated elsewhere. A department consistently under budget with superior individual work results and higher quality of care may result from factors such as effective managerial style, positive employee attitude and commitment, and well-designed processes. Necessarily, control is concerned with the negative; however, improvement control also recognizes and emphasizes the positive.

There are instances when actual performance exceeds (is better than) standards but this is undesirable. For example, it may seem desirable that nursing care hours per patient be below the standard, but evaluation may show this to be unacceptable if quality of care is diminished. Physical plant maintenance expenditures may be below budget, yet this may be undesirable if preventive maintenance is postponed. If actual results and performance are better than standards and expectations but are not desirable or appropriate, the cause should be determined and either the "acceptance" or "required change" control loops should be used in the control process.

CONTROL AND CQI

In HSOs, meeting standards is never the end of the control process. The philosophy of CQI uses continuous inquiry to improve processes and inputs so that outputs can be improved. The control model in Figure 12.2 shows use of CQI in the dash-outlined box. If no improvement of process or inputs is possible, the control loop flows from actual results/performance [1] through to the assessment component [2]. If improvement is possible, change is made to inputs and/or process, and new standards and expectations are developed to replace those used in the assessment component [2].

CONTROL AND PROBLEM SOLVING

As presented in Chapter 10, "Managerial Problem Solving and Decision Making," problem solving depends on information generated by control. The four conditions that initiate problem solving are deviation, opportunity/threat, crisis, and improvement. The most common is deviation, which occurs when individual and organizational work results are found to be inconsistent with those that are desired. Comparison of actual results with prospective standards for inputs, processes, or outputs shows deviation. Problem solving under the condition of deviation is triggered by monitoring and evaluation during control. Problem solving under the condition of improvement improves processes or inputs to positively affect outputs. Information obtained from control is prerequisite to process investigation and improvement activities.

CONTROL CONSIDERATIONS

Several managerial and design considerations are important when control systems are established and maintained.

Managerial Considerations

Managerial questions to be answered when a control system is established or modified are:

1. *Where is control focused?* Control may focus on input (review of resource use); process or conversion (review of efficiency of work systems in converting inputs to outputs); or output (concern for overall organizational results).
2. *What types of measures are used for standards and monitoring results?* Measures used in control depend on focus, quantifiability of results, and the extent to which measures convey accurate, usable, and meaningful information.
3. *Who has authority to establish standards?* A principle of control is that those whose activities are monitored have input but not sole authority to establish standards and monitor results. Checks and balances are universal in accounting systems; for example, cashiers who handle cash do no final audits or reconciliations. Similarly, utilization review and tissue audit are not performed by those providing the services.
4. *How flexible should standards be?* Blind and inflexible use of numerical measures causes distortions. Changes and unforeseen circumstances require that judgment, common sense, and flexibility be used in control systems.
5. *Who has access to control system information?* Controlling requires dissemination of information, but certain information is appropriately restricted to certain levels of management or specific managers.
6. *Who is responsible for intervention?* Just as organizations have a defined authority-responsibility hierarchy, managerial consideration of control includes who is responsible and who intervenes when appropriate.

Design Considerations

There are situations in which control systems cause unintended and undesirable consequences, cost more than they are worth, measure the wrong things, or focus on the wrong points. Design of these systems should include the following considerations to decrease the occurrence of such dysfunctional outcomes and to improve quality:

1. *When possible, control should be prospective.* Control cannot always be forward looking or predictive. Usually, information flows or organizational constraints limit it to being concurrent or retrospective. If available, feedforward control provides information to managers that enables them to anticipate deviation and makes them more effective.
2. *Control should be organizationally realistic and understandable to users.* Control systems must be in harmony with the organization, must realistically fit, and must be understandable. A system that creates barriers or artificial constraints is dysfunctional. For example, control on inventories and supplies is best centralized in materials management. Centralizing access to and control of photocopiers in one office may be unrealistic.
3. *Control should be accurate, timely, and reliable.* In designing control systems, standards and measurements must be accurate and reliable. Making corrections based on inaccurate or unreliable information defeats the purpose of control, as does using obsolete data that do not reflect accurately the current situation.
4. *Control should be significant and/or have economic benefit.* Significant refers to the importance of what is controlled. Economic benefit refers to the cost of control relative to the value of what is controlled. There is little economic benefit to disposal (destruction) control of used syringes. It is beneficial, however, for such reasons as preventing use by drug addicts and protecting those who handle medical waste. Medication control has significant clinical and economic benefits. Conversely, after a box of tissues has been charged to a patient, control of

individual tissue consumption is insignificant and without economic benefit. Costs of control exceed any saving.

5. *Control should be information appropriate.* Too much or too little information is undesirable. Important indicators are lost in the avalanche of paper caused by excessive information. Too little information denies managers the ability to focus on critical elements. Control systems should be designed to give managers sufficient and discriminating information at the right time and in a usable format.

MANAGEMENT INFORMATION SYSTEMS AND CONTROL

HSO managers depend on information. Effective planning, problem solving, and control occur only when managers receive appropriate, accurate, and timely information in the proper format. "The importance of accurate information to support the delivery of health care and the management of the institutions and programs that deliver that care is beyond question."[7] Formal communication mechanisms are established to ensure that information is collected, disseminated, and retrievable on demand. Management information systems (MIS) are such a mechanism.

MIS is a generic term that refers to custom-designed systems that gather, store, format, and report data to and/or make it retrievable by users. The purpose is to "help managers plan, execute, and control the organization's activities."[8] Most traditional information systems are application driven; information is retrieved from discrete files created for specific purposes by units in HSOs. In their design, users specify type and extent of information desired. Historically, MIS design was performed by in-house systems analysts and programmers. "More recently, the trend has been toward increased use of generalized software available from commercial sources or employment of 'turnkey' systems in which a vendor provides software, training of personnel, and system installation."[9]

HSO information systems generally fall into two broad categories. First, administrative and financial systems provide information supporting administrative operations and managerial planning, resource allocation, and control activities. Second, clinical and medical systems provide information to support patient care activities. A survey of 2,400 senior hospital managers rated these as the two most important categories. Others are cost accounting, resource utilization and productivity analysis, and market intelligence.[10] Figure 12.3 shows a hospital information system (HIS)—an MIS application profile.

Types of MIS

The sophistication of information systems ranges from: 1) application reporting systems to 2) data-base management systems to 3) decision support systems. Applications reporting is the most familiar to HSO managers and consists of tailored reports about organizational operations or areas of activity such as payroll, inventory, admission, census, and scheduling.

Rapid technological advances in computer hardware and software have made data-base management systems increasingly common in HSOs. Data from throughout the organization are integrated and consolidated in a single MIS data base accessible by authorized users rather than segregated for specific applications reporting. These systems are inquiry based, and information can be obtained about any application.

An extension of MIS is decision support systems (DSS), which are model based and have statistical and simulation capabilities. They are interactive, which permits managers to ask "what if" questions through on-line terminals.[11] A financial example is: "What would be the effect on profit margin of a 20% increase in Medicare patients?" The applications of DSS are not restricted to administration; clinical applications are evolving in the form of medical decision support systems (MDSS).[12] It is projected "that computer-assisted diagnostic data bases and medical decision support systems will have a significant impact on patient care by the year 1995."[13] Attributes of

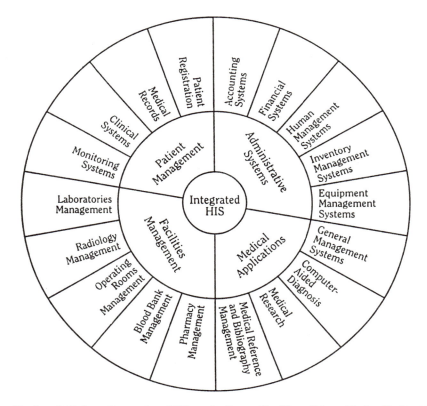

Figure 12.3. The hospital information system (HIS) application profile. (From Zviran, Moshe. Design considerations for integrated hospital information systems. *Hospital & Health Services Administration* 35 [Fall 1990]: 387; reprinted by permission. © 1990, Foundation of the American College of Healthcare Executives. Ann Arbor, MI: Health Administration Press.)

MDSS include clinical algorithms, statistical pattern classification, and hierarchical decision analysis.[14] Such systems also are used to assess and improve quality and achieve control by comparing clinical outcomes with historical results.[15] It is anticipated that future MDSS will provide information enabling physicians to evaluate the merits of and point to changes in treatment protocols.[16]

MIS Uses

Given that control in HSOs depends on information, Austin delineates a number of areas in which MIS can support managers and clinicians:

> *Medical Quality Assurance [Quality Assessment and Improvement].* Clinical information abstracted from patient medical records provides the basic material utilized by health professionals in peer review systems to assess diagnostic and treatment practices within the HSO. One goal of a computerized information system is to make such data readily accessible and retrievable from a central patient data file for purposes of quality assessment and initiation of necessary corrective action.
>
> *Cost Control and Productivity Enhancement.* Health services organizations are under increasing pressure to contain increases in the cost of services. Computerized information systems offer the potential for providing cost analyses and productivity reports for use by management and board members in improving the efficiency of operation. Such systems require the ability to integrate clinical and financial information systems.
>
> *Utilization Analysis and Demand Estimation.* A complete information system should provide current and historical data on utilization of health services. Such data systems serve to assist in current

analysis of the efficiency of utilization of resources and also provide a basis for predicting future demand for services.

Program Planning and Evaluation. Information obtained for the above purposes—quality assurance [quality assessment and improvement], cost control, utilization analysis, and demand estimation—serves as the basic input for management decisions related to evaluation of present programs and services. When combined with projections about future changes in the demographic characteristics of the service population, the information system can provide an important resource for planning future programs and services.[17]

From a control perspective, MIS should:

Provide information that meets specific needs of managers so they can monitor activities at the input, process, and/or output points.

Provide each level of management with specific reports relative to its area of responsibility that contain accurate, relevant, and timely information to improve decisions on control (intervention or change).

Extract and pinpoint critical and high-priority items requiring management's analysis and, perhaps, intervention.

The technological changes occurring in computer hardware and software and their application in MIS are breathtaking. Personal computers (PCs) that have processing capabilities equal to mainframes of a decade ago are only one example. PCs may be dedicated to information processing in a single department[18] or, when linked to networks, may become extensions of mainframes functioning as terminals that are tied into MIS systems.[19] MIS advancements, especially decision support systems, enable managers and clinical staff to make more informed decisions and to more effectively control—monitor inputs, process, and output.

RISK MANAGEMENT AND QUALITY ASSESSMENT AND IMPROVEMENT

Background

Historically, safety programs and measuring the quality of clinical services were separate control activities usually limited to acute care hospitals. In the early 1970s, safety programs began evolving into the broader concept of risk management* (RM) and included proactively managing risk. A comprehensive RM program includes identifying, controlling, and financing risks of all types. Inherent in RM is preventing risk and minimizing the effect of untoward events, should they occur. RM programs are now common in HSOs, especially hospitals.

Both internal and external factors caused these changes. Internally, HSO managers increasingly recognized their ethical duty to provide a safe environment for patients, staff, and visitors, and high-quality clinical services. External stimuli included: 1) the increasing litigiousness in society and court decisions that put greater legal liability on the HSO; 2) federal laws such as the Occupational Safety and Health Act, which mandated the study of hazards in acute care hospitals so that national standards could be set; and 3) the requirements of private organizations such as the Joint Commission on Accreditation of Healthcare Organizations (Joint Commission) and public bodies such as the Department of Health and Human Services, which increasingly emphasized the quality of services and managing risk. Better programs followed as it became apparent that HSOs had to effectively manage the economic costs of all types of risk.

In the 1990s, improving clinical quality (quality assessment and improvement) for patients will be an important part of the expanded concept of RM. The 1992 Joint Commission *Accredita-*

---

*"(R)isk management functions encompass activities in health [services] organizations that are intended to conserve financial resources from loss. Those functions include a broad range of administrative activities intended to reduce losses associated with patient, employee, or visitor injuries; property loss or damages; and other sources of potential organizational liability."[20]

tion Manual for Hospitals (AMH) discontinued use of the terms and methodology of quality assurance (QA) and mandated quality assessment and improvement (QA/I) as an improved, more proactive and effective focus to evaluate and improve quality. The AMH links QA/I and RM, but does not fully integrate them. It requires in standard QA.4.2.2 that: "There are operational linkages between the risk management functions related to the clinical aspects of patient care and safety and quality assessment and improvement functions" and in standard QA.4.2.3 that "Existing information from risk management activities that may be useful in identifying clinical problems and/or opportunities to improve the quality of patient care and/or resolve clinical problems is accessible to the quality assessment and improvement function."[21] Linking QA/I and RM is prudent and will enhance the effectiveness of both. HSOs should be cautious, however, that it does not appear they are more concerned with reducing economic risk than with providing high-quality clinical services.

RM and efforts to improve clinical quality do not have the same set of activities, but there are similarities. Figure 12.4, which includes a Venn diagram, shows the overlap between RM and traditional QA activities, many of which will continue in the new QA/I. Risk financing, employee benefits, and general liability issues have been unique to RM and are likely to remain so. The evolution of QA to QA/I will expand the historic focus of QA beyond clinical activities to include the processes that support them. This change will further diminish distinctions between RM and clinical activities and increase their linkages. Certainly, opportunities to benefit from cooperation will increase. In the meantime,

> (F) or some professionals on both sides, integration means that one function envelops and subsumes the other—a circumstance that would not be in the best interests of either function. . . . *Operational linkages* is a term that is vague enough to allow for a variety of organizational models, reporting relationships, and data flow.[22]

Risk Management

Only 20 years ago even large acute care hospitals probably had only a part-time safety officer, typically someone in the maintenance department with little formal preparation in how to make the facility less hazardous for employees and visitors. Patient safety may have received some special, but limited, attention. RM was undeveloped, and various risks facing the HSO were neither integrated nor handled comprehensively. Insurance was the typical means of protecting HSOs against monetary loss; proactive efforts or programs to reduce risk likely came from insurance companies wanting to decrease their exposure.

Link to Senior Management   Regardless of the extent to which RM is integrated with

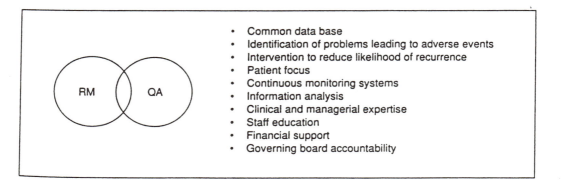

Figure 12.4.   Relationship between risk management and quality assurance. (From Kibbee, P. *Quality assurance, utilization, and risk management,* 1989, 58. Deerfield, IL: National Association of Quality Assurance Professionals, 1989; reprinted by permission.)

QA/I, encouragement and commitment at the highest levels of an HSO are necessary for an RM program to be successful. Governing body support is evidenced by providing adequate resources to the chief executive officer (CEO) for RM activities. This support should be readily available once the economics of prevention are explained. A RM program has a staff rather than a line relationship to the CEO.

RM is coordinated through an interdisciplinary committee, typically chaired by the risk manager. This committee develops policy and provides general oversight. To the extent that RM and QA/I are integrated, this committee will include members of professional staff organization committees and have a more clinical orientation.

The Risk Manager   Typically, risk managers have backgrounds in security, safety, and loss prevention. Experience in law enforcement and investigative techniques also is not unusual. This person may be full or part time; larger HSOs need someone full time. Increasingly, persons with master's degrees in health services management are employed as risk managers.

Risk managers have become increasingly important in HSOs. As the role of the risk manager matured, their duties came to include identifying and analyzing risks; developing, implementing, and monitoring the insurance program; maintaining and distributing a RM manual; reviewing existing and proposed contracts and agreements and consulting with legal counsel; supervising claims reporting; assisting in adjusting losses; developing and maintaining reporting and analysis systems for risk and loss; and attending and giving seminars that will improve personal and organizational RM skills.[23] In the 1990s risk managers may add more financial management responsibilities, such as evaluating equipment purchase agreements and joint venture contracts.[24]

Risk managers depend on the work of various HSO units and departments. Working effectively with persons over whom the risk manager has no line authority necessitates excellent interpersonal skills and an ability to coordinate and integrate disparate sources of information and resources. The risk manager may have the effect of exerting line authority by presenting information that is the basis for senior management decision making, as well as by persuading senior management to take action. The risk manager's influence is, nonetheless, indirect.

Principles of Managing Risk   The steps in managing risk include identifying, evaluating, eliminating, reducing, and transferring risk. Risk is identified in several ways. The most common is to collect and aggregate data about problems so that patterns become foci for action. However, managing risk is not only reactive. It should concentrate on eliminating, reducing, and transferring risk.

Evaluating risk means reviewing and categorizing information about problems over time. This allows the HSO to concentrate efforts where problems are greatest. Evaluating risk should be prospective, too, because it is known, actuarially, that certain types of problems will occur, or have a particular probability of occurring. Prospective, retrospective, and concurrent efforts can use evaluative techniques such as cost-benefit and cost-effectiveness analyses to select the best course of action. Evaluative efforts also aid in identifying strategies to eliminate, reduce, or transfer risk. Safety inspections and audits of various activities and functions (ranging from financial to fire protection) of the HSO are ways to prospectively identify problem areas.

Eliminating or reducing risk (or both) can be achieved in many ways. Examples include sponsoring education and awareness programs for staff; modifying physical plant and structure; enhancing the credentialing process and review of clinical staff activities (QA&I); improving processes and procedures; initiating material management systems; improving patient and staff relations; and hiring qualified personnel in appropriate categories. It is preferable to eliminate risk, but for many types of risk this may be impossible. Therefore, the emphasis must be on minimizing risk.

Corporate reorganization (restructuring) can eliminate certain economic risks. For example, assets of the operating HSO may be leased from the parent corporation; this makes them immune from attachment by successful plaintiffs. Establishing trusts and foundations in a corporate reorganization has the same effect. Putting HSO assets beyond the legal reach of successful plaintiffs has its place and is a legitimate business strategy. Failing to provide a means of compensating persons injured because of interacting with an HSO, however, is socially irresponsible and unethical.

Some risks can be transferred to others. A common example is the "hold harmless" agreement. It requires that a party doing business with an HSO indemnify the HSO for any liability incurred because of that party's negligence. Contracts to purchase equipment commonly include such clauses. Risk transfer clauses should be used in all agreements with subcontractors.

Financing Risk Some risks cannot be eliminated or transferred. The financial viability of the HSO must be protected from them; insurance is the most common way of doing so. Commercial insurance requires that the insured pay a premium. Coverage under the contract of insurance provides specified protection against certain losses for a fixed period. This contract between the HSO (the insured) and the insurer (carrier) puts obligations on the insured, as well. Examples include prompt reporting of problems with potential liability and cooperating in the carrier's investigation and defense of claims. In addition to commercial insurance, HSOs may participate in insurance programs through captive insurance companies that have been established by the state, a trade association, a consortium of HSOs, or by a very large HSO. Rapid increases in premium costs made these variations popular after the malpractice crises in the late 1960s and early 1970s, and in the 1980s, which were discussed in Chapter 4, "Legal Considerations." Because some carriers stopped writing medical malpractice liability insurance, availability also became a factor.

Prior to the 1980s, medical malpractice liability insurance was usually written on an occurrence basis. *Occurrence coverage* protects the insured from a claim regardless of how long after the occurrence it was filed. This resulted in a "long tail"; in other words claims could be brought for an extended period of time, but within the statute of limitations. For example, a newborn infant could bring suit for 21 years plus the statute of limitations. Carriers argued that this made it difficult, if not impossible, to actuarially estimate their risk (exposure), and therefore they could not accurately determine premiums. To avoid this problem, they began to write policies with *claims made coverage*. This meant that the insured must have a policy in effect when the claim is brought, rather than when the insured event occurs, as in occurrence coverage. The effect of this shift on HSOs is not yet fully known, but it seems to have reduced the rate of increase of medical malpractice liability insurance premiums.

Larger HSOs are more able to self-insure by establishing self-insurance programs. Such programs are usually broader than medical malpractice liability and may include financial protection against a broad range of risks, including business interruption, fire and other casualty losses, and bonding for employees with financial responsibilities. Establishing a self-insurance program is much more than simply stating that the HSO is self-insured. Actuarial studies must be done to determine the potential for various types of losses, including special attention to the specific risk from clinical services offered or contemplated. Based on these data, the HSO must establish dedicated reserves to meet expected claims. Usually it takes several years to accumulate the reserves needed for a self-insurance program to be financially viable. In the interim, commercial coverage is necessary. In addition, when the program is fully established, vigilance is necessary to ensure that the fund both is adequate to meet expected claims and is not raided for other purposes. Underfunding or stripping reserves for self-insurance protection can have disastrous consequences.

Even when the self-insurance program is mature, most HSOs carry excess liability and casualty coverage against large claims. For example, an HSO might self-insure for losses up to $3 million; beyond that it may have a policy with a commercial carrier to a total coverage of $20 million. It is important to note that even if an HSO carries only commercial insurance, the policy will likely have a deductible, which is a form of self-insurance. Deductibles must be met from reserves.

Good business practice demands that HSOs protect themselves against a range of financial risks. In addition, it is socially responsible and ethical that they do so. A few have chosen to "go bare" in terms of medical malpractice claims. This means they are neither self-insured nor do they carry commercial insurance. This practice is not uncommon among physicians who have a poor medical malpractice liability record. Assets of these physicians are in a spouse's name or otherwise beyond the reach of plaintiffs. This, too, is socially irresponsible. It is prudent for all HSOs to require members of their clinical staffs to provide evidence of insurance policies that meet established minimum requirements as a condition of having clinical privileges. This is standard practice in acute care hospitals.

Nonclinical staff caregivers and managers should carry personal liability insurance to protect themselves as individuals from legal actions for alleged malpractice. Although rare, individual malpractice policies are becoming more common among registered nurses, for example, and the profession recommends it. Managers should not forget that they, too, are liable for errors and omissions (malpractice) committed in their professional activities. The HSO's umbrella policy covers employees. Nonetheless, the effects of litigation have many nuances for employers and employees. It becomes apparent early in the litigation process that the various parties have substantially different interests. Umbrella policies, which are commonly found in HSOs, do not include employees as named insureds. This means, for example, that legally an individual employee has no voice in a decision to settle a lawsuit. Although not a legal determination, settling suggests an admission of fault. This may be adverse to the employee's interests from the standpoints of professional reputation, licensure, certification, and references. Conversely, a personal policy gives one a much more powerful position. It is important to recall that the Health Care Quality Improvement Act, described in Chapter 4, requires that payments made for the benefit of physicians *and* licensed independent practitioners be reported to the national data bank. This greatly increases the effects of settling a malpractice claim and makes it important for affected parties to have maximum control.

Members of the HSO's governing body are not employees. They should be protected against legal actions for errors and omissions under a directors' and officers' liability policy, a policy that should be provided by the HSO.

The Process of RM   It is crucial that an RM system report circumstances that put HSOs at risk. These can be fire and safety problems, accidents, or any type of negligence. Common to such control systems is a written statement, usually called an incident or occurrence report. Incident or occurrence reports alert risk managers to specific problems and, when aggregated, show problem areas and patterns. Figure 12.5 is a sample occurrence report form. Some states include such reporting as part of QA/I. This protects the reports under state laws that limit legal discovery of information used to improve the quality of care. These laws were passed in the belief that allowing plaintiffs' attorneys access to QA/I information had a chilling effect on physicians' willingness to engage in peer review. Such legal limits reduce the likelihood that a plaintiff will succeed. On balance, however, society's interests are better served by promoting QA/I-related activities.

Analysis of data from reporting systems is used in the feedback loop—it informs the risk manager about problems and suggests steps to correct them. For example, data about falls because patients had excessive waits in getting assistance to use the toilet could be used to support a nursing service request for more staff. Data about postsurgical wound infections could be used to improve the training of staff in central sterile supply, or it could be used to teach correct handwashing techniques to nursing staff. Data about the number of back injuries to staff who move patients could result in training about proper lifting techniques.

Legal counsel should review the RM program. Their advice about the effects of certain ac-

THE GEORGE WASHINGTON UNIVERSITY MEDICAL CENTER

OCCURRENCE REPORT

(READ INSTRUCTIONS ON REVERSE SIDE BEFORE COMPLETING)

| ☐ Inpatient | ☐ Outpatient | ☐ Other | SEX | DATE OF BIRTH |
| ☐ Staff | ☐ Visitor | | ☐ Male ☐ Female | |

OCCURRENCE

Location ▶ _____ Date ▶ _____
Day of Wk. ▶ _____ Time ▶ _____

ADMITTING DIAGNOSIS (IF APPLICABLE)

TYPE OF OCCURRENCE AND/OR RELATED FACTORS

☐ Found on Floor*   *See Reverse Side
☐ Witnessed Fall/Slip
  ☐ Ambulating
  ☐ Sitting
  ☐ From Bed
  ☐ Other

☐ Medication/Transfusion/IV Related*
  ☐ Procedural Error
  ☐ Allergic Drug Reaction/Drug Interaction
  ☐ Transfusion Reaction
  ☐ IV Technique Error

☐ Equipment/Use Related

☐ Infection Control

☐ Complaint
☐ Behavior
☐ AMA/Walkout

☐ Property Loss/Damage
☐ Physical Plant Related

☐ Documentation Related
☐ Communication Related
☐ Policy/Procedure/Practice Variance
☐ Permit/Authorization

☐ Invasive Procedure Complication
☐ Cardiac/Respiratory Arrest in Operative Suite
☐ Surgery Complication
☐ Foreign Body Possibly Retained
☐ Return to Operating Room, Same Admission
☐ Anesthesia Complication
☐ Cancellation of Surgery After Inducing Anesthesia

☐ Other _____

PERSONS INVOLVED

NAME	DEPARTMENT/ADDRESS	PHONE NO.	PROFESSIONAL DESIGNATION TRAINING YEAR (If Applicable)

FACTS

BRIEFLY GIVE THE FACTS OF THE OCCURRENCE. AVOID OPINION OR SPECULATION. INDICATE INVOLVEMENT OF THE ABOVE INDIVIDUALS, APPARENT INJURY/LOSS/DAMAGE, MENTAL STATUS AND PATIENT REACTION, IF ANY.

RESPONSE TO OCCURRENCE

	NAME	TIME	METHOD OF NOTIFICATION	BY WHOM	RESPONSE
PHYSICIAN(S) NOTIFIED					
OTHERS NOTIFIED					
OTHER ACTION TAKEN AND BY WHOM					

DIAGNOSTIC/THERAPEUTIC INTERVENTIONS

	TEST/PROCEDURE	RESULT
☐ NONE INDICATED		
☐ RADIOLOGIC STUDIES ▶		
☐ LABORATORY STUDIES ▶		
☐ SURGERY ▶		
☐ EMERGENCY UNIT REFERRAL ▶		
☐ SUTURES ▶		
☐ OTHER _____ ▶		

COMPLETED BY	DATE	TIME	SUPERVISOR	DATE	TIME

PHYSICIAN FOLLOW-UP

DID OCCURRENCE RESULT IN INJURY? ☐ NO ☐ YES   DESCRIBE _____

Treatment/Observation Prescribed	Indication	Patient Response

FURTHER FOLLOW-UP CARE INDICATED?   ☐ NO
☐ YES, PLEASE SPECIFY ▶ _____

PHYSICIAN'S SIGNATURE ▶ _____ DATE ▶ _____ TIME ▶ _____

GWH-191 (3/85)

Figure 12.5. Sample occurrence report form. (From The George Washington University Medical Center; reprinted by permission.)

tions is indispensable. If counsel are available on site (in-house counsel), it is likely they will be more involved in an RM program than would be retainer counsel. Some HSOs use in-house counsel as the risk manager. Regardless, legal counsel must participate in the program.

The risk manager can minimize loss after injury to patients has occurred by immediately taking four steps. First, if the patient has been discharged, the medical record (including radiographs) should be obtained and absolute custody of it retained by the risk manager. Second, if the patient continues under treatment and the record is active, it should be photocopied (new entries are photocopied on a regular basis) and the copy retained by the risk manager. This standard operating procedure should be known throughout the HSO. Third, meetings should be held with the patient and/or relatives to determine their interest in settling any potential claim. Once the patient or relatives have legal counsel the case becomes much more complex and costly. Fourth, the HSO should do whatever it can to retain the patient's goodwill; above all, insult should not be added to injury. An injured patient who needs additional treatment should never be sent a bill for the extra services. Angry patients are much more likely to sue than are those who believe the HSO did the best it could under the circumstances and acted responsibly.

Efforts at early settlement raise a potential conflict of interest. Patients and their relatives should clearly understand that the risk manager is an HSO employee. Risk managers must never allow a patient to believe that they are an advocate for the patient or acting as legal counsel on the patient's behalf. Honesty and forthrightness succeed far better than other tactics. Fraud or misrepresentation by the risk manager not only are unethical, but will cause a court to set aside any agreement and may result in criminal charges or punitive damages being levied against the HSO.

Assessing and Improving Quality

Early concerns about the quality of clinical practice in HSOs focused on hospitals and were addressed through peer review, which is defined as physician review of the care provided by physicians and other types of caregivers. The American College of Surgeons (ACS) began developing the concept of peer review in 1912. In 1918, it published the *Minimum Standard*, part of which addressed peer review of medical practice: "the (medical) staff (shall) review and analyze at regular intervals their clinical experience in the various departments of the hospital."[25] The work of the ACS was continued by the Joint Commission on Accreditation of Hospitals, now the Joint Commission on Accreditation of Healthcare Organizations (Joint Commission), when it was formed in 1951.

The process of peer review was called medical audit, terminology that was used into the 1960s. Enactment of Medicare codified utilization review, which focused on use of services by beneficiaries. Utilization review did not directly affect quality of care in hospitals, except that judging the appropriateness of admission, use of ancillary services, and length of stay minimized nosocomial (institution-caused) and iatrogenic (physician-caused) problems. The current focus of utilization review in Medicare was discussed in Chapter 2. Medical audit utilization review did not stress solving the problems that were identified.

Efforts to measure quality continued to evolve. In the early 1970s, the Joint Commission required quality assessment activities, a variation of medical audit. In the middle 1970s the term changed to medical care evaluation, but it remained essentially medical audit. By 1980, the concept of quality assurance had become a Joint Commission standard. QA meant that the standards had evolved from problem finding (medical audit) to a more proactive and dynamic concept. QA went beyond identifying and describing problems and stressed problem solving to improve clinical quality. In 1991, the Joint Commission changed QA to quality assessment and improvement (QA/I). This shift to a focus on clinical indicators, combined with applying the principles of continuous quality improvement, is discussed below.

Quality Defined   Historically, quality has been defined as the degree of adherence to standards or criteria. As applied in health services, QA meant using prospectively determined criteria to measure performance, something usually done retrospectively. Newer definitions of quality are discussed in Chapter 11 in the context of CQI. These include conformance to requirements and fitness for use or fitness for need and are customer driven because they focus on customer expectations and do not exclusively reflect criteria or standards developed through professional expertise. It is suggested that quality should be defined as meeting latent needs—identifying "needs" customers may not even know they have but are pleased when the provider identifies and meets them. CQI defines customer broadly to include all those who receive goods or services.

Measuring quality using the concepts of QA required that the HSO establish standards (criteria), typically by using professional judgment. Developing criteria was only the first step, however. Two other elements were necessary: a means of surveillance to identify deviations that required action, and stopping the deviation or minimizing its recurrence—the corrective action. These steps were simple in theory and may have been in practice, as well, depending on what was being measured. Much of the conceptual framework buttressing efforts to measure quality was developed by Avedis Donabedian, a physician. His nomenclature of *structure, process, and outcome* is standard in health services. Structure and process were the major foci of the Joint Commission's QA standards in the 1980s.

Donabedian notes the difficulty of developing a definition of quality medical care and measuring the quality of the interpersonal relationship between physician and patient—a relationship essential to the process of care as well as reflected in the outcome of care. Technical aspects of care are more definable and measurable than are interpersonal relationships.[26] Regardless, however, measuring quality under traditional QA began with criteria, whether developed internally, externally imposed, or a combination of the two.

Donabedian defines *structure* as the tools and resources that providers of care have at their disposal and the physical and organizational settings in which they work.[27] *Process* is the set of activities that go on within HSOs and between practitioners and patients. Here, judgment of quality may be made either by direct observation or by reviewing recorded information. Donabedian considers this means of measuring quality to be largely normative in that the norms come either from the science of medicine or from the ethics and values of society.[28] *Outcome* is a change in a patient's current and future health status that can be attributed to antecedent health care.[29] Donabedian defines outcome broadly to include improvement of social and psychological function in addition to physical and physiological aspects. Also included are patient attitudes, health-related knowledge acquired by the patient, and health-related behavioral change.[30]

Structure, Process, and Outcome Compared   Donabedian concludes that "good structure, that is, a sufficiency of resources and proper system design, is probably the most important means of protecting and promoting the quality of care."[31] He adds that assessing structure is a good deal less important than assessing process and outcome. Comparing process and outcome, Donabedian concluded that neither is clearly preferable. Either may be superior, depending on the situation and what is being measured. Donabedian emphasized that it is critical, however, to know the link between the content of the process and the resulting outcome. Only by knowing this link (preferably at the level of a causal relationship) can what is done or not done in the process be modified to improve the outcome. Achieving a desired outcome without knowing how it was achieved makes replication impossible. Table 12.1 shows the advantages and disadvantages of focusing on process and outcome to measure quality. Outcome indicators in Donabedian's taxonomy focus on the overall outcomes of medical care, such as health status and disability. The approach by the Joint Commission includes, as well, outcomes of specific aspects of the process of care.

Development and application of these theories and concepts of QA reached a peak in the late 1980s. At that point the Joint Commission began to emphasize indicators of the outcomes of the process of care and undertook a major shift to adopting CQI, a process detailed in Chapter 11. At

Table 12.1. Advantages and disadvantages of process and outcome measures of quality

Process		Outcome	
Advantages	Disadvantages	Advantages	Disadvantages
Practitioners have no great difficulty specifying technical criteria for standards of care Even not fully validated standards and criteria can serve as interim measures of acceptable practice Information about technical aspects of care is documented in the medical record and is usually accessible as well as timely—can be used for prevention and intervention Use of this information permits specific attribution of responsibility so that credit or blame can be more easily ascertained and specific corrective action taken	Great weakness in the scientific basis for much of accepted practice and use of prevalent norms as basis for judging quality may encourage dogmatism and perpetuate error Because practitioners prefer to err on the side of doing more than is necessary, there is a tendency toward overly elaborate and costly care; this is reflected in the norms While technical aspects are overemphasized, management of the interpersonal process tends to be ignored, partly because the usual sources of data give little information about the physician-patient relationship	When the scientific basis for accepted practice is in doubt emphasis on outcome tends to discourage dogmatism and helps maintain a more open and flexible approach to management Open and flexible approach may help in development of less costly but no less effective strategies of care Outcomes reflect all the contributions of all the practitioners to the care of the patient and thus provide an inclusive, integrative measure of the quality of care Also reflected in the outcome is the patient's contribution to the care that may have been influenced by the relationship between patient and practitioners; a more direct assessment of the patient-physician relationship can be obtained by including aspects of patient satisfaction among measures of care	Even expert practitioners are unable to specify the outcomes of optimal care, as to their magnitude, timing, and duration When indicators of health status are obtained, it is difficult to know how much of the observed effect can be attributed to medical care Choosing outcomes that have marginal relevance to the objectives of prior care is an ever-present pitfall; even when relevant outcomes are selected, information about many outcomes is often not available in time to make it useful for certain types of monitoring Waiting for a pattern of adverse outcomes can be questioned on ethical grounds Examining outcomes without examining means of attaining them may result in a lack of attention to the presence of redundant or overly costly care

Adapted with permission from Donabedian, Avedis. *Explorations in Quality Assessment and Monitoring.* Vol. I, *The Definition of Quality and Approaches to its Assessment,* 119–122. Ann Arbor, MI: Health Administration Press, 1980.

the highest point of development in the 1991 AMH, the standards prescribed a 10-step process for conducting QA:

1. Assign responsibility for monitoring and evaluation activities;
2. Delineate the scope of care provided by the organization;
3. Identify the most important aspects of care provided by the organization;
4. Identify indicators (and appropriate clinical criteria) for monitoring the important aspects of care;
5. Establish thresholds (levels, patterns, trends) for the indicators that trigger evaluation of the care;
6. Monitor the important aspects of care by collecting and organizing the data for each indicator;
7. Evaluate care when thresholds are reached in order to identify either opportunities to improve care or problems;
8. Take actions to improve care or to correct identified problems;
9. Assess the effectiveness of the actions and document the improvement in care; and
10. Communicate the results of the monitoring and evaluation process to relevant individuals, departments, or services and to the organizationwide quality assurance program.[32]

Despite the focus of steps 8 and 9, it is generally conceded that QA as implemented in the 1980s was less than effective in improving the quality of care. "On the whole, to the extent that quality measurement tools have been developed at all, they tend to unveil the *fact* of flaw, not its *cause*."[33]

The 1992 AMH deleted the 10-step process, but its vestiges are likely to be found well into the 1990s, especially in nonhospital HSOs, as CQI concepts are fully implemented. Equally significant is that the 1992 AMH no longer uses quality assurance; instead, quality assessment and improvement is used. The new focus is a major paradigm shift for all HSOs accredited by the Joint Commission.

Developments for the 1990s   The Joint Commission's shift to a focus on outcome indicators began in 1988. Its "Agenda for Change" began to identify outcome measures for major areas of acute care hospital activity. This followed by about one year the release of hospital mortality data by the Health Care Financing Administration. The first clinical indicators to be developed were hospital-wide care and obstetrical and anesthesia care.[34] In early 1989, 12 key principles of organizational and management effectiveness were announced and pilot testing was undertaken. The purpose was to characterize an acute care hospital's commitment to continuously improve its quality of care. A central aspect is that applying quality improvement relies on identifying and monitoring outcome indicators that assist the hospital in focusing attention for its QA/I activities. By 1991 indicators had been developed for anesthesia, obstetrics, cardiovascular, oncology, and trauma care.[35]

The work of the Joint Commission in developing indicators is being complemented by numerous physician organizations that are developing practice parameters (guidelines). "Practice parameters are a generic term for acceptable approaches to the prevention, diagnosis, treatment, or management of a disease or condition, as determined by the medical profession based on the best medical evidence currently available."[36] Practice parameters are not the same as indicators. Practice parameters are a means for describing what should be done; indicators are a means for measuring. "Once one moves from determining what ought to be done to seeing if or how often it is done, one moves from guidelines [parameters] to indicators."[37]

By 1990, 26 physician organizations had developed practice parameters for their specialties. The American Academy of Pediatrics was the first to do so in 1938.[38] It was not until the late 1970s that such efforts gained momentum. In addition to setting guidelines for physicians, practice parameters are instrumental in setting the legal standard of care, which was described in Chapter 4. Work by the American Society of Anesthesiologists in setting practice parameters for intraoperative monitoring (monitoring during surgery) has been credited with eliminating hypoxic (insufficient oxygen) injury lawsuits and causing a significant reduction in medical malpractice insurance premiums.[39] Table 12.2 shows the preferred practice pattern guide for a comprehensive adult eye evaluation that was developed by the American Academy of Ophthalmology.

Importance of QA/I   The importance of evaluating quality was suggested in Chapter 2. Several reasons should be reiterated, however. HSOs that seek Joint Commission accreditation must have organized, effective QA/I activities. Unaccredited acute care hospitals are not in "deemed status" for purposes of Medicare reimbursement and must meet the conditions of participation established by the Department of Health and Human Services. Accreditors of medical education programs in HSOs usually demand that the HSO be accredited. Insurance carriers that write coverage for HSOs expect them to be accredited, and lending institutions and organizations that rate bond offerings consider accreditation important in their decisions. Chapter 7, "How HSOs Are Organized," details the importance of credentialing the clinical staff, and this activity is indispensable to QA/I. In addition, failing to effectively assess and improve quality increases the probability of adverse medical malpractice judgments because the HSO has not met the legal standard of care.

QA/I is considered important by managerial, clinical, and support staff who want to do their

Table 12.2. Excerpts from "Comprehensive Adult Eye Evaluation" preferred practice pattern guideline

I. Components of Physical Examination
The comprehensive examination consists of an evaluation of the physiological functioning and the anatomic status of the eye, visual system, and its related structures. In general, this will include, but not be limited to, evaluation of the following:

Physiological function:
1. Visual acuity with present correction (the power of the present correction recorded) at distance, and where appropriate, near;
2. Measurement of best corrected visual acuity (with refraction where indicated);
3. Ocular alignment and motility;
4. Pupil; and
5. Intraocular pressure.

Anatomical status:
6. Lids, lashes and lacrimal apparatus, orbit, and other facial features which may be pertinent;
7. Anterior segment: tear film, conjunctiva, sclera, cornea, anterior chamber, iris, lens, posterior chamber; and
8. Posterior segment: vitreous, retina (including posterior pole and periphery), uvea, vessels, and optic nerve.

Examination of anterior segment structures will routinely involve gross and biomicroscopic evaluation prior to dilation. Evaluation of structures situated posterior to the iris will generally require dilatation of the pupil. Posterior segment structures will be routinely examined with an ophthalmoscope.

While it is assumed the ophthalmologist will perform most of the examination, certain aspects of data collection may be conducted by another trained individual under the ophthalmologist's supervision and with his or her review.

II. Timing of Evaluation for "Normal" Patient
When evaluation is entirely normal or only involves optical abnormalities requiring a spectacle prescription, the ophthalmologist will reassure the patient and advise him or her with regard to the appropriate interval for re-examination. All patients are advised to return as soon as possible should ocular symptoms or related problems develop.

In the *absence of symptoms or other indications,* patients should generally be seen for a comprehensive examination within the period indicated below, which takes into account the relationship between their age and race and the risk of asymptomatic or otherwise overlooked disease:

65 years or older	every 1–2 years
40–64 years	every 2–4 years
20–39 years	African-Americans, because of the high incidence and more aggressive course of glaucoma even in the absence of visual or ocular symptoms, should be seen every 3–5 years. Others can be seen less frequently.

Interim examinations may be expected to be performed for discrete purposes, routine refractions, and patient reassurance at more frequent intervals.

From Sommer, Alfred, Jonathan P. Weiner, and Lea Gamble. Developing specialtywide standards of practice: The experience of ophthalmology. *Quality Review Bulletin, 16* (February 1990): 67; copyright 1990 by the Joint Commission on Accreditation of Healthcare Organizations, Oakbrook Terrace, IL; reprinted with permission from the February 1990 *Quality Review Bulletin.*

Note: Do not apply these excerpts without consulting original text. They are taken out of context.

best. They strive to do so because they are professionals who have internalized the motivation to provide high-quality care and be part of an excellent HSO. This includes and necessitates the need to learn what is being done correctly and what is not, as well as how to improve performance.

Figure 12.6 shows the flow of QA/I activities. Data sources (many of which will be outcome indicators) focus the attention of the coordinating body, which may be called the quality assessment and improvement council. The coordinating body sanctions establishment of cross-functional quality improvement teams to investigate processes and recommend changes to improve them. The coordinating body may also establish intradepartmental quality improvement teams, or this may be done by the department itself. In addition, the department may assign individual workers who are process owners to monitor and improve a process. The coordinating body approves major changes and expenditures.

Quality Improvement (QI) and Quality Assurance (QA) Compared[40] As HSOs increasingly use the philosophy and techniques of CQI, it is vital to understand its relationship to the traditional approach of QA. This is especially important during the transition period of the 1990s. As described in Chapter 11, QI (or CQI) necessitates a paradigm shift because it uses powerful

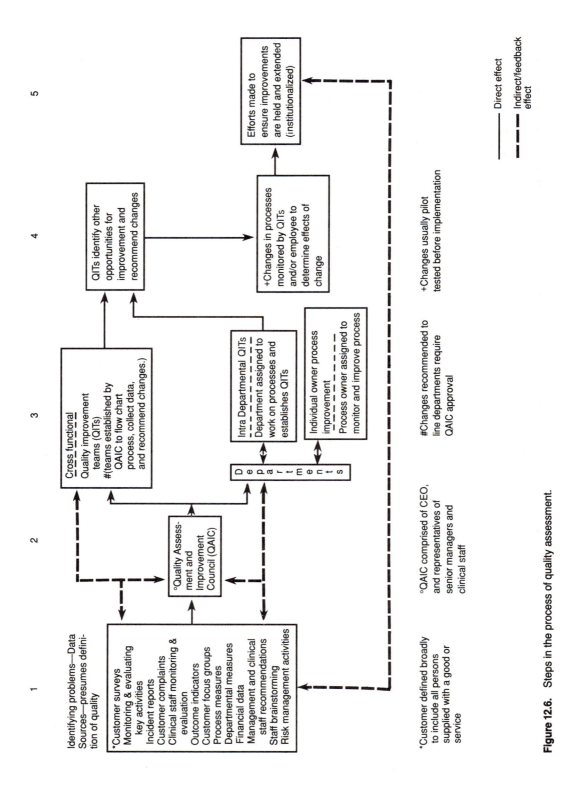

Figure 12.6. Steps in the process of quality assessment.

462

tools supported by a radically different philosophy about relationships between managers and employees.

Some steps and tools in the Joint Commission's 10-step process are similar to QI, but the philosophy and basic approach are different. Most differences are obvious, even with a brief description (Table 12.3). Conceptually, some bear further attention: the focus on why versus who; focusing on all processes to improve fitness for use; efforts to improve processes rather than solve problems; and assumptions about the irreducibility of problems. Despite some anecdotes or case experience to the contrary, QA is typically seen as a negative process. It focuses on the "who" of problem identification and solution; being found in the middle of a problem is risky for caregivers and others participating in the process. QI seeks the why of a problem or inefficiency; even those directly involved in a process are not the focus. In this regard, QI has adopted the view of W. Edwards Deming, whose theories were described in Chapter 11, that 85%–94% of problems are the fault of the process; only the small percentage remaining are caused by the people working in it.

Typically, QA exclusively measured the quality of clinical practice, which has been the Joint Commission's focus. QI looks at clinical practice, but is equally concerned with the myriad of processes and systems that support delivery of clinical services, as well as those that are administrative such as admitting and patient accounts. Clinical and administrative aspects of many processes cannot be easily separated, and QI will look at integrated or cross-functional processes as well as those that are intradepartmental. Improvements in an HSO's support and administrative areas increase quality there and positively affect clinical areas because of greater organization-wide quality consciousness and because, without exception, these areas affect clinical services. An example is admitting. Inefficient intradepartmental or interpartmental admitting processes directly and indirectly affect patient care.

Another important difference is that QI focuses on improving processes, whereas QA focused on solving problems. Traditionally, for QA this meant dealing with the unusual or unique—what Deming calls special causes—and, as suggested in the 10-step process, QA investigated indicators that exceeded thresholds. Similar to QA's focus, managers spend much of their time "fighting fires." There are times when putting out fires is necessary, but doing so does not improve processes and does not increase efficiency or effectiveness. Putting out a fire only returns the process, more or less, to the state it was in before the fire started. There is a school of thought in the QI movement that asserts that unique and unusual results or outcomes should be ignored

Table 12.3. Characteristics of QI versus QA

QI	QA
"Why" focused (positive)	"Who" focused (negative)
Prospective	Retrospective
Internally directed	Externally directed
Follows patients	Follows organizational structure
Involves the many	Delegated to the few
Integrated analysis	Divided analysis
Bottom up	Top down
Proactive	Reactive
Employee focused	Management focused (directing)
Full staff involvement	Limited staff involvement
Process based	Event based
Process approach	Inspection approach
Quality is integral activity	Quality is separate activity
Focus on all processes to improve fitness for use	Focus on meeting clinical criteria
Focus on improving processes	Focus on solving problems
Makes no assumption about irreducibility of problems	Assumes problems/numbers of problems reach irreducible number

unless they pose a danger and that attention should be exclusive to process improvement. HSO managers cannot ignore unusual or unique events that affect patients, but the effort spent on them should be minimized because the real gain comes from improving processes to reduce variation, error rates, and other inefficiencies.

Assumptions that have been made about the irreducibility of problems are the most insidious dimension of the philosophy of QA and have probably been responsible for delaying improvement in quality of care. This in no way diminishes the work of persons in QA during the 1980s—they were hampered by its conceptual framework and the limited tools it provided.

Psychologically, it is crucial that "good enough" is no longer acceptable; QI rejects it. An element of "good enough" is suggested when HSOs compare outcome indicators or other performance measures with their own criteria, or with external criteria. Criteria and indicators are important as a starting point and to gain a macro-level understanding of outcomes produced by an HSO or from a process. The fact is that organizations in which CQI has been implemented improve quality by reducing waste, rework, and redundancy, not by accepting a place within the herd. Until a systematic search for the root causes of medication errors has been done using the tools of QI, for example, no one knows what the irreducible level of medication errors is.

Despite the differences in philosophy and process between QI and QA and the extent of the paradigm shift that is occurring, QI and QA have complementary elements. For example, QA monitoring of clinical indicators is the basis for prioritizing processes to be improved, using QI tools and techniques.

In the final analysis, improving clinical (and managerial) quality in HSOs requires change. If Deming is correct that only 6%–15% of problems result from causes within the worker's control, it is up to management to change processes so staff can improve quality. Traditionally, however, managers have assumed that poor quality occurs because employees *choose* to perform suboptimally. Managers must shed this viewpoint.

What must be remembered, especially with the increased emphasis on outcome indicators, is that understanding the link between process and outcome is crucial. Unless it is known how the outcome was produced, desired outcomes cannot be purposefully replicated, nor can a process be changed to prevent undesired outcomes.

Final Comments

Readers should have a clear sense of the importance of measuring the quality of clinical and managerial performance and managing risk. These processes have an important place in the control function of managers in HSOs. Making changes is more difficult in HSOs, where much that is done is a personal service rendered by clinical staff who are, in many cases, independent contractors. For the manager, this requires attention to interpersonal skills and an ability to work with and through people. Maintaining quality of care for patients and protecting employees and visitors depend largely on these skills.

Improving quality (and minimizing risk) is part of the manager's control function described previously and shown in the control model in Figure 12.2. In terms of clinical practice, the purpose is to improve the quality of care. Size, organizational complexity, severity of patient illness, and intensity of service necessitate that acute care hospitals have sophisticated RM programs and make extensive efforts to improve quality. Increasingly, similar programs are found in all HSOs. Pragmatically, there are no differences between the type of statistical quality control used in industry and that which can be applied to many HSO activities. Even the methodologies used in clinical areas are remarkably alike.

It is platitudinous, but true nonetheless, to say that managers must be part of the solution or they will remain a part of the problem. Managers should be unwilling to accept an attitude anywhere in the HSO that what is being done is "good enough."

CONTROL METHODS

Managers use numerous methods and techniques to monitor and control inputs, processes, and/or outputs. RM and QA are examples of structured, programmatic control methods. Others are budgeting, case-mix accounting, operational-activity and financial ratio analysis, and network programming.

Budgeting

One of the most common methods for control is the use of budgets. They serve a dual purpose. First, they are numerical expressions of plans,[41] and, second, they become control standards against which results are compared.[42] Types of budgets and time frames vary. Most, such as operating expense and revenue budgets, are made for one year; capital expenditure budgets, however, may be multiyear.[43]

Budgeting depends on planning and forecasting. Individual cost centers or departments forecast the volume of service they expect to deliver, workload demand, and resources needed in the next budget period. Cost centers are organizational units in which there is a well-defined relationship between inputs and outputs. Examples are surgery, nursing service, clinics, laboratories, pharmacy, diagnostic testing, dietary, patient billing, medical records, and maintenance. Based on expected work loads, revenue budgets can be derived for those units with which revenues can be associated; examples are the emergency department, clinics, diagnostic testing, pharmacy, and surgery. For all departments, including those in which revenues cannot be directly associated, such as nursing service, social services, maintenance, and administration, operating expense budgets are derived that reflect the amount and types of resources necessary to perform the projected work load.

Operating expense budgets include two types: direct and indirect. Direct expenses are those that are incurred by a cost center or a department and can be specifically attributed to it. They include labor and nonlabor components. Human resource requirements must be converted to dollars paid for salary and wages. Nonlabor expenses are supplies and equipment. Indirect expenses include overhead costs throughout the institution, such as general facility maintenance, building depreciation, utilities, and management staff not identified with specific cost centers. They are usually allocated among cost centers on some basis such as space occupied, number of employees, or volume of output. Usually cost centers have control only over their direct expenses.

Operating budgets can be fixed or variable.[44] Fixed budgets represent a resource commitment to a cost center or department for the budget period. They are based on planned work load. Variable budgets recognize that as volume, work load, or service demands change, so will resource need. Often, hybrid fixed-variable operating budgets are developed. They separate costs into fixed and variable components, with the latter changing as work load increases or decreases.

Budgets force managers to be aware of how input resources are used and the associated costs for staff, materials, equipment, or supplies. Preparing a budget requires managers to think about the cost and amount of resources that will be consumed and used in conversion. Also, budgets are standards against which results can be compared. Typically, budget reports are prepared monthly to compare actual expenditures for the month and the year to date with the amount budgeted. Variances that indicate deviations of actual from budgeted amounts can be identified and used for control purposes.

A sample hospital pharmacy budget that reports inpatient and outpatient revenues and direct operating expenses for the month of May is presented in Table 12.4. It shows actual, budget, budget variance, and percentage of actual to budget amount information for the current month and the year to date. (Variance is the difference between planned budgeted revenues/expenditures and actual revenues/expenditures for a given period.) Budget reports such as these enable managers to

Table 12.4. Sample pharmacy revenue and expense budget, month ending May 31 and year to date

Description	Current month					Current year to date				
	Month actual	Month fixed budget	Month budget variance	% of budget	Over/under	Year-to-date actual	Year-to-date fixed budget	Year-to-date variance	% of budget	Over/under
Revenues										
Inpatient	$1,071,522	$821,038	$250,484	30.5	ov	$11,764,145	$9,852,467	$1,911,678	19.4	ov
Outpatient	938,405	742,145	196,260	26.4	ov	9,764,407	8,905,737	858,670	9.6	ov
TOTAL	$2,009,927	$1,563,183	$446,744	28.6	ov	$21,528,552	$18,758,204	$2,770,348	14.8	ov
Expenses										
Wages and salaries	$77,503	$69,003	$8,500	12.3	ov	$904,207	$837,662	$66,545	7.9	ov
Costs of drugs sold	172,765	110,917	61,848	55.8	ov	1,915,048	1,331,010	584,038	43.9	ov
Cost of hemophilia drugs	350,861	283,542	67,319	23.7	ov	3,724,591	3,402,500	322,091	9.5	ov
Intravenous solutions	31,201	22,912	8,289	36.2	ov	273,882	274,941	(1,059)	(0.4)	un
Purchased service	1,152	1,263	(111)	(8.8)	un	15,416	15,300	116	0.8	ov
Pharmacy overhead	4,211	2,548	1,663	65.3	ov	35,477	30,600	4,877	15.9	ov
TOTAL	$637,693	$490,185	$147,508	30.0	ov	$6,868,621	$5,892,013	$976,608	16.6	ov
Revenues minus expenses	$1,372,234	$1,072,998	$299,236	27.9	ov	$14,659,931	$12,866,191	$1,793,740	13.9	ov

exercise greater control over resource use and determine if department activity such as revenue generation is meeting projections.

Case–Mix Accounting

HSOs typically control resource consumption and conversion through the budget process at cost center or department level. This vertical form of budgeting in which direct and indirect costs are identified and monitored has limitations, however. The most important is that it does not accurately identify true final costs associated with patient care outcomes. Prospective or output-based pricing (i.e, diagnosis-related groups [DRGs]) caused HSOs to develop a new control technique known as horizontal budgeting, which identifies and monitors costs within and across cost center and departmental lines and those associated with specific final outputs.[45] The goal of horizontal budgeting, which is commonly known as case-mix accounting, is to present a complete financial picture of the costs of treating individual patients grouped into similar classes (case-mix or DRG) on the basis of resource use.[46]

Industry has used horizontal cost-finding and allocation systems for years.[47] By analyzing input—labor, materials, and equipment—and indirect and overhead costs throughout the organization and associating them with different products or services, standard costs by type of output can be determined. Control is exercised by comparing actual costs of final output with prospectively determined standard costs. Analysis of variance allows inferences to be drawn about appropriateness of input consumption and efficiency of conversion.

Before case-mix accounting, HSOs had difficulty defining end products (services) and the costs associated with producing them and had few incentives to do so. A unit of service such as patient day is a poor output measure because it fails to reflect variations in resource use resulting from factors such as admission type or severity of medical problems (e.g., acuity level). For example, providing care for a high-risk premature infant requires very different resources from various cost centers than does care for a full-term infant not at risk. Also, nursing service resources necessary to care for severely ill rather than convalescing patients differ, although the intermediate output measure, patient day, is the same.

Case-mix accounting gives HSOs an allocation process that identifies true costs associated with final outputs by type and severity of case. DRGs are such a classification. Once standard costs by type of final output are identified, operating expense and/or revenue budgets can be prepared on the basis of expected number of patients by type of case. Throughout the budget period, interim reports providing information comparing actual costs to budget projections by case type enable managers to more effectively monitor and control use of input resources. Such reports also enable them to analyze the net contribution (profitability) of cases by specific types (i.e., relationship of true costs to revenues regardless of whether payment is prospective or based on charges). In short, a case-mix cost allocation system that identifies costs associated with final, as opposed to intermediate, outputs provides managers with more accurate information about true costs and thus improves their ability to control input use and the conversion processes that generate outputs.

Ratio Analysis

The language common to all organizations is numerically expressed data. For example, HSOs are described by number and type of beds, by number of employees and type, and by size and specialty mix of members of the professional staff organization; they are evaluated, in part, by number of patients admitted, procedures performed, and expenditures. Managers use similar data to control (monitor) the HSO's functioning and how well it is done. This may be done by comparing any activity to predetermined standards, or by ratio analysis. The latter involves evaluating the relationship between two pieces of data that may be expressed as an index or percentage. They are simple measures and typically occur in two modes; point specific and longitudinal. The analysis is generally applied to two areas, operational-activity and financial status.[48]

Operational-Activity Analysis   Operational-activity analysis is a control method that involves the evaluation of any activity—input, process, or output variable—that is of interest to the manager and that can be expressed numerically. Control charts are one form of operational-activity analysis. Control charts have predetermined standards—upper and lower control limits—that can be developed for any form of unit volume or measurable product or service attribute. Chapter 11 includes a control chart for patient waiting time in the admitting department (see Figure 11.6). Other types of control charts include portion size of meals, age of blood in the blood bank, or time to answer incoming phone calls.

Another method for operational-activity analysis is through use and evaluation of nonfinancial indices expressed as ratios or percentages. Managers can design any type of operational-activity ratio (or percentage index) to meet specific control needs as long as it can be expressed in numerical terms. Such ratios are valuable in controlling because they can be used as point-specific input, conversion, and output standards and as indicators of improvement; and they can be tracked and compared longitudinally to show trends. The variety and derivations of such ratios are endless. Three broad categories are performance-utilization ratios, input-to-output ratios, and key indicator ratios.

Performance-utilization ratios provide index information about specific activities such as inventory turnover by area (dietary services, pharmacy, general stores, laboratory), inventory dollar value per occupied bed, percentage of readmissions, and personnel turnover and absenteeism by area or type of employee. Ratios also yield information about capacity utilization such as average length of stay, percentage occupancy, and efficient use of space and time (surgical suites, clinics, emergency department, radiology). Finally, they can provide indices of specific process outputs usually expressed in patient days or some other common denominator; for example, radiographs per admission, laboratory tests per patient day, clinic visits per day, and pounds of laundry processed per occupied bed.

Input-to-output ratios are indicators of resource consumption. They relate specific measures of resource use to units of output. Examples include the whole range of labor hours per unit of service, such as nursing hours per patient day, radiographs per radiology technician hour, and square feet cleaned per housekeeping hour. Another type of input-to-output ratio is cost of supplies per patient day.

Key indicator ratios fall outside the previous two groups, but are important to control. Incident ratios yield inferences about quality. Examples are patient incidents and injuries per 100 patient days, percentage of incomplete medical records 24 hours after discharge, gross and net death rates, anesthesia deaths per 10,000 surgical procedures, infection rates, and percentage of normal tissue removed in operative procedures. Other key indicator ratios include patient mix by type of payor, average age of clinical staff or mix by specialty, and patient origin by service area segment.

Data analysis services that provide comparative operational-activity analyses are available from vendors. The most widely known vendor is Hospital Administrative Services (HAS), a subsidiary of the American Hospital Association (AHA). Table 12.5 presents one sample of the many reports available from HAS/MONITREND II™. In this case, it is an executive summary report for an anonymous medium-sized not-for-profit hospital (the anonymous hospital has between 200 and 299 beds). The top half of the table shows average utilization and revenue ratios for the previous 3 months in the reporting hospital and compares them with those of other hospitals of similar size (200–299 beds) nationally and statewide and with those of selected rural referral centers. The bottom portion contains longitudinal information for the reporting hospital only that compares utilization and revenue ratios for the current month, for the prior 3 months, and for the same

Table 12.5. MONITREND II hospital report with worked hours—level 3

	Hospital indicator	Executive summary—Group data					
		A 101 Hospitals Ind	Qtr	B 14 Hospitals Ind	Qtr	C 53 Hospitals Ind	Qtr
Utilization							
Occupancy percent	59.53	64.06	2	62.16	2	60.90	2
Average daily census	167.29	165.10	3	116.95	4	130.07	3
Average length of stay	6.52	6.61	2	6.56	2	6.34	3
Medicare percent all patient days	61.11	54.04	3	54.04	4	53.89	4
Medicare average length of stay	8.34	8.70	2	8.34	2	7.95	3
Medicare case-mix index	1.34	1.25	4	1.21	4	1.23	4
Hospital case-mix index	0.93	1.01	2	0.95	2	0.96	2
Revenue data							
Inpatient revenue per patient day	851.42	1052.35	1	978.38	2	931.77	2
Inpatient revenue per discharge	5547.09	6908.90	1	6836.71	2	5869.10	2
Med surgical/card revenue/ICU day	558.75	778.20	1	694.46	2	708.23	1
Inpatient revenue/acute care day	223.12	328.89	1	249.35	2	293.49	1
Inpatient revenue/subacute care day	298.99	304.87	2	331.32	2	301.30	2
Outpatient revenue percent	24.82	26.26	2	20.76	4	28.26	2
Inpatient revenue percent	73.45	71.53	3	76.45	2	69.71	3
Deductions from revenue PCT	35.91	35.20	3	35.56	3	30.22	4
Contract allow % of total revenue	28.77	27.79	3	25.87	4	24.70	4
Charity care PCT of total revenue							

		Executive summary—Internal trend data				
	Apr 1991	3 Mth ending Mar 1991	3 Mth ending Mar 1990	Percent change	3 Mth ending Mar 1989	Percent change
Utilization						
Occupancy percent	58.68	59.53	66.14	−9.99	62.49	−4.74
Average daily census	164.90	167.29	184.52	−9.34	182.48	−8.32
Average length of stay	6.39	6.52	6.90	−5.31	7.13	−8.56
Medicare percent all patient days	63.13	61.11	61.61	−0.81	65.74	−7.04
Medicare average length of stay	8.70	8.34	9.06	−7.95	8.98	−7.13
Medicare case-mix index	1.22	1.34	1.22	9.84	1.22	9.84
Hospital case-mix index	0.87	0.93				
Revenue data						
Inpatient revenue per patient day	876.91	851.42	780.85	9.04	785.74	8.36
Inpatient revenue per discharge	5604.72	5547.09	5387.77	2.96	5605.23	−1.04
Med surgical/card revenue/ICU day	581.54	558.75	559.03	−0.05	539.53	3.56
Inpatient revenue/acute care day	226.26	223.12	225.27	−0.95	215.59	3.49
Inpatient revenue/subacute care day	296.07	295.99	295.05	0.32	300.75	−1.58
Outpatient revenue percent	27.50	24.82	22.46	10.51	18.51	34.09
Inpatient revenue percent	70.72	73.45	75.88	−3.18	79.88	−8.05
Deductions from revenue PCT	35.85	35.91	36.38	−1.29	38.49	−6.70
Contract allow % of total revenue	29.84	28.77	29.98	−4.04	32.77	−12.21
Charity care PCT of total revenue					0.25	

From *MONITREND II hospital report.* Chicago: American Hospital Association, 1991; reprinted by permission. Copyright American Hospital Association, May 1991.

A, National—200 thru 299 beds. B, Oklahoma—100 thru 299 beds. C, Rural referral centers. Ind, indicator.

3 months for each of the preceding 2 years. Such data services are valuable because reports are very extensive and the HSO can choose the other institutions to be used for comparison. Furthermore, point-specific as well as longitudinal information useful for controlling the HSO's activities is readily available to managers.

This discussion of performance-utilization, input-output, and key indicator ratio groupings is not exhaustive, but it does illustrate that ratios can be derived by comparing any two sets of numbers. When used in control, ratio analysis should address two issues. First, does the ratio make sense? Some do, many do not—the ratio of maintenance expenditures per Medicare patient day is meaningless. Managers must evaluate the underlying derivation of the ratio, what it measures, and its meaning. Second, judgment must be used in interpreting results. Particularly important is assessing the many causes of single-point deviation (that occurring at one point) or longitudinal deviation (change over time). Ratios are only one of many indicators that show how actual results deviate from desired results at the input, process, or output points. The cause of the deviation must be investigated, understood, and corrected, if necessary. Blind use without evaluation may result in inappropriate conclusions and intervention and, perhaps, undesirable consequences.

Financial Analysis If data expressed in numerical terms represent the common language of organizations, their lifeblood is finance as it relates to the value of resources. Financial ratio analysis is the process of calculating and evaluating various indices that measure the HSO's financial status: its risk exposure, activity, and profitability.[49] The accepted conventions for these measures are typically grouped into four categories, as summarized in Table 12.6:[50]

Liquidity ratios are risk measures that refer to the HSO's ability to meet short-term obligations. Included are current ratio, acid test, and collection period.

Capital structure ratios are also risk measures. They reflect the ratio of debt (borrowed funds) to total capital structure and, in the case of investor-owned HSOs, the proportion of debt to owners' investment (equity). Generally, higher debt ratio(s) mean greater leverage and higher risk. Other risk-measuring ratios include times interest earned and cash flow to debt.

Activity ratios are turnover measures that reflect asset utilization. In a sense, this is the degree to which various categories of assets generate revenues. Those presented in Table 12.6 compare operating revenues to total, fixed, and current assets and to inventories.

Profitability ratios are indicators of the HSO's performance expressed in financial terms. Particularly critical measures are deductibles (allowances for contractual adjustments and uncollectible accounts), operating margin, nonoperating revenue contribution, and return on assets. A measure important to investor-owned HSOs is return on equity (operating income plus interest divided by stockholders' equity).

Data analysis services are available from vendors, as are operating-activity ratios. Table 12.7 is a sample HAS/MONITORED II™ executive summary financial report for a medium-sized hospital. The top portion of the table compares selected financial indicators for the previous 3 months with those of hospitals of similar size nationally and statewide and with those of selected referral centers. The bottom portion contains longitudinal information for the reporting hospital only that compares profitability, liquidity, and activity ratios for the current month, for the prior 3 months, and for the same 3 months for each of the preceding 2 years.

As with operational-activity ratio analysis, control by using financial ratios requires an understanding of what ratios mean and judgment in interpreting results. Two other points are important. First, meaningful financial ratio analysis incorporates longitudinal assessment (i.e., comparing the same ratio over time). For example, in Table 12.7, the hospital's current ratio ranged between 3.330 and 3.680 during the past 2 years. This is consistent with the 3.442 ratio for simi-

Table 12.6. Common financial ratios used for control

LIQUIDITY

1. Current $= \dfrac{\text{Current Assets}}{\text{Current Liabilities}}$

2. Acid Test $= \dfrac{\text{Cash + Marketable Securities}}{\text{Current Liabilities}}$

3. Collection Period $= \dfrac{\text{Net Accounts Receivable}}{\text{Average Daily Operating Revenue}}$

4. Average Payment Period $= \dfrac{\text{Current Liabilities}}{(\text{Total Operating Expenses } - \text{ Depreciation}) \div 365}$

CAPITAL STRUCTURE

5. Long-Term Debt to Fixed Assets $= \dfrac{\text{Long-Term Debt}}{\text{Net Fixed Assets}}$

6. Long-Term Debt to Equity $= \dfrac{\text{Long-Term Debt}}{\text{Unrestricted Fund Balance}}$

7. Times Interest Earned $= \dfrac{\text{Net Income + Interest}}{\text{Interest}}$

8. Debt Service Coverage $= \dfrac{\text{Net Income + Depreciation + Interest}}{\text{Principal Payment + Interest}}$

9. Cash Flow to Debt $= \dfrac{\text{Net Income + Depreciation}}{\text{Total Liabilities}}$

ACTIVITY

10. Total Asset Turnover $= \dfrac{\text{Total Operating Revenue}}{\text{Total Assets}}$

11. Fixed Asset Turnover $= \dfrac{\text{Total Operating Revenue}}{\text{Net Fixed Assets}}$

12. Current Asset Turnover $= \dfrac{\text{Total Operating Revenue}}{\text{Current Assets}}$

13. Inventory Turnover $= \dfrac{\text{Total Operating Revenue}}{\text{Inventory}}$

PROFITABILITY

14. Mark-up $= \dfrac{\text{Gross Patient Revenue}}{\text{Operating Expenses}}$

15. Deductible $= \dfrac{\text{Allowances for Contractual Adjustments and Uncollectible Accounts}}{\text{Gross Patient Revenue}}$

16. Operating Margin $= \dfrac{\text{Operating Income}}{\text{Operating Revenue}}$

17. Nonoperating Revenue Contribution $= \dfrac{\text{Nonoperating Revenue}}{\text{Net Income}}$

18. Return on Assets $= \dfrac{\text{Operating Income + Interest}}{\text{Total Assets}}$

COMPOSITE

19. Viability Index $= \dfrac{[\text{Total Liabilities}]}{[\text{Total Assets}]} \times \dfrac{[\text{Operating Expense}]}{[\text{Operating Revenue}]} \times \dfrac{1}{\text{Current Ratio}} \times 4.0$

From Cleverley, William O. Financial ratios: Summary indicators for management decision-making. *Hospital & Health Services Administration* 26 (Special Issue, 1981): 30–31; reprinted by permission. © 1981, Foundation of the American College of Healthcare Executives. Ann Arbor, MI: Health Administration Press.

Table 12.7. MONITREND II Hospital report with worked hours—level 3

		Executive summary—Group data					
	Hospital indicator	A 101 Hospitals Ind Qtr		B 14 Hospitals Ind Qtr		C 53 Hospitals Ind Qtr	
Profitability							
Nonoperating revenue ratio							
Liquidity							
Current ratio	3.498	2.257	3	3.442	3	3.015	3
Quick ratio	1.622	1.908	2	2.669	1	2.413	1
Acid test	0.334	0.323	3	0.636	2	0.363	2
Days net revenue in net A/R	60.554	79.652	1	79.955	L	77.914	1
Days gross revenue in gross A/R	82.167	73.756	4	83.926	2	77.842	3
Days gross revenue in allow for uncollectable	43.350	16.793	4	29.276	3	23.083	H
Days exp in accounts payable	31.900	34.978	2	37.706	2	33.270	2
Operating days cash on hand	16.374	15.326	3	31.976	2	18.948	2
Average payment period	49.019	55.083	2	41.351	3	44.789	3
Activity							
Asset turnover	0.083	0.077	3	0.068	3	0.083	2
Current asset turnover ratio	0.194	0.259	2	0.211	2	0.261	1
Fixed asset turnover ratio	0.148	0.159	2	0.113	3	0.155	2
Inventory per ADJ occupied bed	2496.857	3876.668	2	6236.821	1	4603.624	2
Inventory turnover ratio	6.850	5.235	3	3.355	3	4.432	3

		Executive summary—Internal trend data				
	Apr 1991	3 Mth ending Mar 1991	3 Mth ending Mar 1990	Percent change	3 Mth ending Mar 1989	Percent change
Profitability						
Nonoperating revenue ratio						
Liquidity						
Current ratio	3.330	3.498	3.680	−4.95	3.488	0.29
Quick ratio	1.627	1.622	1.879	−13.68	1.761	−7.89
Acid test	0.490	0.334	0.259	28.96	0.225	48.44
Days net revenue in net A/R	54.910	60.564	71.189	−14.93	83.628	−27.58
Days gross revenue in gross A/R	76.945	82.167	83.250	−1.30	85.452	−3.84
Days gross revenue in allow for uncollectable	41.721	43.350	37.959	14.20	33.944	27.71
Days exp in accounts payable	37.381	31.900	50.410	−36.72	42.022	−24.09
Operating days cash on hand	25.013	16.374	12.132	34.97	13.103	24.96
Average payment period	51.010	49.019	46.766	4.82	58.211	−15.79
Activity						
Asset turnover	0.084	0.083	0.081	2.47	0.074	12.16
Current asset turnover ratio	0.192	0.194	0.197	−1.52	0.168	15.48
Fixed asset turnover ratio	0.151	0.148	0.139	6.47	0.133	11.28
Inventory per ADJ occupied bed	2576.580	2496.867	1959.917	27.40	2630.469	−5.08
Inventory turnover ratio	6.623	6.850	7.945	−13.78	5.769	18.74

From *MONITREND II hospital report.* Chicago: American Hospital Association, 1991; reprinted by permission. Copyright American Hospital Association, May 1991.

A, National—200 thru 299 beds. B, Oklahoma—100 thru 299 beds. C, Rural referral centers. Ind, indicator.

lar-sized hospitals in the state. Second, ratio deviation only shows that results differ from expectations. It is a sensing clue—a signal that causes must be identified. For example, an increase in total asset turnover (operating revenue divided by total assets) from previous years may be caused by many factors: increased admissions and occupancy, or depreciation charges against the asset base that exceed the value of new facility and or equipment acquisitions. Generally, an increasing total asset turnover indicates better utilization of capacity—more efficient use of the hospital's facilities and equipment. Similarly, a decrease in total asset turnover may be due to fewer admissions and lower occupancy, or an increase in facility and equipment assets resulting from an increase in beds or the acquisition of new equipment. Regardless of the direction of the ratio, if the cause of deviation is identified and understood, ratio analysis has done its job.

Network Programming

There are two procedural network programming methods, the performance evaluation review technique (PERT) and the critical path method (CPM), that are helpful to managers in planning, scheduling, and controlling work. They are used most often in large projects such as building programs. However, they can be applied to small tasks such as scheduling departmental work.

PERT involves identifying the sequence of work and developing three estimates of completion times for each activity in the sequence: an optimistic, a pessimistic, and a probabilistic expected time.[51] Diagramming (sequencing) activities on a time axis allows the three different time requirements for the project to be determined. This improves scheduling, allocating resources, and control of project completion.[52] Developing the network requires identifying specific tasks, their relationships, and how they will be completed in terms of equipment, human resources, and other inputs.

The critical path method is similar to PERT. It focuses on work and project activities and their sequencing; however, it uses only one estimated time. In CPM, a circle denotes activity completion and an arrow denotes allocation and consumption of resources to complete the activity and its sequence relationship to others. Using the information in Table 12.8, a network drawing for a nursing station remodeling project is presented in Figure 12.7. It shows sequencing and relationship of activities, time for completing each, total project completion time (which is 16 days), and the critical path, which is A → B → C → D → F → G → H → I → J.

CPM is valuable as a control method because the manager identifies activities or tasks as well as resources involved in work projects and graphically shows their interrelationships. This information permits identification of three items important to control. First is the critical path that shows the activities that must be closely monitored and controlled to ensure timely completion. Delaying any activity in the critical path delays the entire project. Second, identifying slack time is meaningful from a resource allocation perspective. Review of Table 12.8 and Figure 12.7 indi-

Table 12.8. Nursing station remodeling project

Activity	Description	Immediate predecessor	Time (days)
A	Construct temporary nursing station (NS) work area in a vacant room	—	1
B	Move NS records, phones, etc., to temporary facility	A	1
C	Remove (gut) original NS counter, desks, etc.	B	1
D	Construct new NS shell	C	3
E	Install electrical wiring	D	2
F	Install heating and air-conditioning ducts	D	4
G	Install drywall	E, F	2
H	Install floor	G	2
I	Paint	H	1
J	Replace equipment from temporary NS work area	I	1

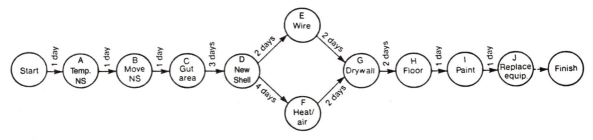

Figure 12.7. CPM network: nursing station remodeling project. (Critical path = A → B → C → D → F → G → H → I → I → J.)

cates that activity E (install wiring) has slack time of 2 days. The implication is that a 2-day delay will not affect the critical path and project completion. Finally, "crash" times can be determined. They yield information enabling cost-benefit decisions to be made in allocation and use of resources. For example, if activity F (install heating and air-conditioning ducts) could be completed in 2 compared to 4 days, the entire project could be completed 2 days sooner because activity F is part of the critical path. The manager can weigh the costs of allocating more resources to this activity against the benefits of completing the project 2 days sooner.

USE OF ANALYTICAL TECHNIQUES IN RESOURCE ALLOCATION

Converting inputs to outputs requires allocation and use of resources. One dimension of control is determining if such allocation and use are appropriate and meet expectations. One dimension of CQI is improving processes to more efficiently use resources. It is imperative that HSO managers understand the wide range of analytical techniques available as they make decisions about allocating resources, using resources, and improving processes.

Analytical techniques are methods or procedures that systematically arrange and permit evaluation of information in a specific fashion. They help managers focus on important considerations and judge them against criteria. Results are expressed in objective terms. The problem-solving model in Chapter 10 (see Figure 10.4) shows that analytical techniques are useful in evaluating and selecting alternatives, especially those concerning resource allocation. It should be remembered that nonquantitative considerations are important when evaluating alternatives, and that only when both nonquantitative and quantitative measures are included do effective problem solving and decision making occur. Analytical techniques are the predominant means for deriving objective information.

Analytical techniques can be used to evaluate the allocation and use of resources for new projects and improvement of existing processes. Those techniques described in the following sections are volume analysis (with and without revenue as a variable), capital budgeting, cost-benefit analysis, and simulation. Volume analysis with revenue as a variable is used to evaluate economic viability of an alternative, such as adding a service or buying equipment. When revenue is not a variable, volume analysis can be used to evaluate alternatives with different fixed and variable cost characteristics. It can be used to evaluate the resource implications of improving an existing process. Capital budgeting is a ranking method used to compare several proposed alternatives. Cost-benefit analysis identifies the resource consequences of a proposed alternative compared to the current situation. Finally, simulation yields "what if" information about the resource consequences of changes in existing situations—such as adding staff to decrease patient waiting time or modifying the flow of a process—without actually making a change. Analytical techniques not included here, but which are also used, are decision matrix analysis, inventory analysis, linear programming, queuing, network analysis, and statistical techniques such as regression, forecasting, and hypothesis testing. Table 12.9 provides brief descriptions of some of these techniques.

Greater familiarity with quantitative techniques can be acquired in the rich literature on operations research, management science, and quantitative analysis. Useful bibliographies of journal articles with specific applications of quantitative techniques to health services have been compiled by Fries[53] and Smith-Daniels and colleagues.[54]

Volume Analysis with Revenue

Volume analysis with revenue as a variable is often called break-even analysis.[55] It is one of the simplest analytical techniques available to evaluate the economic viability of a proposed alternative involving resource allocation. In order to use such analysis, identifiable costs and identifiable revenue must be available. Important components of volume analysis with revenue as a variable are:

> Identifiable revenues measured by price or charge (P) per unit of output or service (X) (e.g., charge per emergency department, outpatient, or office visit; per laboratory test, electrocardiogram, or radiograph; or per day of hospital or nursing facility stay)
>
> Identifiable fixed costs (FC)—costs that do not vary with output or volume (e.g., associated capital costs for facility and equipment lease or depreciation, utilities, and minimum staffing levels)
>
> Identifiable variable costs (VC)—costs that vary with output or volume (supplies, materials, medications, additional staff beyond minimum levels, overtime)

Three variants of volume analysis yield different results depending on which variables are known. The *break-even model* determines economic viability of an alternative. If fixed and variable costs and price/charge per unit of output/service are known, the break-even model determines the volume of output/service (X) needed to break even. It should be noted that type of provider reimbursement (fixed such as DRG, cost based, or charges) and payor mix significantly complicate the use of volume analysis. Breaking even occurs when total revenue (price per unit of service times volume) equals total costs (fixed plus variable). The general formula is (solve for X):

$$\text{Break-even point} = \frac{FC + VC(X)}{P(X)}$$

or

$$(P)(X) - VC(X) = FC$$
$$(P - VC)X = FC$$
$$X = \frac{FC}{P - VC}$$

A second variant of volume analysis is determining the *net (positive or negative) contribution* (NC) that results from an alternative when price or charge, total volume, and fixed and variable costs are known. Positive net contribution (NC) occurs when total revenue (volume times price) exceeds total costs (fixed plus variable); net contribution is negative when total costs exceed total revenue. The general formula is (solve for NC):

$$P(X) = FC + VC(X) + NC$$

or

$$NC = P(X) - [FC + VC(X)]$$

The third variant of volume analysis is to use it as a *price- or charge-setting model*. If fixed and variable costs and volume are known, the technique yields the price or charge per unit of output/service required to meet end-result criteria ranging from breaking even (where total reve-

Table 12.9. Quantitative techniques for decision analysis

Technique	Linear programming	Queuing theory	Network analysis	Regression analysis
Description	This technique attempts to optimize the distribution of scarce resources among competing activities. This is accomplished by the maximization or minimization of a dependent variable, which is a function of several independent variables that are subject to a set of restraints, i.e., limited resources. This method is capable of being executed manually, but is very adaptable to solution by a computer.	Queuing theory is the study of the probabilities associated with the length of a waiting line and the time an individual must wait in the queuing system. This information is used to achieve a balance between the cost of waiting for a service and the cost associated with providing this service. "Cost in a medical setting invariably includes elements defined by 'good medical care' which are, at best, difficult to quantify but must be included with monetary cost to obtain the proper solution." In queuing theory the waiting line may be organized on a first-in-first-out basis, a random basis, or by some other priority technique. The waiting line can have a finite or infinite calling population and it is assumed that the average service rate is greater than the average arrival rate for a single-channel single-server queuing model.	Network analysis is characterized by a network of events and activities. Activities are defined as the actual performance of tasks, while events represent the start of completion of an activity. Events do not consume time. This technique allows the determination of probabilities of meeting specified deadlines; identifies bottlenecks in the project; evaluates the effect of shifting resources from a noncritical activity to a critical activity and vice versa and enables the manager to evaluate the effect of a deviation of the actual time requirement for an activity from what had been predicted. Specific network analysis models include Critical Path Methods (CPM), Program Evaluation and Review Techniques (PERT), and Graphical Evaluation and Review Techniques (GERT). The difference between these systems lies in their different abilities to analyze complex network systems.	This is a technique that derives a mathematical equation to describe or express the relationship between the data of two or more variables over a period of time. The variable to predict in this equation is referred to as the dependent variable. The other variables in the equation are called independent variables or predicting variables. The basic measure of the relationship between the dependent variable and the independent variable(s) is depicted by a regression line, which is computed by the method of least squares. This will result in an equation, based upon historical data, that will predict the future behavior of the dependent variable. This technique is used primarily for the purpose of forecasting and control.
Hospital Applications	Physician, nurse, and patient scheduling problems; purchasing problems associated with hospital supplies and equip-	Determination of the most effective serving system for food service operations, outpatient clinic operations, admission	Hospital planning and control efforts associated with building or research and development projects or the determination	Used to forecast dependent variables such as number of hospital admissions, inpatient days, outpatient visits, average daily

	ment; hospital transportation problems and assignment problems.	operations, telephone switchboard operations, etc. In each of these situations, queuing theory balances the cost of an individual waiting with the cost of additional facilities that would be incurred in order to prevent the individual from waiting.	of flow allocations through a health care system, such as a mass screening facility.	census, cost per patient day, etc., and to control deviations from the planned costs associated with each of these variables.
Data Required	Manager must express desires in a unidimensional objective function; data that pertain to an objective function expressed in terms of maximization of benefits or minimization of costs, set of constraints, variables, and alternative courses of action.	Average number of arrivals per a unit of time; the average service time per arrival; the number of waiting lines, the number of waiting line phases, and the number of persons in the waiting line.	Data that pertain to the determination of project activities and events; determination of optimistic, pessimistic, and most likely time estimates with associated mean activity times and time required for an activity in terms of probability distribution and associated parameters.	Historical data compiled either daily, monthly, quarterly or annually with respect to the dependent and independent variables of the problem.
Advantages	Optimum use of productive factors; potential to increase decision quality; highlights problem bottlenecks; forces objectivity and quantification.	Description of the probabilities that a waiting line will contain a certain number of individuals; the expected length of the waiting line and the expected waiting time for the individual.	Determination of longest time paths through a network; identification of the relative frequency of occurrence of different paths; evaluation of program changes.	Provides accurate forecasts of dependent variables in a three-month to two-year time frame. Allows management to analyze deviations from the planned program changes.
Disadvantages	Inability to represent several goals/objectives in a unidimensional objective function; costs associated with data upkeep; homogeneous values in constraints; assumption of linearity.	Assumption that both arrival and service completion lines follow a Poisson distribution; upkeep of data.	Accurate time forecasts for activities.	Cost of data upkeep: assumption of linearity; the assumption that no causal relationship exists between the variables.

nue equals total costs) to attaining a specific net positive contribution (*NC*). When *NC* is set at the value desired—which may be zero—the general formula is (solve for *P*):

$$P(X) = FC + VC(X) + NC$$

or

$$P = \frac{FC + VC(X) + NC}{X}$$

HSOs encounter many situations with identifiable cost and revenue attributes in which volume analysis can be applied. Examples are acquiring new equipment (magnetic resonance imager, laboratory diagnostic equipment); expanding facilities (new beds, parking deck); adding new services (neonatology, open heart surgery); and embarking on new ventures (emergency care center, ambulatory surgery center, physicians' office building). Depending on known variables, or assumptions about them, volume analysis can determine economic viability. Will the project break even? Will it have a net positive or negative contribution? Volume analysis also can be used as a price-setting model to meet specific criteria (i.e., break even or yield a net positive contribution). Figure 12.8 provides an example: a freestanding satellite urgent care center is proposed by a hospital. Fixed costs (building and equipment depreciation, minimum staffing levels) are $600,000 per year. Variable costs (supplies and materials) per patient visit are assumed to be $20. The average price/charge per patient visit is $80. Volume analysis can be used to determine what number of patient visits per year (or per day) will be necessary to break even. This is determined as follows (solve for *X*):

$$
\begin{aligned}
P(X) &= FC + VC(X) \\
\$80(X) &= \$600,000 + 20(X) \\
\$60(X) &= \$600,000 \\
X &= \frac{\$600,000}{\$60} \\
&= 10,000
\end{aligned}
$$

Thus, to break even, 10,000 patient visits per year (28 per day) will be necessary.

If other information (knowledge about competition, population in the service area) is available, the decision maker can judge whether it is reasonable to expect 10,000 patient visits per year (28 per day) and determine the economic viability of the project. If only 8,000 patient visits may be expected each year, the net (negative) contribution would be $- \$120,000$ as indicated in Figure 12.8. Algebraically, this is determined as follows (solve for *NC*):

$$
\begin{aligned}
P(X) &= FC + VC(X) + NC \\
\$80(8,000) &= \$600,000 + \$20(8,000) + NC \\
\$60(8,000) &= \$600,000 + NC \\
\$480,000 &= \$600,000 + NC \\
NC &= \$480,000 + (-\$600,000) \\
NC &= -\$120,000
\end{aligned}
$$

Similarly, if volume were 11,000 patient visits per year, net (positive) revenue would be $60,000.

Volume Analysis without Revenue

HSOs often have alternative situations that do not have an identifiable revenue attribute but do have volume and fixed and variable cost attributes. Volume analysis without revenue is useful to evaluate and compare cost consequences of alternatives with each other. It may be used in situations in which there is no revenue, when revenue is indeterminate, or when revenue is the same for all alternatives. Since revenue is not a variable, the analysis focuses on fixed and variable cost trade-offs among volume alternatives.

Figure 12.9 illustrates the concept. Renting one of two copying machines is under considera-

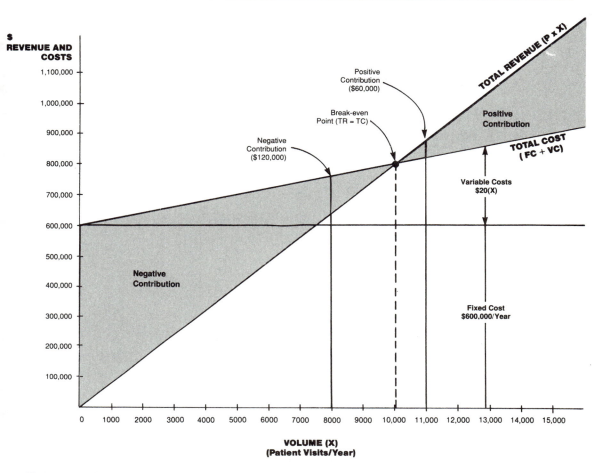

Figure 12.8.   Urgent care center volume analysis.

tion. Machine A is slow (10 copies per minute) and leases for $200 per month (fixed cost). Machine B is faster (30 copies per minute) and leases for $600 per month. Machine A has lower fixed cost than B ($FC_a < FC_b$); however, the variable cost of staff waiting at the machine while photocopying is higher ($VC_a > VC_b$). Given the different fixed and variable cost attributes, the preferred alternative is different at various volume levels. If volume were X_1, machine A is preferred because total costs are lower ($TC_{a1} < TC_{b1}$). If volume were X_2, machine B is preferred ($TC_{b2} < TC_{a2}$). Alternative preference is thus dependent on the extent to which there are fixed and variable cost trade-offs relative to volume.

Volume analysis without revenue is powerful because it focuses on the relationship of cost components to volume alternatives. Applications include equipment replacement and machine/technology-people substitution. As larger portions of HSO revenue are prospectively determined, alternative evaluation from a cost trade-off perspective becomes important.

Capital Budgeting

Capital budgeting commonly refers to several techniques to evaluate, compare, and rank multiple investment alternatives or to compare single alternatives to a given criterion such as rate of return. The degree of sophistication ranges from simply determining payback period to complex evaluations of revenue and cost streams that are discounted to net present value.[56]

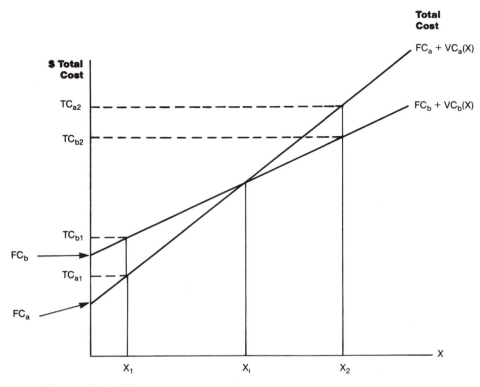

Figure 12.9.   Volume analysis without revenue.

Payback is an uncomplicated capital budgeting technique because it does not consider the net present value of revenue and cost streams for investment alternatives under consideration. It simply determines the years needed to recoup an initial investment and yields a gross index of the desirability of investment alternatives. In any comparison of multiple investment alternatives, the one with the shortest payback period (lowest index) is preferred. There are distorted results if revenue and cost streams are dissimilar and the useful life of alternatives differs appreciably. Type of provider payment and payor mix also affect analysis. A more precise ranking index is the net present value of alternatives.

In payback analysis, necessary components for each alternative are:

Identifiable annual revenue generated
Identifiable annual costs
Identifiable investment and salvage value

The payback technique has two basic elements. The first is net investment—initial cost minus salvage value. The second is annual net benefit from the investment, if selected. Net benefit is determined by revenues generated minus operating expenses. Dividing net investment by net benefit determines the number of years to return the cost of the investment. The general formula for the payback period is:

$$\text{Payback period} = \frac{\text{(Cost of the proposed investment)} - \text{(Salvage value)}}{\text{(Revenue generated from investment)} - \text{(Operating expenses)}}$$

It should be noted that payback is used predominantly to rank and compare multiple investment alternatives—whether to acquire personal computers for managers or fetal monitoring equipment—or alternatives for the same use—which vendor's personal computers to acquire. If investment, cost, and revenue streams are discounted to present value (and assuming a given rate of interest), a new present value index similar to the payback index can be used to rank alternatives. Applications in HSOs generally involve equipment or facility expansion alternatives such as adding or replacing equipment, building a parking deck or an office building, or expanding facilities.

Cost-Benefit Analysis

Conceptually, cost-benefit analysis, which is "an evaluation of the relationship between benefits and costs of a particular project or program,"[57] is similar to payback analysis. However, unlike payback analysis—a capital budgeting technique—cost-benefit analysis may be used whether or not there is an identifiable revenue stream. Used widely to evaluate government programs, such as the cost-benefit of infant immunization or federally-supported prenatal care, cost-benefit analysis can also be applied to HSOs. "A proposal to convert the heating plant of a hospital from oil to coal involves the same type of analysis."[58]

Cost-benefit analysis has wide applicability in almost all areas of an HSO's operations and can readily be used in making process improvement decisions. It almost always involves comparing a proposed alternative to an existing situation and need not (although it may) have a revenue component.

Important components in analysis are:

Identifiable imputed or actual costs associated with the proposed alternative and the existing situation

Identifiable changes in productivity (and imputed value of the productivity) associated with the proposed alternative and the existing situation

Identifiable changes in revenue associated with the proposed alternative and the existing situation (this variable is not required to perform the analysis)

Other considerations that may not be quantifiable

Costs, which may be actual or imputed, may include capital expenditures for equipment, space, employees, and materials and supplies. Net benefit is the marginal difference between the components listed above for the proposed alternative (PA) and the existing situation (ES). That is, net benefit equals PA − ES for the above components. If the net benefit is positive, this suggests that the proposed alternative is preferred. However, other nonquantifiable considerations, such as the impact of the proposed alternative relative to the existing situation on customer satisfaction, may suggest that the existing situation is preferred. In this instance, the decision maker must evaluate the importance of the nonquantifiable considerations and whether they outweigh the quantifiable results.

Applications of cost-benefit analysis exist in virtually every area and operational activity of HSOs. Examples include evaluating the cost versus benefit of using disposable versus nondisposable tableware in the cafeteria, word processing versus a manual system, computer system upgrading, owning or leasing a phone system, or contract versus in-house housekeeping services. Applications can occur in any situation with identified and/or imputed costs and benefits (which may be revenue based but more often are cost-saving based) associated with a proposed alternative relative to an existing situation.

Table 12.10 shows an application of cost-benefit analysis. A nursing facility is considering use of disposable tableware (plates, cups, utensils)—the proposed alternative—rather than continuing to use nondisposable items—the existing situation. Costs associated with implementing the proposed alternative are shown in part A of Table 12.10. Marginal benefits of the alternative are presented in part B. Annual costs associated with using disposable tableware are $46,000.

Table 12.10. Cost-benefit analysis: disposable tableware

A. Costs		
1. Annual cost of disposable dishes, cups, and utensils		$45,000
2. Annual cost of trash disposal		1,000
		$46,000
B. Benefits		
1. Annual reduction in costs for replacing nondisposable dishes, cups, and utensils if disposables used		$ 7,000
2. Annual savings in washing detergent and water if disposable used		5,000
3. Annual savings in wages and fringes due to need for 2.5 fewer FTE cafeteria personnel (to wash tableware) if disposables used		36,500
4. Annual savings in repair/depreciation cost of dishwashing equipment		1,000
5. Imputed annual value of dishwashing area space if used for other purposes (expansion of kitchen, storage)		2,000
		$51,500

Net benefit = benefits − costs
= $51,500 − $46,000
= $5,500

Marginal benefits (i.e., reducing costs from the present situation) are $51,500, resulting in a net benefit of $5,500. Consequently, objective analysis shows that use of disposables is advantageous. However, other nonquantifiable considerations that will affect the decision are employee and visitor perception of and attitude about disposables, institutional image, and sanitary implications.

Simulation

Simulation is one of the most powerful analytical tools available to health services managers in making resource allocation decisions and in determining if and how processes can be improved. It enables managers to ask "what if" questions and review the implications and consequences of alternatives without altering the present situation.

Simulation involves constructing a detailed, computer-based mathematical model representing situations and variables. The model has detailed rules that each variable follows as it interacts with the "system," which may be a work process such as diagnostic testing or surgery and recovery. (The simulation literature uses the term "system" to denote such a process, and that term is used here.) The simulation model replicates and reflects variables in the system, and it is constructed using mathematical expressions of relationships, attributes, and probability distributions of events derived from empirical observations of the system. The model is activated by use of a random number generator to represent events, such as admission, arrival for service, a particular type of surgical case, and length of stay.

Simulation models are dynamic. When variables, rules, or assumptions are changed, the model produces the consequences of that change. When no change is made in the relationships of variables in the model (static state), simulation can forecast the effect of increased demand on the system and suggest what resource allocation and capacity changes are needed to meet the desired level of quality. In a dynamic state, variable relationships can be changed, "what if" questions can be asked, and the results will indicate whether and how systems can be improved to enhance the quality of product or service.

Simulation is applicable to any activity that involves scheduling and service rates and capacity constraints, for both physical plant and staffing.[59] Examples are admissions,[60] operating room,[61] emergency department,[62] diagnostic testing, clinics, ancillary services, bed planning,[63] and nurse staffing.[64]

To solve a capacity problem and to increase patient satisfaction, a simulation study was conducted in a large not-for-profit teaching hospital to determine the appropriate allocation of beds among services.[65] The hospital had underutilized beds in one surgical unit (surgery B) and overutilized beds in orthopedics. A simulation model was developed to ask "what if" questions about reallocating beds between the services and to determine the effect on the average number of patients waiting for admission, percentage of patients admitted to the service, and number of patients who could not be admitted. Figures 12.10 and 12.11 show effects on bed utilization and average number of patients waiting for admission to the service, respectively, as the simulation model reallocated beds. The model indicated average patient waiting time was lowest and bed utilization most effective for both types of patients with 44 orthopedic beds (versus 33) and 37 surgery B beds (versus 48). The information on (re)allocating beds provided by simulation improved the effectiveness of resource use and quality by substantially decreasing patient waiting time.

In another simulation, managers of a 500-bed acute care hospital were concerned about the quality of patient service, specifically complaints about waiting times in radiology.[66] The simulation model depicted arrival, processing, and waiting times for eight types of inpatients and outpatients. Procedures tracked included fluoroscopy, radioisotope scanning, computed tomography (CT) scan, and ultrasound. Distributions of arrival rates by type of patient and service times by type of procedure were constructed by observing the actual system. The simulation determined the effects of various capacity changes on queues and patient waiting time. Figure 12.12 shows the results of simulating changes in capacity—increasing the number of radiologists (note the scale is reversed and the x axis should be read right to left). Patient waiting time before the start of service decreased substantially (approximately 22 minutes for all four procedures) when capacity was

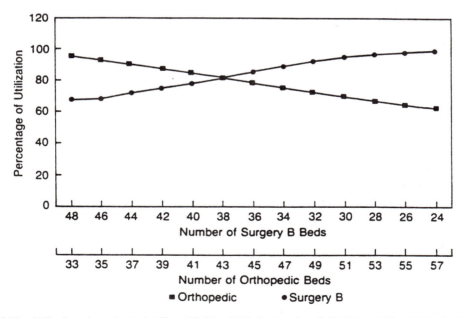

Figure 12.10. Utilization of service beds. (From Klafehn, Keith A., Jonathon S. Rakich, and Paul J. Kuzdrall. The use of simulation as an aid in hospital decision making. *Hospital Topics* 67 [March/April 1989]: 10; reprinted by permission of the Helen Dwight Reid Educational Foundation. Published by Heldref Publications, 4000 Albemarle St., N.W., Washington, D.C. 20016. Copyright © 1989.)

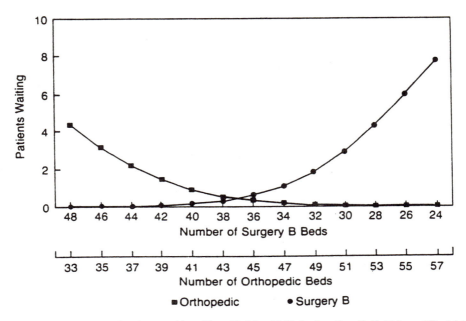

Figure 12.11. Average number of patients waiting. (From Klafehn, Keith A., Jonathon S. Rakich, and Paul J. Kuzdrall. The use of simulation as an aid in hospital decision making. *Hospital Topics* 67 [March/April 1989]: 10; reprinted by permission of the Helen Dwight Reid Educational Foundation. Published by Heldref Publications, 4000 Albemarle St., N.W., Washington, D.C. 20016. Copyright © 1989.)

increased from 5 to 6 radiologists. Increasing the number of radiologists provided the largest marginal gain for all capacity configurations. Only a modest decrease in waiting time (about 6 minutes) occurred when a seventh radiologist was added.[67] This simulation provided "what if" information useful in deciding if and how to alter a capacity-bound process. Such information enables managers to make more informed resource allocation and use decisions.

The power of simulation as an analytical technique in resource allocation and utilization and in process improvement is evident. To the extent that health services managers are generally familiar with it and the other techniques presented here, they can positively affect the quality of output, improve the processes that generate it, and make more informed resource allocation decisions.

SUMMARY

The management function of control involves gathering information about and monitoring HSO activities, comparing actual and expected results, and intervening with corrective action as appropriate by introducing change in inputs or process. Control depends on planning. Preestablished standards and expectations of performance and results are based on organizational plans and objectives. The three control monitoring points are outputs, where control is retrospective; processes, where it may be concurrent; and inputs, where control may be prospective. The control model in Figure 12.2 integrates CQI and uses a systematic approach to control in HSOs. The positive control loop, in which desirable organizational work results/performance exceed standards/expectations, suggests the CQI philosophy—determine why good results occur, replicate them elsewhere, and encourage continued improvement.

Control depends on information. Effective management information systems are critical if managers are to plan, solve problems, control, and appropriately allocate and use resources. De-

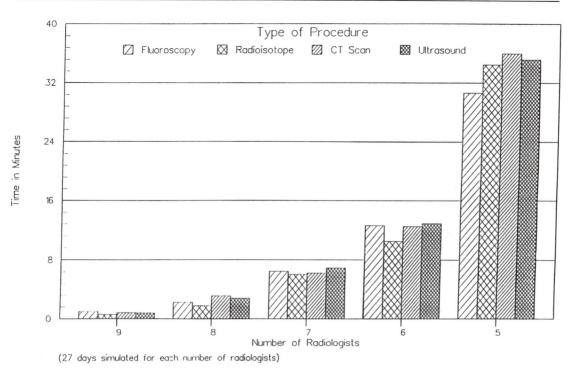

Figure 12.12. Patient wait time by procedure (excludes processing time); average wait time for greater than zero. (Based on data from: Klafehn, Keith A., Paul J. Kuzdrall, Jonathon S. Rakich, and Alan G. Krigline. Application of simulation in hospital resource allocation and utilization. *Journal of Management Science & Policy Analysis* 8 [Spring/ Summer 1991]: 346–356.)

cision support systems and their extension, medical decision support systems, permit managers and clinicians greater control over the HSO's activities and the quality of care.

Risk management is a structured, programmatic control method important in HSOs. Quality assessment and improvement has elements of control and is partially or fully integrated with risk management. The methodology and philosophy of QA/I, however, focuses on improving processes and thereby avoids the inspection approach inherent in most traditional control activities.

Control is not happenstance. Budgeting is the most prevalent of the traditional control methods. Budgets are numerical plans that show the resources available for the HSO's activities and plans. Other important control methods presented are operational-activity analysis and financial ratio analysis. Network programming, a method particularly pertinent to scheduling projects, is described.

Converting inputs to outputs requires that resources be allocated and their use controlled. The final section of this chapter presents analytical techniques used in resource allocation: volume analysis, capital budgeting, cost-benefit analysis, and simulation. Cost-benefit analysis is especially useful in many areas of the HSO without assignable revenue. Simulation is a powerful tool for investigating how systems (i.e., processes) can be improved. The ability to ask "what if" questions without having to actually change the system allows managers to understand theoretically the effects of changes in activities such as traffic and materials flow, capacity design, staffing patterns, patient service and waiting times, and reallocation of beds among services. Based on the simulated results, resources can be allocated or reallocated, thereby ensuring greater control over their effective use.

DISCUSSION QUESTIONS

1. Define control. What are the major elements of control?
2. What are the three monitoring and two intervention points for control? Why is MIS important to control?
3. Review the control model in Figure 12.2 and give examples of situations for each of the control loops. What are the similarities between the control model (Figure 12.2) and the problem-solving model (Figure 10.4) presented in Chapter 10?
4. How does CQI relate to control? Specifically, what control point is its focus and how does this affect the control model (see Figure 12.2)?
5. Describe the purpose, structure, and process of risk management and quality assessment. Why are both important to HSOs from a control perspective?
6. What are the duties of risk managers? Where do they fit into the HSO's structure?
7. Identify several difficulties *and* several benefits of working with members of the clinical staff to improve quality. Suggest considerations that managers should keep in mind when working with clinical staff on improving quality.
8. Contrast traditional quality assurance (QA) with quality improvement (QI) as formulated by W. Edwards Deming. How are they complementary? Different?
9. Identify control methods presented in this chapter. Why are budgets and ratio analysis so important? How does each relate to the control model in Figure 12.2?
10. Identify the analytical techniques for resource allocation that were presented in this chapter. Explain how and why they are useful.

CASE STUDY 1: ADMITTING DEPARTMENT

Shelley York is supervisor of the admitting department at Newhealth, a health maintenance organization. Three clerks—Shemenski, Turner, and Underwood—report to her. All are responsible for processing patients. Using a sampling method for monitoring productivity, York obtained the following data for a 2-hour period:

Clerk	Patients processed
Shemenski	14
Turner	16
Underwood	11

Each clerk is expected to process seven patients per hour.

Questions

1. What should York do?
2. What is the control point (input, process, or output)?
3. What kind of information should York obtain relative to Turner and Underwood? What might be some of the "causes" for the deviations?

CASE STUDY 2: CENTRALIZED REPRODUCTION

Carey Snook saw Ted Rath drinking coffee in the cafeteria. "I thought you guys in management services were up to your eyeballs in productivity improvement projects," Snook said as he walked over to sit down with Rath.

"We are," Rath said. "In fact, we have so much work and so many project deadlines coming up, we've had to work Saturdays."

Snook responded, "Then how come you're goofing off by wasting time and drinking coffee?"

"I'm not wasting time," said Rath, "I'm waiting."

"For what?" said Snook.

"For some layout prints to be reproduced. We're in the middle of a systems analysis project. We're redesigning the outpatient department layout and work process flow. I can't continue with the project until I get the template layout drawings copied in central reproduction. Our secretary took them over there 20 minutes ago and they won't be ready for another 20 minutes. So, I'm waiting. This happens about three times a week to each of the three of us in my department."

Rath continued, "We used to have a Xerox machine in our department. Well, some people were caught reproducing personal documents. This probably cost the hospital about $10 a week, so they centralized all reproducing equipment to save money on use and have fewer machines. Now we have to walk our materials way over there to the central building and wait until it's our turn to have them reproduced."

"I guess the biggest gripe I have is with Smith, head of centralized reproduction. Sometimes it takes 10 minutes to convince Smith that the reproduction job is hospital business and is important. Smith really seems to like the authority. Anyway, take this isometric drawing I have here; I bet Smith will think it's my 6-year-old daughter's homework assignment. I wonder how long it will take me to convince Smith it is job related."

"Want some more coffee?" asked Snook.

Questions

1. What is the focus of control in this situation?
2. What dysfunctional results have occurred from centralizing reproduction?

CASE STUDY 3:   BARRIERS TO AN EFFECTIVE QA/I PROGRAM

District Hospital is a 260-bed, public, general acute care hospital owned by a special tax district. Its service area includes five communities with a total population of 180,000 in a southeastern coastal state in one of the nation's fastest growing counties. It is one of three hospitals owned by the special tax district. The seven other hospitals in District Hospital's general service area make the environment highly competitive.

District Hospital has a wide range of services and a medical staff of 527 from most specialties. The emergency department (ED) is a major source of admissions. Last year, 26,153 patients visited the ED and 3,745, or 14.3%, were admitted. This was 42% of admissions. Some admissions were sent to the ED by private physicians and some came by ambulance, but most were self-referred.

The hospital chief executive officer, W. G. Lester, noted that the number of visits to the ED was decreasing. Over a 3-year period they had declined from a high of 29,345 to the current low of 26,153. Only part of this reduction seemed attributable to competition. Lester was also concerned about an increasing number of complaints about the quality of emergency services. These complaints related to excessive waiting time, poor attitudes of physicians, and questions about the quality of care. Investigation found that many complaints were justified, but the causes of these problems were difficult to discern.

Registered nurses (RNs) employed in the ED want a larger role in triaging and treating patients, but the dominance of ED physicians limits the RNs' duties and frustrates other staff as well. This is manifested by high turnover, low morale, and difficulty in attracting and retaining a quality nursing staff.

Another factor is the emergency medical technician (EMT) program started in the county a few years ago. The EMTs are an important community medical resource and are very influential in deciding to which hospital ED patients will be transported. It will be necessary for District Hospital, through the ED physicians, to actively participate in training and managing the EMT program if District Hospital is to receive its share of emergency patients. ED physicians have refused to participate in teaching or directing the program, however. In fact, they often alienate the EMTs.

Lester is concerned, too, that the position of full-time director of emergency medicine at District Hospital has been vacant for 4 years. Residency programs in emergency medicine are producing physicians who are seeking positions with higher salaries and better working conditions than those at District Hospital.

There has been little turnover among the four physicians who staff the ED: two retired general surgeons and two foreign medical graduates trained in family practice. The ED physicians lack a clear commitment to District Hospital. They are employed in a variation of the Alexandria Plan—each contracts separately with the hospital. District Hospital bills ED patients and collects the physicians' fees: moneys above the guaranteed minimum are paid to them pro rata. They participate in District Hospital's fringe benefits and are covered by its professional liability insurance.

One ED physician, Dr. Balck (a retired surgeon), recognizes the progress being made nationally in emergency medicine. She made several unsuccessful attempts to move District Hospital in the same direction. With great effort she instituted programs on intradepartmental education and mandatory attendance at approved courses in emergency medicine. Quality assessment and improvement activities were done perfunctorily. Also, she had tried to obtain full recognition of the ED.

The members of the professional staff organization (PSO) seem satisfied with the situation. Its executive committee did not understand the changing status of emergency medicine. As evidence of its unwillingness to grant full recognition to the department, the PSO has consistently denied its requests for full departmental status.

Questions

1. Use the problem-solving methodology described in Chapter 10 to define the problem facing Lester. Which alternative solution do you prefer? Why?
2. Describe the relationship between inpatient census and ED admissions. Outline a strategy to educate the members of the ED physician staff as to the relationship and importance of the ED to the financial good health of District Hospital.
3. Use the concept of QA/I and the principles of CQI to outline a basic program to improve quality in the ED.
4. Analyze the role of the EMTs and their relationship with District Hospital. What should be the role of ED physicians and staff at District Hospital in terms of educating the EMTs? What are the negative aspects of this educational activity? Is there a potential conflict of interest?

CASE STUDY 4: DON'S RISK MANAGEMENT

Don Phelps is the director of engineering at Sunrise Village, a large life-care community located in a rural area on the West coast. Phelps has a staff of 19, including those who maintain and repair heating, ventilation, and air conditioning (HVAC) and electrical and plumbing. There are several utility repairmen who do carpentry, locksmithing, and general maintenance. The grounds are maintained by two full-time employees, supplemented by high school students in the summer.

Senior management at Sunrise feels lucky to have Phelps on its staff. Phelps is a baccalaureate mechanical engineer and has done graduate work in electrical engineering. He is dedicated, hardworking, and genuinely concerned that his department perform efficiently.

Sunrise self-insures for all risks, including liability, up to $1 million. It has an excess liability insurance policy to $5 million. Last year the excess liability carrier recommended that Sunrise develop a risk management program, but provided little specific information on how to do it. Phelps thinks such a program is a good idea.

Phelps has some data on visitor and resident accidents, but has had no time to do anything with them. He has no data on the quality of care provided in the skilled nursing unit at Sunrise, but he knows there have been several "incidents" in the past few years. He knows, too, that one of the reasons Sunrise began to self-insure was that there had been dramatic premium increases in its liability coverage because of three large settlements paid by their previous insurance carrier.

Senior management asked Phelps to organize a risk management program, but he isn't sure where to start.

Questions

1. Should Sunrise have a risk management program? Why?
2. Outline the steps Phelps should take in establishing a risk management program. Which types of persons should help him?
3. Identify and describe the types of links, including data collection, that should be present among quality assessment and improvement and risk management.
4. Incident or occurrence reporting is considered an important part of a risk management program. Why do staff often regard it as negative? What can be done to change this perception?

CASE STUDY 5:   THE ARRAY MACHINE

An equipment acquisition proposal was being considered by a large hospital laboratory. The Array machine would enable the hospital to perform autoimmunity tests (for immunoglobulins IgG, IgM, and IgA, and complements C3 and C4) in-house rather than sending them to a reference laboratory. As a result, test turnaround time would be decreased by 2 days. The machine costs $50,000, with a useful life of 5 years. The depreciation schedule would be $10,000 per year.

The hospital's volume for the five autoimmunity tests is one of each test per day. Having the tests done by the reference laboratory costs the hospital an average of $10 per test. The hospital's average charge to patients is $20 per test. If the Array machine were acquired and the autoimmunity tests done in-house, the costs of reagents used would average $2 per test.

The Array machine can run a maximum of 40 patient samples and perform 20 different tests on each sample every 2 hours. Except in extraordinary circumstances, tests would be run Monday through Saturday.

The machine requires approximately 1 hour of technician time (valued at $15/hour) each day to calibrate it, to conduct a test run for control purposes, and to perform general maintenance. This is a fixed cost since it does not vary by volume. Technician set-up time to run tests is negligible. Beyond the five autoimmunity tests the lab wants to perform in house, the machine can also perform apolipoprotein cardiac profiles that are currently done on equipment in the clinical chemistry department. The Array machine can provide a quantitative measure and not just the positive or negative indicator that the clinical chemistry department's current equipment gives.

Questions

1. How many autoimmunity tests per year will have to be performed on the Array machine to break even?
2. Given present volume, would there be an annual net contribution and, if so, how much?
3. If half the patients have Medicare (DRG reimbursement includes all tests), would the lab break even on the equipment? If not, should the equipment be acquired anyway?

NOTES

1. Austin, Charles J. *Information systems for hospital administration*, 34. Ann Arbor, MI: Health Administration Press, 1988.

2. Higgins, James M. *The management challenge: An introduction to management*, 568. New York: Macmillan Publishing Company, 1991.

3. Pearce, John A., II, and Richard B. Robinson, Jr. *Management*, 581. New York: Random House, 1989.
4. Pearce and Robinson, *Management*, 586.
5. Van Fleet, David D. *Contemporary management*, 444. Boston, MA: Houghton Mifflin Company, 1991.
6. Pearce and Robinson, *Management*, 584.
7. Boxerman, Stuart B. Technological glitter can't replace IS basics. *Journal of Health Administration Education* 8 (Winter 1990): 37.
8. Pearce and Robinson, *Management*, 657.
9. Austin, Charles J. Information technology and the future of health services delivery. *Hospital & Health Services Administration* 34 (Summer 1989): 159.
10. Jones, V. Brewster, and L. Clark Taylor. Expectations and outcome skills of a generalist health care administrator. *Journal of Health Administration Education* 8 (Winter 1990): 46.
11. Stamen, Jeffrey P. Decision support systems help planners hit their targets. *Journal of Business Strategy* 11 (March/April 1990): 30.
12. Martin, James B. The environment and future of health information systems. *Journal of Health Administration Education* 8 (Winter 1990): 19.
13. Austin, Information technology, 161.
14. Austin, Charles J. Commentary on "Clinical data systems: Management imperative for tomorrow." *Journal of Health Administration Education* 6 (Spring 1988): 345.
15. Jelinek, Richard C., and Matthew M. Person, III. Clinical data systems: Management imperative for tomorrow. *Journal of Health Administration Education* 6 (Spring 1988): 341.
16. Raco, Robert, Christine Shapleigh, and Donald Cook. Decision support in the 1990s. *Computers in Healthcare* 10 (December 1989): 27.
17. Austin, *Information Systems*, 11.
18. Chown, Ed. *Hospital departmental operations: A guide for trustees and managers*, 95. Ottawa, Ontario: Canadian Hospital Association, 1988.
19. Christensen, William W., and Eugene I. Stearns. *Microcomputers in health care management*, 7–8. Rockville, MD: Aspen Publishers, Inc.
20. Harpster, Linda Marie, and Margaret S. Veach, eds. *Risk management handbook for health care facilities*, 378. Chicago: American Hospital Association, 1990.
21. Joint Commission on Accreditation of Healthcare Organizations. *Accreditation manual for hospitals, 1992*, 142, 143. Oakbrook Terrace, IL: 1991.
22. Harpster and Veach, *Risk management*, 107.
23. Sielicki, Adam P., Jr. Current philosophy of risk management. *Topics in Health Care Financing* 9 (Spring 1983): 1–7.
24. Taravella, Steve. The rise of risk management. *Modern Healthcare* 20 (October 8, 1990): 37.
25. American College of Surgeons. *The minimum standard*. 1918.
26. Donabedian, Avedis. *Explorations in quality assessment and monitoring*. Vol. II, *The criteria and standards of quality*. Ann Arbor, MI: Health Administration Press, 1982.
27. Donabedian, Avedis. *Explorations in quality assessment and monitoring*. Vol. I, *The definition of quality and approaches to its assessment*, 81. Ann Arbor, MI: Health Administration Press, 1980.
28. Donabedian, *Explorations*, Vol. I, 79–89.
29. Donabedian, *Explorations*, Vol. I, 83.
30. Donabedian, *Explorations*, Vol. I, 83.
31. Donabedian, *Explorations*, Vol. I, 82.
32. Joint Commission on Accreditation of Healthcare Organizations. *Accreditation manual for hospitals, 1991*, 218. Oakbrook Terrace, IL: 1990.
33. Berwick, Donald M., A. Blanton Godfrey, and Jane Roessner. *Curing health: New strategies for quality improvement*, 11. San Francisco: Jossey-Bass Publishers, 1990.
34. Joint Commission on Accreditation of Healthcare Organizations. *Agenda for change* 2 (June 1988): 3, 4. Oakbrook Terrace, IL.
35. Joint Commission, *Accreditation manual, 1992*, Appendix D, 225–232.
36. Kelly, John T., and James E. Swartwout. Development of practice parameters by physician organizations. *QRB* 16 (February 1990): 54.
37. Marder, Robert J. Relationship of clinical indicators and practice guidelines. *QRB* 16 (February 1990): 60. (This article defines practice parameters and indicators and discusses their uses and relationships.)
38. Kelly and Swartwout, Development of practice, 55.
39. Kelly and Swartwout, Development of practice, 55.
40. This section is adapted from Darr, Kurt. Quality improvement and quality assurance compared. *Hospital Topics* 69 (Summer 1991): pp. 4–5.
41. Esmond, Truman H., Jr. *Budgeting for effective hospital resource management*, 26. Chicago: American Hospital Association, 1990.
42. Neumann, Bruce R., James D. Suver, and William N. Zelman. *Financial management: Concepts and applications for health care providers*, 2nd ed., 269. Owings Mills, Md: National Health Publishing/AUPHA Press, 1988.
43. Those interested in further reading about budgeting in HSOs are referred to: Berman, Howard J., Lewis E. Weeks, and Steven F. Kukla. *The financial management of hospitals*, 6th ed., chpt. 17. Ann Arbor, MI: Health Administration Press, 1986; Broyles, Robert W., and Michael D. Rosko. *Fiscal management of healthcare institutions*, chpts. 15, 16. Owings Mills, MD: National Health Publishing, 1990; Cleverley, William O. *Handbook of health care accounting and finance*, Vol. I and II, chpts. 13, 14. Rockville, MD: Aspen Systems Corporation, 1982. Cleverley, William O. *Essentials of health care finance*, chpt. 10. Rockville, MD: Aspen Publishers, Inc., 1986; Esmond, *Budgeting for effective*; Herkimer, Allen G., Jr. *Understanding health care budgeting*. Rockville, MD: Aspen Publishers, Inc., 1988; Neumann, Suver, and Zelman, *Financial management*, chpt. 8.
44. Esmond, *Budgeting for effective*, 28–29.
45. Smith, C. Thomas. Hospital management strategies for fixed-price payment. *Health Care Management Review* 11 (Winter 1986): 24.
46. Examples for orthopedic DRGs are provided in Stier, Margaret M., and Alan H. Rosenstein. Scrutiny of resource use can increase efficiency. *Healthcare Financial Management* 44 (November 1990): 28–31. Excellent reviews of the impact of DRGs on hospitals are provided in Balinsky, Warren, and Jodi L. Starkman. The impact of DRGs on the health care industry. *Health Care Management Review* 12 (Summer 1987): 61–74; Crawford, Myra, and Myron D. Fottler. The impact of diagnosis-related groups and prospective pricing systems on health care management. *Health Care Management Review* 10 (Fall 1985): 73–84; Fetter, Robert B. Diagnosis-related

groups: Understanding hospital performance. *Interfaces* 21 (January-February 1991): 6–26; and Smith, Howard L., and Myron D. Fottler. *Prospective payment: Managing for operational effectiveness*. Rockville, MD: Aspen Systems Corporation, 1985.

47. Counte, Michael A., and Gerald L. Glandon. Managerial innovation in the hospital: An analysis of the diffusion of hospital accounting systems. *Hospital & Health Services Administration* 33 (Fall 1988): 371.

48. Those interested in additional reading about ratio and financial analysis in HSOs should consult Berman, Weeks, and Kukla, *Financial management*, chpt. 22; Cleverley, *Handbook of health*, chpt. 23; Cleverley, *Essentials of health*, chpt. 6; *and* Neumann, Suver, and Zelman, *Financial management*, chpt. 3.

49. For application of financial ratio analysis in merged and consolidated hospitals, see Mullner, Ross M., and Ronald M. Andersen. A descriptive and financial ratio analysis of merged and consolidated hospitals: United States, 1980–1985. In *Advances in health economics and health services research*, edited by Richard M. Scheffler and Louis F. Rossiter, Vol.7, 57. Greenwich, CT: JAI Press, Inc., 1987; for comparisons of solvent hospitals and those in financial distress, see U.S. Department of Health and Human Services. *Financially distressed hospitals: A profile of behavior before and after PPS*, 8–9. Publ. No. PHS 90-3467. Washington, D.C.: U.S. Government Printing Office, 1990; for applications comparing financial ratios of Catholic and all other hospitals, see Cleverley, William O. Ten financial management principles for survival. *Hospital Progress* 69 (March 1988): 36–41, 104; and for application of financial ratios to hospitals by geographic region, see Cleverley, William O. *Hospital industry analysis report, 1980–1984*. Oak Brook, IL: The Healthcare Financial Management Association, 1985.

50. Cleverley, William O. Financial ratios: Summary indicators for management decision making. *Hospital & Health Services* Administration 26 (Special Issue, 1981): 30–31. See also Berman, Weeks, and Kukla, *Financial management*, 664–665.

51. Vonderembse, Mark A., and Gregory P. White. *Operations management: Concepts, methods, and strategies*, 579. St. Paul, MN: West Publishing Company, 1991.

52. Cleverley, *Handbook of health*, chpt. 44.

53. Fries, Brant E. Bibliography of operations research in health-care systems. *Operations Research* 24 (September-October 1976): 801–814; Fries, B. Bibliography of operations research in health-care systems: An update. *Operations Research* 27 (March-April 1979): 408–419.

54. Smith-Daniels, Vicki L., Sharon B. Schweikhart, and Dwight E. Smith-Daniels. Capacity management in health care services: Review and future directions. *Decision Sciences* 19 (Fall 1988): 889–919.

55. For examples, see Cleverley, *Essentials of health*, 208–209; Fogarty, Donald W., Thomas R. Hoffmann, and Peter W. Stonebraker. *Production and operations management*, 719–724. Cincinnati, OH: South-Western Publishing Co., 1989; Hy, Ronald John. *Financial management for health care administrators*, 90–91. New York: Quorum Books, 1989; Vonderembse and White,

Operations management, 254–259; and Weiss, Howard J., and Gershon, Mark E. *Production and operations management*, 64–72. Boston, MA: Allyn and Bacon, Inc., 1989.

56. Further reading about capital budgeting analytical technique in HSOs can be found in: Berman, Weeks, and Kukla, *Financial management* chpt. 18; Broyles and Rosko, *Fiscal management*, chpt. 13; Cleverley, *Handbook of health*, chpt. 8; Cleverley, *Essentials* of health, chpt. 13; and Neumann, Suver, and Zelman, *Financial management*, chpt. 12.

57. Ziebell, Mary T., and Don T. DeCoster. *Management control systems in nonprofit organizations*, 913. San Diego: Harcourt Brace Jovanovich, 1991.

58. Anthony, Robert N., and David W. Young. *Management control in nonprofit organizations*, 4th ed., 413. Homewood, IL: Irwin, 1988.

59. An excellent review of the literature concerning the application of simulation and other operations research techniques to health care is found in Smith-Daniels, Schweikhart, and Smith-Daniels, Capacity management. For classic reviews of applications, see Stimpson, David H., and Ruth H. Stimpson. *Operations research in hospitals: Diagnosis & prognosis*, chpt. 2. Chicago: Hospital Research and Educational Trust, 1972; and Valinsky, David. Simulation. In *Operations research in health care: A critical analysis*, edited by Larry J. Shuman, R. Dixon Speas, Jr., and John P. Young, 114–176. Baltimore, MD: The Johns Hopkins University Press, 1975.

60. Hancock, Walter M., and Paul F. Walter. The use of admission simulation to stabilize ancillary workloads. *Simulation* 43 (August 1984): 88–94.

61. Kwak, N.K., Paul J. Kuzdrall, and Homer H. Schmitz. The GPSS simulation of scheduling policies for surgical patients. *Management Science* 22 (May 1976): 982–989.

62. Klafhen, Keith A., and Debbie Owens. A simulation model designed to investigate resource allocation in a hospital emergency room. In *Proceedings of the 11th annual symposium on computer applications in medical care* (November 1987): 676–679.

63. Dumas, Barry M. Simulation modeling for hospital bed planning. *Simulation* 43 (August 1984): 69–78; Vassilacopoulos, G. A simulation model for bed allocation to hospital inpatient departments. *Simulation* 45 (November 1985): 233–241.

64. Hashimoto, Fred, Staughton Bell, and Sally Marshment. A computer simulation program to facilitate budgeting and staffing decisions in an intensive care unit. *Critical Care Medicine* 15 (March 1987): 256–259.

65. Klafehn, Keith A., Jonathon S. Rakich, and Paul J. Kuzdrall. The use of simulation as an aid in hospital management decision making. *Hospital Topics* 67 (March/April 1989): 6–12.

66. Klafehn, Keith A., Paul J. Kuzdrall, Jonathon S. Rakich, and Alan G. Krigline. Application of simulation in hospital resource allocation and utilization. *Journal of Management Science & Policy Analysis* 8 (Spring/Summer 1991): 346–356.

67. Klafehn, Kuzdrall, Rakich, and Krigline, Application of simulation, 351.

BIBLIOGRAPHY

Austin, Charles J. Commentary on "Clinical data systems: Management imperative for tomorrow." *Journal of Health Administration Education* 6 (Spring 1988): 344–354.

Austin, Charles J. *Information systems for hospital administration.* Ann Arbor, MI: Health Administration Press, 1988.

Austin, Charles J. Information technology and the future of health services delivery. *Hospital & Health Services Administration* 34 (Summer 1989): 157–165.

Balinsky, Warren, and Jodi L. Starkman. The impact of DRGs on the health care industry. *Health Care Management Review* 12 (Summer 1987): 61–74.

Berman, Howard J., Lewis E. Weeks, and Steven F. Kukla. The financial management of hospitals, 6th ed. Ann Arbor, MI: Health Administration Press, 1986.

Berwick, Donald M., A. Blanton Godfrey, and Jane Roessner. *Curing health: New strategies for quality improvement.* San Francisco: Jossey-Bass Publishers, 1990.

Boxerman, Stuart B. Technological glitter can't replace IS basics. *Journal of Health Administration Education* 8 (Winter 1990): 36–40.

Broyles, Robert W., and Michael D. Rosko. *Fiscal management of healthcare institutions.* Owings Mills, MD: National Health Publishing, 1990.

Chown, Ed. *Hospital departmental operations: A guide for trustees and managers*, Ottawa, Ontario: Canadian Hospital Association, 1988.

Cleverley, William O. *Essentials of health care finance.* Rockville, MD: Aspen Publishers, Inc., 1986.

Cleverley, William O. Financial ratios: Summary indicators for management decision making. *Hospital & Health Services Administration* 26 (Special Issue, 1981): 26–47.

Cleverley, William O. *Handbook of health care accounting and finance*, Vol. I and II. Rockville, MD: Aspen Systems Corporation, 1982.

Cleverley, William O. Ten financial management principles for survival. *Hospital Progress* 69 (March 1988): 36–41.

Counte, Michael A., and Gerald L. Glandon. Managerial innovation in the hospital: An analysis of the diffusion of hospital accounting systems. *Hospital & Health Services Administration* 33 (Fall 1988): 371–384.

Crawford, Myra, and Myron D. Fottler. The impact of diagnosis-related groups and prospective pricing systems on health care management. *Health Care Management Review* 10 (Fall 1985): 73–84.

Darr, Kurt. Quality improvement and quality assurance compared. *Hospital Topics* 69 (Summer 1991): 4–5.

Donabedian, Avedis. *Explorations in quality assessment and monitoring.* Vol. I, *The definition of quality and approaches to its assessment.* Ann Arbor, MI: Health Administration Press, 1980.

Donabedian, Avedis. *Explorations in quality assessment and monitoring.* Vol. II, *The criteria and standards of quality.* Ann Arbor, MI: Health Administration Press, 1982.

Dumas, Barry M. Simulation modeling for hospital bed planning. *Simulation* 43 (August 1984): 69–78.

Esmond, Truman H., Jr. *Budgeting for effective hospital resource management* Chicago: American Hospital Association, 1990.

Fetter, Robert B. Diagnosis-related groups: Understanding hospital performance. *Interfaces* 21 (January-February 1991): 6–26.

Fogarty, Donald W., Thomas R. Hoffmann, and Peter W. Stonebraker. *Production and operations management.* Cincinnati, OH: South-Western Publishing Co., 1989.

Fries, Brant E. Bibliography of operations research in health-care systems. *Operations Research* 24 (September-October 1976): 801–814.

Fries, Brant E. Bibliography of operations research in health-care systems: An update. *Operations Research* 27 (March-April 1979): 408–419.

Hancock, Walter M., and Paul F. Walter. The use of admission simulation to stabilize ancillary workloads. *Simulation* 43 (August 1984): 88–94.

Harpster, Linda Marie, and Margaret S. Veach. *Risk management handbook for health care facilities.* Chicago: American Hospital Association, 1990.

Hashimoto, Fred, Staughton Bell, and Sally Marshment. A computer simulation program to facilitate budgeting and staffing decisions in an intensive care unit. *Critical Care Medicine* 15 (March 1987): 256–259.

Helmer, F. Theodore, William H. Kucheman, Edward B. Oppermann, and James D. Suver. Basic management science techniques for decision analysis. *Hospital & Health Services Administration* 27 (March/April 1982): 58–71.

Herkimer, Allen G., Jr. *Understanding health care budgeting.* Rockville, MD: Aspen Publishers, Inc., 1988.

Higgins, James M. *The management challenge: An introduction to management.* New York: Macmillan Publishing Company, 1991.

Hy, Ronald John. *Financial management for health care administrators.* New York: Quorum Books, 1989.

Jelinek, Richard C., and Matthew M. Person, III. Clinical data systems: Management imperative for tomorrow. *Journal of Health Administration Education* 6 (Spring 1988): 337–343.

Joint Commission on Accreditation of Healthcare Organizations, *Accreditation manual for hospitals, 1992.* Oakbrook Terrace, IL: 1991.

Jones, V. Brewster, and L. Clark Taylor. Expectations and outcome skills of a generalist health care administrator. *Journal of Health Administration Education* 8 (Winter 1990): 41–52.

Kelly, John T., and James E. Swartwout. Development of practice parameters by physician organizations, *QRB* 16 (February 1990): 54–57.

Klafehn, Keith A., Paul J. Kuzdrall, Jonathon S. Rakich, and Alan G. Krigline. Application of simulation in hospital resource allocation and utilization. *Journal of Management Science & Policy Analysis* 8 (Spring/Summer 1991): 346–356.

Klafehn, Keith A., Jonathon S. Rakich, and Paul J. Kuzdrall. The use of simulation as an aid in hospital management decision making. *Hospital Topics* 67 (March/April 1989): 6–12.

Marder, Robert J. Relationship of clinical indicators and practice guidelines. *QRB* 16 (February 1990): 60.

Martin, James B. The environment and future of health information systems. *Journal of Health Administration Education* 8 (Winter 1990): 11–24.

Mullner, Ross M., and Ronald M. Andersen. A descriptive and financial ratio analysis of merged and consolidated hospitals: United States, 1980–1985. In *Advances in health economics and health services research*, edited by Richard M. Scheffler and Louis F. Rossiter, Vol. 7., 41–58. Greenwich, CT: JAI Press, Inc., 1987.

Neumann, Bruce R., James D. Suver, and William N. Zelman. *Financial management: Concepts and applications for health care providers*, 2nd ed. Owings Mills, MD: National Health Publishing/AUPHA Press, 1988.

Pearce, John A. II, and Richard B. Robinson, Jr. *Management*. New York: Random House, 1989.

Smith, C. Thomas. Hospital management strategies for fixed-price payment. *Health Care Management Review* 11 (Winter 1986): 21–26.

Smith, Howard L., and Myron D. Fottler. *Prospective payment: Managing for operational effectiveness*. Rockville, MD: Aspen Systems Corporation, 1985.

Smith-Daniels, Vicki L., Sharon B. Schweikhart, and Dwight E. Smith-Daniels. Capacity management in health care services: Review and future directions. *Decision Sciences* 19 (Fall 1988): 889–919.

Van Fleet, David D. *Contemporary management*. Boston, MA: Houghton Mifflin Company, 1991.

Vassilacopoulos, G. A simulation model for bed allocation to hospital inpatient departments. *Simulation* 45 (November 1985): 233–241.

Vonderembse, Mark A., and Gregory P. White. *Operations management: Concepts, methods, and strategies*. St. Paul, MN: West Publishing Company, 1991.

Weiss, Howard J., and Gershon, Mark E. *Production and operations management*. Boston, MA: Allyn and Bacon, Inc., 1989.

Zviran, Moshe. Design considerations for integrated hospital information systems. *Hospital & Health Services Administration* 35 (Fall 1990): 377–393.

VI / Managing People in Health Services Organizations

13 / Motivation

*A grand theory of motivation is not likely to
even be considered in the 1990s.*
The Economist[1]

Managers in health services organizations (HSOs) may be adept at planning and organizing human and physical resources, but unless they can motivate people to work effectively to achieve organizational goals, true success will be elusive. This chapter and the three chapters that follow deal with the critically important managerial topic of getting people to do what must be done. This is the directing function of management; if done badly, the functions of planning, organizing, staffing, and controlling cannot be carried out effectively.

Motivation is covered in this chapter, leadership in Chapter 14, communication in Chapter 15, and organizational dynamics and change in Chapter 16. These topics are intertwined in that they all involve various aspects of how managers get work done through people. Part VII examines topics related to the staffing function, including personnel/human resources management and labor relations, in Chapters 17 and 18. The six chapters in these parts explain how health services managers manage the organization's vitally important human resources.

To appreciate the complexity and importance of managing human resources in HSOs, readers will recall from Chapter 1 that it is only through people that work occurs. Managers accomplish work through people by integrating structure, tasks/technology, and people, as shown in the conversion component of the managment model presented in Figure 1.6. Thus, successful managing depends on the manager's ability to get other people to do what needs to be done.[2]

THE CONCEPT OF MOTIVATION

Critical to the manager's ability to get other people to make significant contributions to the HSO's objectives are the answers to questions such as: Why do people act as they do? How does one person obtain the cooperation of others? The answers to such questions involve many variables, but a key element is the concept of motivation. The first step in fully appreciating the role of motivation in effective management is to realize that it is a means of understanding the way people behave in organizations,[3] and that much, although certainly not all, of what is known about motivation is generalizable. A second important step is to consider the various types of behaviors an HSO needs from its members. Greenberger et al. categorize them as:

> *Entering the Organization.* Crucial to the survival of the organization is the ability to attract good people. This statement implies two things. First, adequate numbers of employees must be motivated to join the organization. Second, these employees must have the needed skills and abilities, or at least the aptitude or potential, to respond positively to formal and informal training. Custodians, physicians, technicians, nurses, administrators, and others need to be motivated to choose your organization from among many other options as they graduate from school or leave another employer. Some organizations are better than others at the recruiting function. In fact, many hospitals employ nurse and/or physician recruiters exactly for this reason. Many things contribute to this ability, and the inability to motivate competent people to join is harmful to any organization.
>
> *Remaining in the Organization.* An organization must attract personnel; then it must motivate people to continue their employment relationship with the organization. When employees are motivated to seek employment elsewhere . . . the turnover may have tremendous direct and indirect costs to the organization, including quality of patient care. Many hospitals invest money and time in

attempts to curb tremendous rates of turnover, and it is essential that these resources be allocated in ways that will most efficiently and appropriately motivate retention. Again, as with motivating people to enter the organization, the goals of retention are twofold. A critical mass of people must be maintained, and those who are most motivated to remain within the organization will, hopefully, be the best employees.

Attendance. Employees must be motivated to come to work regularly, punctually, and predictably. Poor attendance creates staffing problems, quality-of-care problems, frustrations, cost overruns, and other negative repercussions. What seems to be a simple issue—getting people to come to work—is often a source of administrative headaches.

Performance. Job performance is typically conceptualized along the dimensions of quantity of output (productivity) and/or quality of work. Good attendance rates by themselves do not ensure high or even adequate levels of performance. Employees hired to do a job are expected to do it well. Moreover, to the extent that tasks are interdependent, the performance of one employee may positively or negatively affect the performance of others. In HSOs, performance is even more critical than in many other organizations, because poor performance may be not only financially costly but also dangerous. Clearly, it is essential to motivate organizational members toward high levels of individual, group, departmental, and organizational performance.

Citizenship Behaviors. Quantity and quality of job performance are not the only dimensions of behavior that employees exhibit or fail to exhibit while at work. Katz and Kahn discuss a much wider array of behaviors that are not an explicit part of the job description but that loyal, committed organizational members might be motivated to exhibit: cooperation; altruism; making positive statements about work; protecting fellow employees and organizational property; avoiding waste, complaints, and arguments; and generally going above and beyond the call of duty.[4] Such prosocial, pro-organizational gestures might be referred to as citizenship behaviors,[5] because they probably make the manager's job easier and contribute to smoother departmental and organizational functioning. Citizenship behaviors are perhaps less obvious and measurable than job performance per se, but they are of value to any organization.[6]

HSO managers must motivate all these categories of behaviors. The list suggests the extensive and pervasive role of motivation in managing organizations. The concept of motivation is at once simple and complex. Motivation is simple because it is now known that behavior is goal directed and is induced by increasingly well-understood forces, some of which are internal to the individual and others of which are external. Motivation is complex because mechanisms that induce behavior include very complicated and individualized needs, wants, and desires that are shaped, affected, and satisfied in ways that differ for every individual.

MOTIVATION MODELED AND DEFINED

Why does one person work harder than another? Why is one more cooperative than another? In part, these differences occur because people have varying needs and act differently to satisfy them. People's needs are, in effect, deficiencies that cause them to undertake a pattern of behavior intended to fill the deficiency. For example, at a very simple level human needs are physiological. A hungry person needs food, is driven by hunger, and is motivated to satisfy the need (overcome the deficiency). Other needs are more complex; some are psychological (e.g., the need for self-esteem) and others are sociological (e.g., the need for social interaction). In short, "Needs are energizers or triggers of behavioral responses."[7]

This information is the basis for the motivation process model shown in Figure 13.1, which suggests that the motivation process is cyclical. It begins with an unsatisfied need (need deficiency) and ends after the individual assesses the results of efforts to satisfy the need. In between, the person searches for ways to satisfy the need, chooses a course of action, and exhibits goal-directed behavior intended to remove or reduce the need deficiency.

The model is oversimplified, but it does contain the essential elements of the human motivation process. It also suggests definitions of motivation. One is that "*motivation is the internal drive to satisfy an unsatisfied need.*"[8] Another is that "*motivation is the stimulus of behavior.*"[9] Figure 13.1 suggests, too, that goal-directed behavior intended to remove or diminish need defi-

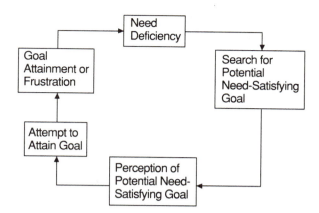

Figure 13.1. The motivation process. (From Aldag, Ramon J., and Timothy M. Stearns. *Management,* 2d ed., 407. Cincinnati, OH: South-Western Publishing Co., 1991; reprinted by permission. Copyright 1991 by South-Western Publishing Co. All rights reserved.)

ciencies is fundamental to the motivation cycle. An important addendum to these definitions is that the direction, intensity, and duration of motivation may be influenced by factors outside the individual, such as the ability of managers and the HSO to satisfy an individual's needs. By combining these definitions and the addendum, it may be concluded that motivation: 1) is driven by unsatisfied needs, 2) results in goal-directed behaviors, and 3) is influenced by factors that may be internal or external to the individual.

Motivation is a key determinant of individual performance in organizations and is of obvious importance to achieving an HSO's objectives. Applying the above conclusions about motivation to enhance the contributions of people to an HSO is one of the most important tasks managers face. Motivation is a key variable in people's level of performance, but it is only one of many. Intelligence, physical and mental abilities, and previous experiences also determine performance. In addition, the nature of the work environment is important in determining performance. Good equipment and pleasant surroundings facilitate high levels of performance. Without motivation, however, none of these variables will lead to excellent performance.

Managers vary widely in their effective use of knowledge about human motivation.[10] This variation results partly from the different views managers hold about the basic nature of people in work situations and how managers relate to people they manage because of these views. Before examining underlying theories about motivation, it is useful to consider how attitudes managers hold about people affect efforts to motivate them. This is the context in which managers motivate others to do an HSO's work.

MANAGERIAL ATTITUDES AND MOTIVATION

A generation ago, Douglas McGregor postulated two opposing views held by managers on the nature of human beings. The negative view was labeled *Theory X* and the positive view *Theory Y.*[11] The central tenet of McGregor's writings is that managers' views of human beings are based on assumptions they make about human nature, and that their behavior toward people is, in turn, largely influenced by these assumptions.

Organizations whose management is characterized by highly centralized direction and control use methods that are rooted in the long and successful experience of religious and military organizations. The line of authority or command in such organizations runs from the top down through the layers of the organization along with delegation of authority. Full and detailed accountability goes up the line from bottom to top. Such organizations tend to have autocratic and authoritarian management styles. McGregor argues that this approach to management arose from several assumptions about the nature of human beings. The assumptions made by Theory X managers were:

1. The average human being has an inherent dislike of work and will avoid it if possible.
2. Because of this human characteristic of dislike of work, most people must be coerced, controlled, directed, and threatened with punishment to get them to put forth adequate effort toward the achievement of organizational objectives.
3. The average human being prefers to be closely directed, wishes to avoid responsibility, has relatively little ambition, wants security above all.[12]

In contrast, assumptions held by the more positive Theory Y managers about human nature were:

1. The expenditure of physical and mental effort in work is as natural as play or rest. The average human being does not inherently dislike work. Depending upon controllable conditions, work may be a source of satisfaction (and will be voluntarily performed) or a source of punishment (and will be avoided if possible).
2. External control and the threat of punishment are not the only means for bringing about effort toward organizational objectives. People will exercise self-direction and self-control in the service of objectives to which they are committed.
3. Commitment to objectives is a function of the rewards associated with their achievement. The most significant of such rewards, e.g., the satisfaction of their ego and self-actualization needs, can be direct products of efforts directed toward organizational objectives.
4. The average human being learns under proper conditions not only to accept but to seek responsibility. Avoidance of responsibility, lack of ambition, and emphasis on security are generally consequences of experience, not inherent human characteristics.
5. The capacity to exercise a relatively high degree of imagination, ingenuity, and creativity in the solution of organizational problems is widely, not narrowly, distributed in the population.
6. Under conditions of modern organizational life, the intellectual potentialities of the average human being are only partly utilized.[13]

Theory X and Theory Y managers reflect the different attitudes managers have about people. They are important in considering how motivation theory is applied. A Theory Y manager sees motivating as creating an organizational climate in which people can fulfill their needs while performing work that meets the HSO's needs. Theory Y assumptions are applicable to HSOs because they reflect the belief that it is most effective to *work with* people rather than *use* them. This means that workers are involved in decisions that govern their workplace and work.

Ouchi[14] developed a view of management that he calls Theory Z—an obvious extension of McGregor's terminology. Theory Z is distinguished by implicit recognition that the major challenge for managers lies in creating an environment in which all workers understand that organizational objectives are *best* met by meeting the needs and objectives of individuals. The central premise of Theory Z is that involved workers are critical to quality and productivity gains.

Shortell, who believes that Theory Z is especially important in HSOs, writes that:

Involvement is brought about through development of trust, subtlety, and intimacy, which form the basic building blocks of the Theory Z organization. . . . Through development of these factors, it is possible to develop an involved group of participants who share a relatively common culture conducive to high-quality, productive work.[15]

Ouchi[16] described five attributes of Theory Z organizations: 1) lifetime employment relationships, 2) investment in organization-specific skills, 3) balance between explicit and implicit decision criteria (Is a decision correct in terms of quantitative variables and in terms of the more qualitative or implicit criteria such as the organization's philosophy?), 4) participative decision making, and 5) a holistic view of people (less emphasis on superior-subordinate relationships among people in the organization). It is well known that the Japanese have developed these attributes to a high degree in many of their organizations, with remarkable success. Figure 13.2

RELATIONSHIPS BETWEEN BASIC CHARACTERISTICS OF THEORY Z

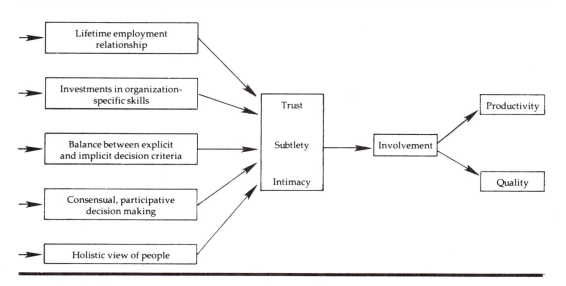

Figure 13.2. Relationships between basic characteristics of Theory Z. (From Shortell, Stephen M. Theory Z: Implications and relevance for health care management. *Health Care Management Review* 7 [Fall 1982]: 9; reprinted by permission.)

illustrates how the attributes lead to trust, subtlety, and intimacy, and to more involved workers who contribute to productivity and quality gains.

The key point of the Theory X/Theory Y dichotomy and of Theory Z is that managers' *attitudes* about people and the *assumptions* managers make about people's nature and their approach to work shapes how managers seek to motivate employees. In fact, all contemporary motivation theories integrate in one way or another McGregor's observation about the importance of managers' attitudes about people in determining their approach to motivation. The following discussion shows there is no undisputed and comprehensive theory about motivation or how managers effect it in the workplace.[17]

MOTIVATION THEORIES

Because human motivation is not well understood, a confusing diversity of theories has been developed to explain it. The quotation at the beginning of this chapter suggests the lack of a grand theory of motivation and that none is likely to emerge soon. At present, there is disagreement as to how motivation occurs in people, as well as about its causes. Significant research continues, and eventually motivation may be completely understood. Until then, however, knowledge about motivation will remain piecemeal. One consequence of incomplete knowledge is that many competing theories are vying to explain motivation. Another consequence is that students of management theory must absorb many theories and much related information to understand motivation. The most important motivation theories can be divided into two broad categories: *content theories* and *process theories*.

Content theories focus on the internal needs and desires that initiate, sustain, and eventually terminate behavior. They focus on *what* motivates people. In contrast, process theories seek to explain *how* behavior is initiated, sustained, and terminated. Combined, these theories define variables that explain motivated behavior and show how they interact and influence each other to produce certain behavior patterns. Table 13.1 summarizes examples of the most important theoretical developments in both categories from a managerial perspective. It serves as an outline for the discussion of content and process theories of motivation that follows.

CONTENT THEORIES

The process of motivation shown in Figure 13.1 begins with a need deficiency—an unfulfilled need. Content theorists seek to determine how managers motivate people by studying their needs (e.g., *what* motivates them). Content theories focus on identifying human needs and helping people understand the things and behaviors that can satisfy them. Perhaps the most widely recognized content theory of motivation—and certainly one of the most important—was developed by Abraham Maslow half a century ago.[18]

Maslow's Hierarchy of Needs

Maslow, a psychologist, formulated a theory of motivation that stressed two fundamental premises. The first is that human beings are wanting beings whose needs depend on what they already have. In Maslow's view, only needs not yet satisfied influence behavior; an adequately fulfilled need is not a motivator. His second premise is that people's needs are arranged in a *hierarchy*. Once a need is fulfilled, another emerges and demands fulfillment. Maslow's need theory stressed the idea that, within the hierarchy, "higher" needs become dominant only after "lower" needs are satisfied. Figure 13.3 illustrates Maslow's need hierarchy.

From lowest to highest order, the five categories of needs identified by Maslow are:[19]

1. *Basic physiological needs* This category includes basic survival needs such as air, food, and water.

Table 13.1.   Managerial perspective of content and process theories of motivation

Theoretical base	Theoretical explanation	Founders of the theories	Managerial application
Content	Focuses on factors within the person that energize, direct, sustain, and stop behavior. These factors can only be inferred.	Maslow—five-level need hierarchy Alderfer—three-level hierarchy (ERG) Herzberg—two major factors called hygiene-motivators McClelland—three learned needs acquired from the culture: achievement, affiliation, and power	Managers need to be aware of differences in needs, desires, and goals because each individual is unique in many ways.
Process	Describes, explains, and analyzes how behavior is energized, directed, sustained, and stopped.	Vroom—an expectancy theory of choices Adams—equity theory based on comparisons that individuals make Locke—goal-setting theory that conscious goals and intentions are the determinants of behavior Skinner—reinforcement theory concerned with the learning that occurs as a consequence of behavior	Managers need to understand the process of motivation and how individuals make choices based on preferences, rewards, and accomplishments.

Adapted from Gibson, James L., John M. Ivancevich, and James H. Donnelly, Jr., *Organizations: Behavior, structure, processes,* 7th ed., 102. Homewood, IL: Irwin. Copyright © 1991, Irwin.

2. *Safety and security needs* Once survival needs are met, attention is turned to ensuring continued survival by protecting oneself against physical harm and deprivation.

3. *Affection and social activity needs* This third level relates to people's social and gregarious nature. This is a breaking point in the hierarchy because here it moves away from the physical or quasi-physical needs of the first two levels. This level reflects people's need for association or companionship, for belonging to groups, and for giving and receiving friendship and affection.

4. *Esteem and status needs* Need for self-respect or self-esteem results from awareness of one's importance to others.

5. *Self-realization needs* This highest level of needs includes developing one's potential. It is evidenced by the need to be creative and the need to have opportunities for self-expression and self-fulfillment.

Probably because of its great intuitive appeal, as well as the ease with which most people can understand it, Maslow's theory has been widely adopted. However, it is only a theory. Maslow offered no significant empirical substantiation. In a remarkable bit of candor he wrote of his concern that his theory was "being swallowed whole by all sorts of enthusiastic people, who really should be a little more tentative in the way that I am."[20]

Numerous studies have failed to validate the theory exactly as Maslow specifies it,[21] but they have found that people have numerous needs and seek to fulfill them. In this sense, Maslow's work contributes important insight into the nature of motivation, and especially into how need deficiencies influence actions to fill them. This is consistent with the motivation process model in Figure 13.1. Most importantly, Maslow's theory provided a conceptual framework that could be used to build and test more sophisticated theories about needs and how they affect human behavior.

Alderfer's ERG Theory

Building on Maslow's theoretical base, an improved theory was developed by Clayton Alderfer, who agrees with Maslow that each individual's needs are arranged in a hierarchy.[22] In Alderfer's view, however, the hierarchy of needs is more accurately conceptualized as having only three

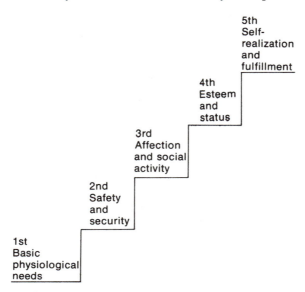

Figure 13.3. Hierarchy of human needs. (From Maslow, Abraham H. A theory of human motivation. *Psychological Review* 50 [July 1943]: 370–396.)

distinct categories, not five as Maslow had hypothesized. The three are *existence needs, relatedness needs,* and *growth needs*—thus the title of the ERG theory of motivation.[23] Alderfer's three categories of human needs can be described as follows:

1. *Existence needs* These include material and physical needs—needs that can be satisfied by such things as air, water, money, and working conditions.
2. *Relatedness needs* These include all needs that involve other people—needs satisfied by meaningful social and interpersonal relationships. Relatedness needs include anger and hostility, as well as more positive needs such as friendship.
3. *Growth needs* These include all needs involving creative efforts—needs satisfied by an individual through creative or productive contributions.

Alderfer's ERG theory is similar to Maslow's hierarchy of needs. Alderfer's existence needs are similar to Maslow's physiological and safety needs; his relatedness needs are similar to Maslow's affection and social activity category; and his growth needs are similar to the esteem and self-realization needs identified by Maslow. The theories differ, however, in an important respect: the manner in which needs predominate in influencing behavior.

Maslow theorizes that unfulfilled lower level needs are predominant and that the next higher level of needs is not activated until the predominant (unmet lower level) need is satisfied. He calls this the *satisfaction-progression* process. In contrast, Alderfer argues that his three categories of needs form a hierarchy only in the sense of increasing abstractness, or decreasing concreteness: as an individual moves from existence to relatedness to growth needs, the means to satisfy the needs become less and less concrete. In Alderfer's theory, people focus first on needs that are satisfied in relatively concrete ways; then they focus on needs that are satisfied more abstractly. This is similar to Maslow's idea of satisfaction-progression. However, Alderfer proposes that a *frustration-regression* process is also present in determining which category of needs predominates at any time. By this he means that someone frustrated in efforts to satisfy growth needs might regress and focus on satisfying more concrete relatedness or even more concrete existence needs. In Alderfer's view, the coexistence of the satisfaction-progression and the frustration-regression processes leads to a cycling between categories of needs.

An example will clarify Alderfer's concept of cycling between categories of needs. Take the case of Jennifer Smith, a young registered nurse. Smith is a single parent of two children and is concerned about the security of her position and her pay, although she finds the social interactions with co-workers rewarding. She is an excellent nurse who enjoys her work. When a vacancy occurred for the head nurse position on her unit, she considered the opportunities this presented for professional growth and development, as well as for a higher salary. Ms. Smith applied for the position and looked forward to the challenges, if she would be promoted.

However, a more experienced and equally qualified nurse was promoted. Smith's disappointment showed and she became concerned about her future. Several co-workers noticed her reaction and made special efforts to ease her disappointment. They told her that other opportunities would come up and with a little more experience she would be promoted. The newly promoted head nurse was sensitive to this situation and made a point of telling Smith what a valuable contribution she was making. After a few weeks Smith returned to the level of enjoyment of her work she felt before this episode. In terms of needs, Smith has cycled from having existence and relatedness needs predominate, to predominance of the growth needs represented by the promotion, and then back to predominance of relatedness needs, all in a few weeks. In other words, she experienced a satisfaction-progression process *and* a frustration-regression process.

Another important part of Alderfer's ERG theory and another way in which it differs from Maslow's theory lies in his view that when individuals satisfy their existence and relatedness needs, those needs become less important. The opposite is true for growth needs, however; as growth needs are satisfied they become increasingly important. People who become more creative and productive raise their growth goals and are dissatisfied until the new goals are reached. In the case of Jennifer Smith described above, this means that when she becomes a head nurse she will want to become a nursing supervisor, then a nursing service director, and so on.

Herzberg's Two-Factor Theory

Frederick Herzberg takes a different approach to the study of what factors motivate human behavior in the workplace. He starts with questions of what satisfies or dissatisfies people about their work, assuming that the answers are keys to understanding what motivates people. Because he seeks the factors that motivate people, his is also a content theory of motivation. His research was first published in the late 1950s[24] and later updated,[25] and recently has been restated and defended.[26] The original research involved 200 engineers and accountants who were asked to recall a time when they felt exceptionally good about their jobs. Other questions determined why they felt satisfied and whether these feelings affected performance, personal relationships, and well-being. Finally, the events that returned their attitudes to "normal" were identified. A second set of interviews asked the same people to describe incidents that made them feel exceptionally negative about their jobs—instances in which negative feelings were related to some event on the job.

Herzberg and associates conclude that job satisfaction consists of two separate and independent dimensions, and they postulate a "two-factor" theory of motivation. They argue that one set of factors, called *satisfiers* or *motivators,* result in satisfaction when they are adequate. The other factors, termed *dissatisfiers* or *hygiene factors,* cause dissatisfaction when they are deficient.

Hygiene Factors (Dissatisfiers) Absence of some job conditions can dissatisfy employees. However, presence of the same conditions does not necessarily lead to a high degree of motivation. Herzberg calls these conditions hygiene (or maintenance) factors, since they are necessary to maintain a reasonable level of satisfaction. Managers who eliminate factors that create job dissatisfaction do not necessarily increase motivation. Many of Herzberg's hygiene factors had been thought by managers to be motivators, but they are actually more potent dissatisfiers when absent. Herzberg identifies 10 hygiene or maintenance factors:

1. Organizational policy and administration
2. Technical supervision
3. Interpersonal relations with supervisor
4. Interpersonal relations with peers
5. Interpersonal relations with subordinates
6. Salary
7. Job security
8. Personal life
9. Work conditions
10. Status

Motivational Factors (Satisfiers) In Herzberg's theory the presence of other job conditions tends to build high levels of motivation and job satisfaction. However, the absence of these conditions does not prove to be highly dissatisfying. Herzberg identifies six motivational factors or satisfiers:

1. Achievement
2. Recognition
3. Advancement
4. The work itself
5. The possibility of growth
6. Responsibility

Impact of the Two-Factor Theory A comparison of the Herzberg and Maslow models shows them both to be content theories—they theorize about what motivates human behavior. In fact, Herzberg's theory is largely based on Maslow's needs hierarchy, as Figure 13.4 illustrates. The key difference between the Herzberg and Maslow theories is that Herzberg proposes two distinct influences in the workplace. Hygiene factors affect job dissatisfaction, and motivators affect job satisfaction. Herzberg states that managers must improve or control hygiene factors to minimize dissatisfaction; satisfaction depends on other factors. Figure 13.5 illustrates this distinction. In it, the motivators shown are typically *intrinsic* factors (e.g., part of the job) and the hygiene factors are *extrinisic* (e.g., controlled by the manager or someone else in the organization). This distinction must be remembered in the design and redesign of jobs in HSOs.[27]

Herzberg's two-factor theory made a major contribution to understanding the dynamics of job satisfaction. Earlier theories viewed job satisfaction (people's attitudes toward their jobs) as unidimensional. Job satisfaction was at one end of a continuum, with job dissatisfaction at the other. Herzberg shows that two distinct continua affect job satisfaction: one affects dissatisfaction and the other satisfaction. The opposite of satisfaction is not dissatisfaction—it is no satisfaction. The opposite of dissatisfaction is not satisfaction—it is no dissatisfaction. If managers are to effectively motivate people they must be concerned with one set of factors to minimize dissatisfaction *and* another to help people achieve satisfaction.

Herzberg's two-factor theory extends the understanding of motivation, but it is not without flaws or critics.[28] One criticism is that the research methodology used individual story telling in response to questions. This methodology is very susceptible to personal attribution biases—when things go well people take the credit in terms of intrinsic factors, but they are likely to blame failure on extrinsic factors.

Such criticism notwithstanding, Herzberg's two-factor theory caused managers to think more carefully about the role of intrinsic factors in achieving job satisfaction and about their own role in enhancing opportunities for intrinsic satisfaction. Herzberg's work is responsible for the job enrichment movement in the United States. In his view, job enrichment "seeks to improve both task efficiency and human satisfaction by means of building into people's jobs, quite specifically, greater scope for personal achievement and recognition, more challenging and responsible work, and more opportunity for individual advancement and growth."[29]

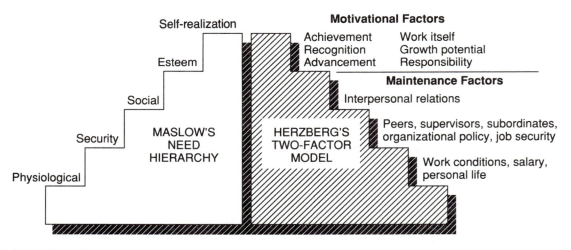

Figure 13.4. Comparison of the Maslow and Herzberg models. (Adapted from Donnelly, James H., Jr., James L. Gibson, and John M. Ivancevich. *Fundamentals of management,* 7th ed., 313. Homewood, IL: BPI-Irwin, 1990; reprinted by permission.)

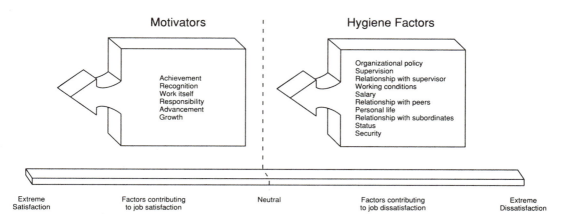

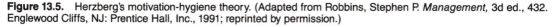

| Extreme Satisfaction | Factors contributing to job satisfaction | Neutral | Factors contributing to job dissatisfaction | Extreme Dissatisfaction |

Figure 13.5. Herzberg's motivation-hygiene theory. (Adapted from Robbins, Stephen P. *Management,* 3d ed., 432. Englewood Cliffs, NJ: Prentice Hall, Inc., 1991; reprinted by permission.)

McClelland's Learned Needs Theory

Another important contribution to *content* theory was made by David McClelland.[30] McClelland's theory, called the *learned* or *acquired needs theory,* posits that people learn their needs through life experiences; they were not born with them. This theory builds on the much earlier work of Henry Murray,[31] who theorized that people acquire an individual profile of needs by interacting with their environment. McClelland was also influenced by the work of John Atkinson.[32] Both McClelland and Atkinson suggest that people have three sets of needs:

1. *Need for achievement* The need to excel, achieve in relation to standards, accomplish complex tasks, and resolve problems
2. *Need for power* The need to control or influence how others behave and to exercise authority over others
3. *Need for affiliation* The need to associate with others, to form and sustain friendly and close interpersonal relationships, and to avoid conflict

McClelland theorizes that people are not born with these needs. Instead, they are learned or acquired as people grow and develop, which occurs through unique experiences. For example, children learn the need to achieve because of encouragement and reinforcement of autonomy and self-reliance by adults who influence their early years. McClelland also suggests that everyone has all three sets of needs, but that one set predominates and affects a person's decisions and behaviors. This point is important because it relates to how well people "fit" particular work situations.

For example, Holt notes that "achievers do not always make the best managers because organizations are based on diffused authority and group activities, and achievers are often uncomfortable in situations of group responsibility and control."[33] In contrast, people who are predominantly influenced by a need for power are generally better suited to be managers because they are comfortable with executive decision making and are likely to aggressively control work activities in their areas of responsibility.

People most heavily influenced by a need for affiliation might not make good managers because they have difficulty making decisions and taking actions that interfere with social compatibility, even when such decisions are vital to organizational effectiveness. Holt correctly observes that "few affiliators are happy or successful in line management and executive positions, where emotionally difficult decisions must often be made, such as disciplining employees, enforcing policies, and retrenching outdated technologies."[34] Nonetheless, such people are vital to HSOs because so much depends on effective teamwork. Affiliators are adept at bringing together groups or individuals with diverse interests and viewpoints, coordinating interdependent tasks, and helping solve conflicts. Therefore, people with strong affiliation needs are valuable in HSOs.

People with high achievement needs might fit well in many positions in HSOs, especially those with extensive and rigorous demands for excellence. In McClelland's view, certain characteristics identify people with high needs for achievement:[35]

1. A clear desire for personal responsibility
2. A strong preference for quick and concrete feedback on their performance
3. The ability to derive intrinsic satisfaction from doing a job well or solving problems (For these people, monetary and material rewards received for their achievement are more a type of feedback than ends in themselves.)
4. A tendency to set moderately difficult (in contrast to easy or difficult) performance goals (This characteristic surprises managers who assume that people with high levels of need for achievement would set high goals for themselves or relish having their superiors do so. Instead, people with high achievement needs prefer goals that lie within their capabilities.)

Reflecting McClelland's theory and research, Gibson, Ivancevich, and Donnelly offer a useful prescription for actions by managers interested in developing a positive high need for achievement in people they supervise:

1. Arrange job tasks so that employees receive periodic feedback on performance, providing information that enables them to make modifications or corrections.
2. Point out to employees models of achievement. Identify and publicize the accomplishments of achievement heroes, the successful people, the winners, and use them as models.
3. Work with employees to improve their self-image. People [with high need for achievement] like themselves and seek moderate challenges and responsibilities.
4. Introduce realism into all work-related topics: promotion, rewards, transfer, development opportunities, and team membership opportunities. Employees should think in realistic terms and think positively about how they can accomplish goals.[36]

The Content Theories Summarized

The common thread of the four content theories is the focus on *what needs* motivate human behavior. Each defines human needs differently, but each holds that managers motivate people by helping them identify and meet their needs in the workplace. The synopsis of each content theory in Table 13.2 compares the key points. None is a complete model of human motivation. It is not sufficient to understand what motivates people; managers must also understand the processes by which behavior is initiated, directed, sustained, and terminated. The content theories provide a conceptual foundation for research intended to explain *how* individuals are motivated. This research led to development of a number of process motivation theories.

PROCESS THEORIES

Process theorists focus on how individuals' expectations and preferences for outcomes associated with their performance actually influence performance. A key element in the process theories of motivation examined here is that people are decision makers who weigh the personal advantages and disadvantages of their behavior. Following the outline presented in Table 13.1, Vroom's expectancy theory, Adams' equity theory, Locke's goal setting theory, and Skinner's reinforcement theory are the major models of processes by which motivation occurs. Each theory concerns *how* motivation occurs in human beings.

Table 13.2. Comparison of four content theories of motivation

Content motivation theories	Assumptions made	How motivation is measured	Practical application value	Problems and limitations
Maslow's need hierarchy	Individuals attempt to satisfy basic needs before directing behavior toward higher-order needs.	Maslow, as a clinical psychologist, used his patients in asking questions and listening to answers. Organizational researchers have relied on self-report scales.	Makes sense to managers and gives many a feeling of knowing how motivation works for their employees.	Does not address the issue of individual differences, has received limited research support; and fails to caution about the dynamic nature of needs—needs change.
Alderfer's ERG theory	Individuals who fail to satisfy growth needs become frustrated, regress, and refocus attention on lower-order needs.	Self-report scales are used to assess three need categories.	Calls attention to what happens when and if need satisfaction does not occur; frustrations can be a major reason why performance levels are not attained or sustained.	Not enough research has been conducted; available research is self-report in nature, which raises the issue of how good the measurement is. Another issue is whether individuals really have only three need areas.
Herzberg's two-factor theory	Only some job features and characteristics can result in motivation. Some of the characteristics that managers have focused on may result in a comfortable work setting, but do not motivate employees.	Asks employees in interviews to describe critical job incidents.	Talks in terms that managers understand. Identifies motivators that managers can develop, fine-tune, and use.	Assumes that every worker is similar in needs and preferences; fails to meet scientific measurement standards; has not been updated to reflect changes in society with regard to job security and pay needs.
McClelland's learned needs	The needs of a person are learned from the culture (society); therefore, training and education can enhance and influence a person's need strength.	Thematic Apperception Test (TAT), a projective technique that encourages respondents to reveal their needs.	If a person's needs can be assessed, then management can intervene through training to develop needs that are compatible with organizational goals.	Interpreting the TAT is difficult; the effect that training has on changing needs has not been sufficiently tested.

From Gibson, James L., John M. Ivancevich, and James H. Donnelly, Jr. *Organizations: Behavior, structure, processes*, 7th ed., 118. Homewood, IL: Irwin. Copyright © 1991, Irwin.

Vroom's Expectancy Theory

Acknowledging the content theorists who preceded him, Victor Vroom, in the early 1960s, theorized that people are not only driven by their needs, but they make choices about what they will and will not do to fulfill their needs based on three conditions: 1) the person must believe that effort to perform at a particular level will make the desired performance or behavior more likely,

2) the desired performance or behavior must lead to some concrete outcome or reward, and 3) the person must value the outcome.[37] Figure 13.6 shows the three central components and the relationships in the expectancy theory model.

Expectancy is what individuals perceive to be the probability that their efforts will lead to a desired level of performance. The person must believe that effort will cause something to happen. If it is believed that more effort will lead to improved performance, expectancy will be high. If, in a different situation, the same person believes that trying harder will not improve performance, the expectancy that effort will lead to performance will be low.

Instrumentality is the probability perceived by individuals that their performance will lead to desired outcomes or rewards. If a person believes that better performance will be rewarded, the instrumentality of performance to reward will be high. Conversely, if the person believes that improved performance will not be rewarded, the instrumentality of improved performance will be low.

Outcomes are listed only once in Figure 13.6, but they play two important roles in the expectancy theory. "Level of performance" (in the center of Figure 13.6) actually represents an outcome of the "Individual effort to perform." Vroom calls this a first-order outcome. Examples of first-order outcomes include productivity, creativity, absenteeism, quality of production, or other behaviors that result from the individual's effort to perform. The "Outcomes" component listed on the right side of Figure 13.6 is a second-order outcome that results from attainment of first-order outcomes. That is, these outcomes are the reward (or punishment) associated with performance. Examples include merit pay increases, esteem of co-workers, supervisory approval, promotion, and flexible work schedules.

Crucial to Vroom's expectancy theory is the concept that people have preferences for outcomes. Vroom terms the value an individual attaches to a particular outcome its *valence*. When people have a strong preference for a particular outcome it receives a high valence; similarly, a lower preference for an outcome yields a lower valence. People have valences for both first- and second-order outcomes. For example, someone might prefer a merit pay increase over a more flexible work schedule (second-order outcomes). Individuals might prefer to produce quality work (a first-order outcome) because they believe this will lead to a merit pay increase (a second-order outcome), which might be high on the person's list of preferences or which, in Vroom's terminology, would be assigned a high valence.

These three components of the expectancy theory (expectancy, instrumentality, and valence for outcomes) can be combined into an equation to express the motivation to work:

$$\text{Motivation} = \text{Expectancy} \times \text{Instrumentality} \times \text{Valence}$$
or
$$M = E \times I \times V$$

It is important to note that because the equation is multiplicative, a low value assigned to any variable will yield a low result. For example, if a person is certain that effort will lead to performance (an E value of 1.0 is assigned) and is certain that performance will lead to reward (an I value of 1.0 is assigned) but does not have a very high valence or preference for the reward involved (a V value of 0.5 is assigned), the result ($1.0 \times 1.0 \times 0.5 = 0.5$) is low, indicating that motivation is low. For motivation to be high, expectancy, instrumentality, and valence values must all be high.

For the manager, Vroom's expectancy explains a great deal about motivated behavior. For motivated behavior to occur, three conditions must be met:

1. The person must have a high expectancy that effort and performance are actually linked.
2. The person must have a high expectancy that performance will lead to outcomes or rewards.
3. The person must have a preference for (assign a high valence value to) the outcomes that result from effort. This is true both for first- and second-order outcomes.

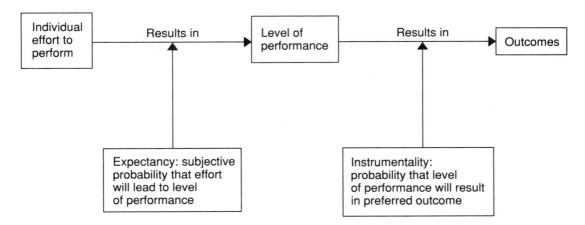

Figure 13.6. Simplified model of expectancy theory.

Managers who know what their workers prefer in terms of second-order outcomes for their efforts and performance have an advantage in developing effective motivation strategies. It is important to remember that implicit in Vroom's model is the fact that individuals have different preferences about outcomes. The design of motivation programs must reflect this fact—they must be flexible enough to address differences in individual preferences regarding the rewards of work.

Adams's Equity Theory

An important extension of expectancy theory came from recognizing that, in addition to preferences as to the rewards associated with performance, individuals also assess the degree that potential rewards will be *equitably* distributed within the organization. Equity theory posits that people calculate the ratios of their efforts to the rewards they receive and compare them to the ratios they believe exist for people in similar situations. People do this because they are motivated by a strong desire to be treated fairly.

J. Stacy Adams developed and tested his *equity theory of motivation* in the early 1960s.[38] Adams theorizes that people judge equity with the following equation:

$$\frac{O_p}{I_p} = \frac{O_o}{I_o}$$

Where:
   O_p is the person's perception of the outcomes he or she is receiving.
   I_p is the person's perception of his or her inputs.
   O_o is the person's perception of the outcomes some comparison person (or comparison other) is receiving.
   I_o is the person's perception of the inputs of the comparison other.

This formulation suggests that equity exists when an individual's perception of the ratio of inputs (efforts) to outcomes (rewards) received is equivalent to that of some "comparison other" or referent. Conversely, inequity exists when the ratios are not equivalent.

It is noteworthy that perception, not reality, is considered in this equation. Furthermore, there are options as to the comparison others or referents in the equation. These options include persons in similar circumstances (co-workers or someone whose circumstances are thought to be similar); a group of people in similar circumstances (e.g., all registered nurses in the HSO); or the perceiving person under different circumstances (e.g., earlier in the position or circumstances when the person worked in another HSO). Choice of referent is a function of information available as well as perceived relevance. Finally, it is important to note that there may be many different inputs and outcomes. Inputs are what people believe they contribute to their jobs, such as experience, time, effort, dedication, and intelligence. Outcomes are what they believe they get from their jobs, such as pay, promotion, status, esteem, monotony, fatigue, and danger.

Equity theorists point out that people are interested in distributive fairness—getting what they believe they deserve for their work. Even with all the variables involved in making comparisons, people consider equity regularly. Extensive research supports this view.[39] Robbins notes that:

> Equity theory recognizes that individuals are concerned not only with the absolute rewards they receive for their efforts, but also with the relationship of these rewards to what others receive. They make judgments concerning the relationship between their inputs and outcomes and the inputs and outcomes of others. . . . When people perceive an imbalance in their inputs-outcomes ratio relative to those of others, they experience tension. This tension provides the basis for motivation as people strive for what they perceive as equity and fairness.[40]

People in a situation they perceive to be inequitable use many methods to restore equity. They might

> *Increase* their performance and work to justify higher rewards when they perceive a positive inequity—when their pay, for instance, seems too high by comparison with others.
> *Decrease* their performance and work to compensate for lower rewards when they perceive a negative inequity—when their pay, for instance, seems too low by comparison with others.
> *Change* the compensation they receive (usually when they perceive that rewards are too low) through legal or other action, or by inappropriate behavior such as misappropriation or theft.
> *Modify* their comparisons—for example, by persuading low performers who are receiving equal pay to increase their efforts or by discouraging high performers from exerting so much effort.
> *Distort* reality and psychologically rationalize that the perceived inequities are justified.
> *Leave* the inequitable situation—by quitting the organization or by changing jobs or careers—because they think inequities will not be resolved.[41]

Except for the first, each mechanism used to restore equity presents serious problems for the manager and the HSO.

Equity theory makes an important contribution to understanding human motivation because it shows that motivation is significantly influenced by absolute *and* by relative rewards. It also shows that if people perceive inequity, they act to reduce it. Thus, it is important that managers minimize inequities—real and perceived—in the workplace.

Locke's Goal-Setting Theory

Another process theory, one enjoying increased popularity recently, derives from the work of Edwin Locke.[42] Locke observes that:

> A cardinal attribute of the behavior of living organisms is goal-directedness. It may be observed at all levels of life: in the assimilation of food by an amoeba, in the root growth of a tree or a plant, in the stalking of prey by a wild animal, and in the activities of a scientist in a laboratory.[43]

Building on the pervasiveness of the "goal-directedness" of human behavior, Locke proposed a *goal-setting theory* to explain motivation. In his view, goal setting is a cognitive process through which conscious goals, as well as intentions about pursuing them, are developed. Goals and intentions developed in this way become primary determinants of behavior.[44] Thus, in Locke's theory of motivation, the intent to work toward goals they have established is an important part of peoples' motivation.[45]

Recent research confirms the importance of goals in motivation.[46] Latham and Locke state that:

> We believe that goal setting is a simple, straight-forward and highly effective technique for motivating employee performance. It is a basic technique, a method on which most other methods depend for their motivational effectiveness. The current popular technique of behavior modification, for example, is mainly goal setting plus feedback, dressed up in academic terminology.[47]

Other studies confirm Locke's original theory that goal specificity (the degree of quantitative precision of the goal) and goal difficulty (the level of performance required to reach the goal) are important to motivation.[48] In fact, it is now clear, as Latham and Baldes noted some time ago, that "The setting of a goal that is both specific and challenging leads to an increase in performance because it makes it clearer to the individual what he/she is supposed to do."[49]

Finally, understanding the role of goals in motivation has been enhanced by research that shows the relationship of goal acceptance by a person to that person's performance. One line of research shows that acceptance of goals significantly increases performance.[50] Another line of research shows that people are more likely to accept goals (other than those they set for themselves), especially difficult goals, when they participate in establishing them.[51]

The most widely adopted method of using goal-setting theory to enhance the contributions of individuals in organizations is management by objectives (MBO). Peter Drucker coined the phrase and conceptualized MBO as a process by which everyone in an organization participates in developing specific, attainable, measurable personal objectives (goals).[52] When MBO works, individual objectives mesh with and support attainment of overall organizational objectives.

Figure 13.7 shows MBO applied in HSOs and illustrates the process of establishing objectives (goals) for everyone by having all manager-subordinate pairs *jointly* establish objectives. Jointly developed goals can have the desired degrees of specificity and difficulty to maximize their usefulness in motivating behavior. Participating in development of the goals increases their acceptability to those persons trying to achieve the objectives.

Skinner's Reinforcement Theory

Reinforcement theory is a counterpoint to the goal-setting theory of motivation, which holds that an individual's goals and intentions about pursuing them drive behavior. Establishment of goals and intentions by people is a cognitive activity that occurs mostly internally, although using a process like MBO subjects individual goals and intentions to negotiation. By contrast, *reinforcement theory* holds that behavior is associated with externally imposed consequences learned from experience.

Reinforcement theory suggests that consequences of behavior are *reinforcers*, and when positive consequences immediately follow an act the act will likely be repeated. The converse is true for negative consequences. At the heart of reinforcement theory is *operant conditioning*, the concept that people learn through experience what to do or not do to assure positive consequences or avoid negative ones. Operant conditioning's most widely read and quoted theorist is B.F. Skinner, who theorizes that reinforcement concepts explain all human behavior.[53] Figure 13.8 illustrates Skinner's conceptualization of how reinforcement theory motivates human behavior.

In this model, someone responding to a *stimulus* makes a *response*. The response or behavior triggers *consequences*, which can be positive or negative and which will affect *future responses*. People learn from the consequences of previous experiences. When faced with the same stimulus—or one that is similar—they follow one of two paths. If the consequences of previous responses were positive or desirable, the person is likely to respond in the same manner (shown as path 4 in Figure 13.8). If previous consequences were negative or undesirable, the person will likely follow path 5 in Figure 13.8, which represents a new response.

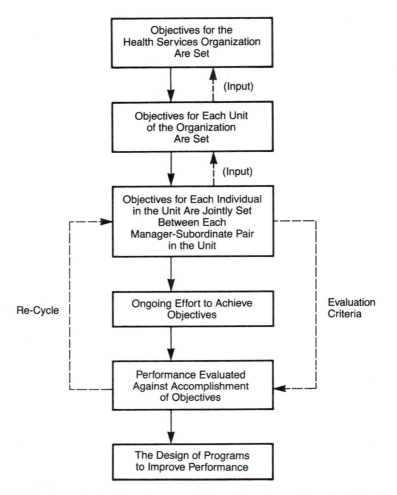

Figure 13.7. The MBO process in a health services organization. (From Longest, Beaufort B., Jr. *Management practices for the health professional,* 4th ed., 67. Norwalk, CT: Appleton & Lange, 1990; reprinted by permission.)

For managers, the key concept in reinforcement theory is that people repeat behavior that is rewarded and avoid behavior that is punished, and that managers encourage preferred behaviors by reinforcing them. *Positive reinforcement* is achieved by doing something positive after preferred behavior is exhibited. Merit pay linked to desired behavior or expressions of approval, especially when visible to co-workers, are positive reinforcers.

Conversely, managers must not reward undesired behavior. *Nonreinforcement,* or withholding positive reinforcement for a previously learned response, can be used to eliminate undesired behavior. Workers can learn to make demands when managers repeatedly agree to them. Managers can gradually end this behavior by refusing to agree to demands. Workers learn that unwarranted demands are not met and will stop making them.

Punishment differs from nonreinforcement. Punishment is an undesirable consequence of a behavioral response, or removal of a desirable consequence. In the case of workers making unreasonable demands, for example, managers might be able to change this behavior by punishing it with an undesirable consequence such as a letter of reprimand. Or, managers might punish behav-

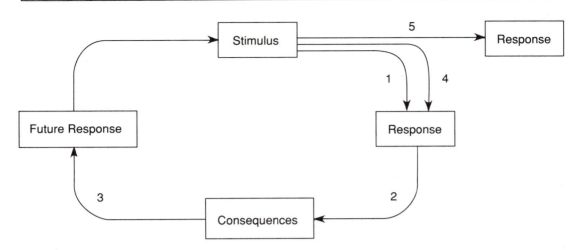

Figure 13.8. The reinforcement theory of motivation. (From *Beyond freedom and dignity* by B.F. Skinner. Copyright © 1971 by B.F. Skinner. Reprinted by permission of Alfred A. Knopf, Inc.)

ior by withholding or removing a desirable consequence, such as ending social interactions. As Aldag and Stearns note:

> Most managers don't like to punish others. And punishment is likely to embitter employees, leading to dissatisfaction and perhaps to turnover. Further, managers who use punishment frequently may find that their subordinates obey their orders only when they are present. When they are absent, the employees may secretly rebel. Finally, since punishment only stops undesirable behavior, the task of increasing desired behavior remains.[54]

Even so, punishment is widely used to alter behavior inside and outside the workplace. Sometimes, it is the only means available. Generally, however, reinforcement theory works best when it focuses on positive reinforcement of desired behaviors or nonreinforcement of undesired behaviors, and not on punishment, to change human behavior.

TOWARD INTEGRATING THE THEORIES OF MOTIVATION

Theories examined in this chapter are divided into content theories and process theories. Each theory explains important aspects of the phenomenon of human motivation. It is unfortunate when theories are pitted against one another in the literature or the workplace as proponents seek to convince others that their theory is the correct one, or at least that it best explains motivation. It is more productive to view the diversity of theories underpinning motivation as part of a large, incomplete puzzle. Each is significant, and they are more useful combined than separate.

One of the best efforts to integrate motivation theories was that of Lyman Porter and Edward Lawler.[55] Figure 13.9 adapts and extends their integrative model. This model emphasizes relationships among effort, performance, rewards, and satisfaction. It also adds an important point to the previous discussion: individuals' performance is related to their abilities as well as to the constraints of a situation. For example, no amount of effort offsets inability to perform the work. Furthermore, situational constraints such as inadequate budgets for technology or training impede performance. With these additions, and recognizing that the model does not capture all intricacies of the theories examined, Porter and Lawler's work goes far to integrate motivation theories into a meaningful whole.

The integrative model emphasizes differences in people and that they are motivated differently. For example, it is now understood that people have different reward preferences and expec-

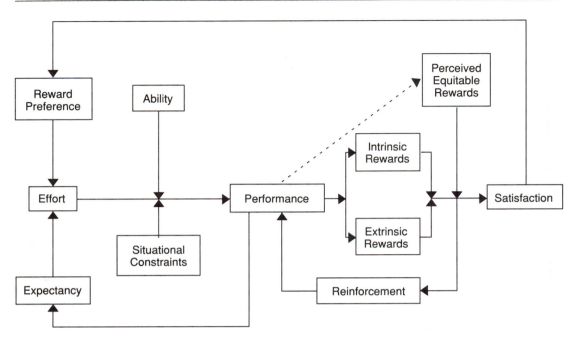

Figure 13.9. A model of motivation integrating content and process theories. (Adapted from Porter, Lyman W., and Edward E. Lawler, III. *Managerial attitudes and performance*, 165. Homewood, IL: Richard D. Irwin, 1968; reprinted by permission.)

tancies regarding the linkages between their efforts and performance and rewards. When the theorizing about motivation is done, managers must apply theory to real people in real settings. This is especially challenging in HSOs because workers have diverse educational, social, and economic backgrounds. Motivational strategies successful for the laundry manager might fail if used by the chief of surgery or the director of a clinical department. People are unique, and they differ in basic mental abilities, personality, interests, level of aspiration, energy, education, and experience. This makes it difficult for managers, especially in large units, to create an environment in which all workers can satisfy their needs.

Finally, Figure 13.9 suggests that performance causes satisfaction. This contrasts with the traditional view that satisfaction causes performance. Until recently it was an article of faith that satisfied workers were productive. Some theory, supported by limited research, suggests that this relationship is opposite—performance leads to satisfaction.[56] Other research, however, shows that broad performance measures such as helping co-workers with job-related problems, making constructive suggestions, and protecting organizational assets seem to be directly influenced by job satisfaction.[57]

The subject of motivation is extraordinarily complex, and current motivation theory does not permit unequivocal statements about how people are motivated or how the phenomenon occurs. Theories are regularly challenged and modified; sometimes they are discarded.

SUMMARY

Motivation is an internal drive to satisfy an unsatisfied need and results in goal-directed behavior. It can be influenced by factors internal and external to the person. An important factor in applying motivation theory in HSOs is the attitude managers have toward those to be motivated. McGregor's Theory X/Theory Y dichotomy is a way to understand how managers' attitudes about people affect efforts to motivate them. Ouchi's Theory Z is explained; its premise is that involved workers are critical to quality and productivity gains.

Four content theories of motivation are presented: Maslow's hierarchy of needs theory, Alderfer's ERG theory, Herzberg's two-factor theory, and McClelland's learned needs theory. Four process theories of motivation are also presented: Vroom's expectancy theory, Adams's equity theory, Locke's goal-setting theory, and Skinner's reinforcement theory. How these theories build on one another, differ, and are complementary is described. An integrative model is introduced to tie the content and process theories of motivation together.

DISCUSSION QUESTIONS

1. Describe five types of behavior an HSO needs from its members.
2. Use the motivation process model in Figure 13.1 to identify an example of a need deficiency you have experienced. Review the goal you established and pursued to fulfill this need deficiency. Was the goal attained? Was the need fulfilled?
3. What is the relationship between a manager's view of human nature and the approach the manager might take to motivate the people supervised?
4. Compare and contrast McGregor's Theory X and Theory Y. How do they relate to Ouchi's Theory Z?
5. How does Herzberg's two-factor theory of motivation relate to Maslow's need hierarchy model of motivation?
6. Discuss McClelland's approach to motivation. What categories of needs do people have according to McClelland?
7. How do process theories of motivation differ from content theories?
8. Draw a general model of expectancy theory. Use this model to discuss how expectations relate to performance.
9. Define equity theory. How are people in the workplace likely to react to perceived inequities?
10. Discuss the relationship of MBO to Locke's goal-setting theory of human motivation.

CASE STUDY 1: A POTENTIAL CONFLICT

Brad Smith is director of the laboratory at Memorial Hospital. With a professional staff of 67, the laboratory is large, complex, and very busy. Smith does an excellent job, but just keeping up with demands of the job requires considerable evening and weekend work. He intends to obtain a master's degree (part-time in the evening) and use it as a stepping stone to a higher level management position in the health field. With an outstanding undergraduate record and excellent scores on the Graduate Management Admission Test (GMAT), he was easily admitted into the program, but twice the demands of his job prevented him from beginning graduate studies.

Smith earns a good salary, but his responsibility for a young and growing family means he has no choice but to continue to work and attend school only part time.

Questions

1. Why does Brad Smith want to attend graduate school? What needs could it help him fulfill?
2. Is there another way these needs could be satisfied?
3. Does Memorial Hospital have any responsibility to Brad Smith in this situation? How could the hospital help him?

CASE STUDY 2: THE YOUNG ASSOCIATE'S DILEMMA

Jane O'Hara faced a serious choice. Five years after receiving her master's degree in health administration from a prestigious midwestern university, she was advancing quickly in a large accounting firm. She was receiving assignments with some of the firm's most important clients and her salary had increased steadily. She was certain that she made at least $10,000 more per year than classmates working in hospitals. The only thing that bothered her about her position, besides the travel, was a nagging feeling that she wanted to become the chief executive officer (CEO) of a large hospital.

One of O'Hara's clients was a large eastern teaching hospital that had a vice president for finance who was about 5 years from retiring. He was set in his ways; O'Hara judged him to be about a decade behind the sophisticated financial management techniques in her "bag of tools." She was surprised when he offered her a position as his assistant—with a strong hint that he wanted to groom a replacement. The salary was about what she made with the accounting firm, and the hospital position had slightly better fringe benefits.

When she discussed the offer with her managing partner, he showed a resigned interest in learning what it would take to retain her. Over the next several weeks the firm developed a counteroffer that included a $7,000 salary increase and a clear indication that she was "pegged" for a partnership position in a few years.

O'Hara took a long weekend to consider her choice.

Questions

1. Identify and describe the motivation variables present here.
2. Would these two positions permit O'Hara to fulfill different needs? If so, what are they?
3. What would you do if you were O'Hara? Why?

CASE STUDY 3:   CLOCKWORK

At present, your organization requires all employees except department heads and above to use a time clock. Categories below this level are paid only for hours recorded on their time cards. Certain professional employees, including registered dietitians, social workers with master's degrees, and medical technologists, have asked to be removed from the rigorous controls of the time clock.

Questions

1. What factors prompted these employees to make their request?
2. What might happen if the request is not granted?
3. If the request were granted, how would other employees react?

CASE STUDY 4:   BILL'S PROMOTION

Community Hospital had an opening for a dietary supervisor. Kathy Harris applied, and her background was judged to be suitable by the human resources department and the director of dietary services.

A few days after Harris started she had problems. The previous dietary supervisor had been discharged and most of the dietary aides assumed that Bill Warner would be promoted to the position. The director of dietary services told Harris that Warner had been considered but was thought to be too young for that much responsibility.

It soon became evident that, while Warner was cooperative, many employees were not. Dietary services employees unhappy with an assignment would tell Harris that if Warner had been appointed such problems would not occur. Many comments were made as Harris continued her duties. Some were very embarrassing. One suggested she had friends in senior management who gave her the job out of friendship rather than because she was competent.

Then Harris got an idea. Since Warner was close to the employees, she delegated authority to him to coordinate daily job assignments. Warner was delighted and did an excellent job. As a result, Harris had less contact with individual dietary services employees, and she began to depend on Warner in these relationships. Warner was apparently happy and the employees were satisfied. One day, Warner suggested to Harris that he be given a raise to reflect his new responsibilities. Since he was doing an effective job she requested that his job description be reviewed by human resources and that he be given a promotion and pay raise. However, the vice president for human resources denied the request because "Harris had had no approval for the action she had taken in the first place."

Questions

1. If you were Kathy Harris, what would you do?
2. In dealing with Warner, was Harris using Theory X or Y? Discuss.
3. How does a promotion policy affect employee motivation?
4. What problems now exist in motivating Warner?
5. What should the director of the dietary department do?

CASE STUDY 5: WHAT NEEDS ARE MOST IMPORTANT TO YOU?[58]

This exercise will give you an opportunity to assess the needs that are most important to have fulfilled by your work.

Instructions: Rank your responses for each of the following questions. The response that is most important or most true for you should receive a 5; the next should receive a 4; the next a 3; the next a 2; and the least important or least true should receive a 1.

Example
The work I like best involves:

A 4 Working alone.
B 3 A mixture of time spent with people and time spent alone.
C 1 Giving speeches.
D 2 Discussion with others.
E 5 Working outdoors.

1. Overall, the most important thing to me about a job is whether or not:
   A ___ The pay is sufficient to meet my needs.
   B ___ It provides the opportunity for fellowship and good human relations.
   C ___ It is a secure job with good employee benefits.
   D ___ It allows me freedom and the chance to express myself.
   E ___ There is opportunity for advancement based on my achievements.

2. If I were to quit a job, it would probably be because:
   A ___ It was a dangerous job, such as working with inadequate equipment or poor safety procedures.
   B ___ Continued employment was questionable because of uncertainties in business conditions or funding sources.
   C ___ It was a job people looked down on.
   D ___ It was a one-person job, allowing little opportunity for discussion and interaction with others.
   E ___ The work lacked personal meaning to me.

3. For me, the most important rewards in working are those that:
   A ___ Come from the work itself—important and challenging assignments.
   B ___ Satisfy the basic reasons why people work—good pay, a good home, and other economic needs.
   C ___ Are provided by fringe benefits—such as hospitalization insurance, time off for vacations, security for retirement, etc.

D __ Reflect my ability—such as being recognized for the work I do and knowing I am one of the best in my organization or profession.

E __ Come from the human aspects of working—that is, the opportunity to make friends and to be a valued member of a team.

4. My morale would suffer most in a job in which:
   A __ The future was unpredictable.
   B __ Other employees received recognition, when I didn't, for doing the same quality of work.
   C __ My co-workers were unfriendly or held grudges.
   D __ I felt stifled and unable to grow.
   E __ The job environment was poor—no air conditioning, inconvenient parking, insufficient space and lighting, primitive toilet facilities.

5. In deciding whether or not to accept a promotion, I would be most concerned with whether:
   A __ The job was a source of pride and would be viewed with respect by others.
   B __ Taking the job would constitute a gamble on my part, and I could lose more than I gained.
   C __ The economic rewards would be favorable.
   D __ I would like the new people I would be working with, and whether or not we would get along.
   E __ I would be able to explore new areas and do more creative work.

6. The kind of job that brings out my best is one in which:
   A __ There is a family spirit among employees and we all share good times.
   B __ The working conditions—equipment, materials, and basic surroundings—are physically safe.
   C __ Management is understanding and there is little chance of losing my job.
   D __ I can see the returns on my work from the standpoint of personal values.
   E __ There is recognition for achievement.

7. I would consider changing jobs if my present position:
   A __ Did not offer security and fringe benefits.
   B __ Did not provide a chance to learn and grow.
   C __ Did not provide recognition for my performance.
   D __ Did not allow close personal contacts.
   E __ Did not provide economic rewards.

8. The job situation that would cause the most stress for me is:
   A __ Having a serious disagreement with my co-workers.
   B __ Working in an unsafe environment.
   C __ Having an unpredictable supervisor.
   D __ Not being able to express myself.
   E __ Not being appreciated for the quality of my work.

9. I would accept a new position if:
   A __ The position would be a test of my potential.
   B __ The new job would offer better pay and physical surroundings.
   C __ The new job would be secure and offer long-term fringe benefits.
   D __ The position would be respected by others in my organization.
   E __ Good relationships with co-workers and business associates were probable.

10. I would work overtime if:
    A __ The work is challenging.
    B __ I need the extra income.

C __ My co-workers are also working overtime.
D __ I must do it to keep my job.
E __ The organization recognizes my contribution.

Scoring Directions: Place the values you gave A, B, C, D, and E for each question in the spaces provided in the scoring key. Notice that the letters are not always in the same place for each question. Then add up each column and obtain a total score for each of the motivational levels.

Scoring Key						
Question 1	A	C	B	E	D
Question 2	A	B	D	C	E
Question 3	B	C	E	D	A
Question 4	E	A	C	B	D
Question 5	C	B	D	A	E
Question 6	B	C	A	E	D
Question 7	E	A	D	C	B
Question 8	B	C	A	E	D
Question 9	B	C	E	D	A
Question 10	B	D	C	E	A
TOTAL SCORE					
	I	II	III	IV	V
	MOTIVATION LEVELS				

The five motivation levels are as follows:

Level I   Physical needs
Level II   Safety needs
Level III Social needs
Level IV Esteem needs
Level V   Self-realization needs

Those levels that received the highest scores are the most important needs identified by you in your work. The lowest show those needs that have been relatively well satisfied or de-emphasized by you at this time.

NOTES

1. All about people. *The Economist* 312 (July 29, 1989): 50–60.

2. Keys, Bernard, and Thomas Case. How to become an influential manager. *The Executive* 4 (November 1990): 38–51; Turnipseed, David L. Evaluation of health care work environments via a social climate scale: Results of a

field study. *Hospital & Health Services Administration* 35 (Summer 1990): 245–262.

3. Ulrich, Dave, and Dale Lake. Organizational capability: Creating competitive advantage. *The Executive* 5 (February 1991): 77–92.

4. Katz, Daniel, and Robert L. Kahn. *The social psychology of organizations.* New York: John Wiley & Sons, 1966.

5. Bateman, Thomas S., and Dennis W. Organ. Job satisfaction and the good soldier: The relationship between affect and employee citizenship. *Academy of Management Journal* 26 (December 1983): 587–595.

6. Greenberger, David, Stephen Strasser, Roy J. Lewicki, and Thomas S. Bateman. Perception, motivation, and negotiation. In *Health care management: A text in organization theory and behavior,* edited by Stephen M. Shortell and Arnold D. Kaluzny, 2nd ed., 102–103. New York: John Wiley & Sons, 1988.

7. Gibson, James L., John M. Ivancevich, and James H. Donnelly, Jr. *Organizations: Behavior, structure, processes,* 7th ed., 99. Homewood, IL: Richard D. Irwin, Inc., 1991.

8. Higgins, James M. *The management challenge: An introduction to management,* 423. New York: Macmillan Publishing Company, 1991.

9. Holt, David H. *Management: principles and practices,* 2d ed., 422. Englewood Cliffs, NJ: Prentice Hall, 1990.

10. Mountain, G.A., P.C.W. Bowie, and A.R. Dabbs. Preliminary report on nurse job satisfaction on wards for the elderly, mentally ill. *Health Services Management Research* 3 (March 1990): 22–30.

11. McGregor, Douglas T. *The human side of enterprise.* New York: McGraw-Hill, 1960.

12. McGregor, *Human side,* 33–34, Copyright © 1960. Reprinted by permission of McGraw-Hill, Inc.

13. McGregor, *Human side,* 47–48, Copyright © 1960. Reprinted by permission of McGraw-Hill, Inc.

14. Ouchi, William G. *Theory Z: How American business can meet the Japanese challenge.* Reading, MA: Addison-Wesley, 1981.

15. Shortell, Stephen M. Theory Z: Implications and relevance for health care management. *Health Care Management Review* 7 (Fall 1982): 8.

16. Ouchi, *Theory Z.*

17. Vroom, Victor H., and Arthur G. Jago. *The new leadership: Managing participation in organizations.* Englewood Cliffs, NJ: Prentice Hall, 1988.

18. Maslow, Abraham H. A theory of human motivation. *Psychological Review* 50 (July 1943): 370–396; Maslow, Abraham H. *Motivation and personality,* 2d ed. New York: Harper & Row, 1970.

19. Maslow, Theory of human motivation.

20. Maslow, Abraham H. *Eupsychian management,* 56. Homewood, IL: Dorsey-Irwin, 1965.

21. Hall, Douglas T., and Khalil E. Nongaim. An examination of Maslow's need hierarchy in an organizational setting. *Organizational Behavior and Human Performance* 3 (February 1968): 12–35; Lawler, Edward E., III, and J. Lloyd Suttle. A causal correlational test of the need hierarchy concept. *Organizational Behavior and Human Performance* 7 (April 1972): 265–287; Wahba, Mahmoud A., and Lawrence G. Bridwell. Maslow reconsidered: A review of research on the need hierarchy theory. In *Motivation and work behavior,* edited by Richard M. Steers and Lyman W. Porter, 4th ed., 51–67. New York: McGraw-Hill Book Company, 1987.

22. Alderfer, Clayton P. A new theory of human needs. *Organizational Behavior and Human Performance* 4 (May 1969): 142–175; Alderfer, Clayton P. *Existence, relatedness, and growth: Human needs in organizational settings.* New York: Free Press, 1972.

23. Alderfer, *Existence.*

24. Herzberg, Frederick, Bernard Mausner, and Barbara Snyderman. *The motivation to work.* New York: John Wiley & Sons, Inc., 1959.

25. Herzberg, Frederick, Bernard Mausner, and Barbara Snyderman. *The motivation to work,* 2d ed. New York: John Wiley & Sons, Inc., 1967.

26. Herzberg, Frederick. One more time: How do you motivate employees? *Harvard Business Review* 87 (September-October 1987): 109–117.

27. Hernandez, S. Robert, Cynthia Carter Haddock, and Jose B. Quintana. The relationship between technology and task design in hospital nursing units. *Health Services Management Research* 3 (July 1990): 137–148; Mottaz, Clifford J. Work satisfaction among hospital nurses. *Hospital & Health Services Administration* 33 (Spring 1988): 57–74; Thomas, Kenneth W., and Betty A. Velthouse. Cognitive elements of empowerment: An "interpretive" model of intrinsic task motivation. *Academy of Management Review* 15 (October 1990): 666–681; Wetzel, Kurt, Donna E. Soloshy, and Daniel G. Gallagher. The work attitudes of full-time and part-time registered nurses. *Health Care Management Review* 15 (Summer 1990): 79–85.

28. House, Robert J., and Lawrence A. Wigdor. Herzberg's dual-factor theory of job satisfaction and motivation: A review of the evidence and a criticism. *Personnel Psychology* 20 (Winter 1967): 369–389; Whitset, David A., and Eric K. Winslow. An analysis of studies critical of the motivator-hygiene theory. *Personnel Psychology* 20 (Winter 1967): 391–416.

29. Paul, William J., Jr., Keith B. Robertson, and Frederick Herzberg. Job enrichment pays off. *Harvard Business Review* 47 (March-April 1969): 61.

30. McClelland, David C. *The achieving society.* Princeton, NJ: Van Nostrand, 1961; McClelland, David C. *Power: The inner experience.* New York: Irvington Publishers, 1975; McClelland, David C. *Human motivation.* Glenview, IL: Scott, Foresman, 1985.

31. Murray, Henry A. *Explorations in personality.* New York: Oxford University Press, 1938.

32. Atkinson, John W. *An introduction to motivation.* New York: Van Nostrand, 1961; Atkinson, John W., and Joel O. Raynor. *Motivation and achievement.* Washington, D.C.: Winston, 1974.

33. Holt, *Management,* 429–430.

34. Holt, *Management,* 430.

35. McClelland, *Human motivation.*

36. Gibson, Ivancevich, and Donnelly, *Organizations,* 116.

37. Vroom, Victor H. *Work and motivation.* New York: Wiley, 1964.

38. Adams, J. Stacy. Toward an understanding of inequity. *Journal of Abnormal and Social Psychology* 67 (November 1963): 422–436; Adams, J. Stacy. Inequity in social exchanges. In *Advances in experimental social psychology,* edited by Leonard Berkowitz, Vol. 2. New York: Academic Press, 1965.

39. Walster, Elaine H., G. William Walster, and Ellen Berscheid. *Equity: Theory and research.* Boston: Allyn & Bacon, 1978; Mowday, Richard T. Equity theory predictions of behavior in organizations. In *Motivation and*

work behavior, edited by Richard M. Steers and Lyman W. Porter, 4th ed., 89–110. New York: McGraw-Hill Book Company, 1987.

40. Robbins, Stephen P. Management, 3d ed., 438. Englewood Cliffs, NJ: Prentice Hall, 1991.

41. Holt, Management, 433–434.

42. Locke, Edwin A. Toward a theory of task motivation and incentives. Organizational Behavior and Performance 3 (May 1968): 157–189; Locke, Edwin A. The ubiquity of the technique of goal setting in theories of and approaches to employee motivation. In Motivation and work behavior, edited by Richard M. Steers and Lyman W. Porter, 4th ed., 111–120. New York: McGraw-Hill Book Company, 1987.

43. Locke, Edwin A. Purpose without consciousness: A contradiction. Psychological Reports 24 (June 1969): 991.

44. Wood, Robert E., and Edwin A. Locke. Goal setting and strategy effects on complex tasks. In A theory of goal setting and task performance, edited by Edwin A. Locke and Gary P. Latham, 293–319. Englewood Cliffs, NJ: Prentice Hall, 1990.

45. Tubbs, Mark E., and Steven E. Ekeberg. The role of intentions in work motivation: Implications for goal-setting theory and research. Academy of Management Review 16 (January 1991): 180–199.

46. Mento, Anthony J., Robert P. Steel, and Ronald J. Karren. A meta-analytic study of the effects of goal setting on task performance: 1966–1984. Organizational Behavior and Human Decision Processes 39 (February 1987): 52–83.

47. Latham, Gary P., and Edwin A. Locke. Goal-setting—a motivational technique that works. In Motivation and work behavior, edited by Richard M. Steers and Lyman W. Porter, 4th ed., 132. New York: McGraw-Hill Book Company, 1987.

48. Naylor, James C., and Daniel R. Ilgen. Goal setting: A theoretical analysis of a motivational technique. In Research in organizational behavior, edited by Barry M.

49. Latham, Gary P., and J.J. Baldes. The practical significance of Locke's theory of goal setting. Journal of Applied Psychology 60 (February 1975): 124.

50. Erez, Miriam, and Frederick H. Kanfer. The role of goal acceptance in goal setting and task performance. Academy of Management Review 8 (July 1983): 454–463.

51. Erez, Miriam, P. Christopher Earley, and Charles L. Hulin. The impact of participation on goal acceptance and performance: A two-step model. Academy of Management Journal 28 (March 1985): 50–66; Schwartz, Robert H. Coping with unbalanced information about decision-making influence for nurses. Hospital & Health Services Administration 35 (Winter 1990): 547–559.

52. Drucker, Peter F. The practice of management. New York: Harper & Brothers, 1954.

53. Skinner, B.F. Science and human behavior. New York: Free Press, 1953; Skinner, B.F. Beyond freedom and dignity. New York: Alfred Knopf, 1971.

54. Aldag, Ramon J., and Timothy M. Stearns. Management, 2d ed., 432. Cincinnati, OH: South-Western Publishing Co., 1991.

55. Porter, Lyman W., and Edward E. Lawler, III Managerial attitudes and performance. Homewood, IL: Richard D. Irwin, 1968.

56. Lawler, Edward E. III, and Lyman W. Porter. The effect of performance on job satisfaction. Industrial Relations 7 (October 1967): 20–28.

57. Organ, Dennis W. A reappraisal and reinterpretation of the satisfaction-causes-performance hypothesis. Academy of Management Review 2 (January 1977): 46–53; Bateman and Organ, Job satisfaction.

58. From Manning, George, and Kent Curtis. Human behavior: Why people do what they do, 17–20. Cincinnati, OH: Vista Systems/South-Western Publishing Co., 1988; reprinted by permission. Copyright 1988 by South-Western Publishing Co. All rights reserved.

BIBLIOGRAPHY

Adams, J. Stacy. Inequity in social exchanges. In Advances in experimental social psychology, edited by Leonard Berkowitz, Vol. 2. New York: Academic Press, 1965.

Aldag, Ramon J., and Timothy M. Stearns. Management, 2d ed. Cincinnati, OH: South-Western Publishing Co., 1991.

Alderfer, Clayton P. Existence, relatedness, and growth: Human needs in organizational settings. New York: Free Press, 1972.

Alderfer, Clayton P. A new theory of human needs. Organizational Behavior and Human Performance 4 (May 1969): 142–175.

Atkinson, John W. An introduction to motivation. New York: Van Nostrand, 1961.

Atkinson, John W., and Joel O. Raynor. Motivation and achievement. Washington, DC: Winston, 1974.

Bateman, Thomas S., and Dennis W. Organ. Job satisfaction and the good soldier: The relationship between affect and employee citizenship. Academy of Management Journal 26 (December 1983): 587–595.

Donnelly, James H., Jr., James L. Gibson, and John M. Ivancevich. Fundamentals of management, 7th ed. Homewood, IL: BPI-Irwin, 1990.

Drucker, Peter F. The practice of management. New York: Harper & Brothers, 1954.

Erez, Miriam, P. Christopher Earley, and Charles L. Hulin. The impact of participation on goal acceptance and performance: A two-step model. Academy of Management Journal 28 (March 1985): 50–66.

Gibson, James L., John M. Ivancevich, and James H. Donnelly, Jr. Organizations: Behavior, structure, processes, 7th ed. Homewood, IL: Irwin, 1991.

Greenberger, David, Stephen Strasser, Roy J. Lewicki, and Thomas S. Bateman. Perception, motivation, and negotiation. In Health care management: A text in organization theory and behavior, edited by Stephen M. Shortell and Arnold D. Kaluzny, 2nd ed., 81–141. New York: John Wiley & Sons, 1988.

Hernandez, S. Robert, Cynthia Carter Haddock, and Jose B. Quintana. The relationship between technology and task design in hospital nursing units. Health Services Management Research 3 (July 1990): 137–148.

Herzberg, Frederick. One more time: How do you motivate employees? Harvard Business Review 87 (September-October 1987): 109–117.

Herzberg, Frederick, Bernard Mausner, and Barbara Snyderman. *The motivation to work,* 2d ed. New York: John Wiley & Sons, Inc., 1967.

Higgins, James M. *The management challenge: An introduction to management.* New York: Macmillan Publishing Company, 1991.

Holt, David H. *Management: Principles and practices,* 2d ed. Englewood Cliffs, NJ: Prentice Hall, 1990.

Katz, Daniel, and Robert L. Kahn. *The social psychology of organizations.* New York: John Wiley & Sons, 1966.

Latham, Gary P., and Edwin A. Locke. Goal-setting—a motivational technique that works. In *Motivation and work behavior,* edited by Richard M. Steers and Lyman W. Porter, 4th ed., 120–134. New York: McGraw-Hill Book Company, 1987.

Lawler, Edward E. III, and Lyman W. Porter. The effect of performance on job satisfaction. *Industrial Relations* 7 (October 1967): 20–28.

Lawler, Edward E., III, and J. Lloyd Suttle. A causal correlational test of the need hierarchy concept. *Organizational Behavior and Human Performance* 7 (April 1972): 265–287.

Locke, Edwin A. Purpose without consciousness: A contradiction. *Psychological Reports* 24 (June 1969): 991–1009.

Locke, Edwin A. Toward a theory of task motivation and incentives. *Organizational Behavior and Performance* 3 (May 1968): 157–189.

Locke, Edwin A. The ubiquity of the technique of goal setting in theories of and approaches to employee motivation. In *Motivation and work behavior,* edited by Richard M. Steers and Lyman W. Porter, 4th ed., 111–120. New York: McGraw-Hill Book Company, 1987.

Longest, Beaufort B., Jr. *Management practices for the health professional,* 4th ed. Norwalk, CT: Appleton & Lange, 1990.

Maslow, Abraham H. *Eupsychian management.* Homewood, IL: Dorsey-Irwin, 1965.

Maslow, Abraham H. *Motivation and personality,* 2d ed. New York: Harper & Row, 1970.

Maslow, Abraham H. A theory of human motivation. *Psychological Review* 50 (July 1943): 370–396.

McClelland, David C. *The achieving society.* Princeton, NJ: Van Nostrand, 1961.

McClelland, David C. *Human motivation.* Glenview, IL: Scott, Foresman, 1985.

McGregor, Douglas T. *The human side of enterprise.* New York: McGraw-Hill, 1960.

Mottaz, Clifford J. Work satisfaction among hospital nurses. *Hospital & Health Services Administration* 33 (Spring 1988): 57–74.

Mountain, G.A., P.C.W. Bowie, and A.R. Dabbs. Preliminary report on nurse job satisfaction on wards for the elderly, mentally ill. *Health Services Management Research* 3 (March 1990): 22–30.

Mowday, Richard T. Equity theory predictions of behavior in organizations. In *Motivation and work behavior,* edited by

Richard M. Steers and Lyman W. Porter, 4th ed., 89–110. New York: McGraw-Hill Book Company, 1987.

Naylor, James C., and Daniel R. Ilgen. Goal setting: A theoretical analysis of a motivational technique. In *Research in organizational behavior,* edited by Barry M. Staw and Larry L. Cummings, Vol. 6, 95–140. Greenwich, CT: JAI Press, 1984.

Organ, Dennis W. A reappraisal and reinterpretation of the satisfaction-causes-performance hypothesis. *Academy of Management Review* 2 (January 1977): 46–53.

Porter, Lyman W., and Edward E. Lawler, III. *Managerial attitudes and performance.* Homewood, IL: Richard D. Irwin, 1968.

Robbins, Stephen P. *Management,* 3d ed. Englewood Cliffs, NJ: Prentice Hall, 1991.

Schwartz, Robert H. Coping with unbalanced information about decision-making influence for nurses. *Hospital & Health Services Administration* 35 (Winter 1990): 547–559.

Skinner, B.F. *Beyond freedom and dignity.* New York: Alfred Knopf, 1971.

Thomas, Kenneth W., and Betty A. Velthouse. Cognitive elements of empowerment: An "interpretive" model of intrinsic task motivation. *Academy of Management Review* 15 (October 1990): 666–681.

Tubbs, Mark E., and Steven E. Ekeberg. The role of intentions in work motivation: Implications for goal-setting theory and research. *Academy of Management Review* 16 (January 1991): 180–199.

Turnipseed, David L. Evaluation of health care work environments via a social climate scale: Results of a field study. *Hospital & Health Services Administration* 35 (Summer 1990): 245–262.

Ulrich, Dave, and Dale Lake. *Organizational capability.* New York: John Wiley & Sons, Inc., 1990.

Vroom, Victor H. *Work and motivation.* New York: Wiley, 1964.

Vroom, Victor H., and Arthur G. Jago. *The new leadership: Managing participation in organizations.* Englewood Cliffs, NJ: Prentice Hall, 1988.

Wahba, Mahmoud A., and Lawrence G. Bridwell. Maslow reconsidered: A review of research on the need hierarchy theory. In *Motivation and work behavior,* edited by Richard M. Steers and Lyman W. Porter, 4th ed., 51–67. New York: McGraw-Hill Book Company, 1987.

Walster, Elaine H., G. William Walster, and Ellen Berscheid. *Equity: Theory and research.* Boston: Allyn & Bacon, 1978.

Wetzel, Kurt, Donna E. Soloshy, and Daniel G. Gallagher. The work attitudes of full-time and part-time registered nurses. *Health Care Management Review* 15 (Summer 1990): 79–85.

Wood, Robert E., and Edwin A. Locke. Goal setting and strategy effects on complex tasks. In *A theory of goal setting and task performance,* edited by Edwin A. Locke and Gary P. Latham, 293–319. Englewood Cliffs, NJ: Prentice Hall, 1990.

14 / Leadership

*Leaders do not have to be great men or women
by being intellectual geniuses or omniscient
prophets to succeed, but they do need to have the
"right stuff" and this stuff is not equally present
in all people. Leadership is a demanding,
unrelenting job with enormous pressures and
grave responsibilities. It would be a disservice to
leaders to suggest that they are ordinary people
who happened to be in the right place at the
right time. Maybe the place matters, but it takes
a special kind of person to master the challenges
of opportunity.*

Kirkpatrick and Locke[1]

Effective leadership is essential if a health services organization (HSO) is to provide high-quality patient care and succeed financially. Leadership is vital because some people determine, initiate, coordinate, influence, and oversee the work of others. Some lead, others follow. The quality of leadership is crucial to how work gets done in an HSO. In turn, the quality of work is integral to how well the HSO performs and how well its mission is achieved.

In relation to performance, leadership should be viewed in two distinct ways. One reflects the fact that throughout the organization, but especially at middle and lower levels, managers directly supervise people. This establishes "supervisor-subordinate" relationships, and good leadership skills and techniques are essential to properly manage them.[2] Leadership in these relationships is really a *transactional* process in which the needs of followers are met if they perform to the leader's expectations.[3] The leader enters a transaction with followers in which each receives something of value. This conception of leadership is examined carefully in this chapter because supervisor-subordinate relationships are so pervasive in HSOs.

In addition, another leadership role is increasingly important. This one is played by the HSO's top manager—the chief executive officer (CEO)—in providing institutional leadership. Here, the leadership task is rather different. Stevens describes it as managers/leaders at the institutional level having a "critical role as the conscience of the enterprise."[4] More specifically, the institution-level leader is concerned with issues such as:

Developing an internal consensus on organizational priorities;
Enlisting internal and external support for the organization's purposes;
Selecting an optimal service and patient mix;
Locating responsibility for the organization's direction and performance;
Developing effective planning strategies;
Selecting competitive strategies to pursue;
Managing conflicts between economic and professional interests;
Negotiating reimbursement with third parties and the government.[5]

Burns and Becker note that, to address such issues, CEOs must:

Engage in the promotion of organizational values, the resolution of moral questions, the invocation of various symbols, the management of internal and external coalitions, the assessment of environmental constraints, and the search for opportunities and choices within those constraints.[6]

In addition to transactional leadership, effective leaders at the top of an organization also engage in what Burns[7] calls *transformational* leadership. Transformational leaders have a vision for the organization and motivate followers to help realize the vision. Bass[8] characterizes such leaders as having the ability to develop and instill a common vision and to stimulate determined adherence to that vision. Zuckerman points out that CEOs play key roles "in providing strategic direction and vision to the organization, serving as the keeper of the corporate values, and assuring that the organization achieves its mission."[9]

Because of their importance to the success of the HSO, both transactional and transformational leadership are examined here. Research and theories about leadership and leaders can be divided into two schools. Some research examines managers as supervisors and the part leadership plays in these supervisor–subordinate relationships—a focus on transactional leadership. Other research and theories focus on top-level managers, particularly their relationship with their organizations, and between managers and the external environments of their organizations—the leader's transformational role. These two foci are very important to HSO managers, although their relative importance varies with the organizational level of managers. This chapter incorporates elements of both.

LEADERSHIP MODELED AND DEFINED

Leadership is a complex, multidimensional concept that is defined in different ways, although most definitions suggest it is a process of *influencing* people to achieve particular goals. Cartwright and Zander[10] describe leadership as the acts and activities of one person that contribute to performance by others. Fiedler and Chemers[11] describe leadership as an "unequal influence and power relationship" in which followers accept the leader's right to make certain decisions for them. Holt describes leadership as "the process of influencing others to behave in preferred ways to accomplish organizational objectives."[12] Blake and Mouton[13] explain leadership as the managerial activity through which managers maximize productivity, stimulate creative problem solving, and promote morale and satisfaction among those who are led. In Jago's[14] view, leadership is a process that uses noncoercive influence as a means of directing and coordinating the activities of the members of a group toward attaining the group's objectives. Bass notes that "leadership occurs when one group member modifies the motivation or competencies of others in the group."[15] In one of the most comprehensive definitions of leadership, Yukl defines it as "influence processes involving determination of the group's or organization's objectives, motivating task behavior in pursuit of these objectives, and influencing group maintenance and culture."[16]

These definitions include many interrelated ideas: groups, organizations, goals/objectives, influence, and acceptance. In sum, they suggest that the leader's role is to determine what is to be accomplished by a group or organization and influence others to contribute to achieving that goal. At the level of supervisor–subordinate relationships, leadership focuses on what a specific group is to accomplish. At the level of institutional leadership, the focus is on what the organization is to accomplish. These ideas further suggest that those being led—the followers—must accept the leader's role and influence over them. As Bass states, "Leaders are agents of change, persons whose acts affect other people more than other people's acts affect them."[17]

The definitions of leadership fit institutional leadership *and* supervisor-subordinate relationships because leadership for both means determining what is to be accomplished and influencing others to contribute to the goal. However, the scale and focus are different for the two levels of leadership. At one level they are more transactional and at the other more transformational.

Managers at the supervisor-subordinate level lead relatively small groups of people, and the groups tend to be more homogeneous in purpose, and as individuals, than the HSO staff as a whole. Thus, the groups are generally easier to lead. Larger numbers and more diversity magnify the challenge of leadership. In supervisor–subordinate relationships, leadership focuses on what occurs between—or the exchanges between—individual supervisors and their subordinates in terms of influencing one another. Figure 14.1 illustrates the leadership process between supervisors and subordinates.

In contrast, institutional leadership focuses on various decisions and activities that affect the entire HSO, including those intended to ensure survival and overall health. As McLaughlin and Kaluzny describe it, the role of institutional leaders is to "manage culture and to allocate resources."[18] As is discussed in Chapter 1, an HSO's culture is the ingrained pattern of shared beliefs, values, behaviors, and assumptions, with symbols and rituals, that are acquired over time by members. Culture is the historically developed sense of the "institution's legacy."[19] Other examples of the activities of leaders at the institutional level include establishing goals, inculcating values in the HSO, building interorganizational coalitions, interpreting and responding to various challenges and opportunities presented to the HSO from the external environment, and acting to alter constraints put on the HSO by the external environment.

Much as with the discussion of motivation in Chapter 13, the study of leadership has followed several paths, no one of which has produced a definitive theory of effective leadership. The earliest studies of leadership focused on power and its sources and uses. Much of what was learned is important to understanding leadership because, by definition, leadership involves one person influencing others, and power is the ability to influence others. Power and influence alone, however, are not fully explanatory. Another approach was based on the proposition that traits, skills, abilities, or characteristics inherent in some persons explain why they are better leaders. In yet another approach, researchers sought to explain leadership by first understanding behavior associated with successful leaders. An integrative approach to the study of leadership focuses on how the leader, the followers, and the situation in which they find themselves interact and work. Such situational approaches to the study of leadership have advanced understanding of this phenomenon in important ways.

These approaches to the study of leadership (power, traits and skills, leadership behavior, and situational) all contribute to understanding leadership, and the key theories, findings, and conceptualizations developed in each are examined in this chapter. The reader is cautioned that this way of organizing the chapter was chosen because it provides a framework to cover a great deal of material coherently, not because the different approaches are to be seen as competing explanations of leadership, even though this was the case when much of the original work was done. Yukl notes:

> Leadership research has been characterized by narrowly focused studies with little integration of findings from the different approaches. The research on leader power has not examined leadership behavior except for explicit influence attempts, and there has been little concern for traits except ones that are a source of leader influence. The trait research has shown little concern for direct measurement of leadership behavior or influence, even though it is evident that the effects of leader traits are mediated by leadership behavior and influence. The behavior research has seldom included leader traits or power, even though they influence a leader's behavior. Finally, situational theories examine how the situation enhances or nullifies the effects of selected leader behaviors or traits, rather than taking

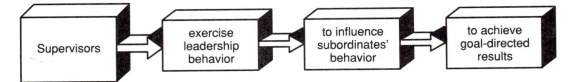

Figure 14.1. Leadership at the supervisor-subordinate level. (Adapted from Holt, David H. *Management: Principles and practices,* 2d ed., 451. Englewood Cliffs, NJ: Prentice Hall, 1990; used by permission. Copyright © 1990, Prentice Hall, Inc.)

a broader view of the way traits, power, behavior, and situation interact to determine leadership effectiveness.[20]

This suggests that one can only understand leadership by integrating several theories or conceptual approaches. These are covered below, and the chapter concludes with an integrative model of leadership.

POWER AND INFLUENCE

Two concepts are critical to understanding leadership in an organizational context. *Influence* is the effect someone has on others that causes them to change their behavior and/or motivation. "Influence is simply the process by which people successfully persuade others to follow their advice, suggestion, or order."[21] The essence of leadership is the ability to influence followers. *Power* is the potential to exert influence. More power means more potential to influence others. These definitions implicitly focus on people—leaders and followers—but it should be noted that power often derives from the leader's control over inanimate things, such as all types of resources, including information.

Sources of Power

If power is the potential to influence, and the ability to influence is critical to effective leadership, it is useful to understand how leaders acquire power. Leaders must be interested in understanding and using the various sources of power available to them. French and Raven[22] developed what is regarded as the classic scheme for categorizing the various bases of power. They suggested five distinct bases of interpersonal power: legitimate, reward, coercive, expert, and referent.

Legitimate power is power derived from a person's position in an organization. It is also called formal power or authority and exists because organizations find it advantageous to assign certain powers to individuals so they can do their jobs effectively. All managers have some degree of legitimate power or authority based on their position.

Reward power is based on the leader's ability to reward desirable behavior. Reward power stems partly from the "legitimate power" granted to the leader by the organization. In other words, managers by virtue of their positions are given control over certain rewards to buttress their legitimate power. Rewards include pay increases, promotions, work schedules, recognition of accomplishments, and status symbols such as office size and location.

Coercive power is the opposite of reward power and is based on the leader's ability to punish or prevent someone from obtaining desired rewards. As described in Chapter 13, rewards and punishments are powerful motivational tools, although HSO leaders are generally better served by reward power than by coercive power.

Expert power derives from having knowledge valued by the organization, such as expertise in problem solving or critical tasks. Expert power is personal to the person who has the expertise. Thus, it is different from legitimate, reward, and coercive power, which are prescribed by the organization, even though persons may be granted these forms of power because they possess expert power. For example, persons with expert power often rise to management positions in their areas of expertise. It is also noteworthy that in organizations in which work is highly technical or professional, such as a typical HSO, expert power alone makes some people very powerful. For example, the power of the clinical staff is based on medical knowledge and skills. Physicians with scarce expertise, such as transplant surgery, gain more power than physicians whose expertise is more readily replaceable. Expert power is not reserved for those with clinical or technical skills, however. The ability and knowledge to effectively manage increasingly complex HSOs is itself a source of power for those with the expertise.

Referent power results when some persons engender admiration, loyalty, and emulation to the extent that they gain the power to influence others. At the level of institutional leadership this is sometimes called charismatic power. Charismatic leaders typically have a vision for the organizations they lead, strong convictions about the correctness of the vision, and great self-confidence about their ability to realize the vision, and are perceived by their followers as agents of change.[23]

It is rare for a leader to gain sufficient power to heavily influence followers simply from referent or charismatic power. If referent power is to be significant at the supervisor-subordinate level it must be developed over a long period of close interaction in which the leader demonstrates friendliness, concern for the needs and feelings of followers, and fairness toward them. Charismatic leaders are rare at the institutional level. As with expert power, referent power cannot be given by the organization as can legitimate, reward, and coercive power.

The five bases of power are not necessarily independent and can be complementary. Leaders who use reward power wisely strengthen their referent power. Conversely, leaders who abuse their coercive power will quickly weaken or lose referent power. Effective leaders are those who translate power into influence, understand the sources of their power, and act accordingly. For example, if a person's power is expertise, it is dangerous to try to lead in areas outside that expertise. As Morlock and colleagues note, effective leaders "understand—at least intuitively—the costs, risks, and benefits of using each kind of power and are able to recognize which to draw on in different situations and with different people."[24]

Persons who effectively use power(s) and translate those powers into influence or use them to lead are distinguished by their interpersonal and political skills. Access to power is not enough. One must know how to use power to influence others. Mintzberg recognizes this important fact and attributes success in use of power largely to the leader's political skills, defined as:

> The ability to use the bases of power effectively—to convince those to whom one has access, to use one's resources, information, and technical skills to their fullest in bargaining, to exercise formal power with a sensitivity to the feelings of others, to know where to concentrate one's energies, to sense what is possible, to organize the necessary alliances.[25]

Yukl's comprehensive model of the sources of power in an organization includes the importance of political skills to the effective exercise of power (Table 14.1). He notes:

> Power is derived in part from the opportunities inherent in a person's position in the organization; this "position power" includes legitimate authority, control over resources, control over information, control over punishments, and ecological control. Power also depends on attributes of the interpersonal relationship between [leader and follower]; this "personal power" includes relative task expertise, friendship and loyalty, and a leader's charismatic qualities. Finally, power depends upon some political processes ("political power") such as controlling key decisions, forming coalitions, and co-opting opponents.[26]

Table 14.1 shows that people in organizations have many sources of power: positional, personal, and political. Depending on circumstances, the power from these sources is available in

Table 14.1. Sources of power in organizations

Position power	Formal authority
	Control over resources and rewards
	Control over punishments
	Control over information
	Ecological control
Personal power	Expertise
	Friendship/loyalty
	Charisma
Political power	Control over decision processes
	Coalitions
	Co-optation

Adapted from Yukl, Gary A. *Leadership in organizations,* 2d ed., 14. Englewood Cliffs, NJ: Prentice Hall, 1989; used by permission. © 1989, Prentice Hall, Inc.

different degrees to leaders in the HSO. For example, at the level of departments, where leadership is primarily through supervisor-subordinate relationships, managers have power to influence or lead because they have formal authority over the department and people in it; have some control over resources, rewards, punishments, and information (position power); and have more expertise in the work of the department than others in the department (personal power derived from expertise). Such managers may have little political power, but this is not a problem if position and personal power sources are sufficient to lead the department. In contrast, CEOs who lead at the institutional level derive power from the same menu of sources, but in a different mix. For example, the CEO possesses considerable political power by control of decision processes in the HSO, the ability to form coalitions of key decision makers, or the ability to co-opt opponents. The CEO may have considerable charisma, extremely loyal assistants, and deep friendships with key physicians and board members, all of which provide the CEO with considerable personal power. The CEO's positional power can be great in terms of control over resources and information available in the HSO. Finally, as Mintzberg[27] points out, the CEO may be in a strong position to control the *access* of others to the sources of power in the organization. This is an important source of power in itself.

LEADER TRAITS AND SKILLS

The link between interpersonal and political skills and the fact that some personal characteristics such as expertise and personal charisma are important bases of power suggest that certain traits and skills are associated with effective leaders. Most studies of leadership in the first half of the 20th century sought to find leader traits in physical characteristics, personality, and ability. They theorized that it was possible to identify traits that distinguished leaders and followers, or successful and unsuccessful leaders. These studies focused on traits associated with effective leaders in business organizations, but they also looked at leaders in government, the military, and religious organizations. To prove the *trait theory* of leadership, the researchers had to find traits that *all* leaders had in common. The many different traits studied included physical characteristics such as height, weight, and appearance, and personality traits such as alertness, originality, integrity, and self-confidence, as well as intelligence or cleverness.

None of the hundreds of studies conducted in search of universal leader traits was successful. A landmark review of the subject by Stogdill in 1948 analyzed all the major studies of leader traits and concluded that "A person does not become a leader by virtue of the possession of some combination of traits . . . the pattern of personal characteristics of the leader must bear some relevant relationship to the characteristics, activities, and goals of the followers."[28] This conclusion was useful in later research that studied leadership in the context of specific situations.

Stogdill's conclusion discouraged additional research to identify universal leader traits. However, industrial psychologists interested in improving the selection of managers continued to search for traits *associated* with effective leaders. They used improved methodologies and added administrative and technical abilities to the traits of intelligence and personality studied earlier. Many of these studies showed strong associations between certain traits and leader effectiveness. Interestingly, Stogdill confirms his original negative assessment of efforts to identify universal leader traits in his review of these later, more sophisticated studies. Stogdill does conclude, however, that it is possible to develop a trait profile that characterizes successful leaders:

> The leader is characterized by a strong drive for responsibility and task completion, vigor and persistence in pursuit of goals, venturesomeness and originality in problem solving, drive to exercise initiative in social situations, self-confidence and sense of personal identity, willingness to accept consequences of decision and action, readiness to absorb interpersonal stress, willingness to tolerate frustration and delay, ability to influence other persons' behavior, and capacity to structure social interaction systems to the purpose at hand.[29]

The idea that traits, whether of intelligence, personality, or ability, are associated with leader effectiveness continues to be assessed. There is no longer a search for universal leader traits, but the traits associated with leader effectiveness continue to be refined. Table 14.2 shows traits associated with leader effectiveness using the categories of "Intelligence," "Personality," and "Abilities." Table 14.3 is a list of traits and skills that most frequently characterize successful leaders.

Kirkpatrick and Locke describe contemporary thought about the role of leader traits in determining institution-level leadership effectiveness:

> While research shows that the possession of certain traits alone does not guarantee leadership success, there is evidence that effective leaders are different from other people in certain key respects. Key leader traits include: drive (a broad term which includes achievement, motivation, ambition, energy, tenacity, and initiative); leadership motivation (the desire to lead but not to seek power as an end in itself); honesty and integrity; self-confidence (which is associated with emotional stability); cognitive ability; and knowledge of the business. There is less clear evidence for traits such as charisma, creativity, and flexibility. We believe that the key leader traits help the leader acquire necessary skills; formulate an organizational vision and an effective plan for pursuing it; and take the necessary steps to implement the vision in reality.[30]

Others agree that the leader's ability to articulate a meaningful organizational vision is important. Connors goes further and states that the major concern about leadership in the health services field "is the lack of a vision, an agreement on what we want to end up with as far as a more rational, a more humane, a more affordable system."[31]

Partly because the search for universal leader traits was unsuccessful and partly because researchers became interested in other variables, the study of leadership and leaders shifted from traits to behavior in the 1950s, a shift that continued well into the 1960s. The studies in leader behavior have added another dimension to understanding leadership.

LEADER BEHAVIOR

Research into behavioral theories of leadership raised the exciting possibility that if leader behavior explained leadership effectiveness, then leadership could be *taught*. Education may not increase intelligence levels or change personality profiles, but behavior can be learned. Robbins notes:

> The difference in trait and behavioral theories, in terms of application, lies in their underlying assumptions. Trait theories maintained that leaders are born: Either you have it or you don't! On the other hand, if specific behaviors identified leaders, then we could teach leadership—we could design programs to implant these behavioral patterns in individuals who desired to be effective leaders. This was surely a more exciting avenue, since it meant that the supply of leaders could be expanded. If training worked, we could have an infinite supply of effective leaders.[32]

The promise of the behavioral approach was further enhanced when two major universities, Ohio State University and the University of Michigan, undertook major leadership research in the late 1940s to understand behavior that contributes to effective leadership. Most behavioral studies

Table 14.2.   Traits associated with leadership effectiveness

Intelligence	Personality	Abilities
Judgment	Adaptability	Ability to enlist cooperation
Decisiveness	Alertness	Cooperativeness
Knowledge	Creativity	Popularity and prestige
Fluency of speech	Personal integrity	Sociability (interpersonal skills)
	Self-confidence	Social participation
	Emotional balance and control	Tact, diplomacy
	Independence (nonconformity)	

Adapted from Bass, Bernard M. *Handbook of leadership*, 75–76. New York: Free Press, 1982; used by permission.

Table 14.3. Traits and skills found most frequently to be characteristic of successful leaders

Traits	Skills
Adaptable to situations	Clever (intelligent)
Alert to social environment	Conceptually skilled
Ambitious and achievement-oriented	Creative
Assertive	Diplomatic and tactful
Cooperative	Fluent in speaking
Decisive	Knowledgeable about group task
Dependable	Organized (administrative ability)
Dominant (desire to influence others)	Persuasive
Energetic (high activity level)	Socially skilled
Persistent	
Self-confident	
Tolerant of stress	
Willing to assume responsibility	

From Yukl, Gary A. *Leadership in organizations,* 2d ed., 176. Englewood Cliffs, NJ: Prentice Hall, 1989; reprinted by permission. © 1989, Prentice Hall, Inc.

of leadership are based on the pioneering work done in the leadership studies conducted at these two universities.

Ohio State University Leadership Studies

One of the most comprehensive and widely used behavioral theories of leadership was developed by researchers at Ohio State University, who identified two categories of leader behavior that they thought explained effective leadership at the supervisor-subordinate level. These categories are "consideration" and "initiating structure"[33] and are described by Yukl:

> *Consideration* is the degree to which a leader acts in a friendly and supportive manner, shows concern for subordinates, and looks out for their welfare. Some examples include: doing personal favors for subordinates, finding time to listen to subordinates' problems, backing up or going to bat for a subordinate, consulting with subordinates on important matters before going ahead, being willing to accept surbordinate suggestions, and treating a subordinate as an equal.
> *Initiating structure* is the degree to which a leader defines and structures his or her own role and the roles of subordinates toward attainment of the group's formal goals. Some examples include: criticizing poor work, emphasizing the importance of meeting deadlines, assigning subordinates to tasks, maintaining definite standards of performance, asking subordinates to follow standard procedures, offering new approaches to problems, coordinating the activities of subordinates, and seeing that subordinates are working up to capacity.[34]

Early research described these patterns as at opposite ends of a continuum. Using the concept of a continuum raised the question of which pattern most enhanced leader effectiveness. Empirical answers were ambiguous until later, reconceptualized research showed that these different patterns of leader behavior could both be exhibited by the same leader and in various combinations in different situations.

The premise of research based on this reconceptualization was that leaders who scored high on *both* patterns of behavior were most effective, which was defined as achieving high subordinate performance and satisfaction. The premise was not supported in all situations, however. Reinterpretation of the findings led to the conclusion that the combination of initiating structure and consideration behaviors that produces leadership effectiveness is dependent on the situation in which leadership is exercised.[35]

University of Michigan Leadership Studies

The studies at Ohio State University were complemented by parallel research at the University of Michigan.[36] Extensive interviews of leaders and followers in a variety of organizations identified distinct styles of leadership, which were called "job centered" behaviors and "employee centered" behaviors. More recently, these behaviors have been called "task-oriented" behaviors and "relationship-oriented" behaviors.[37] The leader behaviors identified at the University of Michigan are similar to those identified at Ohio State University: job-centered or task-oriented behaviors correspond to the initiating structure category and employee-centered or relationship-oriented behaviors correspond to the consideration category.

In the University of Michigan studies, leaders who were employee or relationship oriented emphasized interpersonal relations, took a personal interest in the needs of their subordinates, and readily accepted differences among group members. These leaders were considerate, supportive, and helpful with subordinates. In contrast, job- or task-oriented leaders emphasized technical or task aspects of the job, were more concerned with accomplishing the group's tasks than anything else, and regarded group members as a means to this end. These leaders spent their time planning, scheduling, coordinating, and closely supervising the work of the group's members.

As was true at Ohio State University, researchers at the University of Michigan first believed that job-centered (or task-oriented) leader behaviors and employee-centered (or relationship-oriented) leader behaviors were mutually exclusive and at opposite ends of a continuum. As their research progressed, however, they also found that leaders could exhibit either set of behaviors, or a combination of them.

Fundamentally, this mutual reinforcement of the results of the leadership behavior studies added to their credibility, and the research programs at the University of Michigan and Ohio State University developed the intellectual foundation for later theories and formal studies that sought to explain effective leadership styles. The main thrust was to identify the optimal mix of leader behaviors to achieve effectiveness.

Likert's System 4 Management Model

An important theory explaining the relative effectiveness of various leadership styles was developed by Rensis Likert.[38] He participated in the University of Michigan leadership research program and was influenced by findings about the relationship of task-oriented and relationship-oriented behaviors to leadership effectiveness. He concentrated on relationship behaviors almost exclusively because he believed that a key element in effective leadership at the level of supervisor-subordinate was the degree to which leaders allow followers to influence their decisions.

Figure 14.2 is a schematic of Likert's model of the ways leaders relate to followers on the dimension of follower participation in decisions about their work. He calls this model *System 4 management* because it contains four distinct systems of interpersonal relationships.

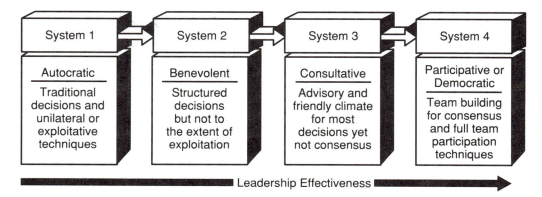

Figure 14.2. Likert's System 4 management model. (Adapted from Likert, Rensis. *Past and future perspectives on system 4,* 3–5, 9. Ann Arbor, MI: Rensis Likert Associates, 1977; used by permission.)

Likert considers *participative leadership* or *democratic leadership* styles superior to *autocratic leadership* styles in terms of their contribution to productivity and follower satisfaction. In his model, System 1 leaders are autocratic and rely on authority granted by the organization as the basis for their leadership. Such leaders show little confidence or trust in their followers. System 2 leaders are more benevolent toward followers, although they utilize highly authoritarian approaches. System 3 leaders consult with followers about decisions. Leaders using this system of interpersonal relationships stop short of permitting full participation in decisions.

In Likert's view, System 4 leaders give followers full participation in decision making. They endorse open channels of communication and other behaviors that ensure a high level of reciprocal influence between leader and followers and use group methods of supervision rather than close, one-to-one supervision of followers. System 4 leaders show high levels of confidence and trust in followers in most matters. The chief benefit of System 4 leadership, according to Likert, is that it encourages acceptance of decisions and commitment to them, both of which contribute directly to productivity and follower satisfaction.[39]

Likert's views on the benefits of participatory leadership stimulated substantial research on its effects. Miller and Monge[40] provide a good meta-analytical review of this research for readers who want more detail. It is sufficient to say that the advantages of a participative leader style are well supported. Many of them are important in HSOs:

1. There is a tendency for followers to identify with the organization more closely. This enhances motivation, especially in such citizenship behaviors as cooperation, protecting fellow employees and organization property, avoiding waste, and generally going beyond the call of duty. If people have some voice in their jobs, they tend to be more enthusiastic in performing them. Since a large percentage of health services employees are professionally trained, this style may be particularly applicable in HSOs.
2. Participation can be a means to overcome resistance to change. Those who participate in decisions that cause change will understand the changes and be less likely to resist them.
3. Participation can enhance personal growth and development of organization members. By participating in decisions, followers gain from experience in decision making. They get better and better at the process.
4. Participation enables a wider range of ideas and experiences to be brought to bear on a problem. Often followers who are close to a situation and familiar with it can solve problems related to the situation better than the leaders in those situations.
5. Participation can increase organizational flexibility because followers gain a wider range of experience about the job situation.

Certain managerial guidelines improve use of a participative approach to leadership. Following these guidelines is recommended because it is likely that HSO managers cannot achieve their goals without significant participative decision making.[41] For example, the participative leadership style is critical to the success of activities designed to improve the quality of patient care. An HSO's professional employees will not tolerate being left out of decisions in this area. The following points can be helpful in practicing participative leadership:

1. People who are permitted to participate in decisions should have expertise and skill in the matters under consideration, or the expertise must first be developed before they can effectively participate in decisions.
2. The cost of possible error should be considered. When others participate, do they raise or lower the risk that mistakes will be made?
3. Avoid quick shifts in leadership style. Followers should be prepared for any change in style to reduce skepticism and to build confidence.

4. Followers must be willing to participate. Some people do not want the responsibility that participation entails. Furthermore, the climate of respect between manager/leader and subordinates/followers should be such that followers are not afraid to voice opinions.

5. Finally, the participative style of leadership must be used with sincerity and integrity. Specifically, the manager/leader who frequently asks subordinates/followers to participate, while having no intention of following their recommendations, will soon lose support and acceptance. Once mistrust arises, followers may never view the participative style as legitimate. This does not mean leaders can never reject followers' recommendations. It means, however, that if those recommendations are rejected, the manager must adequately explain the decision to do so.

Blake and McCanse's Leadership Grid®

Another model that depicts the variety of leadership styles was developed by Robert Blake and Jane Mouton[42] and revised by Blake and McCanse.[43] Their model uses two variables of leadership orientation: *concern for people* and *concern for production*. These are attitudinal dimensions of leadership theory, as distinct from the behavioral dimensions identified in the Ohio State University and University of Michigan studies.

The Blake and McCanse Leadership Grid® has been a significant tool for helping people understand variation in leadership styles (Figure 14.3). The grid is formed by the axes of concern

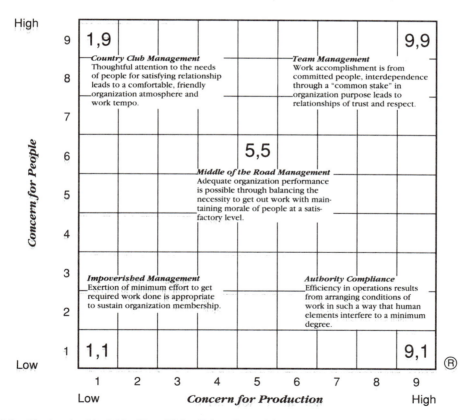

Figure 14.3. The Leadership Grid®. (From Blake, Robert R., and Anne Adams McCanse. *Leadership dilemmas— grid solutions,* 29. Houston: Gulf Publishing Company, 1991. (The Grid® designation is the property of Scientific Methods, Inc., and is used here with permission.)

for people and concern for production. By plotting various locations on the grid formed by these variables, Blake and McCanse identified five leadership styles. Table 14.4 shows their typical characteristics.

Blake and McCanse[44] took the position that the 9,9 style is *universally* the most effective leader orientation, just as Likert had done regarding System 4 leaders. The position that there is "one best way" to lead troubled other researchers, who always found exceptions. As distinct models of leader behavior were developed, especially in the University of Michigan and Ohio State University research, it became apparent that what works best in one situation *may not* work best in another. Missing from existing leadership theories were variables that explained why the most appropriate leadership behavior varied by situation.

It should be noted that the importance of situational variables is only clear cut in hindsight. It must be remembered that researchers pursuing both trait theories and behavioral theories began with the premise that it was important to discover the set of traits characteristic of all successful leaders or the behavioral style of leadership that explained leadership effectiveness. It was only after much work had been done that researchers realized there was neither one set of traits nor a specific behavioral style and that situational variables were needed. One model bridges the pure behavioral theories and the emerging situational theories. It deserves special recognition for this important role and is considered next.

Tannenbaum and Schmidt's Continuum of Leader Decision-Making Authority

Another example of the theories or models that have been developed to explain the many leadership styles available to managers is a continuum developed by Tannenbaum and Schmidt[45] (Figure 14.4). Their model has two polar ends with varying amounts of decision-making authority shared by managers/leaders and subordinates/followers, and shows alternative ways for managers/leaders to approach decision making, depending upon how much participation they want from subordinates/followers. Styles on the left are more authoritarian, and those on the right more participative.

Tannenbaum and Schmidt provide descriptions of the various styles presented in Figure 14.4, indicating the degree of decision-making authority held by the manager. Below these de-

Table 14.4. The major Leadership Grid. styles

1,1	Impoverished Management. This type of leadership is often referred to as laissez-faire leadership. Leaders in this position have little concern for people or productivity, avoid taking sides, and stay out of conflicts. They do just enough to get by.
1,9	Country Club Management. Managers in this position have great concern for people and little concern for production. They try to avoid conflicts and concentrate on being well liked. To them the task is less important than good interpersonal relations. Their goal is to keep people happy. (This is a soft Theory X approach and not a sound human relations approach.)
9,1	Authority–Compliance. Managers in this position have great concern for production and little concern for people. They desire tight control in order to get tasks done efficiently. They consider creativity and human relations to be unnecessary.
5,5	Middle of the Road Management. Leaders in this position have medium concern for people and production. They attempt to balance their concern for both people and production, but are not committed to either.
9,9	Team Management. This style of leadership is considered to be ideal. Such managers have great concern for both people and production. They work to motivate employees to reach their highest levels of accomplishment. They are flexible and responsive to change, and they understand the need to change.

Adapted from Blake, Robert R., and Anne Adams McCanse. *Leadership dilemmas—Grid solutions.* Houston, Gulf Publishing Company, 1991; used by permission.

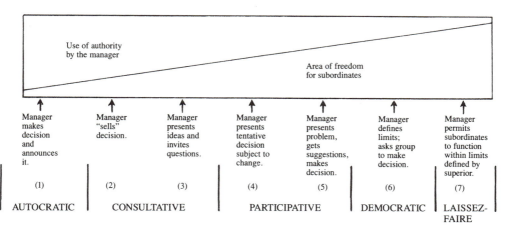

Figure 14.4. Continuum of leader decision-making authority. (From Tannenbaum, Robert, and Warren H. Schmidt. How to choose a leadership pattern. *Harvard Business Review* 51 [May–June 1973]: 162–180; reprinted by permission. Copyright © 1973 by the President and Fellows of Harvard College; all rights reserved.)

scriptions have been added commonly used labels describing the basic leadership behaviors being exhibited along the continuum, from autocratic to laissez-faire. Each style is described here.

Autocratic leaders (style 1 in the model) are those who make decisions and announce them to their followers. The role of subordinates is to carry out orders without an opportunity to materially alter decisions already made by the manager/leader.

Consultative leaders "sell" decisions to their followers by carefully explaining the rationale for the decision and its effect on the followers—style 2 in the model. Style 3 leaders permit slightly more subordinate involvement—the leader presents decisions to followers but invites questions so that understanding and acceptance are enhanced.

Participative leaders present tentative decisions that will be changed if subordinates can make a convincing case for a different decision—style 4 in the model. Style 5 leaders present a problem to subordinates, seek their advice and suggestions, and then make the decision. This leadership style makes greater use of participation and less use of authority than do the autocratic and consultative styles.

Democratic leaders—style 6—define the limits of the situation and problem to be solved and permit followers to make the decision.

Laissez-faire leaders—style 7—permit followers to function within limits set by the *leader's* superior. The manager/leader does not interfere and participates in decision making with no more influence than other members of the group. Leader and follower roles are indistinguishable in this style.

Tannenbaum and Schmidt describe possible leadership styles much as do Likert, Blake, and McCanse, and others who searched for the *best* style. Here the similarity ends, however, and the importance of Tannenbaum and Schmidt's contribution to understanding leadership effectiveness results from their conclusion that the best style depends on the particular situation. In their view, the choice of a style should be based on forces internal to the manager/leader (e.g., value system, confidence in subordinates/followers, and tolerance for ambiguity and uncertainty); forces within subordinates/followers (e.g., expectations, need for independence, ability, knowledge, and experience); and forces in the situation (e.g., type of organization, nature of the problem to be solved or the work to be done, and time pressure).[46] No single leader decision-making authority style is correct all the time. Managers must adapt and change to fit the situation.

An autocratic style might be appropriate in an operating room because work activity must be performed immediately, perhaps under crisis conditions. However, if physicians who are autocratic in the operating room become HSO managers, a very different style may be necessary, especially when other professionals are supervised. Subordinates' characteristics—training, education, motivation, and experience—influence the leader authority style. If subordinates are skilled professionals, the manager may readily seek their opinions and use a consultative or participative style. Similarly, the work being performed can determine which style is appropriate. If it is routine, clerical, and must have a specific sequence flow, the manager may be more consultative than democratic in determining what, how, and when work will be performed. However, if work is creative and flexible and other departments do not rely on timely completion, the manager may use a participative or democratic style. Certainly, the business office manager will use a different leader authority style than the manager of a medical research department.

The Tannenbaum and Schmidt model identifies a set of leadership styles, couples this with the concept that certain factors dictate choosing one over the others, and provides a bridge between early behavioral theories of leadership and the more sophisticated situational or contingency theories of leadership described next. The best style can only be determined after evaluating the situation, including the work environment, what is to be done, the nature of followers, the personality of the manager, and the organizational climate.

SITUATIONAL THEORIES OF LEADER TRAITS AND BEHAVIOR

When traits or particular behavior could not fully explain leader effectiveness and when it was found that behavior appropriate in one circumstance produced failure in others, researchers turned to situational influences. Many *situational* or *contingency* theories of leadership resulted from this research. These theories share an effort to explain how leader traits or behavior influence leadership effectiveness from situation to situation.

From among the many models or theories,[47] four of the most important are described here: the Fiedler model, Hershey and Blanchard's situational model, the Vroom-Yetton participation model, and House and Mitchell's path-goal theory. The Fiedler model shows that the situation moderates or influences the relationship between leader *traits* and leadership effectiveness. The other three describe how the situation influences the relationship between leader *behavior* and effectiveness.

Fiedler's Contingency Theory

Fiedler's research focuses on specifying situations in which certain leader traits would be particularly effective.[48] He calls his theory "contingency" because of his hypothesis that effective leadership is contingent upon whether the elements in a particular situation in which leadership is being exercised fit particular traits of the leader.

Fiedler hoped to identify leader traits that fit particular situations and could be used to improve leader effectiveness. Leadership could be improved by: 1) changing leader traits to fit situations, 2) selecting leaders whose traits fit particular situations, 3) moving leaders in organizations to situations that fit their traits, or 4) changing situations to better fit leader traits. Fiedler's theory can be appreciated by understanding the leader traits he examines and the way he assesses situations. His interest is in whether a leader is more task or relations motivated.

House and Baetz[49] describe these traits in terms of which of two sets of needs are dominant in a leader's personality. The *task-motivated* personality is more concerned about task success and task-related problems. Such persons are motivated primarily by achieving task objectives and are not motivated to establish good relationships with followers unless the work is going well and there are no serious task-related problems. In contrast, the *relations-motivated* personality is more concerned with good leader–follower relations, is motivated to have close interpersonal relationships, and will act in a considerate, supportive manner when relationships need to be improved. For such persons, achievement of task objectives is important only if the primary affiliation motive is adequately satisfied by good personal relationships with followers.

Unlike the behavioral styles of leadership (consideration and initiating structure) examined earlier, Fiedler considers task and relations motivations to be polar opposites. He measures these two traits in leaders by using the *least preferred co-worker* (LPC) score, which asked leaders to think of the present or past co-worker with whom they least liked to work. The LPC questionnaire has a number of attribute sets, such as pleasant-unpleasant, with an 8-point rating scale (Figure 14.5). The LPC score is the sum of the ratings for the attribute sets. A high score reflects a leader who is primarily relations motivated; a low score reflects a leader who is primarily task motivated. The reason for using the LPC score to measure a personality trait is described by Jago:

> Interpreting your LPC score hinges on the assumption that your description of your co-worker says more about *you* than about the person you have described. In essence, it is assumed that everyone's least preferred co-worker is about equally "unpleasant" and that differences in descriptions of these

Think of the person with whom you can work least well. This may be someone you work with now or someone you knew in the past. It does not have to be the person you like least well but should be the person with whom you had the most difficulty in getting a job done. Describe this person as he or she appears to you.

Pleasant	8 7 6 5 4 3 2 1	Unpleasant
Friendly	8 7 6 5 4 3 2 1	Unfriendly
Rejecting	1 2 3 4 5 6 7 8	Accepting
Helpful	8 7 6 5 4 3 2 1	Frustrating
Unenthusiastic	1 2 3 4 5 6 7 8	Enthusiastic
Tense	1 2 3 4 5 6 7 8	Relaxed
Distant	1 2 3 4 5 6 7 8	Close
Cold	1 2 3 4 5 6 7 8	Warm
Cooperative	8 7 6 5 4 3 2 1	Uncooperative
Supportive	8 7 6 5 4 3 2 1	Hostile
Boring	1 2 3 4 5 6 7 8	Interesting
Quarrelsome	1 2 3 4 5 6 7 8	Harmonious
Self-assured	8 7 6 5 4 3 2 1	Hesitant
Efficient	8 7 6 5 4 3 2 1	Inefficient
Gloomy	1 2 3 4 5 6 7 8	Cheerful
Open	8 7 6 5 4 3 2 1	Guarded

Figure 14.5. Fiedler's LPC scale. *Note:* LPC score is the sum of the answers to these 16 questions. High scores indicate a relationship orientation; low scores, a task orientation. (From Fiedler, Fred E., and Martin E. Chemers. *Leadership and effective management.* Glenview, IL: Scott, Foresman and Company, 1974; reprinted by permission.)

co-workers actually reflect differences in an underlying personality trait among the people doing the describing.[50]

According to Fiedler's theory, the relationship between a leader's LPC score and leadership effectiveness depends on a complex situational variable called *situational favorability*. Favorability is determined by three aspects of a situation:

1. *Leader–member relations* (It is important to note that Fiedler's contingency model relates specifically to a leader and a work group, hence the use of the term "member." This also means the theory is directly applicable to leadership at the supervisor–subordinate interface rather than to institution- level leadership.) This aspect of the situation refers to the extent to which the leader has the support and loyalty of group members and the members are friendly and cooperative. One way of measuring leader–member relations is by asking the group members to respond to a set of attribute questions (e.g., friendly–unfriendly) about the leader to indicate whether or not they accept and endorse the leader. A high score indicates good leader–member relations, while a low score indicates the opposite. Good leader–member relations imply that the leader is able to obtain compliance with minimum effort, whereas poor leader–member relations imply compliance with reservation and reluctance, if at all.

2. *Task structure* This aspect of the situation refers to the extent to which the task can be performed by following a detailed set of standard operating procedures. A structured task is a job situation that has specific instructions and standard procedures provided for its completion. In contrast, an unstructured task has only vague and inexplicit procedures without step-by-step guidelines.

3. *Position power* This aspect of the situation refers to the extent to which the leader has authority (including reward, coercive, and legitimate power) to evaluate the performance of followers (group members) and reward or punish them.

Figure 14.6 shows how the style of effective leadership varies with the situation. The reader should examine this figure closely because it contains a number of pieces of information that are relevant to the Fiedler contingency theory of leadership. The bottom portion shows combinations of the three situational favorability aspects: leader–member relations (good–poor), the task structure (structured–unstructured), and the manager's position power (strong–weak). The result is eight unique combinations that Fiedler calls octants.

For example, octant 1 shows good leader–member relations, a structured task, and a leader with strong position power. Octant 8 shows poor leader–member relations, an unstructured task, and a leader with weak position power. An intermediate octant, such as number 4, shows good leader–member relations, an unstructured task, and a leader with weak position power. In Fiedler's schema to measure the favorability of particular situations for leaders, octant 1 is most favorable, and octant 8 least favorable.

With a way to measure certain leader traits and to scale the favorability of the situations faced by leaders, Fiedler tested the relationships. His results are shown in the upper portion of Figure 14.6, where it can be seen that relationship-motivated leaders (high LPC scores) do well (relative to task-motivated leaders) in moderately favorable situations. Conversely, task-motivated leaders (low LPC scores) do relatively well in situations that are either very favorable or very unfavorable.

Fiedler attributes success of relationship-motivated leaders in situations with intermediate favorability to the leader's nondirective, permissive approach; a more directive approach could cause anxiety in followers, conflict in the group, and lack of cooperation.[51] He attributes success of the task-motivated leader in very favorable situations to the fact that because the leader has power, formal backing, and a well-structured task, followers are ready to be directed in their tasks. He attributes success of the task-motivated leader in very unfavorable situations to the fact that, without the leader's active and aggressive intervention and control, the group might fall apart.

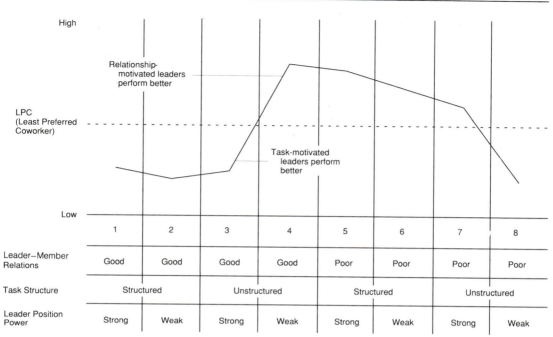

Figure 14.6. How the style of effective leadership varies with the situation. (From Fiedler, Fred E., and Martin E. Chemers. *Leadership and effective management,* 80. Glenview, IL: Scott, Foresman and Company, 1974; reprinted by permission.)

Complex theories have ample room for criticism, and Fiedler's is no exception.[52] Most research, however, supports the model.[53] Fiedler's work has a special place because it represents the first comprehensive attempt to incorporate situational variables directly into a leadership theory. This new dimension was refined in many subsequent studies. Furthermore, his model has considerable utility in management practice, especially in suggesting to managers the importance of systematically assessing their position power, leader–member relations, and task structures in relationship to their leadership effectiveness.

Hershey and Blanchard's Situational Leadership Model

Paul Hershey and Kenneth Blanchard have developed a leadership model that attempts to explain effective leadership as interplay among: 1) the leader's *relationship behavior* (extent to which leaders maintain personal relationships with followers through open communication and by exhibiting socioemotional supportive behaviors and actions toward them), 2) the leader's *task behavior* (extent to which leaders organize and define roles of followers and guide and direct them), and 3) the followers' *readiness level* (readiness to perform a task or function or to pursue an objective).[54] The leader behaviors used by Hershey and Blanchard are similar to the initiating structure and consideration behaviors identified in the Ohio State University studies discussed earlier.

While recognizing that many situational variables, such as leader, followers, superiors, peers, organization, nature of the job, and time, affect leadership effectiveness, the Hershey and Blanchard model focuses on followers as the key situational variable—specifically on their readiness to perform. The central premise is that the "leadership style a person should use with individuals or groups depends on the readiness level of the people the leader is attempting to influence."[55] Even though their model focuses on only one situational variable, Hershey and Blanchard call it the *situational leadership model.*

To appreciate the situational leadership model requires an understanding of how it uses leadership styles, as well as the concept of follower readiness. Hershey and Blanchard assume that the relative presence (high–low) of task and relationship behaviors can be used to identify four distinct leadership styles (S1–S4) as follows:

S1 or *Telling* (high task–low relationship)—the leader makes the decision. The leader defines roles and tells followers what, how, when, and where to do various tasks, emphasizing directive behavior.

S2 or *Selling* (high task–high relationship)—the leader makes the decision and then explains it to followers. The leader provides both directive behavior and supportive behavior.

S3 or *Participating* (low task–high relationship)—the leader and followers share decision making. The main role of the leader is to encourage and assist followers in contributing to sound decisions.

S4 or *Delegating* (low task–low relationship)—the followers make the decision. The leader provides little direction or support.

Follower readiness in the situational leadership model is not a personal characteristic or trait. Readiness refers to how ready a person is to perform a particular task. Readiness is assessed by two factors, ability and willingness, which Hershey and Blanchard define:

Ability is the knowledge, experience, and skill that an individual or group brings to a particular task or activity.

Willingness is the extent to which an individual or group has the confidence, commitment, and motivation to accomplish a specific task.[56]

Hershey and Blanchard use the ability of followers and their willingness (divided into commitment/motivation and confidence) to develop a four-stage continuum of follower readiness, from low (R1) to high (R4):

R1: Followers are unable *and* unwilling to take responsibility for performing a task, or they are unable to take and feel insecure about taking responsibility.

R2: Followers are unable but willing to do job tasks—they are motivated but lack appropriate skills—or they are unable but feel confident if the leader provides guidance.

R3: Followers are able but unwilling to do what the leader wants, or they are able to but feel insecure about doing what the leader wants.

R4: Followers are able and willing to do what is asked of them, or they both are able and feel confident about their ability to do what is asked of them.

Figure 14.7 integrates the four leadership styles identified by Hershey and Blanchard (Telling, Selling, Participating, and Delegating) with the four levels of follower readiness to suggest that effectiveness results when the leader's style matches followers' readiness. The model suggests that, as followers reach high levels of readiness (R4), the leader responds by decreasing task *and* relationship behaviors. At R4, the leader need do very little because followers are willing and able to take responsibility. At the lowest level of follower readiness (R1), followers need explicit direction because they are unable and unwilling to take responsibility. At moderate or intermediate levels (R2 and R3), different leadership styles are needed. At R2, where the followers are unable but willing, the leader must exhibit high levels of task and relationship behaviors. High task behavior compensates for followers' lack of ability, and high relationship behavior may help get them to psychologically "buy into" the leader's wishes. At R3, where followers are able but unwilling or insecure, a leadership style incorporating high levels of relationship behaviors may help overcome unwillingness or insecurity among followers.

Hershey and Blanchard stress that their situational leadership model is *not* a theory. They

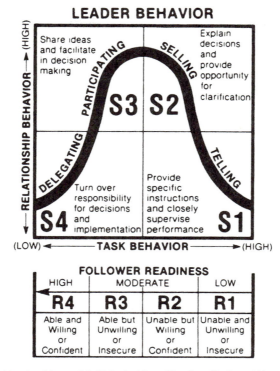

LEADER BEHAVIOR

Figure 14.7. The situational leadership model. (Adapted from Hershey, Paul, and Kenneth H. Blanchard. *Management of organizational behavior,* 5th ed., 171. Englewood Cliffs, NJ: Prentice Hall, 1988; used by permission.)

define a theory as an explanation of why something happens, and describe a model as "a pattern of already existing events that can be learned and therefore repeated."[57] The distinction is important because, as a theory, situational leadership is largely untested.[58] As a model, however, it illustrates that leaders must be concerned about the readiness of their followers to be led and that the level of readiness can be affected by actions of the leader.

Vroom–Yetton Model

Victor Vroom and Phillip Yetton developed a model to prescribe the most appropriate leadership style(s) for various situations.[59] It is based on analyses of how leader decision-making behavior affects the quality of the decision making in problem-solving situations, based in part on the degree of acceptance by followers. This model was previously presented in Chapter 10 (Figure 10.6) with a focus on problem-solving styles. It is presented here (see Figure 14.8) with a focus on leadership styles. As originally developed, the model features a decision tree and questions to guide users.[60] A revised version[61] replaces decision rules with mathematical functions and is so complex that microcomputer software is needed to fully understand it. The earlier version is presented here to explain the model's logic and use.

The Vroom-Yetton model assumes that five leader behaviors can be used: two types of autocratic decision making (AI and AII), two types of consultation (CI and CII), and one behavior that represents joint decision making by leader and followers as a group (GII). These leader behaviors are defined as:

> AI. You [the leader] solve the problem or make the decision yourself, using information available to you at the time.
> AII. You obtain the necessary information from your subordinates, then decide the solution to the

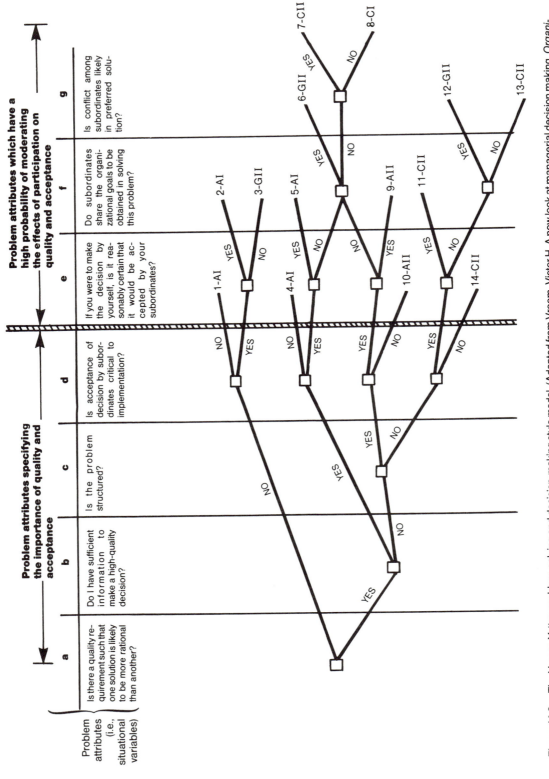

Figure 14.8. The Vroom-Yetton problem-solving and decision-making style model. (Adapted from Vroom, Victor H. A new look at managerial decision making. *Organizational Dynamics* 1 [Spring 1973]: 70; used by permission. Copyright © 1973. American Management Association, New York. All rights reserved.)

problem yourself. You may or may not tell your subordinates what the problem is in getting the information from them. The role played by your subordinates in making the decision is clearly one of providing necessary information to you, rather than generating or evaluating alternative solutions.

CI. You share the problem with the relevant subordinates individually, getting their ideas and suggestions, without bringing them together as a group. Then you make the decision, which may or may not reflect your subordinates' influence.

CII. You share the problem with your subordinates as a group, obtaining their collective ideas and suggestions. Then you make the decision, which may or may not reflect your subordinates' influence.

GII. You share the problem with your subordinates as a group. Together you generate and evaluate alternatives and attempt to reach agreement (consensus) on a solution. Your role is much like that of a chairperson. You do not try to influence the group to adopt "your" solution, and you are willing to accept and implement any solution which has the support of the entire group.[62]

Figure 14.8 illustrates the model's seven contingency questions ($a-g$ across the top of the figure) and a decision tree to direct a leader to situation-dependent prescribed leader behavior. The leader chooses from among five behaviors (AI, AII, CI, CII, or GII) and is guided by answering questions in the sequence $a-g$.

The Vroom-Yetton model is supported by work done by many researchers.[63] Hershey and Blanchard conclude that, in addition to wide acceptance, the Vroom-Yetton model has great practical value because it demonstrates that "leaders have the ability to vary their styles to fit the situation. This point is critical to acceptance of situational approaches to leadership."[64]

House-Mitchell Path-Goal Theory of Leadership

Like the other situational or contingency approaches described above, the path-goal theory of leadership attempts to predict the leadership behaviors that will be most effective in particular situations. Robert House calls his theory path-goal because he believes that "The motivational function of the leader consists of increasing personal payoffs to subordinates for work-goal attainment and making the path to these payoffs easier to travel by clarifying it, reducing roadblocks and pitfalls, and increasing the opportunities for personal satisfaction en route."[65] House and Terence Mitchell (who helped develop the theory further) note that:

> According to this theory, leaders are effective because of their impact on subordinates' motivation, ability to perform effectively and satisfaction. The theory is called path-goal because its major concern is how the leader influences the subordinates' perceptions of their work goals, personal goals and paths to goal attainment. The theory suggests that a leader's behavior is motivating or satisfying to the degree that the behavior increases subordinate goal attainment and clarifies the paths to these goals.[66]

This theory relies on the results of the Ohio State University and University of Michigan leadership studies and on the expectancy theory of motivation described in Chapter 13. That discussion stated that *expectancy* is the perceived probability that effort will affect performance; *instrumentality* is the perceived probability that performance will lead to outcomes; and the value attached to an outcome by a person is its *valence*. The expectancy model suggests that "people are satisfied with their jobs if they think they lead to things that are highly valued, and they work hard if they believe that effort leads to things that are highly valued."[67] House and Mitchell identify the role leadership plays by noting that followers are "motivated by leader behavior to the extent that this behavior influences expectancies."[68]

Aldag and Stearns describe path-goal theory in terms of expectancy theory by noting that "the path-goal theory sees the leader as having three motivational functions. The leader can increase valences associated with work-goal attainment, instrumentalities of work-goal attainment, and the expectancy that effort will result in work-goal attainment."[69]

Path-goal theory is a situational theory because its basic premise is that the effect of leader behavior on follower performance and satisfaction depends on the situation, specifically including follower/subordinate characteristics and task characteristics. Restated, different leader behaviors are best for different situations. According to House and Mitchell,[70] there are four categories of leader behavior; each is best suited to a particular situation:

Directive leadership describes the behavior of the leader who tells followers what they must do, tells them how to do it, requires that they follow rules and procedures, and schedules and coordinates the work. This is similar to initiating structure in the Ohio State University studies.

Supportive leadership describes the behavior of the leader who is friendly and approachable and exhibits consideration for the status, well-being, and needs of followers. This is similar to consideration in the Ohio State University studies.

Participative leadership describes the behavior of the leader who consults with followers, asks for opinions and suggestions, and considers them.

Achievement-oriented leadership describes the behavior of the leader who establishes challenging goals for followers, expects excellent performance, and exhibits confidence that followers will meet expectations.

House believes all four styles of behavior can and should be used by leaders as the situation dictates, and that effective leaders match styles to situations, which can vary along two dimensions. One dimension is the nature of the people being led. Followers may or may not have the ability to do the job. They differ, too, as to the perceived degree of control they have over their work. They may feel controlling or controlled. The second dimension of situational variance is the nature of the task, which may be routine and one with which follower/subordinates have prior experience, or may be new and ambiguous and one with which followers/subordinates will need help if they are to perform it well.

Figure 14.9 illustrates how the four leader behavior styles are matched to subordinate characteristics and the nature of the task in order to produce leader effectiveness. Leaders face different situations, and the path-goal theory suggests that effective leaders diagnose the situation and match behavior to it. Higgins describes the logic used in the diagnosis/matching effort:

> Directive leadership would be used when people have low levels of training and the work they are doing is partly routine and partly ambiguous. Supportive leadership would be used if people are doing highly routine work and the subordinates have been doing this work for some period of time. Achievement-oriented leadership would be used if people are doing highly innovative and ambiguous work and the subordinates already have a high level of knowledge and skill. Participative leadership would be used if the work people are doing possesses medium levels of ambiguity and subordinates have medium levels of experience doing it.[71]

House and Mitchell do not intend that the path-goal theory be more than a tentative explanation of the motivational effects of leader behavior, and they do not include all relevant variables. Formal studies based on the theory have concentrated on only two hypotheses:

Directive leadership contributes to the satisfaction of followers if they are engaged in ambiguous (unstructured) tasks and contributes to the dissatisfaction of followers if they are engaged in clear (structured) tasks.

Supportive leadership will have its most positive effect on follower satisfaction when followers are engaged in clear (structured) tasks.

Research generally supports these hypotheses,[72] but hypotheses for participative leadership and achievement-oriented leadership are not as fully tested. Despite limited validation of much of the path-goal theory, it is a useful construct because it merges leadership and motivation theories. It provides a pragmatic framework valuable to managers trying to match their leader behaviors to subordinate/follower characteristics and task characteristics.

Finally, path-goal theory is useful because it illustrates *substitutes* for leadership. For exam-

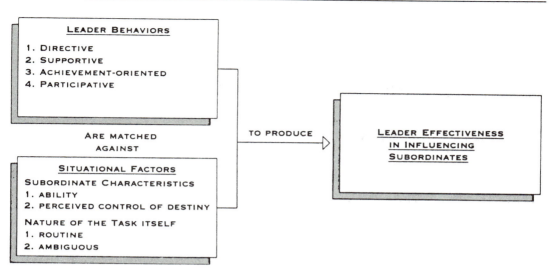

Figure 14.9. Path-goal theory of leadership. (Reprinted with the permission of Macmillan Publishing Company from *The management challenge: An introduction to management* by James M. Higgins. Copyright © 1991 Macmillan Publishing Company, Inc.

ple, if being an effective leader means clarifying the path to a follower goal, the existence of clear organizational rules and plans are a partial substitute for leadership. Substitutes for leader behaviors are anything that clarifies role expectations, motivates employees, or satisfies employees. This phenomenon is significant for HSOs because much of their workforce is highly professionalized and has a body of knowledge with standard practices to guide their work. To the extent that these factors reduce the need for leaders to guide the work, they are a substitute for leadership.

TOWARD INTEGRATING THEORIES OF LEADERSHIP

This chapter describes many approaches to understanding leadership: power, traits and skills, leadership behavior, and situational or contingency theories. These approaches have yielded numerous models, each seeking to explain leadership effectiveness. Individually, however, none of the theories or models fully explains leadership. Levey suggests, "We will probably never be able to achieve a truly elegant and rigorous general theory of leadership."[73]

It is possible, however, to integrate different theories to illustrate the processes and interactions involved in leadership effectiveness. One of the most comprehensive models or frameworks of leadership was developed by Yukl.[74] Figure 14.10 is an adaptation of his model. The model suggests that leadership contributes to the end results of performance and goal attainment. Furthermore, it shows that results are partly determined by complex interactions among leader traits and skills, personal power of the leader, leadership behaviors, and situational variables mediated or influenced by intervening variables. The presence of intervening variables in this model shows that leadership is only one determinant of organizational performance.

The model illustrates the most important interactions among key variables in effective leadership. For example, it shows that leader behavior is influenced by leader traits and skills, power, and situational requirements, as well as by information about intervening variables and results of previous leadership behaviors. In this sense, leader behaviors are simultaneously dependent and independent variables. They influence and are influenced by intervening variables and results. The model also shows how a leader's personal power is determined by results, by the leader's traits and skills, and by situational variables such as the type and extent of position authority possessed by the leader.

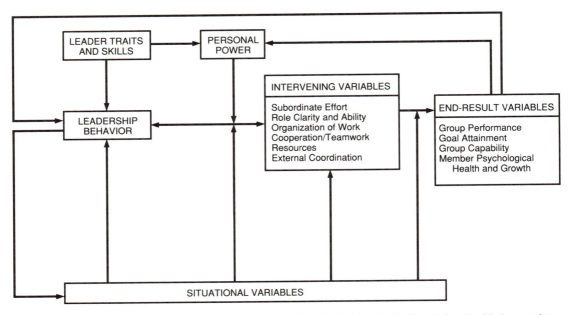

Figure 14.10. Integrating conceptual framework of leadership. (Adapted from Yukl, Gary A. *Leadership in organizations,* 2d ed., 269. Englewood Cliffs, NJ: Prentice Hall, 1989; used by permission. Copyright © 1989, Prentice Hall, Inc.)

While Yukl's model illustrates many of the interactions and reciprocal influence processes in leadership, it remains incomplete. Yukl may be his own harshest critic when he says:

> Unfortunately, few researchers consider all these variable sets simultaneously. The dominant tendency is to study one or two variable sets and ignore the others. Moreover, researchers usually include only one or two variables within a variable set in the same study. . . . Until more integrative research is conducted, it will not be possible to develop the sketchy conceptual framework into a full-fledged leadership theory.[75]

The model is also limited because it does not distinguish leadership at the level of supervisor-subordinate relationships from leadership at the institutional level, especially the CEO's role. While this model integrates thinking about leadership at both levels, its structure requires that the user infer this distinction. This limitation is important because the levels of leadership must be differentiated.

Leadership at the supervisor–subordinate interface is transactional because it involves exchanges between leader and followers. Leadership at the institutional level is more often transformational.[76] Transformational leadership has gained considerable attention recently because it is necessary to revitalizing organizations, including HSOs, and to providing them with strategies and capabilities to meet the future. Significant attention to the role of leadership in transforming or revitalizing organizations is a recent phenomenon,[77] but it is often what people mean when they speak of leadership. When an organization is thought to have done well because of "good leadership," this generally means that decisions about mission and structure, stakeholders, service mix, quality, and adoption of new technologies were good, not that leaders got extra performance from the staff, were helpful in planning staff tasks, or taught staff new skills. The key point is that leadership at the supervisor–subordinate interface *and* at the institutional level is important. Thus, the integrative model presented in Figure 14.10 applies to both levels.

The model suggests that leadership effectiveness at the supervisor–subordinate interface results from interactions among variables including leader traits and skills, leader power, and leader behavior—all selected to fit situational variables and all mediated or influenced by intervening variables that include two describing follower attributes (effort and ability), two describing work group attributes (organization and cooperation), and two describing the larger organizational context (resources and coordination). It can be concluded that there is no one best way for leaders to be effective in all circumstances at the supervisor – subordinate level. Each requires custom-blended traits, skills, power, and behaviors to meet the demands of situational and intervening variables.

At the institutional leadership level, particularly for the CEO, matters are even more complex. First, everything the model suggests about the complexity of leadership at the supervisor-subordinate interface is true for institutional leadership. Effective leadership here also requires blending traits, skills, power, and behaviors to meet the situation. However, as Burns and Becker suggest, CEOs working to be transformational leaders face several unique issues:

1. *Moral Issues.* The need for commonly held values and principles that define the organization's mission and resolve conflicts among competing, but legitimate, ends.
2. *Symbolic Issues.* The need for symbols and stances that legitimatize the organization's claims for support from internal and external coalitions and that provide a sense of organizational stability and self-control.
3. *Proactive Issues.* The need for long-term planning and strategic responses to maintain organizational autonomy within turbulent environments.[78]

Successfully addressing such issues, especially absent widely accepted conceptual and empirical underpinnings for transformational leadership or even a well-integrated model of such leadership, is a challenge for institutional-level leaders. Those who meet the challenges of transformational leadership effectively will be leaders who can take information and insights from many sources, customize them to their situation, and integrate them for themselves.

Successful leaders at the institutional level will perform several interrelated activities. They will have to develop a clear vision for the HSO. They will have to use their legitimate, expert, and referent power to assure that important stakeholders inside and outside the organization consider this vision. Leaders who effectively articulate and communicate their visions will have a distinct advantage in having them considered. Conger observes:

> While we have learned a great deal about the necessity of strategic vision and effective leadership, we have overlooked the critical link between vision and the leader's ability to powerfully communicate its essence. In the future, leaders will not only have to be effective strategists, but rhetoricians who can energize through the words they choose. The era of managing by dictate is ending and is being replaced by an era of managing [leading] by inspiration. Foremost among the new leadership skills demanded of this era will be the ability to craft and articulate a message that is highly motivational.[79]

Finally, successful institutional leaders will select and exhibit leadership behaviors that mobilize widespread commitment to their vision for the institution among followers and that maximize the contributions of followers to realizing the vision.

SUMMARY

Leadership is a process of influencing people to achieve particular goals. The leader determines what is to be accomplished by a group or organization and influences others to contribute to accomplishing that purpose. Leadership at the supervisor – subordinate interface is distinguished from leadership at the institutional level.

Various approaches to the study of leadership are described. Power and influence in relation to leadership, including the sources of a leader's power, are covered. Theories of leadership based on leader traits and skills, including intelligence, personality, and ability, are reviewed. The important research into leader behavior conducted at Ohio State University and the University of Michigan is presented as a prelude to reviewing the main behavioral models of leadership: Likert's System 4 model, Blake and McCanse's Managerial Grid®, and Tannenbaum and Schmidt's continuum of leader decision-making authority model. Four key situational theories of leader traits and behaviors are reviewed: Fiedler's contingency theory, Hershey and Blanchard's situational leadership model, the Vroom-Yetton model, and the path-goal theory of leadership developed by House and refined by House and Mitchell.

How these theories of leadership build on one another, differ, and are complementary is described. Particular emphasis is given to situational theories of leadership, and an integrative model of leadership is used to link current information about leadership at the level of supervisor-subordinate relationships and at the level of institutional leadership, where CEOs are increasingly expected to play transformational leadership roles.

DISCUSSION QUESTIONS

1. Distinguish between the roles of leaders at the level of supervisor-subordinate relationships and those at the level of institutional leadership.
2. How are the terms "groups," "organizations," "goals/objectives," "influence," and "acceptance" related to leadership?
3. What are the sources of a leader's power? Which source is most important?
4. Name four broad conceptual approaches to the study of leadership. How are these approaches interrelated?
5. Outline the key contributions made to the understanding of leadership by the Ohio State University leadership studies and the University of Michigan leadership studies.
6. Some have argued that leaders are born, not made, and that all great leaders have certain common traits. Discuss this viewpoint about leadership.
7. Briefly describe the five models of leader behavior presented in this chapter.
8. Briefly describe the four situational models of leadership presented in this chapter.
9. Distinguish between transactional and transformational leadership.
10. Assume that you have been invited to give a lecture on leadership effectiveness. What three key points would you emphasize?

CASE STUDY 1:   CHARLOTTE COOK'S PROBLEM

Charlotte Cook is a registered nurse (RN) who has three licensed practical nurses (LPNs) (Sally, John, and Betty) reporting to her during the day shift at Longview Nursing Home. She is 48 years old and has worked for Stanley George, the CEO, for 10 years.

Cook is confronted with a leadership problem. Sally, who has worked for Cook for 5 years, is 40 years old, cooperative, dependable, skilled, and an excellent performer. In fact, Cook has such confidence in Sally that she often puts her in charge when she leaves the floor.

John, who is 28, transferred from the evening shift 2 months ago after working there for 1 year. The CEO told Cook that he was transferring John because John could not get along with the new RN supervisor on that shift. The new RN is 2 years younger than John and they had a personality clash. In fact, rumors circulated that John disliked the new RN because she was not satisfied with either John's performance or his attitude. Furthermore, that RN's predecessor and John were very close socially, she was not demanding of John, and she often made exceptions for him. The other second-shift LPNs resented this and would have nothing to do with John.

Betty is 30 years old and has worked for Cook for the year she has been at Longview. Her performance is acceptable, she requires some direct supervision, and she and Cook have a good relationship.

Four weeks ago John began complaining to Sally and Betty. He criticized Mr. George and Ms. Cook and was generally "anti-everything" about Longview and its staff, particularly the new second-shift RN and Cook. He was uncooperative, often did his job poorly, and gossiped constantly with the patients. Cook has noticed that John always seems to be with Betty during their free time and that Betty tends to side with him. Cook feels that if the situation is ignored, matters could get worse.

Presume that LPNs are difficult to recruit and retain and that Cook does not want to discharge John, at least for the present.

Questions

1. How should Cook change the leadership style she uses with Sally when she interacts with John?
2. How should Cook approach and interact with Sally?
3. What should Cook do if John does not change?
4. Did Mr. George do the correct thing in transferring John?
5. What could Mr. George have done to remedy the situation at the time he transferred John?

CASE STUDY 2:   THE PRESIDENTIAL SEARCH

Memorial Hospital is a 500-bed teaching hospital located in a thriving, growing sun-belt city. In recent years, other hospitals in the area have cut into Memorial's market share. The outgoing president has been preoccupied with issues of a deteriorating physical plant and loss of medical staff to other area hospitals.

The board of trustees formed an ad hoc search committee to find a new hospital president. The committee plans to use a national executive search firm but wants to develop a clear picture of the person who will lead the institution back to preeminence in the city before talking with the search firm.

Mr. Adams, a hospital trustee and president of a large financial services company, is chair of the ad hoc committee. He has convened the committee to develop a list of capabilities the president should possess so it can provide this information to the search firm.

Assume you are a member of this committee.

Questions

1. What capabilities should the new president possess? Rank them in order.
2. Should this person be more skilled at the supervisor-subordinate interface or at institutional leadership? How will the committee distinguish between the two?
3. Some committee members point out that the situation at Memorial is unique; therefore, finding a person who was successful at another hospital will not guarantee success at Memorial. What would be your position on this issue?

CASE STUDY 3:   IS LEADERSHIP THE ISSUE?

There are 22 hospitals in a large eastern city. Each is independent of the others, except that three of the largest are affiliated with the local medical school. The others range in size from 180 beds to 600 beds; about half are sponsored by religious organizations. There is one large public hospital, and three hospitals are investor owned. The rest are not-for-profit community hospitals.

The state planning commission has argued for years that there are excess beds and overutilization of services in the community and that this could be relieved through merger and consolidation among some of the hospitals. All the hospitals have resisted this strategy and continue to be autonomous.

Questions

1. What role should the hospital CEOs play in addressing the question of merger or consolidation to solve the excess bed problem? Who else should play a role? Is this a "leadership" problem?

2. Assume you are one of the hospital CEOs and that you want your institution to merge with one or more of the other hospitals. What problems do you face? How could these problems be overcome?

3. A local paper ran a series on the issue, culminating with a harsh editorial that challenged hospital leaders to meet to discuss merger or consolidation as a way to solve the excess bed problem. Assume you are one of the CEOs and that you want to convene such a meeting. How would you approach other CEOs to arrange this meeting? How might they respond? Why?

CASE STUDY 4: "YOU DIDN'T TELL ME!"

Metropolitan Hospital is large and complex; it has 500 beds with 1,500 FTE employees and a professional staff organization of 400. As part of a comprehensive analysis of communication at Metropolitan, a consulting firm called Management Strategies, Inc., surveyed all employees. The results of one question troubled the CEO. The question was: "Does your immediate superior tell you about changes well in advance of their implementation so that you are prepared for them?"

The responses (in percentages) were:

	Always	Often	Sometimes	Seldom	Never
Senior managers	90	8	2		
Middle-level managers (department heads)	78	12	10		
First-line managers	65	25	10		
Nonmanagers	40	20	18	12	10

Questions

1. What do these results show? Why?
2. What reasons could explain these results?
3. What steps should the CEO take based on these results?

CASE STUDY 5: SUPERVISORY BEHAVIOR QUESTIONNAIRE[80]

Instructions: This questionnaire is part of an activity designed to explore supervisory behaviors. It is not a test; there are no right or wrong answers.

Think about supervisors (managers) you have known or know now, and then select the *most effective* supervisor and the *least effective* supervisor (effective is defined as being able to substantially influence the effort and performance of subordinates).

Read each of the following statements carefully. For the *most effective* supervisor, place an X over the number indicating how true or how untrue you believe the statement to be. For the *least effective* supervisor, place a circle around the number indicating how true you believe the statement to be.

Most effective X
Least effective . . . . . O

	Definitely Not True	Not True	Slightly Not True	Uncertain	Slightly True	True	Definitely True

1. My supervisor would compliment me if I did outstanding work. 1 2 3 4 5 6 7

2. My supervisor maintains definite standards of performance. 1 2 3 4 5 6 7

3. My supervisor would reprimand me if my work was consistently below standards. 1 2 3 4 5 6 7

4. My supervisor defines clear goals and objectives for my job. 1 2 3 4 5 6 7

5. My supervisor would give me special recognition if my work performance was especially good. 1 2 3 4 5 6 7

6. My supervisor would "get on me" if my work were not as good as he or she thinks it should be. 1 2 3 4 5 6 7

7. My supervisor would tell me if my work were outstanding. 1 2 3 4 5 6 7

8. My supervisor establishes clear performance guidelines. 1 2 3 4 5 6 7

9. My supervisor would reprimand me if I were not making progress in my work. 1 2 3 4 5 6 7

Supervisory Behavior Questionnaire Scoring Sheet

Instructions: For each of the three scales (A, B, and C), compute a *total score* by summing the answers to the appropriate questions and then subtracting the number 12. Compute a score for both the most effective and the least effective supervisors.

Question Number	Most Effective	Least Effective	Question Number	Most Effective	Least Effective	Question Number	Most Effective	Least Effective
2.	+ ( )	+ ( )	1.	+ ( )	+ ( )	3.	+ ( )	+ ( )
4.	+ ( )	+ ( )	5.	+ ( )	+ ( )	6.	+ ( )	+ ( )
8.	+ ( )	+ ( )	7.	+ ( )	+ ( )	9.	+ ( )	+ ( )
Subtotal			Subtotal			Subtotal		
	( ) − 12	( ) − 12		( ) − 12	( ) − 12		( ) − 12	( ) − 12
Total Score			Total Score			Total Score		
	A	A		B	B		C	C

Next, on the following graph, write in a large "X" to indicate the total score for scales A, B, and C for the most effective supervisor. Use a large "O" to indicate the scores for the least effective supervisor.

A. Goal Specification Behavior

```
|  |  |  |  |     |  |  |  |  |
-9 -7 -5 -3 -1    +1 +3 +5 +7 +9
```

B. Positive Reward Behavior

```
|  |  |  |  |     |  |  |  |  |
-9 -7 -5 -3 -1    +1 +3 +5 +7 +9
```

C. Punitive Reward Behavior

```
|  |  |  |  |     |  |  |  |  |
-9 -7 -5 -3 -1    +1 +3 +5 +7 +9
```

Questions

1. Describe the profile of attributes or characteristics of the most effective supervisor reflected in the A, B, and C scales above.
2. Describe the profile of attributes or characteristics of the least effective supervisor reflected in the A, B, and C scales above.

NOTES

1. Kirkpatrick, Shelly A., and Edwin A. Locke. Leadership: Do traits matter? *The Executive* 5 (May 1991): 59.
2. Kaluzny, Arnold D. Revitalizing decision-making at the middle management level. *Hospital & Health Services Administration* 34, (Spring 1989): 39–51.
3. Burns, James M. *Leadership*. New York: Harper & Row, 1978.
4. Stevens, Rosemary A. The hospital as a social institution, new-fashioned for the 1990s. *Hospital & Health Services Administration* 36 (Summer 1991): 172.
5. Burns, Lawton R., and Selwyn W. Becker. Leadership and managership. In *Health care management: A text in organization theory and behavior*, edited by Stephen M. Shortell and Arnold D. Kaluzny, 2d ed., 143. New York: John Wiley & Sons, 1988.
6. Burns and Becker, *Leadership*, 143.
7. Burns, *Leadership*.
8. Bass, Bernard M. *Leadership and performance beyond expectations*. New York: Academic Press, 1985.
9. Zuckerman, Howard S. Redefining the role of the CEO: Challenges and conflicts. *Hospital & Health Services Administration* 34 (Spring 1989): 35–36.
10. Cartwright, Dorwin, and Alvin Zander. *Group dynamics: Research and theory*. New York: Harper and Row Publishers, 1968.
11. Fiedler, Fred E., and Martin E. Chemers. *Leadership and effective management*, 4. Glenview, IL: Scott, Foresman and Co., 1974.
12. Holt, David H. *Management: Principles and practices*, 2d ed., 450. Englewood Cliffs, NJ: Prentice Hall, Inc., 1990.
13. Blake, Robert R., and Jane S. Mouton. *The versatile manager: A grid profile*. Homewood, IL: Richard D. Irwin, 1981.
14. Jago, Arthur G. Leadership: Perspectives in theory and research. *Management Science* 28 (March 1982): 315–336.
15. Bass, Bernard M. *Stogdill's handbook of leadership*, 16. New York: Free Press, 1982.
16. Yukl, Gary A. *Leadership in organizations*, 2d ed., 5. Englewood Cliffs, NJ: Prentice Hall, 1989.
17. Bass, *Stogdill's handbook*, 16.
18. McLaughlin, Curtis P., and Arnold D. Kaluzny. Total quality management in health: Making it work. *Health Care Management Review* 15 (Summer 1990): 12.
19. Deal, Terrence E. Healthcare executives as symbolic leaders. *Healthcare Executive* 5 (March/April 1990): 25.
20. Yukl, *Leadership*, 10.
21. Keys, Bernard, and Thomas Case. How to become an influential manager. *The Executive* 4 (November 1990): 38.
22. French, John R. P., and Bertram H. Raven. The basis of social power. In *Studies of social power*, edited by Dorwin Cartwright, 150–167. Ann Arbor, MI: Institute for Social Research, 1959.
23. Conger, Jay A., Rabindra Kanungo, and Associates. *Charismatic leadership: The elusive factor in organizations*. San Francisco: Jossey-Bass, 1988.
24. Morlock, Laura L., Constance A. Nathanson, and Jeffrey A. Alexander. Authority, power, and influence. In *Health care management: A text in organization theory and behavior*, edited by Stephen M. Shortell and Arnold D. Kaluzny, 2d ed., 268. New York: John Wiley & Sons, 1988.
25. Mintzberg, Henry. *Power in and around organizations*, 26. Englewood Cliffs, NJ: Prentice Hall, 1983.
26. Yukl, *Leadership*, 14–15.
27. Mintzberg, *Power*.
28. Stogdill, Ralph M. Personal factors associated with leadership. *Journal of Psychology* 25 (January 1948): 64.
29. Stogdill, Ralph M. *Handbook of leadership: A survey of the literature*, 81. New York: Free Press, 1974.
30. Kirkpatrick and Locke, Leadership, 48.
31. Connors, Edwards J. Reflections on leadership in health care. *Hospital & Health Services Administration* 35 (Fall 1990): 314.
32. Robbins, Stephen P. *Management*, 3d ed, 462. Englewood Cliffs, NJ: Prentice Hall, 1991.
33. Stogdill, Ralph M., and Alvin E. Coons, Eds. *Leadership behavior: Its description and measurement*. Research Monograph No. 88. Columbus: Bureau of Business Research, Ohio State University, 1957.
34. Yukl, *Leadership*, 75.
35. Gibson, James L., John M. Ivancevich, and James H. Donnelly, Jr. *Organizations: Behavior, structure, processes*, 7th ed. Homewood, IL: Irwin, 1991.

36. Katz, David, and Robert L. Kahn. Some recent findings in human relations research. In *Readings in social psychology,* edited by Guy E. Swanson, Theodore M. Newcomb, and Robert E. Hartley. New York: Holt, Rinehart & Winston, 1952.
37. Higgins, James M. *The management challenge: An introduction to management.* New York: Macmillan Publishing Company, 1991.
38. Likert, Rensis. *New patterns of management.* New York: McGraw-Hill, 1961; Likert, Rensis. An integrating principle and an overview. In *The great writings in management and organizational behavior,* edited by Louis E. Boone and Donald D. Bowen, 216–238. New York: Random House, 1987.
39. Likert, *New patterns*; Likert, Integrating principle.
40. Miller, Katherine I., and Peter R. Monge. Participation, satisfaction, and productivity: A meta-analytic review. *Academy of Management Journal* 29 (December 1986): 727–753.
41. Nutt, Paul C. How top managers in health organizations set directions that guide decision making. *Hospital & Health Services Administration* 36 (Spring 1991): 57–75.
42. Blake, Robert R., and Jane S. Mouton. *The managerial grid III: The key to leadership excellence.* Houston: Gulf Publishing Company, 1985.
43. Blake, Robert R., and Anne Adams McCanse. *Leadership dilemmas—grid solutions.* Houston: Gulf Publishing Company, 1991.
44. Blake and McCanse, *Leadership dilemmas.*
45. Tannenbaum, Robert, and Warren H. Schmidt. How to choose a leadership pattern. *Harvard Business Review* 51 (May–June 1973): 162–180.
46. Tannenbaum and Schmidt, How to choose.
47. Yukl, *Leadership.*
48. Fiedler, Fred E. A contingency model of leadership effectiveness. In *Advances in experimental social psychology,* edited by Leonard Berkowitz. New York: Academic Press, 1964; Fiedler, Fred E. *A theory of leadership effectiveness.* New York: McGraw-Hill, 1967.
49. House, Robert J., and M. Baetz. Leadership: Some empirical generalizations and new research directions. In *Research in organizational behavior,* edited by Barry M. Staw, Vol. I. Greenwich, CT: JAI Press, 1979.
50. Jago, Leadership, 322.
51. Fiedler, *Theory of leadership.*
52. Schriesheim, C.A., and Steven Kerr. Theories and measures of leadership: A critical appraisal of current and future directions. In *Leadership: The cutting edge,* edited by J.G. Hunt and Lars L. Larson, 9–45. Carbondale, IL: Southern Illinois University Press, 1977.
53. Peters, Lawrence H., Darnell D. Hartke, and John T. Pohlman. Fiedler's contingency theory of leadership: An application of the meta-analysis procedures of Schmidt

and Hunter. *Psychological Bulletin* 97 (March 1985): 274–285.
54. Hershey, Paul, and Kenneth H. Blanchard. *Management of organizational behavior: Utilizing human resources,* 5th ed. Englewood Cliffs, NJ: Prentice Hall, 1988.
55. Hershey and Blanchard, *Management,* 171.
56. Hershey and Blanchard, *Management,* 175.
57. Hershey and Blanchard, *Management,* 170.
58. Robbins, *Management*; Yukl, *Leadership.*
59. Vroom, Victor H., and Phillip W. Yetton. *Leadership and decision making.* Pittsburgh: University of Pittsburgh Press, 1973.
60. Vroom, Victor H. A new look at managerial decision making. *Organizational Dynamics* 1 (Spring 1973): 66–80.
61. Vroom, Victor H., and Arthur G. Jago. *The new leadership: Managing participation in organizations.* Englewood Cliffs, NJ: Prentice Hall, 1988.
62. Vroom and Yetton, *Leadership,* 13.
63. Yukl, *Leadership.*
64. Hershey and Blanchard, *Management,* 116.
65. House, Robert J. A path-goal theory of leader effectiveness. *Administrative Science Quarterly* 16 (September 1971): 324.
66. House, Robert J., and Terence R. Mitchell. Path-goal theory of leadership. *Journal of Contemporary Business* 3 (Autumn 1974): 81.
67. House and Mitchell, Path-goal theory, 81.
68. House and Mitchell, Path-goal theory, 81.
69. Aldag, Ramon J., and Timothy M. Stearns. *Management,* 2d ed., 512. Cincinnati, OH: South-Western Publishing Co., 1991.
70. House and Mitchell, Path-goal theory.
71. Higgins, *Management challenge,* 514.
72. Yukl, *Leadership.*
73. Levey, Samuel. The leadership mystique. *Hospital & Health Services Administration* 35 (Winter 1990): 479.
74. Yukl, *Leadership.*
75. Yukl, *Leadership,* 268–269.
76. Avolio, Brice J., and Bernard M. Bass. Transformational leadership, charisma and beyond. In *Emerging leadership vistas,* edited by James G. Hunt, B. Rajaram Baliga, H. Peter Dachler, and Chester A. Schriesheim, 29–49. Lexington, MA: Lexington Books, 1988.
77. Bass, *Leadership.*
78. Burns and Becker, Leadership, 168.
79. Conger, Jay A. Inspiring others: The language of leadership. *The Executive* 5 (February 1991): 31.
80. From Sims, Henry P., Jr. Patterns of effective supervisory behavior. In *The 1981 annual handbook for group facilitators,* edited by John E. Jones and J. William Pfeiffer, 10th ed., 95–99. San Diego, CA: University Associates, Inc., 1981; reprinted by permission.

BIBLIOGRAPHY

Avolio, Brice J., and Bernard M. Bass. Transformational leadership, charisma and beyond. In *Emerging leadership vistas,* edited by James G. Hunt, B. Rajaram Baliga, H. Peter Dachler, and Chester A. Schriesheim, 29–49. Lexington, MA: Lexington Books, 1988.

Bass, Bernard M. *Leadership and performance beyond expectations.* New York: Academic Press, 1985.

Bass, Bernard M. *Stogdill's handbook of leadership.* New York: Free Press, 1982.

Blake, Robert R., and Anne Adams McCanse. *Leadership dilemmas—grid solutions.* Houston: Gulf Publishing Company, 1991.

Blake, Robert R., and Jane S. Mouton. *The managerial grid III: The key to leadership excellence.* Houston: Gulf Publishing Company, 1985.

Burns, James M. *Leadership.* New York: Harper & Row, 1978.

Burns, Lawton R., and Selwyn W. Becker. Leadership and managership. In *Health care management: A text in organi-*

zation theory and behavior, edited by Stephen M. Shortell and Arnold D. Kaluzny, 2d ed., 142–186. New York: John Wiley & Sons, 1988.

Conger, Jay A. Inspiring others: The language of leadership. *The Executive* 5 (February 1991): 31–45.

Conger, Jay A., Rabindra Kanungo, and Associates. *Charismatic leadership: The elusive factor in organizations.* San Francisco: Jossey-Bass, 1988.

Connors, Edward J. Reflections on leadership in health care. *Hospital & Health Services Administration* 35 (Fall 1990): 309–320.

Deal, Terrence E. Healthcare executives as symbolic leaders. *Healthcare Executive* 5 (March/April 1990): 24–27.

Fiedler, Fred E. A contingency model of leadership effectiveness. In *Advances in experimental social psychology,* edited by Leonard Berkowitz. New York: Academic Press, 1964.

Fiedler, Fred E. *A theory of leadership effectiveness.* New York: McGraw-Hill, 1967.

Fiedler, Fred E., and Martin E. Chemers. *Leadership and effective management.* Glenview, IL: Scott, Foresman and Co., 1974.

French, John R. P., and Bertram H. Raven. The basis of social power. In *Studies of social power,* edited by Dorwin Cartwright, 150–167. Ann Arbor, MI: Institute for Social Research, 1959.

Hershey, Paul, and Kenneth H. Blanchard. *Management of organizational behavior: Utilizing human resources,* 5th ed. Englewood Cliffs, NJ: Prentice Hall, 1988.

House, Robert J. A path-goal theory of leader effectiveness. *Administrative Science Quarterly* 16 (September 1971): 321–339.

House, Robert J., and M. Baetz. Leadership: Some empirical generalizations and new research directions. In *Research in organizational behavior,* edited by Barry M. Staw, Vol. I. Greenwich, CT: JAI Press, 1979.

House, Robert J., and Terence R. Mitchell. Path-goal theory of leadership. *Journal of Contemporary Business* 3 (Autumn 1974): 81–97.

Jago, Arthur G. Leadership: Perspectives in theory and research. *Management Science* 28 (March 1982): 315–336.

Kaluzny, Arnold D. Revitalizing decision-making at the middle management level. *Hospital & Health Services Administration.* 34 (Spring 1989): 39–51.

Keys, Bernard, and Thomas Case. How to become an influential manager. *The Executive* 4 (November 1990): 38–51.

Kirkpatrick, Shelly A., and Edwin A. Locke. Leadership: Do traits matter? *The Executive* 5 (May 1991): 48–60.

Levey, Samuel. The leadership mystique. *Hospital & Health Services Administration* 35 (Winter 1990): 479–480.

Likert, Rensis. An integrating principle and an overview. In *The great writings in management and organizational behavior,* edited by Louis E. Boone and Donald D. Bowen,

216–238. New York: Random House, 1987.

Likert, Rensis. *Past and future perspectives on system 4.* Ann Arbor, MI: Rensis Likert Associates, 1977.

Miller, Katherine I., and Peter R. Monge. Participation, satisfaction, and productivity: A meta-analytic review. *Academy of Management Journal* 29 (December 1986): 727–753.

Mintzberg, Henry. *Power in and around organizations.* Englewood Cliffs, NJ: Prentice Hall, 1983.

Morlock, Laura L., Constance A. Nathanson, and Jeffrey A. Alexander. Authority, power, and influence. In *Health care management: A text in organization theory and behavior,* edited by Stephen M. Shortell and Arnold D. Kaluzny, 2d ed., 265–300. New York: John Wiley & Sons, 1988.

Nutt, Paul C. How top managers in health organizations set directions that guide decision making. *Hospital & Health Services Administration* 36 (Spring 1991): 57–75.

Peters, Lawrence H., Darnell D. Hartke, and John T. Pohlman. Fiedler's contingency theory of leadership: An application of the meta-analysis procedures of Schmidt and Hunter. *Psychological Bulletin* 97 (March 1985): 274–285.

Schriesheim, C.A., and Steven Kerr. Theories and measures of leadership: A critical appraisal of current and future directions. In *Leadership: The cutting edge,* edited by J.G. Hunt and Lars L. Larson, 9–45. Carbondale, IL: Southern Illinois University Press, 1977.

Stevens, Rosemary A. The hospital as a social institution, new-fashioned for the 1990s. *Hospital & Health Services Administration* 36 (Summer 1991): 163–173.

Stogdill, Ralph M. *Handbook of leadership: A survey of the literature.* New York: Free Press, 1974.

Stogdill, Ralph M. Personal factors associated with leadership. *Journal of Applied Psychology* 25 (January 1948): 35–71.

Stogdill, Ralph M., and Alvin E. Coons, Eds. *Leadership behavior: Its description and measurement.* Research Monograph No. 88. Columbus: Bureau of Business Research, Ohio State University, 1957.

Tannenbaum, Robert, and Warren H. Schmidt. How to choose a leadership pattern. *Harvard Business Review* 51 (May–June 1973): 162–180.

Vroom, Victor H. A new look at managerial decision making. *Organizational Dynamics* 1 (Spring 1973): 66–80.

Vroom, Victor H., and Arthur G. Jago. *The new leadership: Managing participation in organizations.* Englewood Cliffs, NJ: Prentice Hall, 1988.

Vroom, Victor H., and Phillip W. Yetton. *Leadership and decision making.* Pittsburgh: University of Pittsburgh Press, 1973.

Yukl, Gary A. *Leadership in organizations,* 2d ed. Englewood Cliffs, NJ: Prentice Hall, 1989.

Zuckerman, Howard S. Redefining the role of the CEO: Challenges and conflicts. *Hospital & Health Services Administration* 34 (Spring 1989): 25–38.

15 / Communication

Someone once said that if we could solve the problems inherent in communications, we would indeed solve most of the problems not only of the organization but of the world.
Schulz and Johnson,
Management of Hospitals and Health Services[1]

The management functions of planning, organizing, staffing, directing, controlling, and decision making depend on effective communication. Without it, decision making would take place in an information vacuum and plans and objectives would go no further than the person who originates them; the health services organization (HSO) would be organized and staffed only as a conglomeration of isolated people and departments; directing people as to what, when, how, or why to do their work would be impossible; and control would be a meaningless exercise without the communication of results to influence future performance. Similarly, all of the managerial roles (interpersonal, informational, and decisional) depend upon effective communication. Managers cannot develop liaison relationships, disseminate information, or negotiate without communicating.

All relationships involving managers in HSOs are information dependent, whether they are internal, such as among managers and between managers and other professionals or members of the governing body, or external, such as relationships with other HSOs or with stakeholders such as patients, insurance companies, and government. The degree to which understanding is transmitted and received effectively through communications plays a key part in accomplishing work results. People communicate facts, ideas, feelings, and attitudes while working and solving problems. If this communication is adequate, the work gets done more effectively and problems are solved more efficiently. In any organized effort, communication is essential for people to work together because it permits them to influence and react to one another.

The importance of communication skills for HSO managers is shown in Table 15.1, which summarizes a study of the competencies that chief executive officers (CEOs) in different types of Canadian HSOs believe they should possess. CEOs were asked to rank the competencies they thought they would need to manage effectively in the future. Communication was ranked in the first five for each category of HSO.

When managers communicate, one of four major functions, or some combination of them, is served. Communication can serve an *information* function, a *motivation* function, a *control* function, and an *emotive* function.[2] Communication provides information people need in order to make decisions. People need information about operating activities, resources, alternatives, and the plans and activities of others in the HSO if they are to make good decisions. The HSO must also provide a great deal of information to external stakeholders, especially potential customers, third-party payors, and regulators, if it is to function effectively within its environment.

As was noted in Chapter 13, "Motivation," motivation is a process internal to the person experiencing it. However, managers can effect motivation in others by informing them about rewards that will result from their performance, by giving them information that builds commitment to the HSO and its objectives, and by using communication skills to help people understand and fulfill their personal needs. Managers also communicate with external stakeholders to influence

Table 15.1. Ranking of managerial competencies by CEOs in order of future importance

Rank	Type of HSO					
	CEOs in teaching hospitals (N = 68)	CEOs in hospitals over 200 beds (N = 84)	CEOs in hospitals under 200 beds (N = 43)	CEOs in mental or rehabilitative hospitals (N = 132)	CEOs in nursing homes over 50 beds (N = 321)	CEOs in medical groups (N = 122)
1	Problem solving/decision making	Organizational/operational skills	COMMUNICATION (public relations)	Problem solving/decision making	Problem solving/decision making	COMMUNICATION (spoken communication, including talking, listening, and public speaking)
2	Health services planning issues	Effecting and managing change	Effecting and managing change	COMMUNICATION (spoken communication, including talking, listening, and public speaking)	Labor relations	Problem solving/decision making
3	COMMUNICATION (spoken communication, including talking, listening, and public speaking)	Proactively affect external government policy	Problem solving/decision making	Effecting and managing change	COMMUNICATION (public relations)	COMMUNICATION (written communication and report writing)
4	Proactively affect external government policy	COMMUNICATION (spoken communication, including talking, listening, and public speaking)	COMMUNICATION (spoken communication, including talking, listening, and public speaking)	COMMUNICATION (public relations)	Personnel administration	COMMUNICATION (public relations)
5	Evaluation methods and control	COMMUNICATION (written communication and report writing)	Evaluation methods and control	Organizational/operational skills	COMMUNICATION (spoken communication, including talking, listening, and public speaking)	Proactively affect external government policy

Adapted from Hastings, John E.F., William R. Mindell, John W. Browne, and Janet M. Barnsley. Canadian health administrator study. *Canadian Journal of Public Health,* 72 (March–April 1981): 48–49.

them to act in ways that benefit the HSO. Examples of desired behaviors include selecting the HSO as a provider of medical services, offering favorable reimbursement levels for services, or establishing favorable regulatory policies. To the extent that communication provides a path by which managers can influence behavior, it serves a motivation function.

Many kinds of communications control the performance of HSOs and those who work in them: activities reports, policies to establish standard operating procedures, budgets, and face-to-face directives are examples. Such communications enhance control when they clarify duties, authorities, and responsibilities.

A final function of communication results from the fact that it is people who communicate, even though they may speak on behalf of the organization. Without exception, they have emotions and feelings such as satisfaction, happiness, sadness, and anger, which must often be expressed. Communication permits this necessary venting to occur among people within the HSO. Emotive communication also assists the HSO to increase acceptance of the organization and its actions both internally and among external stakeholders.

COMMUNICATION DEFINED AND MODELED

Communication can be defined as *the creation or exchange of understanding between sender(s) and receiver(s)*. This definition does not restrict communication to words alone; it includes all methods (verbal and nonverbal) by which meaning is conveyed. Even silence conveys meaning and must be considered part of communicating.

Managers in HSOs must be concerned with two types of communication: that which is internal to the HSO and that which is external and occurs between the HSO and other organizations or outside stakeholders. *Intraorganizational communication* occurs *within* HSOs. In complex HSOs, intraorganizational communication depends on formal channels and networks to transmit information and understanding throughout the organization and on widespread acknowledgment of the existence and effective use of these channels. These channels and networks carry communications multidirectionally: downward, upward, horizontally, and diagonally.

Increasingly, senior managers must be concerned with communication *between* their HSO and other organizations and external stakeholders. This is known as *interorganizational communication*. Examples are marketing the HSO's services or influencing (lobbying) political constituencies in the HSO's external environment.

Both intra- and interorganizational communications are defined as the creation or exchange of *understanding* between sender(s) and receiver(s). Understanding is the key element. Senders want receivers of their messages to understand them. This means receivers must interpret messages exactly as they are intended if communication is to be effective. Unfortunately, complete understanding seldom results because of the many environmental and personal barriers to effective communication. Managers must realize that information can be easily transmitted, but this does not ensure that recipients will understand it. Drucker states the role of the receiver or recipient in the communication process quite specifically:

> It is the recipient who communicates. The so-called communicator, the person who emits the communication, does not communicate. He utters. Unless there is someone who hears, there is no communication. There is only noise. The communicator speaks or writes or sings—but does not communicate. Indeed, he cannot communicate. He can only make it possible, or impossible, for a recipient—or rather, "percipient"—to perceive.[3]

Figure 15.1 is a model of the basic mechanisms of the communication process. Note especially the feedback loop. In intraorganizational communication, where interdependencies among individuals and units are significant, the feedback loop is very important in ensuring that enough information is exchanged to manage effectively these interdependencies. Similarly, interorganizational communication, such as marketing or lobbying, is greatly improved if receivers provide

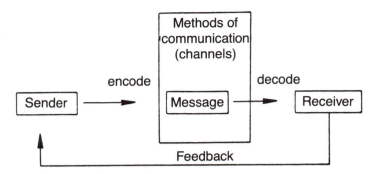

Figure 15.1. Communication process model.

feedback to senders, who can then adjust the message if it is not received as intended. When a sender encodes and transmits a message to a receiver, who decodes the message and indicates understanding by giving feedback, effective two-way communication occurs.

In this model of the communication process, the *sender* is a person or group with ideas, intentions, information, and a purpose for communicating. Senders can be individuals, departments or units of the HSO, or the HSO itself. The sender uses words and symbols to *encode* ideas and information. Words may have different meanings for different people, so care must be taken to communicate in words that are easily understood. These words must be augmented with other symbols if communication is to be effective.

In HSOs, many kinds of symbols have a role in communication. Symbols may be physical things, pictures, or actions. For example, different uniforms permit quick identification of people in the organization. Nurses wear white uniforms, nurse aides may wear yellow, and physicians wear long white coats. These physical symbols communicate identifying information. Pictures or visual representations are another type of symbol. They can be quite efficient and helpful in communicating, and they increase understanding in many situations. Consider how many words would be needed to explain an HSO's organization structure in lieu of an organization chart. Or, imagine the difficulty of communicating all of the information in a computed tomography scan using only words. Finally, action is a symbol that communicates. A smile or a pat on the back has meaning. A promotion or pay increase conveys a great deal to the recipient and to others. Furthermore, lack of action can have symbolic meaning. Davis and Newstrom note:

> Failure to act is an important way of communicating. A manager who fails to praise an employee for a job well done or fails to provide promised resources is sending a message to that person. Since we send messages both by action and inaction, we communicate almost all the time at work, regardless of our intentions.[4]

Actions or inactions that are inconsistent with words transmit contradictory messages. The manager who tells an employee, "I have confidence in your ability, your performance is excellent, and I want to expand your duties by delegating more to you," acts inconsistently by flying into a rage because of a small technical error. The message receiver who says, "I am listening," to the sender and then looks at the clock impatiently or starts to walk away while the conversation is underway sends a mixed message.

The *message* that results from the encoding process can be verbal or nonverbal. Managers seek to serve various purposes with their messages, "such as to have others understand their ideas, to understand the ideas of others, to gain acceptance of themselves or their ideas, or to produce action."[5] Messages can be for intraorganizational audiences and/or for interorganizational audiences.

The *channels* or methods of communication are the means by which messages are transmitted. Channels include face-to-face or telephone conversations involving individual and/or groups of senders or receivers, facsimile messages, letters, memos, policy statements, operating room schedules, reports, electronic message boards, video teleconferences, newspapers, television and radio commercial spots, and newsletters for internal or external distribution. The selection of channels is an important part of the communication process. Effective communication often involves using multiple channels to transmit a message. For example, a major change in an HSO's personnel policy, such as changing the benefit package, might be announced in a letter from the vice president for human resources to all employees, graphically illustrated by posters in key locations, and then reinforced in group meetings where managers explain the policy and answer questions. A decision to lobby the legislature for more generous Medicaid reimbursement might result in messages transmitted through channels such as letters to legislators, direct contact between HSO managers and trustees and legislators, and newspaper advertisements stating the HSO's position. If other HSOs would benefit from the legislation, they might participate, perhaps through an association, to produce and distribute television commercials or use other channels to increase support for their position.

Messages transmitted over any channel must be *decoded* by the *receiver.* Decoding means interpreting the words and symbols in the message. Since decoding is done by the receivers of messages, it is affected by their prior experiences and frames of reference. Decoding involves the receiver's perceptual assessment of both the content of the message *and* the sender, and the context in which the message is transmitted. The fact that messages must be decoded (interpreted) by the receiver raises the possibility that the message the sender intends is not the message the receiver gets. The closer the decoded message is to the one intended by the sender, the more effective the communication.

The best way to determine if messages are received as intended is through *feedback.* "Without feedback, you have a one-way communication process. Feedback makes possible a two-way process, reversing the sender and receiver roles so that information can be shared, recycled, and fine-tuned to achieve an unambiguous mutual understanding."[6] Feedback can be direct or indirect. Direct feedback is the receiver's response to the sender regarding a specific message. Indirect feedback is more subtle and involves consequences that result from a particular message. Internally, indirect feedback on a policy to change the HSO's benefit package might include higher levels of employee satisfaction if the change is liked or increased turnover if the change is disliked. Externally, indirect feedback on attempts to change Medicaid reimbursement might include an increase in rates if the legislature agrees with the HSO, no action if they disagree, or even hostile action if they disagree with the message and/or the methods used to communicate it.

BARRIERS TO EFFECTIVE COMMUNICATION

To more fully reflect the realities of communication within HSOs and between HSOs and their external stakeholders, the model of the communication process shown in Figure 15.1 must be expanded to include certain barriers to effective communication. Figure 15.2 illustrates the presence of environmental and personal barriers. These barriers are ubiquitous and can block, filter, or distort the message as it is encoded and sent and when it is decoded and received.

Environmental Barriers

Environmental barriers are characteristics of the organization and its environmental context that block, filter, or distort communications. Two common examples are *competition for attention* and *time.* These barriers apply to intra- and interorganizational communication. Multiple and simultaneous demands on the sender may cause the message to be packaged inappropriately; such demands may also cause the message to be incorrectly decoded. In such situations, the receiver may hear the message without comprehending it because it is not getting complete attention—the

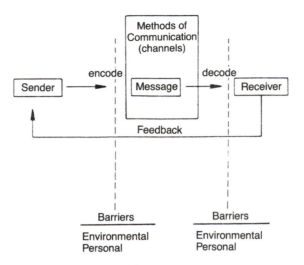

Figure 15.2. Expanded communication process model.

receiver is not really listening. Time may be a barrier to effective communication by giving the sender little opportunity to think through and structure the message to be conveyed, and by giving the receiver too little time to determine its meaning.

Other environmental barriers that can filter, distort, or block a message include the HSO's managerial philosophy, multiplicity of hierarchical levels, and power/status relationships between senders and receivers. *Managerial philosophy* can directly inhibit, as well as promote, effective communication. As a rule, managers who are not interested in promoting intraorganizational communication upward or disseminating information downward will establish procedural and organizational blockages. Requirements that all communication "flow through channels," inaccessibility, lack of interest in employees' frustrations, complaints, or feelings, and insufficient time allotted to receiving information are symptoms of a philosophy that retards communication flow. Furthermore, managers who fail to act on complaints, ideas, and problems signal to those wishing to communicate upward that the effort is unlikely to have much effect and will discourage information flow.

Managerial philosophy also has a significant impact on interorganizational communications with external stakeholders. Differences in philosophy could lead managers of two HSOs to react differently in communicating with external stakeholders in a crisis. For example, knowledge that patients might have been exposed to a dangerous infection while hospitalized in their institutions could lead some managers to cover up the incident, whereas other managers would make wide use of the public media hoping that everyone who might have been exposed would come forth to be tested. Varying reactions to similar events reflect different managerial philosophies about communicating. This topic is addressed at greater length below.

Multiple levels in an organization hierarchy, and especially among organizations in a multi-organizational arrangement, tend to cause message distortion. As the message is transmitted up or down through people at many levels, it is likely that each will interpret the message according to a personal frame of reference and vantage point. When multiple links exist in the communication chain, information can be filtered, dropped, or added, and emphasis can be rearranged as it is retransmitted. As a result, a message sent through many levels is likely to be distorted or even totally blocked. For example, very often a message sent from the CEO to employees through several layers of the organization is received in quite a different form than that originally sent. Or, a report prepared for the CEO that passes through the hierarchy may not reach its destination because it is lying on a desk and is, in essence, blocked.

Power/status relationships can also distort or inhibit transmission of a message. A discordant superior–subordinate relationship can dampen the flow and content of information. Furthermore, an employee's past experiences may inhibit communicating because of fear of reprisal, negative sanctions, or ridicule. For example, it is not unusual to find that the result of poor superior-subordinate rapport is that the subordinate does not inform the superior that something is wrong or that a plan will not work. Power/status communication barriers are prevalent in HSOs where many professionals interact and status relationships create a complex situation. How often does the head nurse with 20 years of experience tell a new medical resident that a procedure or treatment thought to be appropriate and about to be ordered is not efficacious? How is the nurse's message encoded—bluntly or obliquely? Status and role conflicts, particularly among professionals, can be a major barrier to effective communication.

A final environmental barrier that may cause a breakdown in communication occurs when messages require the use of *specific terminology* unfamiliar to the receiver or when messages are especially *complex*. Each profession has its own jargon. HSO managers may use terminology that is very different from those responsible for direct care. Both may use terminology unfamiliar to external stakeholders. Communications between people who use different terminology can be ineffective simply because people attribute different meanings to the same words. When a message is both complex and contains terminology unfamiliar to the receiver, it is especially likely that misunderstanding will occur.

Personal Barriers

Another set of potential barriers—personal barriers—exists when people communicate. These barriers arise from the nature of people, especially in their interaction with others. When people encode and send messages or decode and receive them, they tend to do so according to their frames of reference or beliefs. They may also consciously or unconsciously engage in selective perception. Their communications may also be influenced by emotions such as fear or jealousy.

The sum of socioeconomic background and previous experiences that represent an individual's *frame of reference* shapes how messages are encoded and decoded, or even whether communication is attempted. For example, someone whose cultural background is "don't speak unless spoken to" or "never question elders" may be inhibited in communicating. Naive people accept all communication at face value without filtering out erroneous information or bragging. By contrast, aggressiveness in disseminating self-edifying information can result in transmitting a message that is distorted for personal gain. Furthermore, unless one has had the same experiences as others, it is difficult to completely understand their messages. The wealthy may have difficulty understanding the concerns of people without health insurance. Those who have never experienced pain or childbirth or witnessed death may be unable to fully understand messages about these experiences.

Closely related to one's frame of reference are *beliefs, values,* and *prejudices.* They can cause messages to be distorted or blocked in either transmission or reception. This occurs because people and their personalities and backgrounds differ; they have preconceived opinions and prejudices in areas such as politics, ethics, religion, union versus management, sex, race, and lifestyle. These biases, beliefs, and values filter and distort communication.

Selective perception is one of the most difficult personal barriers to overcome, for both the sender and the receiver. People tend to screen derogatory information and amplify words, actions, and meanings that flatter them—there is a tendency to filter out the "bad" of a message and retain the "good." Selective perception can be conscious or unconscious. When it is conscious, often because one fears the consequences of the truth, intentional distortion results. For example, supervisors whose units have high turnover may fear the consequences of this fact if their superiors notice it. They might amplify the argument that turnover is due to low wages over which they have no control (or responsibility), or delete, alter, or minimize the importance of this information in reports to their superiors.

Sometimes *jealousy,* especially when coupled with selective perception, may result in conscious efforts to filter and distort incoming information, transmit misinformation, or both. For example, the manager with an extremely able assistant who routinely makes that manager look good may tend to block or distort information that would reveal the truth of the situation to superiors. Sometimes as simple a thing as petty personality differences, the feeling of professional incompetence or inferiority, or raw greed can lead to jealousy, resulting in communication distortion.

Two other potential personal barriers to communication arise because people receiving messages have a tendency to evaluate the source (the sender) and because people often prefer the status quo. Both of these personal barriers to effective communication are common in HSOs. Receivers often *evaluate the source* to decide whether to filter out or discount some of the message. However, this can lead to bias on the parts of communicators. For example, a hostile union-management atmosphere may cause employees to ignore messages from management, or managers may ignore messages from physicians with whom they frequently disagree. Source evaluation may be necessary to cope with the barrage of communication received by people in HSOs, but one must recognize the hazard that legitimate messages will be misunderstood.

The *status quo* barrier results from a conscious effort by the sender or receiver to filter out information either in sending, receiving, or retransmitting that would upset the present situation. Internally, conditions that promote fear of sending bad news or a lack of candor among participants can lead to the erection of this barrier. This barrier to effective communication may also exist when communicators in an HSO do not want to upset the status quo with important external stakeholders and react by transmitting messages that are explicitly designed to protect the status quo.

A final personal barrier to effective communication is a *lack of empathy* on the part of communicators. Having empathy means being sensitive to the frames of reference or emotional states of other people in the communication relationship. Such sensitivity promotes understanding. Empathy helps the sender decide how to encode a message for maximum understanding and helps the receiver interpret its meaning. For example, subordinates who empathize with their superiors may discount an angry message because they are aware that extreme pressure and frustration can cause such messages to be sent even when they are not warranted.

Similarly, a sender who is sensitive to the receiver's circumstance may decide how best to encode a message or that it is better left unsent. For example, if the receiver is having a bad day, a reprimand may be interpreted as stronger than it is. Or, if a receiver has just emerged from a traumatic experience such as family illness or financial setback, the empathetic sender might decide to delay bad news until later, if possible. Managers who are concerned about an HSO's community image might delay announcing a generous across-the-board wage increase or a large price increase just after a major local employer announces a plant closing because of a bad economy.

Managing Barriers to Effective Communication

Awareness that environmental and personal barriers to effective communication exist is the first step in minimizing their impact, but positive actions are needed to overcome them. Although the specific steps necessary to overcome the barriers depend on circumstances, several general guidelines can be suggested.

Environmental barriers are reduced if receivers and senders ensure that attention is given to their messages and that adequate time is devoted to listening to what is being communicated. In addition, a management philosophy that encourages open and free flow of communications is constructive. Reducing the number of links (levels in the hierarchy or steps between the HSO as a sender and external stakeholders as receivers) through which messages pass reduces opportunities for distortion. The power/status barrier is more difficult to eliminate because it is affected by interpersonal and interprofessional relationships. However, consciously tailoring words and symbols so messages are understandable and reinforcing words with actions significantly improves communications among different power/status levels. Finally, using multiple channels to reinforce complex messages decreases the likelihood of misunderstanding.

Personal barriers to effective communication are reduced by conscious efforts of sender and receiver to understand each other's frame of reference and beliefs. Recognizing that people engage in selective perception and are prone to jealousy and fear is a first step toward eliminating or at least diminishing these barriers. Empathy with those to whom messages are directed may be the surest way to increase the likelihood that the messages will be received and understood as intended.

FLOW OF INTRAORGANIZATIONAL COMMUNICATION

Intraorganizational communication in HSOs flows downward, upward, horizontally, and diagonally. Each direction has uses and characteristics. Typically, downward flow is communication between superiors and subordinates; upward communication uses the same channels but in the opposite direction. Horizontal flow is that from manager to manager or from worker to worker. Diagonal flow cuts across functions and levels; this violates the chain of command, but is permitted if speed and efficiency of communication are particularly important.

Downward Flow

The objectives of downward communication flow are to:

1. Give specific task directives about job instructions.
2. Give information about organizational procedures and practices.
3. Provide information about the rationale of the job.
4. Tell subordinates about their performance.
5. Provide ideological information to facilitate the indoctrination of goals.[7]

Downward communication flows through many channels. It commonly consists of information, verbal orders, or instructions given from manager to subordinate on a one-to-one basis. Other channels include speeches to groups of employees or meetings. The myriad written methods, such as handbooks, procedure manuals, newsletters, bulletin boards, and the ubiquitous memorandum, are also channels of downward communication. Computerized information systems contribute greatly to downward flow in many HSOs.

Upward Flow

Objectives of upward communication include providing managers with decision-making information, revealing problem areas, providing data for performance evaluation, indicating the status of morale, and generally underscoring the thinking of subordinates. Upward flow becomes more important with increased organizational complexity and scale. Managers rely on effective upward communication, and they encourage it by creating a climate of trust and respect as integral parts of the organizational culture.[8]

In addition to being directly useful to managers, upward communication flow helps employees satisfy personal needs. It permits those in positions of lesser authority to express opinions and perceptions to those with higher authority; as a result they feel a greater sense of participation. The hierarchical structure (chain of command) is the main channel for upward communication in HSOs. However, Luthans suggests the following supplementation:

1. *The grievance procedure.* Provided for in most collective bargaining agreements [and voluntarily provided in many HSOs], the grievance procedure allows an employee to make an appeal upward beyond [the] immediate superior. It protects the individual from arbitrary action from [a] direct superior and encourages upward communication.

2. *The open-door policy.* Taken literally, this means that the superior's door is always open to subordinates. It is a continuous invitation for a subordinate to come in and talk about anything that is troubling [the subordinate]. Unfortunately, in practice the open-door policy is more fiction than fact. The boss may slap [the] subordinate on the back and say, "My door is always open to you," but in many cases both know the door is really closed. It is a case in which the adage that actions speak louder than words applies.

3. *Counseling, attitude questionnaires, and exit interviews.* The [human resources] department can greatly facilitate upward communication by conducting nondirective, confidential counseling sessions, periodically administering attitude questionnaires, and holding meaningful exit interviews for those who leave the organization. Much valuable information can be gained from these forms of upward communication.

4. *Participative techniques.* Participative-decision techniques can generate a great deal of upward communication. This may be accomplished by either informal involvement from subordinates or by formal participation programs.

5. *The ombudsman.* A largely untried but potentially significant technique to enable management to obtain upward communication is the use of an ombudsman. The concept has been used primarily in Scandinavia to provide an outlet for persons who have been treated unfairly or in a depersonalized manner by large, bureaucratic government. It has more recently gained popularity in American state governments, military posts, and universities. [HSOs have applied this approach to improve communication between *patients* and the organization. If properly applied, it may very well work in the larger, more complex, and more depersonalized HSOs as they seek ways to improve upward communication flows from their employees.][9]

Horizontal and Diagonal Flows

Unhindered downward and upward communication are insufficient for effective organizational performance. In complex HSOs, especially those subject to abrupt demands for action and reaction, horizontal flow must also occur. This is especially true when care is rendered to a patient by a variety of staff from several departments. Their work must be coordinated in order to meet patient needs, even in a setting that often limits upward and downward communication. The concept of an acute care hospital as a matrix organization, as described in Chapter 6, "Concepts of Organization Design," illustrates the value of horizontal communication and coordination in HSOs. The popularity of horizontal communication is increased by the simple fact that people in organizations enjoy it. It provides a direct connection to parts of the organization with which they do not communicate through downward and upward flows.

The prevalence of committees in HSOs can be attributed to a need for horizontal communication. Committees and quality circles (see Chapter 10) are a way for representatives of different organizational units at similar levels to discuss common concerns and potential problems face to face and to coordinate activities. Committees are useful boundary-spanning devices. However, as every past and present committee member knows, there are some disadvantages to this form of horizontal communication. Committees tend to be time consuming and expensive, and their decisions are often compromises that may be ineffectual solutions to problems. Despite their disadvantages, committees are the main formal mechanism for horizontal communication in HSOs.

The least used channel of communication in HSOs is diagonal flow. Even so, diagonal flows are common. For example, diagonal communication occurs when the director of a hospital pharmacy alerts a nurse in medical intensive care about a potential adverse reaction between two medications ordered for a patient. Diagonal flows violate the usual pattern of upward and downward communication flows by cutting across departments, and they violate the usual pattern of horizontal communication because the communicators are at different levels in the organization. Yet, such communication is important in HSOs.

Communication Networks

Downward, upward, horizontal, and diagonal communication can be combined into patterns called *communication networks*. A communication network is "a system of decision centers interconnected by communication channels."[10] Figure 15.3 illustrates the five common networks: chain, Y, wheel, circle, and all-channel. The *chain network* is the standard format for communicating upward and downward and follows line authority relationships. An example is a staff nurse who reports to a head nurse, who reports to a nursing supervisor, who reports to the vice president for nursing, who reports to the HSO's president.

The *Y pattern* (turned upside down) shows two people reporting to a superior who reports to two others. An example is two staff pharmacists who report to the pharmacy director, who reports to the vice president for professional affairs, who reports to the president. The *wheel pattern* shows a situation in which four subordinates report to one superior. There is no interaction among subordinates, and all communications are channeled through the manager at the center of the wheel. This pattern is rare in HSOs, although elements of it can be found in the situation in which four vice presidents report to a president if the vice presidents have little interaction among themselves. Even though this network pattern is not used routinely, it may be used in circumstances in which urgency or secrecy is required. For example, the president with an emergency might communicate with vice presidents in a wheel pattern because time does not permit using other modes. Similarly, if secrecy is important, such as during an investigation of possible embezzlement, the president may require that all relevant communication with the vice presidents be kept confidential for a period of time.

The *circle pattern* allows communicators in the network to communicate directly only with two others, but since each communicates with another communicator in the network, the effect is that everyone communicates with everyone and there is no central authority or leader. The *all-channel network* is a circle pattern except that each communicator may interact with every other communicator in the network.

Communication networks vary along several dimensions, and none is best in all situations. The wheel and all-channel networks tend to be fast and accurate compared with the chain or Y-pattern networks, but the chain or Y-patterns promote clear-cut lines of authority and responsibility. The circle and all-channel networks enhance morale among those in the networks better than other patterns because everyone is equal in the communication activity, but these patterns result in relatively slow communication. This is a serious problem if an immediate decision is needed or an action must be taken quickly. Managers must choose networks to fit the various communication situations they face.

Informal Communication

Coexisting with formal communication flows and networks in HSOs are *informal* communication flows, which have their own networks. Informal flows and networks result from the interpersonal relationships of organization members. The common name for informal communication is "grapevine," a term that arose during the Civil War, when telegraph lines were strung between trees much like a grapevine.[11] Messages transmitted over those flimsy lines were often garbled. As a result, any rumor was said to come from the grapevine.

By definition, the grapevine, or informal flow of communication, consists of channels that result from the interpersonal relationships of organization participants. Informal communication flows in an organization are as natural as the patterns of social interaction that develop in all organizations. Like the informal organization (see Chapter 6), informal communication flows coexist with the formal patterns established by management. Grapevines are facts of organization life. Their impact is less clear cut. "The grapevine accomplishes so much positively and so much

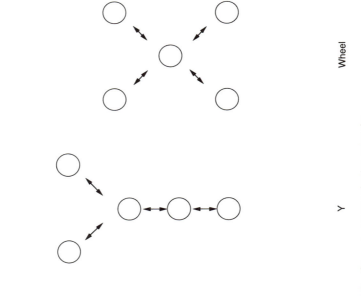

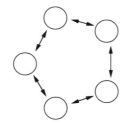

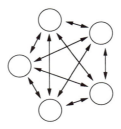

Chain Y Wheel Circle All-Channel

Figure 15.3. Common communication networks.

negatively that it is difficult to determine whether its net effects are positive or negative. Undoubtedly its effects vary among work groups and organizations."[12]

There is no doubt that informal communication channels can be and routinely are misused in HSOs, especially in transmitting rumors. For example, a male registered nurse who realizes he is being passed over for promotion in favor of a more qualified female might start a rumor that the vice president for nursing dislikes male nurses and that she has said she "would not have one as a supervisor." Although untrue, this rumor could cause others to think that the vice president discriminates against male nurses.

Yet, properly managed informal communication flows can be useful. Downward flows move through the grapevine much faster than through formal channels. In an HSO much of the coordination among units occurs through informal give-and-take in informal horizontal and diagonal flows. In the case of upward flow, informal communication can be a rich source of information about performance, ideas, feelings, and attitudes. Because of their potential usefulness and pervasiveness, managers should try to understand informal communication flows and use them to advantage.

Similarly to formal communication flows, informal flows follow certain predictable patterns and form identifiable networks. Figure 15.4 illustrates four common patterns that the grapevine can take. The *single strand* pattern is how many people think the grapevine works. Instead, it is more likely to be a *cluster* pattern.

> Managers occasionally get the impression that the grapevine operates like a long chain in which A tells B, who tells C, who then tells D, and so on, until 20 persons later, Y gets the information—very late and very incorrect. [See the single strand network in Figure 15.4.] Sometimes the grapevine may operate this way, but it generally follows a different pattern. [See the cluster network in Figure 15.4.] Employee A tells three or four others (such as C, D, and F). Only one or two of these receivers will then pass the information forward, and they usually will tell more than one person. Then as the information becomes older and the proportion of those knowing it gets larger, it gradually dies out because not all those who who receive it repeat it. This network is a *cluster chain*, because each link in the chain tends to inform a cluster of other people instead of only one person.[13]

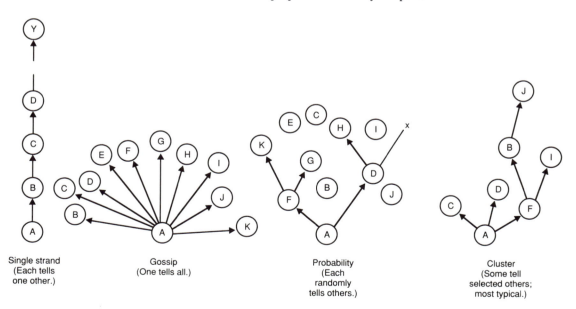

Single strand   Gossip   Probability   Cluster
(Each tells   (One tells all.)   (Each   (Some tell
one other.)   randomly   selected others;
                                                      tells others.)   most typical.)

Figure 15.4. Grapevine networks. (From Davis, Keith, and John W. Newstrom. *Human behavior at work: Organizational behavior*, 8th ed., 373. New York: McGraw-Hill Book Company, 1989. Reproduced with permission of McGraw-Hill, Inc.)

Informal communication flow is present in every HSO and can aid or inhibit effectiveness. Managers can use this flow to achieve organization objectives. This is done by paying attention to the informal communication flow (even inaccurate rumors reflect some aspects of employees' feelings and views) and by occasionally and selectively using the informal communication flow, especially when speed is critical.

Summary of Intraorganizational Communication

The multidirectional communication flows and the networks they form within HSOs each have a purpose, and each is an important tool for managers. To the extent these flows are planned and designed into the HSO, they are formal communication channels and networks. To the extent they are natural communication between and among people, they are informal communication channels and networks.

Understandable information, whether it flows through formal channels or "up and down hallways, in and out of offices, around water coolers, over transoms, and between friends and colleagues,"[14] is as crucial to the life of an HSO as the circulation of blood is to human life. Figure 15.5 summarizes the key uses of downward, upward, horizontal, and diagonal communication flows in HSOs.

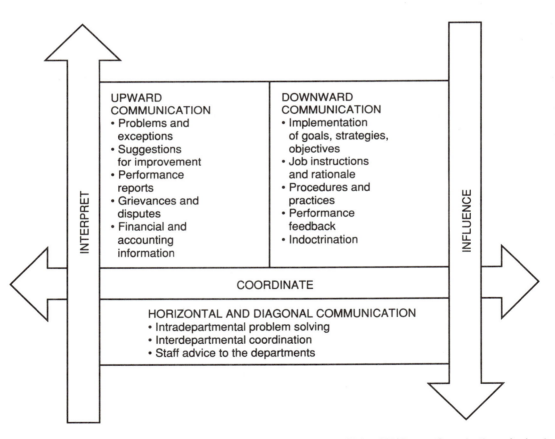

Figure 15.5. Communication flows in HSOs. (From Daft, Richard L., and Richard M. Steers. *Organizations: A micro/macro approach,* 538. Glenview, IL: Scott, Foresman and Company, 1986. Copyright © 1986 by Scott, Foresman and Company. Reprinted by permission of HarperCollins Publishers.)

FLOW OF INTERORGANIZATIONAL COMMUNICATION

HSOs typically maintain relationships with a large and diverse set of external stakeholders.[15] Table 15.2 is a partial list of the types of external stakeholders with which an HSO might interact and communicate. Most of these interorganizational relationships involve a degree of interdependence. An HSO whose mission and objectives affect or are affected by other organizations or stakeholders is interdependent with them.[16]

Managers cannot ignore interdependent others, nor can they be ignored by them. These relationships require active management involvement if the linkages are to be productive. In turn, productive linkages require effective communication. As Pfeffer and Salancik state:

> Linkages arise when communication is most necessary between interdependent others. Linkages also serve as channels for persuasion and negotiation, and in these ways also stabilize interdependent relationships. By exchanging information about each other's activities, the organizations are in a position to plan more predictably. By obtaining commitments from each other, each organization develops certainty about the future course of exchange.[17]

The sheer number and variety of external stakeholders complicates interorganizational communication for HSO managers. Another complication is the nature of relationships. Positive relations between an HSO and stakeholders make it easier to manage the relationship, and communication flows are more effective than when relations are negative. Figure 15.6 uses a large hospital as an example to illustrate the extraordinary diversity of interorganizational relationships that must be maintained by such institutions. The figure also suggests the difficulty of maintaining these relationships when many are negative or neutral at best (the " − " and "0" symbols, respectively, in Figure 15.6). It is important to note that the arrows connecting the hospital with stakeholders go in both directions. Managers in HSOs must be concerned about communication flows to external stakeholders *and* about flows from these stakeholders.

Conceptually, the interdependence between the hospital in Figure 15.6 and its stakeholders can be managed in one of two ways: The hospital can adapt to fit the requirements and expectations of interdependent others or it can alter the interdependent others so that they fit its capabilities and preferences. In practice both occur and both depend on effective communication. Unless what is expected from interdependent others is known and understood, effective adaptation is impossible. Conversely, changing interdependent others requires effective communication from the HSO to the stakeholder, although on occasion the HSO can enlist others in attempts to change

Table 15.2. Organizations and stakeholders with whom HSOs interact and communicate

Accrediting agencies	Insurance companies
Affiliated organizations	Joint venture partners
Alternative health systems	Media
Competitors	Medical staff–hospital joint ventures (MeSHs)
Confederated organizations	Multiorganizational arrangements
Consortia members	Other partners
Consumers	Owners
Consumer representatives (public and private)	Political groups
Employee representatives (unions)	Preferred provider organizations (PPOs)
Financial organizations (bond rating)	Suppliers (including capital, consumables, equipment, and human resources)
Fiscal intermediaries	Third party associations
Foundations	Third party associations
Government (all levels)	Trade associations
Health maintenance organizations (HMOs)	Utilization management companies
Independent practice associations (IPAs)	

Adapted from Beaufort B. Longest, Jr. Interorganizational linkages in the health sector. *Health Care Management Review*, 15 (Winter 1990): 17–28, with permission of Aspen Publishers, Inc., © 1990.

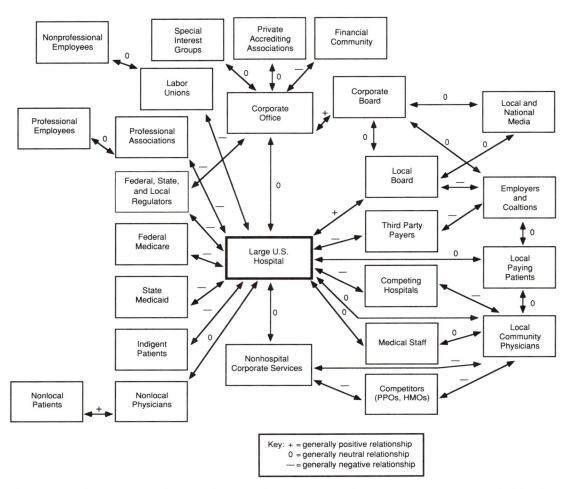

Figure 15.6. Stakeholders in a large hospital. (From Fottler, Myron D., John D. Blair, Carlton J. Whitehead, Michael D. Laus, and Grant T. Savage. Assessing key stakeholders: Who matters to hospitals and why? *Hospital & Health Services Administration* 34 [Winter 1989]: 530. © 1989, Foundation of the American College of Healthcare Executives.)

external stakeholders.* For example, it is likely that the hospital in Figure 15.6 belongs to a state hospital association and to the American Hospital Association. These associations represent many hospitals and lobby government to alter policies in favor of hospitals or to create more favorable environmental contexts for them. Lobbying is, at its heart, communication.

Boundary spanning is the process through which HSOs develop the means of communicating with external stakeholders. *Boundary spanners* are the people who carry out this process.[18] They obtain critical information from external stakeholders that can be used for decision making as the HSO adapts to their preferences and demands. The strategic planning and marketing departments or functions in HSOs are good examples of boundary spanning. Since information is the object of these boundary-spanning activities, communication is critical to their success. Boundary spanners also represent the HSO to external stakeholders. This activity takes many forms, including marketing, public relations, guest or patient relations, government relations, or

*Figure 15.6 was also presented in Chapter 8 (Figure 8.5) to denote the influence of stakeholders relative to strategic planning.

community relations. The common thread in these activities is information. If the HSO is to be effectively represented to its external stakeholders, good communication is necessary.

Boundary-spanning activities are not limited to a few departments or managers. Table 15.3 shows that many managers in HSOs are involved in spanning the boundaries between the organization and its external stakeholders, as well as being responsible for relations with internal stakeholders. In doing so, managers are playing several of the roles Mintzberg[19] identified for them, including figurehead, liaison, monitor, and disseminator (see Figure 1.4 in Chapter 1).

Special Case: Communicating Among Units of Systems

Like many other HSOs, the hospital in Figure 15.6 belongs to a system. The system has a corporate board and the hospital has a local board. This hospital faces the added challenge of communicating effectively with the other organizations in a multiunit system. As described in Chapter 9, "Interorganizational Relationships," systems of HSOs have become common through corporate restructuring (creating several entities to perform medical and nonmedical functions previously done by one corporation) and through active programs of merger and consolidation in the health care industry.

Effectively communicating among units in a system is a demanding management task.[20] Adapting Porter's[21] approach to achieving effective linkages among business units in a diversified corporation suggests ways to manage the task of communication in a system:

Horizontal structure—Using devices that cross unit lines, such as partial centralization and interunit task forces or committees, facilitates communication.

Horizontal systems—Using management systems tailored for the purpose and with a cross-unit dimension in areas such as planning, control, incentives, capital budgeting, and management information systems enhances communication.

Horizontal human resource practices—Using human resource practices that facilitate unit cooperation, such as cross-unit job rotation, management forums, and training, increases the likelihood that managers in one part of the system will understand their counterparts elsewhere in the system and that they will communicate more effectively.

Table 15.3. Hospital executives responsible for particular key stakeholders

Key stakeholders	Responsible managers
Medical staff	CEO, COO, associate administrator, medical staff director
Patients	Director of marketing, director of guest relations
Hospital department managers	COO, associate administrator, assistant administrator, product or service line manager
Professional staff	CEO, COO, associate administrator, human resources director
Board of trustees	CEO, COO, associate administrator
Federal government	Depends on issue
Corporate office	CEO, COO
Nonprofessional staff	Human resources director
Third-party payers	VP for finance, reimbursement manager
Elected public officials	CEO, director of government relations, director of public relations
Political pressure groups	CEO, director of government relations, director of public relations, director of community relations
Local business/industry	CEO
Accrediting/licensing agencies	VP for risk management, director of quality assurance, appropriate department head
Other hospitals	CEO, COO
Media	Director of public relations, director of marketing
Labor unions	Director of human resources

From Fottler, Myron D., John D. Blair, Carlton J. Whitehead, Michael D. Laus, and Grant T. Savage. Assessing key stakeholders: Who matters to hospitals and why? *Hospital & Health Services Administration* 34 (Winter 1989): 542. © 1989, Foundation of the American College of Healthcare Executives.

Horizontal conflict resolution processes—Using management processes that resolve conflicts among units enhances communication. Such processes are different from horizontal structure and systems and relate more to the style of managing a multiunit system. The key is that corporate management installs and operates a system that fairly settles inter-unit disputes. Equitable settlement of disputes facilitates effective communication.

Multiunit systems such as that shown in Figure 15.6 can enhance communication through interlocking boards, which are usually defined as boards with overlapping membership. Interlocking boards provide a stable structure of coordinated activity and communication flow.

Special Case: Communicating When Things Go Badly

Occasionally, things go very badly even in a well-managed HSO. An HSO may lose its accreditation by the Joint Commission on Accreditation of Healthcare Organizations or a state certification because of code violations; serious clinical errors occur, perhaps causing a patient's death; infections break out; or serious financial difficulties arise, perhaps threatening the HSO's existence or raising the specter of major layoffs or closure. As in other large, complex organizations, things can—and do—go wrong in HSOs. When they do, communication with internal and external stakeholders takes on intensified importance. How managers communicate in such circumstances is significant in resolving the problems and in the perception of the HSO held by its stakeholders after the problems are resolved.

For example, a hospital suddenly has a situation wherein a diabetic patient being treated for complications of that disease dies unexpectedly, and the results of blood tests on a sample taken 6 hours before his death show insulin levels 200 times too high. There are several possible explanations, but few are good. The possibilities include a fatal overdose of insulin given by accident or on purpose in a criminal act committed by any of several people. How should the hospital handle this situation? Whose interests are to be protected? What information is to be communicated? To whom? By whom?

There are few hard-and-fast rules to guide managers in communicating with stakeholders under circumstances such as these, although the ethical guidelines described in Chapter 3, "Ethical Considerations," are relevant. However, actions taken in response to a serious problem, and communications made about the actions, can be characterized along a continuum of reactive to proactive.[22] At one end of the continuum, reactive responses include concealing the problem—do and say nothing. Less extreme, but highly reactive, is to admit that a problem may exist (perhaps in response to a reporter alerted by someone), but deny any wrongdoing and take no action to find the cause of the problem or resolve it. Such an obstructionist position could be taken by the HSO regarding further communication about the problem.

A similar reaction is one best labeled defensive. The HSO's managers and spokespersons act and communicate about the problem in a way that complies with the letter of the law. These actions and communications are intended to minimize legal liability, and this is a common response. This partly reflects how expensive responsibility for serious problems involving human health and life can be. However, even when the issues are layoffs, mergers, closures, or problems that do not involve potential lawsuits, a defensive position is commonly taken in communicating with stakeholders who have a legitimate interest in the issue.

Figure 15.7 illustrates these reactive responses and two that are more proactive: accommodation and prevention. Accommodation involves accepting responsibility for the problem and taking aggressive actions to resolve it. In this type of response the actions and communications about them are proactive. Communications are characterized by openness and candor about the problem, its causes, and the actions being taken to resolve it. Prevention is further along the continuum and focuses on taking aggressive and concerted actions to prevent problems from occurring.

Reactive   Proactive

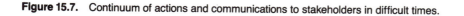

| Concealment (Hide the existence of the problem; no communication.) | Obstruction (Resist communication; disavow any wrongdoing.) | Defense Position (Comply with letter of the law; communicate only favorable, factual information.) | Accommodation (Accept responsibility for the problem; take aggressive actions to resolve it; communicate openly and candidly about the problem and its resolution.) | Prevention (Take aggressive actions to prevent problems from occurring; communicate openly about potential problems and steps to prevent them.) |

Figure 15.7.   Continuum of actions and communications to stakeholders in difficult times.

Continuous quality improvement (see Chapter 11) is an important approach in prevention, as are risk management and quality assessment and improvement programs (see Chapter 12). Communications are characterized by openness and candor, as in accommodation, but they focus on the existence and probabilities of potential problems and the steps that have been taken to prevent them.

HSOs are far better served in managing difficult situations by actions and communications that are proactive rather than reactive. Reactive responses (concealment, obstruction, and, to a large extent, defense positions) imply crisis management and invite the scrutiny of stakeholders. Technically, managers who choose accommodation are reacting to a problem, too, but their response is positive and proactive in that they take responsibility, aggressively seek to resolve the problem, and communicate openly and candidly about the problem and their actions regarding it. Prevention involves aggressive action to avoid problems. Here, managers communicate to stakeholders that problems might occur, but that actions have been taken to prevent them and minimize their impact. No level of effort will prevent all problems from occurring in HSOs, but many can be prevented by careful actions, and their consequences can be managed far more effectively if managers have laid a foundation of understanding and trust with stakeholders by communicating about potential problems and their actions to prevent them or prepare for them.

SUMMARY

Communication is defined as *the creation or exchange of understanding between sender(s) and receiver(s).* Communication is not restricted to words; it includes all methods (verbal and nonverbal) through which meaning is conveyed. The communication process is described in Figure 15.2. Particular attention is given to means of overcoming environmental and personal barriers to effective communication.

Managers in HSOs must be concerned with two basic types of communications: those internal to the HSO and those that are external, such as with other organizations or stakeholders outside the HSO. Communication within HSOs is called intraorganizational communication. Intraorganizational communication in complex HSOs depends on formal channels and networks to transmit information and understanding in all directions and on widespread acknowledgment of the existence and effective use of these channels. The channels carry communications multidirectionally—downward, upward, horizontally, and diagonally—and have characteristics that make them useful for the purposes illustrated in Figure 15.5. Coexisting with formal intraorganizational communication flows is an informal flow that consists of channels and networks (the grapevine) that arise from the interpersonal relationships of HSO staff.

Increasingly, senior managers in HSOs are concerned with communications between their organizations and other organizations and external stakeholders. HSOs are interdependent with external stakeholders, and relationships with them must be carefully managed. Effective formal and informal communication that flows to *and* from these stakeholders are important to successfully managing these relationships. Examples include marketing the HSO's services, monitoring regulatory changes in government agencies, or lobbying for more favorable reimbursement rates for services provided by the HSO. Communication between HSOs and other organizations and stakeholders is called interorganizational communication. Both intra- and interorganizational communications are defined as the creation or exchange of understanding between sender(s) and receiver(s).

DISCUSSION QUESTIONS

1. Draw a model of the communication process. Describe the interrelationships of the parts of the model.
2. Discuss the importance of feedback in communicating.
3. Discuss the various types of communication networks and describe the advantages and disadvantages of each.
4. Discuss the purpose of the downward communication flow in an HSO.
5. Discuss the purpose of the upward communication flow in an HSO.
6. Discuss the role of committees in relation to communication in an HSO.
7. What are barriers to communication? How can they be overcome?
8. Discuss the role of symbols in communication.
9. Think of a situation in which an HSO receives bad press. How might the HSO respond along the reactive-proactive continuum? How should it respond?
10. What are the basic differences between formal and informal communication channels?

CASE STUDY 1: ABC NURSING HOME

As CEO of the ABC Nursing Home, you have been confronted by some behavior and leadership problems with your new director of nursing service. He has been on the job approximately 3 months, and you have had several meetings with him. You have now decided to put some of your thoughts in writing. Following is a letter that you have written to him:

Dear Mr. Jones:

You mentioned to me that you have had a difficult time getting your employees to work as a team. You also mentioned that you feel frustrated because I haven't acted on your suggestions and backed you up. The purpose of this letter is to strongly suggest that you look to yourself as a source of these problems, rather than elsewhere. It is important that you avoid complaining about things that aren't being done for you, and start doing things on your own. Don't always look to others as the source of your problems. Working with people is a difficult challenge, and the upper management must indicate its strength so that a system of sound leadership will permeate the entire organization. You have to stand or fall on your own. You cannot expect the CEO to settle all the problems that arise. You have to develop confidence in yourself and learn to work with your peers and the personnel within your department. If your problems persist, it will be necessary to replace you.

Questions

1. What might Jones do after receiving this letter?
2. How will he feel about this letter and how will he interpret it? What was communicated?
3. Do you think the CEO will be surprised at the effect this letter has on Jones?
4. What other way could the CEO have communicated with Jones?

CASE STUDY 2: THE BUSINESS OFFICE[23]

At 4:45 P.M. on Friday, Mary Hite, an employee in the business office, walked into the office of Henry Staffs, business office manager, and asked to see him privately. Hite told Staffs that she had been elected by the other employees of the business office to speak on their behalf about practices that they wished modified or eliminated. One practice concerned employee evaluations, which they thought were unfair, poorly executed, and used as an excuse for not paying higher salaries. A second practice not accepted well was the arbitrary way management determined employee vacation time. Hite said that one employee was given 2 days' notice before he received his first week of vacation and 5 days' notice before his second week. Staffs listened attentively and told Hite that since it was so late in the day, he would consider these requests the first part of next week. During the following week, Hite noticed that Staffs was out of town and that no action was taken concerning her remarks. However, her fellow employees tended to treat her like a heroine for representing them before Staffs.

When she picked up her check the next Friday afternoon, Hite was shocked to find a discharge notice and 2 weeks' severance pay in the envelope.

Questions

1. What should Staffs have done when Hite came to see him?
2. What messages did Staffs communicate to Hite and the other employees?
3. What will be the outcome of the action he took?
4. Is there any way that Staffs can improve communication in the business office?

CASE STUDY 3:   GOOD WORK IS EXPECTED[24]

A 600-bed general acute hospital, located in a large city in the eastern United States, brought in an outside management consulting firm to analyze its operations. After 5 weeks, the consultants reported to management. One area they investigated was communication between superiors and subordinates. To its dismay, management learned that there were numerous discrepancies between what superiors said and did and what their subordinates said their superiors did. For example, when the consultants conducted a confidential questionnaire survey with 20% of managers and workers, they received the following responses to the question, "Do you tell your subordinates when they do a good job?"

	Top management says of itself	Middle management says of top management	Middle management says of itself	Lower level management says of middle management	Lower level management says of itself	Workers say of lower level management
Always	93%	82%	95%	63%	98%	39%
Often	7	14	5	15	2	23
Sometimes		4		12		18
Seldom				6		11
Never				4		9

Management was quite upset by the findings. As a result, at the next meeting of the governing body, the president proposed that the hospital bring back the consultants to advise them how to deal with this problem. The proposal was accepted unanimously.

When middle and lower level managers learned of this action, they expressed surprise. One noted, "Just because the data indicate poor communication, there is no need to get excited. After all, workers say lots of things that aren't accurate." A fellow colleague explained, "Look, I expect subordinates to do a good job. I only tell them when they are doing a poor one. If I praised them every time they did something right, they'd all have swelled heads. My approach is to say nothing."

Questions

1. What do the responses to the question, "Do you tell your subordinates when they do a good job?" indicate?

2. What do you think of the comments from the two managers? Are they valid?

3. What types of recommendations would you expect from the consultants? Explain.

CASE STUDY 4: THE GROUP HEALTH COOPERATIVE OF PUGET SOUND'S HARD ROCK SELL[25]

The Puget Sound Cooperative in Seattle, Washington, one of the oldest and most respected HMOs, wanted to increase enrollment of young, low-risk subscribers. It was only logical when the newly recruited marketing staff chose the local hard rock music station as their medium and shaped the message accordingly.

"Hey, are you TIRED OF SICK CARE? How about joining THE HEALTH CARE plan?" rasped the announcer.

Within hours after the spot was first aired, an eruption equivalent to that of Mount St. Helen's began in the Seattle medical community. The local medical society was enraged by the implication that doctors not in the HMO made people sick. The cooperative's medical staff was enraged by the degradation of having their services offered on a hard rock station (one wonders why so many of them were listening to it). There was concern that the spots would upset the cooperative's efforts to recruit private physicians in outlying communities into a partnership with it and thus seriously hamper efforts to open these new markets. The spot never surfaced again.

Questions

1. Who were Group Health's stakeholders in this situation?

2. What message was being transmitted to these stakeholders?

3. How should senior management try to communicate with young, low-risk potential subscribers?

NOTES

1. Schulz, Rockwell, and Alton C. Johnson. *Management of hospitals and health services: Strategic issues and performance*, 3d ed., 66. St. Louis: The C.V. Mosby Company, 1990.

2. Scott, William G., and Terence R. Mitchell. *Organization theory: A structural behavioral analysis*, 3. Homewood, IL: Irwin, 1979.

3. Drucker, Peter F. *Management: Tasks, responsibilities, practices*, 483. New York: Harper & Row, 1974.

4. Davis, Keith, and John W. Newstrom. *Human behavior at work: Organizational behavior*, 8th ed., 89. New York: McGraw-Hill Book Company, 1989.

5. Gibson, James L., John M. Ivancevich, and James H. Donnelly, Jr. *Organizations: Behavior, structure, processes*, 7th ed., 540. Homewood, IL: Richard D. Irwin, Inc., 1991.

6. Holt, David H. *Management: Principles and practices*, 2d ed., 483. Englewood Cliffs, NJ: Prentice Hall, 1990.

7. Katz, Daniel, and Robert L. Kahn. *The social psychology of organizations*, 239. New York: John Wiley & Sons, Inc., 1966.

8. Robbins, Stephen P. *Management*, 3d ed. Englewood Cliffs, NJ: Prentice Hall, 1991.

9. Luthans, Fred. *Organizational behavior: A modern behavioral approach to management*, 253. New York: McGraw-Hill Book Co., 1973; used by permission.

10. Scott, William G. *Organization theory*, 165. Homewood, IL: Richard D. Irwin, Inc., 1967.

11. Davis and Newstrom, *Human behavior*, 370.

12. Davis and Newstrom, *Human behavior*, 376.

13. Davis and Newstrom, *Human behavior*, 373–374.

14. Holt, *Management*, 487.

15. Longest, Beaufort B., Jr. Interorganizational linkages in the health sector. *Health Care Management Review* 15 (Winter 1990): 17–28.

16. Freeman, R. Edward. *Strategic management: A stakeholder approach*. New York: Ballinger, 1984.

17. Pfeffer, Jeffrey, and Gerald R. Salancik. *The external control of organizations: A resource dependence perspective*, 146–147. New York: Harper & Row Publishers, Inc., 1978.

18. Aldag, Ramon J., and Timothy M. Stearns. *Management*, 2d ed. Cincinnati, OH: South-Western Publishing Co., 1991.

19. Mintzberg, Henry. *Mintzberg on management: Inside our strange world of organizations*, 6. New York: The Free Press, 1989.

20. Longest, Beaufort B., Jr., and James M. Klingensmith. Coordination and communication. In *Health care management: A text in organization theory and behavior*, edited by Stephen M. Shortell and Arnold D. Kaluzny, 2d ed., 234–264. New York: John Wiley & Sons, 1988.

21. Porter, Michael E. *Competitive advantage: Creating and sustaining superior performance*. New York: The Free Press, 1985.

22. Carroll, Archie B. A three-dimensional conceptual model of corporate performance. *Academy of Management Review* 4 (1979): 497–505; Holt, *Management*, 69–71.

23. From Longest, Beaufort B., Jr. *Business management of health care providers*, Sect. IV, 32–33. Chicago: Hospital Financial Management Association, 1975.

24. Adapted from Hodgetts, Richard M. *Management:*

Theory, process and practice, 258–259. Philadelphia: W.B. Saunders Co., 1979.

25. From Smith, David Barton, and Arnold D. Kaluzny.

The white labyrinth: A guide to the health care system, 2d ed., 115. Ann Arbor, MI: Health Administration Press, 1986.

BIBLIOGRAPHY

Aldag, Ramon J., and Timothy M. Stearns. *Management*, 2d ed. Cincinnati, OH: South-Western Publishing Co., 1991.

Davis, Keith, and John W. Newstrom. *Human behavior at work: Organizational behavior*, 8th ed. New York: McGraw-Hill Book Company, 1989.

Drucker, Peter F. *Management: Tasks, responsibilities, practices*. New York: Harper & Row, 1974.

Freeman, R. Edward. *Strategic management: A stakeholder approach*. New York: Ballinger, 1984.

Gibson, James L., John M. Ivancevich, and James H. Donnelly, Jr. *Organizations: Behavior, structure, processes*, 7th ed. Homewood, IL: Richard D. Irwin, Inc., 1991.

Holt, David H. *Management: Principles and practices*, 2d ed. Englewood Cliffs, NJ: Prentice Hall, 1990.

Katz, Daniel, and Robert L. Kahn. *The social psychology of organizations*. New York: John Wiley & Sons, Inc., 1966.

Longest, Beaufort B., Jr. Interorganizational linkages in the health sector. *Health Care Management Review* 15 (Winter 1990): 17–28.

Longest, Beaufort B., Jr., and James M. Klingensmith. Coordination and communication. In *Health care management: A text in organization theory and behavior*, edited by Stephen M. Shortell and Arnold D. Kaluzny, 2d ed. New York: John Wiley & Sons, 1988.

Luthans, Fred. *Organizational behavior: A modern behavioral approach to management*. New York: McGraw-Hill Book Co., 1973.

Mintzberg, Henry. *Mintzberg on management: Inside our strange world of organizations*. New York: The Free Press, 1989.

Pfeffer, Jeffrey, and Gerald R. Salancik. *The external control of organizations: A resource dependence perspective*. New York: Harper & Row Publishers, Inc., 1978.

Porter, Michael E. *Competitive advantage: Creating and sustaining superior performance*. New York: The Free Press, 1985.

Robbins, Stephen P. *Management*, 3d ed. Englewood Cliffs, NJ: Prentice Hall, 1991.

Schulz, Rockwell, and Alton C. Johnson. *Management of hospitals and health services: Strategic issues and performance*, 3d ed. St. Louis: The C.V. Mosby Company, 1990.

Scott, William G. *Organization theory*. Homewood, IL: Richard D. Irwin, Inc., 1967.

Scott, William G., and Terence R. Mitchell. *Organization theory: A structural behavioral analysis*. Homewood, IL: Irwin, 1979.

Smith, David Barton, and Arnold D. Kaluzny. *The white labyrinth: A guide to the health care system*, 2d ed. Ann Arbor, MI: Health Administration Press, 1986.

It is all around people—in the seasons, in their social environment, and in their own biological processes. Beginning with the first few moments of life, a person learns to meet change by being adaptive.

Davis and Newstrom[1]

As the opening quotation suggests, change is a fact of human life. It is also a fact of organizational life in health services organizations (HSOs). A brief review of Figure 1.6 in Chapter 1, which is a comprehensive model of management for HSOs, reveals the responsibilities of managers. As shown in this model and as indicated in the earlier discussion of control in Chapter 12, when desired outputs are not achieved or when new outputs are sought, managers must change something. Figure 1.6 shows a number of options as to what can be changed.

Inputs can be changed. For example, managers can employ new people with specific education or experience in an effort to achieve a desired output. If such people are not available or if the HSO cannot compete effectively for them with other employers, perhaps the needed change will involve more or different training for current employees. It might also involve the introduction of technology that permits other inputs to be used more effectively. Computerizing much of the information exchanged within an HSO is a good example of such a change.

Managers can also change the organizational structure, the relationships among people who work in the HSO, and the conditions under which they work. Changes in these dimensions can be modest, such as changing job design or work schedules or adding rules and procedures to increase standardization. Or the changes can be more extensive, such as increasing centralization to speed up decision making or combining departments or units to remove vertical layers of the organization and widen spans of control. Such changes make the HSO's organizational structure flatter and less bureaucratic.[2] Sometimes structural changes are even more extensive, as would be the case if the entire structure of an HSO were transformed into a matrix design.

Managers can also change (redefine) outputs. It is senseless to produce an output with no market. A well-managed HSO constantly identifies unmet needs in its service area and responds to them, and this assures a continuous reconsideration of the mix of desired outputs. Using marketing studies to guide it, an HSO might reduce inpatient services and increase ambulatory services or provide industrial medicine services for employers.

Since HSOs do not exist in a vacuum, another option for change is that management alters the HSO's relationships with its external environment and stakeholders. As Jaeger, Kaluzny, and Magruder-Habib note, "The major collective task of any organization is to negotiate an acceptable accommodation with its environment."[3] Changes in inputs, organizational structure, tasks/technology, and outputs (e.g., those described above) can help fit the organization to the opportunities and threats in its external environment. An HSO's managers can also try to change the external environment to make it more closely fit the organization's input requirements and output capabilities. This can be done through marketing an HSO's services (outputs) or lobbying for more resources for production of an input. Seeking to increase federal funding for nurse education is an example of the latter type of activity.

Managers can even change their own functions and roles. They can change the organization's culture, although this usually occurs over a long period of time. Philosophies about how internal and external stakeholders are treated can be changed. Approaches to and methods of motivating, leading, and communicating, as well as problem solving and controlling, can be changed if circumstances require this. Indeed, managers must make changes in HSOs on a continuing basis because the pressures for change are so diverse and numerous.

In this chapter, the pressures for change in HSOs are described. Organizational change is defined and modeled. Several typologies of organizational change are presented to clarify the diversity of change. A four-stage model of the complex process of managing organizational change is described. Finally, the role of managers as change agents is discussed, including the especially difficult change agent role they must play when managing retrenchment.

PRESSURES FOR CHANGE

Substantial and diverse pressures to change come from internal and external sources. A new strategic plan that includes diversifying into new services is a potent *internal driving force* for change. It might stimulate recruiting new people or retraining current personnel. It might stimulate changes in accounting systems or marketing programs. The arrival of a new chief executive officer (CEO) often portends significant organizational changes, sometimes bordering on upheaval. Leadership changes are often followed by significant shifts in strategic direction and the structure of HSOs. They are powerful internal driving forces for change.

The external environments of most HSOs are so dynamic that they exert a constant *external driving force* for change. A growing, declining, or aging population or the plans and actions of competitors have significant implications for an HSO, often requiring it to change. Government policies and regulations exert strong and direct pressure on HSOs. For example, prospective payment that reimburses using diagnosis-related groups (DRGs) for treating Medicare patients changed the basic parameters of how hospitals function because the economic incentives changed. Similarly, National Labor Relations Board (NLRB) rulings can instantly change how HSOs relate to unionized employees. Advances in technology exert a strong force for change on HSOs because they are technology dependent. For example, the dramatic shift from inpatient to outpatient surgery that occurred in the 1980s was largely attributable to better anesthesia, surgical techniques, and postoperative care technologies.

It is important to note that the external forces for change in HSOs are increasing as technology expands, the population ages, and the cost of health services increase. Continued escalation of health care costs, coupled with the fact that many people have inadequate access to health services, is building economic and political pressure that may cause fundamental changes in how health services are organized, delivered, and paid for in the United States.[4]

It is also important to note that the HSO's senior managers are primarily responsible for assessing the external environment and determining what changes are needed, and when. Senior management's perceptions about the external environment facing organizations are a key mechanism for initiating organizational changes.[5] In view of this, great care must be exercised by CEOs and other senior managers in environmental assessment and in interpreting what effects conditions in the environment will have on their organizations. This is no easy task, but the key steps in this process are covered in Chapter 8 in the discussion of strategic planning and environmental assessment.

Perceptions of the environment are influenced by the characteristics of those who observe it, and CEOs are wise to rely on assessments by several people in making decisions about responses to environmental conditions. As Shortell and colleagues note:

> A top management team with a primarily marketing background may be more sensitive to changes in market structure and performance data related to market share than a team with financial or production backgrounds, who may be more sensitive to changes in traditional financial performance indica-

tors or tax and legal changes. Individuals pay selective attention to the environment according to interests and selectively interpret the information they receive.[6]

Managers in HSOs must be able to respond to external and internal pressures for change. These responses can be planned or only piecemeal reactions. A planned approach to change is superior because it helps managers alter the organization's activities in a timely, coordinated, and orderly way. Smith and Kaluzny suggest that "organizations respond to pressure to change by searching for solutions that require limited effort to find and minimal disruption of the status quo."[7] These criteria cause the search for suitable responses to pressures to change to follow a particular course, as outlined in Figure 16.1.

Changes that result from a Search I effort (see Figure 16.1) require only minor repackaging of existing outputs or perhaps better marketing, public relations, or lobbying efforts. In effect, the HSO merely changes its external environment in such a way that pressure for change is reduced to a comfortable level. Changes that result from a Search II effort are often changes in organizational structure or in operating processes and practices, changes that routinely occur in HSOs as they seek to improve performance.

A Search III effort is made when Search I and II efforts are unsatisfactory and involve changing strategic direction, as well as changing products and services. For example, an HSO with declining utilization of inpatient services may have been unable to solve the problem using changes from Search I and II efforts. It might shift strategic direction and offer more outpatient and ambulatory services to offset declining inpatient utilization. Such change is far more involved and disruptive than the comparatively minor changes that resulted from I- and II-level searches.

Finally, at the Search IV level, the organization faces the reality that it will have to change in "extraorganizational" ways. Such changes involve an acute care hospital, for example, merging with a financially stronger organization, converting into a long-term care facility, or, as a last resort, closing.

ORGANIZATIONAL CHANGE DEFINED AND MODELED

In essence, organizational change is "any alteration of activities in an organization"[8] or, as Kaluzny and Hernandez define it, "any modification in operations, structure, or ends of the organization."[9] The simplicity of these definitions can be misleading, however. Holt[10] points out that organizational changes span a broad spectrum and range from an industrywide revolutionary technology, such as occurred in imaging technology, to a small refinement in one job description.

Typologies of Organizational Change

Several typologies of organizational change have been developed to help managers understand the variety and diversity of changes with which they can be involved. Three key examples are described here.

Change Versus Innovation The most basic typology involves nothing more than distinguishing between change and innovation, an important distinction. *Change* occurs when there is any modification in an HSO's established operations, structure, or objectives; innovation is a special kind of change. An *innovative change* occurs when an organization (or a part of it) develops and is the first user of a concept, practice, or physical thing. "Thus all innovation is considered change—but not all change is innovation."[11] As Dunham and Pierce note:

> Because innovation provides more excitement, more challenge, and more uncertainty than most change, managing innovation requires special care. The importance of nurturing support for innovative change and managing the change process systematically is heightened when change involves not only the introduction of something different into the organization but also something new.[12]

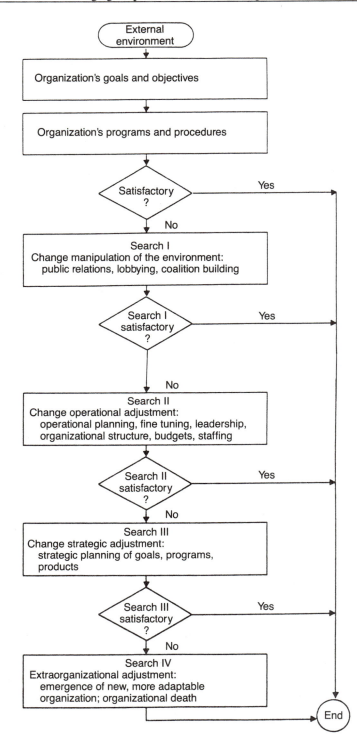

Figure 16.1. Organizational response to pressure to change. (From Smith, David Barton, and Arnold D. Kaluzny. *The white labyrinth: A guide to the health care system*, 2d ed., 184–185. Ann Arbor, MI: Health Administration Press, 1986; reprinted by permission.)

Three Types of Changes Based on Sources   Pelz and Munson[13] expand the simple distinction between change and innovation into three types of change based on the source. They point out that changes in an organization can be *borrowed* (unmodified from elsewhere) or they can be *adapted*. Adapted changes are borrowed and modified to fit the adapting HSO. Also changes in an organization can *originate* there. This type involves much more creativity than borrowed or adapted changes. An adequate borrowed or adapted change is easier to implement (another's experience can be very informative) and is usually less costly than an originated change because someone else has borne the development costs. Wise managers accept the adage that "it makes little sense to reinvent the wheel."

Adaptation and borrowing are the most common sources of change in HSOs—indeed, in all organizations—and reflect the diffusion of innovative changes made elsewhere. The diffusion of medical technologies such as magnetic resonance imaging and lithotripsy have received a great deal of attention, but changes of all kinds are routinely diffused by adaptation or borrowing throughout the health services industry. For example, concepts of corporate restructuring have been widely adapted and borrowed by HSOs. The requirements to remain competitive and to meet accreditation standards of the Joint Commission on Accreditation of Healthcare Organizations assure continued widespread adaptation and borrowing of a wide variety of beneficial changes in HSOs.

This does not mean originated changes are unimportant. There must first be the innovator who develops and first uses a new concept, practice, or physical thing before others can borrow or adapt it. One way to increase the level of creativity in an HSO and enhance the likelihood that it will originate innovations is to hire and sustain creative people. Another is to create a climate in which creativity and innovation are stimulated. Robbins offers the following list of characteristics of such an organizational climate:

1. *Tolerance of risk:* Employees are encouraged to experiment without fear of the consequences should they fail. Mistakes are treated as learning opportunities.
2. *Low external control:* Rules, regulations, policies, and similar controls are kept to a minimum.
3. *Low division of labor:* Narrowly defined jobs create myopia. Diverse job activities give employees a broader perspective.
4. *Acceptance of ambiguity:* Too much emphasis on objectivity and specificity constrains creativity.
5. *Tolerance of conflict:* Diversity of opinions should be encouraged. Harmony and agreement between individuals and/or units are *not* assumed to be evidence of high performance.
6. *Tolerance of the impractical:* Individuals who offer impractical, even foolish, answers to "what if" questions are not stifled. What seems impractical at first might lead to innovative solutions.
7. *Focus on ends rather than means:* Goals should be made clear, and individuals should be encouraged to consider alternative routes toward their attainment. Focusing on ends suggests that there might be several right answers to any given problem.
8. *All-channel communication:* Communication should flow laterally as well as vertically. The free flow of communication facilitates cross-fertilization of ideas.[14]

Just as there are organizational characteristics that encourage innovation and creativity in HSOs, there are behaviors that managers who wish to stimulate creativity and innovation should avoid. For example, Kanter cautions, only slightly tongue-in-cheek, that managers who want to foster creativity should avoid the temptation to:

1. Regard any new idea from below with suspicion—because it's new, and because it's from below.
2. Insist that people who need your approval to act first go through several other levels of management to get their signatures.
3. Ask departments or individuals to challenge and criticize each other's proposals. (That saves you the job of deciding: you just pick the survivor.)
4. Express your criticisms freely, and withhold your praise. (That keeps people on their toes.) Let them know they can be fired at any time.
5. Treat identification of problems as signs of failure, to discourage people from letting you know when something in their area isn't working.

6. Control everything carefully. Make sure people count anything that can be counted, frequently.
7. Make decisions to reorganize or change policies in secret, and spring them on people unexpectedly. (This also keeps people on their toes.)
8. Make sure that requests for information are fully justified, and make sure that it is not given out to managers freely. (You don't want data to fall into the wrong hands.)
9. Assign to lower-level managers, in the name of delegation and participation, responsibility for figuring out how to cut back, lay off, move people around, or otherwise implement threatening decisions you have made. And get them to do it quickly.
10. And above all, never forget that you, the higher-ups, already know everything important about this business.[15]

Such behavior by managers may not eliminate all creativity, but it will greatly diminish this important element in HSOs that wish to be innovators.

Changes Based on Modification of Ends, Means, or Both   Another useful typology of change is based on the fact that any organizational change involves modifying ends, means, or both. Using these variables, Kaluzny and Hernandez[16] identify three types: *technical,* which involves change in means but not ends; *transition,* which involves change in ends but not means; and *transformation,* which involves change in both means and ends. They describe the key characteristics of these three types of change as follows:

> Technical change involves some modifications in the means by which the normal and usual activities of the organization are carried out. This may involve some innovative technology or some programmatic-structural alteration in the design of the organization to meet its designated objectives.
>
> Transition means change in organizational goals but not in the essential means of achieving these goals. The provision of nontherapeutic abortions and the sale of governmental or not-for-profit community hospitals to for-profit systems are examples of transition. In these situations the technology and basic structure (the organizational means) are already available within the institution; however, the intent is to apply these to achieve different objectives (ends).
>
> Transformation is the most extreme form of change. Change occurs in the means the organization uses to reach its ends, and also in the ends themselves. For example, hospitals replace traditional inpatient curative services with provision of preventive health care programs to various employer organizations. They also may diversify their operations to include the building and management of condominiums, office buildings, shopping centers, and retirement homes. Each of these activities involves substantial changes in organizational ends and means. Transformation occurs less frequently than other forms of change, but when it does, it involves a basic modification of overall organizational direction and reflects changes in the means by which organizations accomplish these modified ends.[17]

Final Comments   These typologies of change demonstrate that not all change is alike. It can be innovative change or just change. Changes can be borrowed or adapted from other sources or originated within an HSO. Changes can be technical, transitional, or transformational in nature, depending upon whether they involve ends, means, or both. No matter which type of change is being considered, or the origin of the change, change occurs through a process and managers carry out the change process in HSOs.

The Process of Change Modeled

To manage change effectively, managers must accomplish a series of interrelated activities. They must first recognize the need for change and identify the nature of the change. These two activities are closely related and triggered by internal and external pressures for change. Identification is followed by a series of activities that assure effective planning to implement change. Included are diagnosing the situation by gathering and interpreting information pertinent to success or failure of the change, shaping a general strategy for making the change, and selecting techniques for building support for the change and minimizing resistance. The information gathered in the situational diagnosis and the nature of the general change strategy chosen for implementation aids in selecting these techniques.

The change must then be implemented. The complex act of implementing change involves three interconnected steps that were first identified many years ago by Lewin: unfreezing, changing, and refreezing.[18] The effective and systematic management of change does not end with implementation. The change must be evaluated and the results of this evaluation fed back to inform and guide modification of changes or initiation of further changes. Figure 16.2 contains a schematic model of the process of managing organizational change. The stages in this model are discussed at length in the next section because they show what the manager must do to effectively manage organizational change.

THE PROCESS OF MANAGING ORGANIZATIONAL CHANGE

It is useful to think of managing organizational change as an exercise in problem solving. Recall that problem solving was described in Chapter 10 as a process composed of a series of activities or steps by which managers bring about change. The purpose of problem solving is to introduce change so that actual HSO results or outputs more closely align with those that are desired. The steps in problem solving include:

> Identifying and analyzing a situation that requires a decision
> Identifying and evaluating alternative solutions to address the situation
> Choosing an alternative
> Implementing the alternative
> Evaluating the results after implementation

These problem-solving steps are incorporated into Figure 16.2, which is a highly schematic model of the extremely complex process by which change is managed in HSOs. The four stages are linked in a logical sequence. Success in each depends on successfully completing the previous stage. Viewing the change process as four interrelated stages increases the likelihood of understanding its complexity. Paying attention to each stage increases the probability of effectively managing the process.

In this model, the internal and external pressures for change are treated as triggering mechanisms. That is, the pressures cause managers to respond. The pressure need not be anything more than a manager's own conviction that things always can be done in a better way. This can lead to a continuous assessment of both the need for possible changes and the nature of such changes.

Stage I: Change Identification

As seen in Figure 16.2, the first stage of managing organizational change includes two steps: the manager first must recognize the need for change and then must identify the nature of the change.

Recognize Need for Change Recognizing the need for change is based on information that is often developed while engaged in the function of controlling (see Chapter 12). Financial performance, especially an HSO's operating margin, is always an important source of information about the need for change. Similarly, changes in utilization patterns of HSO services may signal the need for change.

Identify Nature of Change When there is evidence of need for a change, the next step in the change identification stage is to identify the nature of the change. Again, this depends on information. "Sometimes the signals that indicate the need for change suggest the general nature of the change, while at other times they also reveal the specific types of change needed."[19] Often, the information necessary to determine what change is needed is more detailed than the information that signals that a change is required. An example will clarify how information is used in recognizing a need for change and in the more extensive task of identifying the change that is needed.

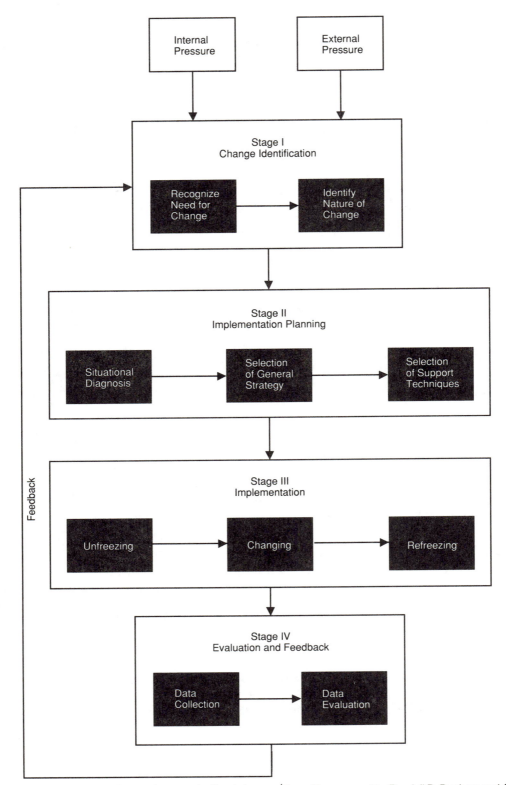

Figure 16.2. The process of managing organizational change. (From *Management* by Randall B. Dunham and Jon L. Pierce. Reprinted by permission of HarperCollins Publishers. Copyright © 1989 by Randall B. Dunham and Jon L. Pierce.)

Information and Change Identification: An Example   Butterworth Hospital's respiratory therapy department had to change because it could not meet all requests for services.[20] Information on the number of missed respiratory therapy sessions was sufficient to reveal the need for change. Determining the nature of the change, however, required more information. To obtain this information, a multidisciplinary team that included members from respiratory therapy and other departments that interacted with it was formed and undertook a series of actions to determine why the department could not meet demand for services. As discussed in Chapter 11, this type of team is often called a quality improvement team.

The team first held a brainstorming session to identify all possible reasons why respiratory therapy could not meet demand. They organized the list into eight categories and developed the *cause-and-effect diagram* shown in Figure 16.3. (Such diagrams are also called *Ishikawa diagrams*, after their developer, or *fishbone diagrams* because of their shape.)

To move beyond mere speculation about possible causes of the problem, the team surveyed members of the respiratory therapy department, who were asked to rank order the reasons for the problem that the team had identified in its brainstorming session. The results of the survey were displayed in a *Pareto diagram*, which lists variables in order of importance. Figure 16.4 shows the six most frequently mentioned reasons why members of the department missed appointments.

Upon examining the Pareto diagram, the team realized that three of the top six reasons given by people who deliver respiratory services at Butterworth Hospital for missed services related to equipment: "equipment availability," "equipment misstocked," and "equipment out of order." The team decided to look more specifically into the equipment problem. By surveying members of the respiratory therapy department again, the team learned that the specific problems were flowmeter and oximeter unavailability and oxygen analyzer downtime. Armed with this information, the team easily identified the changes needed.

This example illustrates both steps in the change identification stage of the process of managing organizational change. As Berwick, Godfrey, and Roessner observe:

> Initially, the team knew only that the respiratory therapy department was not meeting the demand. By the end, they had a clear and specific agenda: solving three specific equipment problems. How had they gotten from here to there? They had followed a very useful pattern in the diagnosis of a problem: the alternating use of *divergent* and *convergent* thinking—alternately accumulating as many ideas as possible and then narrowing them down to the "vital few." They began by brainstorming lots of possibilities (divergent thinking) and then arranging them under eight major sources of flaw (convergent thinking); next they surveyed the entire department for priorities (divergent thinking) and then arranged the survey responses in a Pareto diagram that indicated six major factors (convergent thinking), three of which had to do with a single problem: equipment (convergent thinking).[21]

Stage II: Implementation Planning

As Figure 16.2 shows, Stage II has three steps: a situational diagnosis, selection of a general strategy for implementing change, and selecting techniques to support implementing the change and reducing resistance. The planning stage is a crucial precursor to successful implementation.

Situational Diagnosis   Situational diagnosis is a natural extension of the Stage I information-gathering effort and involves identifying the nature of the change that is needed. In this sense, it overlaps with some Stage I activities. However, situational diagnosis goes beyond the information needed to identify the nature of the change. It includes collecting information about resources available for implementing a change as well as information about the attitudes of key people toward the change. It is necessary to know about resource availability and constraints before choosing a change strategy. Similarly, selection of a change strategy is directly affected by the degree and location of support for—and resistance to—a possible change.

Selection of General Strategy   It is important that managers consider the whole range of general change strategies in their implementation planning. There are many change strategies, but all fit into one of three categories. The strategy can use *power* through coercion or sanctions to

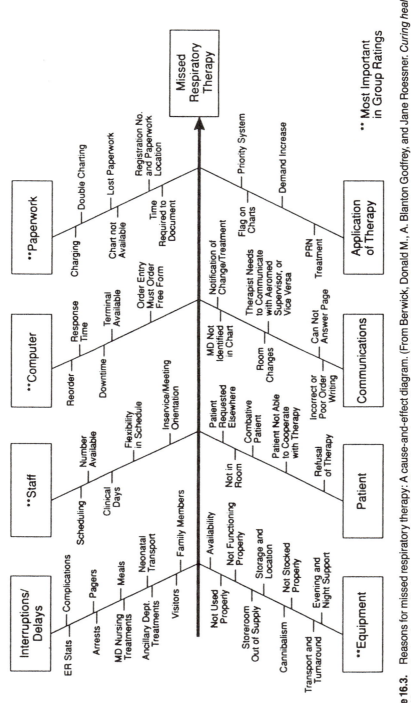
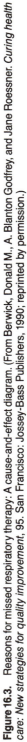

Figure 16.3. Reasons for missed respiratory therapy: A cause-and-effect diagram. (From Berwick, Donald M., A. Blanton Godfrey, and Jane Roessner. *Curing health care: New strategies for quality improvement*, 95. San Francisco: Jossey-Bass Publishers, 1990; reprinted by permission.)

590

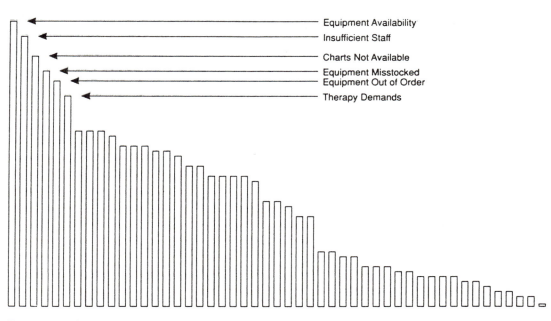

Figure 16.4. Reasons for missed respiratory therapy: A Pareto diagram of survey results. (From Berwick, Donald M., A. Blanton Godfrey, and Jane Roessner. *Curing health care: New strategies for quality improvement*, 96. San Francisco: Jossey-Bass Publishers, 1990; reprinted by permission.)

bring about change. The strategy can use *reason* to lead to rational changes when complete information about the need for change is available. Or, the strategy can take a middle ground and use *reeducation* to improve organizational performance.[22] The reeducation strategy relies on *organizational development* to lead to needed changes. Organizational development is "a specific set of change interventions, skills, activities, tools, or techniques that are used to help people and organizations to be more effective."[23] Table 16.1 contains a list of standard and frequently used organizational development techniques as described by French and Bell.[24]

Another way for managers to think about the change strategies available to them is to consider top-down, bottom-up, or participative strategies that can be used in initiating and implementing changes.[25] In *top-down* strategies, which are power strategies, senior managers determine and announce changes in the HSO; other participants in the organization are expected to accept the changes. Changes in the strategic direction of an HSO often require a top-down initiative, as does quickly adapting to important environmental changes. For example, a change in the reimbursement policy of a major insurance carrier might require an immediate change in HSOs, leaving little time for anything but a top-down edict.

As Holt notes, the top-down approach to change has the advantage of speed by

> requiring only a few people to make timely, comprehensive decisions that can be communicated quickly to lower levels. A top-down change strategy carries great weight and usually reaches deeply into the organization. Its major drawbacks are its disruptiveness, particularly if lower levels don't accept the change, and its tendency to disregard human needs.[26]

In *bottom-up* strategies, the departments or other units of the HSO or even individuals initiate change. For bottom-up strategies to work effectively, organizational development efforts are likely to be required. Some HSOs encourage and reward this type of initiative and creativity. It often takes the form of small groups such as people within a department or in a quality circle identifying a problem and seeking a solution.[27] Table 16.2 provides an overview of the structural

Table 16.1. Frequently used organizational development techniques

Technique	Examples
Organizational diagnoses	Interviews, surveys, group meetings
Team building	Improvement of existing groups; creation of teams for problem solving
Survey feedback	Provision of survey results to members; interpretation of results by members
Education	Classroom training for "sensitivity" skills and interpersonal skills
Intergroup activities	Communication development; conflict reduction
Third-party peace making	Negotiation, mediation by "outsider" for interperson and intergroup conflict
Technostructural/sociotechnical activities	Joint examination of technology, structure, and people systems
Process consultation	Observation of groups in action with immediate feedback on processes observed
Life/career planning	Future oriented—development of personal goals and acquisition of skills to help individuals fit into the organization and the organization match individual needs
Coaching	Nonevaluative feedback to individuals describing how others see them
Planning and goal setting	Training of individuals to improve personal planning and goal-setting effectiveness; emphasis on individual's place in the overall organization

Source: French, Wendell L., and Cecil H. Bell, Jr. *Organizational development: Behavioral science interventions for organization improvement,* 2d ed. Englewood Cliffs, NJ: Prentice Hall, 1978.

components and processes of quality circles. (Chapters 6 and 10 have additional material on quality circles.) The primary advantage of a bottom-up approach to organizational change is that it stimulates creativity in the HSO. It also fosters commitment to implementing the change on the part of those whose initiative led to it. Bottom-up approaches are especially effective when changes involve small parts of the HSO, such as one department, or modest operational changes.

The third category of change strategies is called *participative* strategies. Lawler argues that increasing the level of participation or involvement of employees in decisions about design and management of organizations can reap enormous rewards, including "higher quality products and services, less absenteeism, less turnover, better decision making, and better problem solving—in short, greater organizational effectiveness."[28]

Change that uses higher levels of participation is very different from a top-down approach. Participation suggests the opposite of top-down edicts from senior managers who direct what and how change will be made. However, a higher level of participation is also different from a bottom-up approach. Bottom-up change methods have the goal of an open environment facilitated by effective organizational development efforts that encourage employees to take independent action, "initiating or recommending organizational adaptation."[29]

Participative methods of change implement change through "cooperative efforts, team decision making, and group initiatives."[30] Lawler[31] identifies three categories of approaches to increase employee involvement in organizations: parallel suggestion involvement, job involvement, and high involvement. They vary in the degree to which four features are moved downward in an organization:

(1) information about the performance of the organization, (2) rewards that are based on the performance of the organization, (3) knowledge that enables employees to understand and contribute to

Table 16.2. Overview of structural components and processes of quality circles

DEFINITION: A quality circle is a small group of employees who meet regularly in problem-oriented meetings in which they focus on changes needed to improve morale, productivity, or quality.

BASIC STRUCTURAL COMPONENTS

Circles	3–12 members (generally from same work group) A leader (often the supervisor) A regular meeting time A regular meeting place Access to resource people Access to a management review group
Facilitators	Specially trained to help the leader train the circle, provide group process and problem-solving assistance, and work at the interface of the circle and the remainder of the HSO
Management Review Group	Group of HSO managers who review changes proposed by the circle and make resource allocation decisions
Steering Committee	Group responsible for reviewing and guiding the general direction of the quality circles process in the HSO (usually top management)

Quality Circles Processes

Activity	Locus
1. Objective setting	Circle, organization
2. Problem identification	Circle
Problem analysis	Circle, resource people
Solution generation and selection	Circle
3. Solution approval	Management (if necessary)
4. Solution implementation	Circle, management
5. Follow-up and evaluation	Circle, management
6. Documentation of entire process	Circle recorder, leader
7. Ongoing communication with nonparticipants, other circles	Circle, facilitator

organizational performance, and (4) power to make decisions that influence organizational direction and performance.[32]

When information, rewards, knowledge, and power are concentrated at the top of an HSO, little opportunity for meaningful involvement or participation in change exists elsewhere. Alternatively, when these factors are moved downward, opportunities to participate in managing change are greatly increased.

In *parallel suggestion involvement* approaches to increased participation, employees are encouraged to make suggestions about changes that are needed and about how to implement and manage the changes. Their participation is encouraged through devices such as quality circles, but they have power only to recommend or suggest changes. Decisions are reserved for managers.

Job involvement approaches focus on enriching work so people have more influence over it. In effect, they are empowered to make changes in their own work but nowhere else. This approach does not give employees power to change the structure or operation of an HSO or its strategic direction, but it allows a much greater degree of involvement than does a suggestion approach.

The *high-involvement* approach permits employees to decide about changes in their work, but it also allows input into decisions about changes in the HSO's strategic direction. Employee input is formally sought through such devices as assignment to task forces or project-specific teams. An example is forming a multidisciplinary task force to design a new ambulatory surgery center that will be affiliated with an HSO.

Lawler notes that organizational circumstances determine which approach to increased involvement is best:

The parallel suggestion approach does the least to move power, knowledge, information, and rewards downward, while the high involvement approach does the most. Because they position power, information, knowledge, and rewards differently, these approaches tend to fit different situations and to produce different results. It is not that one is always better than another, but that they are different and, to some degree, competing.[33]

It is Lawler's view that organizations benefit from increased employee involvement in decision making about changes. But, which type is best? In an organization with a traditional hierarchy, well-developed and entrenched management systems, and independent, relatively simple, and repetitive work, suggestion involvement is appropriate. However, in a new organization or a new unit in an existing HSO, in which there is complex and highly interdependent work and managers who value employee involvement, Lawler argues that "it is possible to move to high involvement management and reap the rewards it has to offer."[34] Many HSOs have characteristics that suggest high-involvement approaches are appropriate. The employee empowerment used in the Deming method of continuous quality improvement is one such approach.

Selection of Support Techniques The third step in the implementation planning stage involves selecting the techniques used to develop support for the change and reducing resistance. This step is vital because overcoming resistance is often necessary for successful implementation. In considering useful support techniques, managers must remember that people respond to change in predictable, often negative, ways. Responses are based on their backgrounds, including needs and experiences, and the particular situation in which the change is introduced.

A manager viewing a change as a logical response to a particular problem or opportunity might find that others, looking at the same problem or opportunity and the change made in response to it, are resistant to the change. While the manager might view the resistance as irrational, it may seem perfectly rational to the resistant person, especially if past experiences with change were negative.

Reasons for Resistance to Change Each situation of change is judged according to people's attitudes and feelings, and these determine how they respond to a change. These attitudes and feelings are not the result of chance, but are caused by numerous things. One is personal history, including biological processes, background, and social experiences away from work— what is brought to the work place. A second cause is the work environment itself. For example, if an organization has been very stable it can be doubly difficult to introduce change. When people have adjusted to the status quo and believe it is permanent, inauguration of even minor change is considered revolutionary and disruptive. Conversely, when an organization has a history of frequent change and it is part of the status quo, people expect change and more readily accept it.

There are a many reasons for the often-encountered resistance, including insecurity, possible social loss, economic loss, inconvenience, resentment of control, unanticipated repercussions, union opposition, and threats to influence.[35]

Insecurity is a major source of resistance. The present is known and understood and has been absorbed. There is comfort in the status quo; people have worked out a relationship with it. Any change introduces a degree of uncertainty. Even a seemingly simple change such as moving the photocopying machine can have far-reaching repercussions. To some, such a move is a symbol of management's lack of concern for inconvenienced employees. To others, it means more traffic, noise, and interference around their work area. A third group may see it as more evidence of the autocracy of managers. Change, then, can reduce the current level of satisfaction. People affected by change often do not know what will happen, but past experience may have taught them to expect the worst. In addition, change suggests to employees that they or their methods have been unsatisfactory.

Social losses of various kinds result from change. The mere fact that management seeks to impose a change can be interpreted as evidence that employees lack independence. Change alters informal relationships among people in the HSO, too. Following a change, close friends may have to work in separate rooms or may not be able to interact during work. Complex informal relationships are affected by any change involving people. Established status symbols may be destroyed in the process of reorganizing an HSO. Social acceptance by co-workers may be jeopardized if someone cooperates in a change inaugurated by management that co-workers have rejected. People may be forced to choose between cooperating with management and the friendship of co-workers. Thus, what may seem a desirable and logical change can meet heavy resistance because the price in social relationships is too high.

Economic losses can be inflicted with organizational changes. In many cases, new technology allows more work to be done by the same or even fewer people. Resistance by those affected is understandable. Even without loss of a job or reduced earnings, the change may result in a faster pace of work or increased contributions in other ways.

Inconvenience is a real part of many changes, even when they do not cause economic or social losses. Any change causes some inconvenience, and extra effort is required to adjust to it. Old habits and ways of doing things must be replaced with new practices. Thus, inconvenience stimulates resistance, although if this is the only factor present, the degree of resistance will be related to the degree of inconvenience.

Resentment of control is a normal human reaction to close control of actions and behavior. The degree of control exerted by managers is never more clear cut than during change. People are made sharply aware that they do not fully control their own destinies in the organization.

Unanticipated repercussions accompany many changes. Almost all change has secondary effects, and some unanticipated effects can cause resistance to change. For example, to improve their performance, HSO supervisors can be given training in supervision and leadership. While this may strengthen supervisors, it may have unanticipated secondary repercussions. When the supervisors return from their training, their subordinates, who had worked out a relationship with them, may not know what to expect or how to react to their re-trained supervisors. The most admirable and appropriate action by the newly trained supervisor is likely to be met with a great deal of suspicion, particularly if it is inconsistent with past patterns. It is unlikely that this was the outcome that those who made this change had in mind.

Union opposition can be an especially difficult source of resistance to change. An HSO with unions may find that their representatives occasionally oppose changes suggested by management. Union representatives are not elected to cooperate with management; their role is to protect the union members' interests. Unionized workers are often more comfortable with a contentious union representative than one inclined to cooperate with changes that promote the HSO's interests. It is expected that unions will cause resistance, even where union leaders recognize that proposed changes are good for both groups.

Threats to influence are a final source of resistance to change. In fact, changes that threaten the power base or influence of an individual, a group of people, or a department or unit of the HSO go to the heart of their existence and stimulate some of the strongest resistance to change. For example, changes that threaten the power and influence of physicians in HSOs are routinely and vigorously resisted by them.

All of these factors cause people to resist change in HSOs. The factors often act in combination, and this strengthens the resolve to resist change.

Techniques To Reduce Resistance   Just as there are reasons why people resist change, managers can use a number of approaches to overcome resistance. Basic techniques available to deal with resistance to change are outlined in Table 16.3.

Education and communication are among the most common and useful ways to overcome resistance to change. They involve communicating with the people who will be affected by a change so they are educated about the nature of the change and informed about its implications before it is made. Effective communication about a change and education regarding its implications can turn resistance into support.

Table 16.3. Techniques for reducing resistance to change

Approach	Situational use	Advantages	Drawbacks
Education + Communication	Where there is a lack of information or inaccurate information and analysis.	Once persuaded, people often will help with the implementation of the change.	Can be very time-consuming if many people are involved.
Participation + Involvement	Where the initiators do not have all the information they need to design the change, and where others have considerable power to resist.	People who participate will be committed to implementing change, and any relevant information they have will be integrated into the change plan.	Can be very time-consuming if participators design an inappropriate change.
Facilitation + Support	Where people are resisting because of adjustment problems.	No other approach works as well with adjustment problems.	Can be time-consuming, expensive, and still fail.
Negotiation + Agreement	Where someone or some group will clearly lose out in a change, and where that group has considerable power to resist.	Sometimes it is a relatively easy way to avoid major resistance.	Can be too expensive in many cases if it alerts others to negotiate for compliance.
Manipulation + Co-optation	Where other tactics will not work or are too expensive.	It can be a relatively quick and inexpensive solution to resistance problems.	Can lead to future problems if people feel manipulated.
Explicit + Implicit Coercion	Where speed is essential, and the change initiators possess considerable power.	It is speedy and can overcome any kind of resistance.	Can be risky if it leaves people angry at the initiators.

From Kotter, John P., and Leonard A. Schlesinger. Choosing strategies for change. *Harvard Business Review* 57 (March/April 1979):111; reprinted by permission. Copyright © 1979 by the President and Fellows of Harvard College; all rights reserved.

Participation and involvement in planning for and implementing change can overcome resistance, especially when people who might resist it are encouraged to be involved. Such involvement reduces uncertainty and misunderstanding about a change and its implications and reduces resistance. Participating in decisions about a change provides an opportunity for people to gain a clearer picture of the change and enhances their commitment to successful implementation.

Facilitation and support techniques managers use to help people accept change by facilitating and supporting their adaptation to the change include training programs, granting requests for leave during a painful transition period, or even special counseling sessions for people affected by a change.

Negotiation and agreement are techniques for reducing resistance to change in which managers negotiate with those who resist the change and exchange something of value for reduced resistance. If resistance is centered in a few people or a department, it may be possible to negotiate reduced resistance by giving additional resources or a promise to make a desired change at a later date. In union situations, negotiation about changes is often required by the collective bargaining agreement. A change in how work is performed might mean a new round of negotiations with the union. If a mutually acceptable agreement is reached, the HSO may implement a change but union members receive added compensation or other concessions.

Manipulation and co-optation are sometimes used to reduce resistance to change. It is not recommended, but some managers use devious manipulation in certain situations. Such tactics raise serious ethical problems in HSOs, but they are used and managers should be informed about them. Manipulative techniques include withholding information about the change, releasing false or misleading information, and playing the interests of one person or group off against those of others. Co-optation is manipulation, but it is less devious than other forms. It may be as simple as bringing persons resisting change or who might resist it into planning for the change so they become proponents. However, co-optation may also involve deceit, and this is as unethical as other manipulative strategies.

Explicit and implicit coercion are available to managers, by virtue of their positional power, as techniques to get changes accepted. People can be threatened with loss of their jobs or reduced promotion opportunities in an effort to stop them from resisting change. Acceptance of significant changes in an HSO can be forced on people by the threat of more dire changes (up to and including closing the HSO) if the proposed changes are resisted. Coercion strategies, like manipulation strategies, can easily lead to unethical behavior. The potential for unethical behavior, added to the inevitable anger of people forced into accepting change, means that coercion is an undesirable means of overcoming resistance to change.

Often, the necessary support and resistance-reducing techniques form a "package" of techniques aimed at different people whose resistance must be overcome. Selecting proper techniques, as well as selecting a suitable general change strategy, bears directly on the success of implementing change.

Stage III: Implementation

The implementation stage of managing organizational change presented in Figure 16.2 involves actual use of a new concept, practice, or physical thing. In a successfully implemented change, however, such use occurs more than one time. According to a conceptual framework of how change is implemented developed by Lewin,[36] successful changes occur in three steps: unfreezing the status quo, changing to a new state, and refreezing to make the change permanent. This framework was elaborated by Schein.[37]

Unfreezing   Status quo is a state of equilibrium in which forces supporting a change and forces discouraging it are equal. For change to occur, this equilibrium must be disturbed or "unfrozen." Unfreezing occurs in three ways: 1) supporting forces can be increased, 2) discouraging forces can be decreased, or 3) both can occur. Sometimes all that is needed to unfreeze the status quo is more information about the change being implemented. In HSOs, this information is often provided in the context of education on a new concept, practice, or physical thing. People who understand the advantages of the change over the status quo are more likely to be receptive to the change and to help implement it. They are also more likely to fulfill their responsibilities associated with or growing out of the change.

Changing   In this step change actually occurs. If the change is a physical thing, such as a piece of equipment, it is put in place and people begin using it. If the change is a concept or practice, such as new reporting relationships, a new marketing strategy, or a modified accounting system, it is initiated and people begin using it.

Refreezing   In this step the change is incorporated into the routines of those implementing the change. A new equilibrium is established as people adapt to the change and accept it as the norm. Refreezing makes the change permanent—at least until a future decision that the change is flawed and should be modified or abandoned. Such determinations can be made only through systematic efforts to evaluate the change, as will be seen in the discussion of Stage IV of the process of managing a change.

Actions To Increase Successful Implementation of Change   There is no assurance that a change, no matter how necessary it may be or how carefully its implementation is planned, can be successfully implemented. However, managers can take certain actions to increase the likelihood of a successful outcome. Perhaps the most important is to be certain that people involved in a change understand the situation fully. People who understand the necessity of a change and its details are more likely to adjust to it than people who do not. Managers should provide information as far in advance as possible and include specifics about reasons for the change, its nature and timing, and the expected impact on the HSO and people in it.

It may be useful for a change to be introduced on a trial basis, if feasible. Familiarity gained through experience with a change, as well as assurances that it is not irrevocable, can reduce initial insecurity and increase the likelihood of acceptance. Allowing time for a change to be digested by those involved will also increase ultimate acceptance.

Another useful action for managers when implementing change is to minimize disturbing customs and informal relationships. The culture developed by people at work has real value because it helps them adjust to the workplace and to their role in it. Change almost invariably disrupts the culture. Minimizing disturbance is facilitated by widespread participation in planning and implementing a change. People feel less pressure from changes that they help plan because they understand them better. People are also likely to be more committed to the success of a change if they are involved in planning for and implementing it.

Stage IV: Evaluation and Feedback

The fourth and final stage in the process of managing organizational change (see Figure 16.2) is often given inadequate attention by managers and may be overlooked altogether. Managers must evaluate their actions because they have a responsibility to optimally use resources entrusted to them. All changes involve expending organizational resources such as money and time, which have alternative uses. Systematic evaluation determines if the resources used to implement a change yield benefits such as quality, efficiency, satisfaction, adaptiveness, and survival sufficient to justify them.

In addition, evaluation provides a basis for feedback, which can lead to adjustments in the changes that have been implemented or to a realization that further change is needed. The evaluation and feedback stage involves two steps: data collection and data evaluation.

Data Collection   The purpose for data collection is to determine whether a change has been effectively implemented, whether the objectives established were achieved, and what other changes or modifications might be needed.

Data Evaluation   The second step is evaluating the data collected. Here, managers compare what was accomplished by the change with what was desired. Information that indicates that outcomes do not match objectives provides feedback to the process of managing organizational change so that alterations can be made in the change or alternatives can be developed.

Final Comments

Ideally, the process of managing organizational change unfolds in the four sequential and interrelated stages shown in Figure 16.2. If any stage, or any step within a stage, is inadequately managed, the entire process is jeopardized. In managing the organizational change process, managers are in effect change agents.

MANAGERS AS CHANGE AGENTS

Change in HSOs does not occur without the presence of certain conditions. Key among them are the people who are catalysts and can manage the organizational change process. Such people are called *change agents*. Any manager can be a change agent, and the role of change agent in HSOs is often, but not always, played by managers. Persons who are not managers, such as physicians, nurses, or pharmacists, can also be change agents, especially in regard to technology. On occasion, the role of change agent is played by a consultant from outside the organization who specializes in implementing change.

Requisites to Change

As Peters and Tseng note, requisites to effective organizational change include several that directly involve the change agent:

1. Something has to precipitate change—a happening, development, signal, or an individual has to place the organization in a mold for change.
2. The organization itself must be ready to change, or someone within the organization, the change agent, must convince others that old comfortable ways should be replaced by new untried ways.
3. The proposed new ways either must mesh with or not seriously disturb the existing value system.
4. The change agent must select the approach or combination of approaches necessary to convince others of the need for change (for example, by planting seeds for change through a board-management-medical staff educational process and/or by using task forces and other internal devices to develop ideas and build coalitions).
5. The change agent must create a shared body of values and attitudes—a new consensus where key individuals within an organization reinforce one another in selling the new way and in defending it against inertia, reluctance, or outright opposition.[38]

In their role as change agents, managers are well served by understanding Schein's observations:

1. Any change process involves not only learning something new but also unlearning something that is well integrated into the personality and social relationships of the individual.
2. No change will occur unless the motivation to change is present. Inducing that motivation is often the most difficult part of the change process.
3. Organizational changes in authority structures, processes, and systems occur only through individual change by key members of organizations.
4. Change involves altering attitudes, values, and behavior. The unlearning of present responses can initially be painful and threatening.
5. Change is a multistage process, a complex cycle of behavioral modification that requires a systematic approach.[39]

Schein emphasizes the human element. A change may be a new design for a form, a new piece of technology, or some specific behavior, but *all* organizational change affects people, who must behave differently when change occurs.

The Special Case of Retrenchment

Being a change agent is never easy. It is most difficult when changes involve retrenchment, which is sometimes called downsizing. Retrenchment means reducing an HSO's size or scope of activities. An entire HSO may be downsized, although more frequently only a part is involved. This special change circumstance is noted because it is relatively new in HSOs. Anderson[40] notes that the U.S. health industry has been in a growth phase for at least 100 years and is still accurately characterized as a growth industry. However, within it, individual HSOs must increasingly downsize or retrench.

There are several variations on the basic retrenchment strategy that an HSO might follow: *internal consolidation,* wherein parts of the HSO are melded into a simpler organization; *divestiture,* wherein parts of the HSO and/or subsidiary organizations are sold; and *liquidation,* which is to cease business through bankruptcy or sale of the HSO.

Coddington and Moore point out that downsizing strategies often involve activities in one or more of the following broad classifications:

Staff reductions (that is, layoffs, attrition, transfer of personnel). Downsizing-related staff reductions differ from other staff reductions in three important ways. First, downsizing-related staff reductions usually affect all levels of the organization (from management to nurses to technicians), whereas nondownsizing-related layoffs are often confined to a particular department or service. Second, downsizing-related staff reductions are usually accompanied by an organizational restructuring (that is, a combining of departments) and a reduction in capacity (fewer beds); layoffs not in the context of a downsizing effort are often implemented unilaterally, without corresponding changes in organizational structure. Third, downsizing-related staff reductions tend to be permanent, while traditional layoffs tend to be temporary, in response to a "short-term downturn" in patient volume.

Organizational restructuring, usually consisting of departmental consolidation or elimination. It should be noted that organizational changes—for example, department consolidations—often occur on an interim basis. These short-term actions should not be confused with downsizing-related organizational changes, which are usually permanent.

Plant capacity reduction (reduction of number of beds or operating rooms; closing a wing or floor; sale of excess equipment and supplies).

Conversion of use of facilities (for example, an inpatient operating room to outpatient use, acute care beds into a skilled nursing unit).[41]

A number of problems are associated with downsizing.[42] Among the most serious are: 1) loss of credibility for senior managers; 2) increased in-fighting and "politicking" for position in the retrenched HSO, which increases conflict among first-line and middle-level managers; and 3) decaying motivation and increased voluntary turnover in affected parts of the HSO.

Effective management of these problems is an added burden of managing change caused by retrenchment. There are no magic bullets, but managers can do two things that are especially useful in minimizing these problems:

Management needs to attack directly the ambiguity that organizational retrenchment creates among employees. This is best done by clarifying the organization's strategy and goals. Where is the organization going? What are the organization's future and potential? By addressing these questions, management demonstrates that it understands the problem and has a vision of what the new, smaller organization will look like. Employees want to believe that management is not content to run a "going-out-of-business" sale.

Organizational retrenchment demands that management do a lot of communicating with employees. The primary focus of this communication should be downward—specifically, explaining the rationale for changes that will have to be made. But there should also be an upward communication to give employees an opportunity to vent their fears and frustrations and have important questions answered. Remember that management's credibility is not likely to be high. Additionally, rumors will be rampant. This puts a premium on management making every effort to explain clearly the reasons for, and implications of, all significant changes.[43]

SUMMARY

Significant external and internal pressures drive change in HSOs. When change is needed, managers have many options as to what they might change. Inputs can be changed, as can the HSO's organizational structure, relationships among staff, and conditions of work. In short, managers can change the processes that convert inputs into outputs. Outputs, too, can be changed. Finally, the HSO can try to change its external environment.

All organizational changes involve modifying means, ends, or both. Three types of change are examined: technical (change in means but not ends), transition (change in ends but not means), and transformation (change in both means and ends). Three sources of change are examined: origination, adaptation, and borrowing. No matter the type or source, effective implementation of change in HSOs depends on a complex formal management process.

A four-stage model of the process of managing organizational change is presented in Figure 16.2. Stage I (change identification) has two steps: recognizing need for change and identifying the nature of the change. Both depend on information available to the manager. Stage II (implementation planning) has three steps: situational diagnosis, choosing a general strategy for implementing change, and selecting techniques to support implementation and reduce resistance. Change strategies that rely on power, reason, and reeducation are examined, and special attention is given to the role of organizational development as a reeducation strategy. Change strategies that involve top-down, bottom-up, and participative approaches also are examined. In selecting support techniques, it is emphasized that people resist change for specific reasons, and an array of techniques for reducing resistance to change is presented. These techniques are summarized in Table 16.3.

Stage III (implementation) of the model for managing the organizational change process includes three steps: unfreezing the status quo or equilibrium state, changing to a new state, and refreezing to make the change permanent. A number of specific actions that managers can take to ensure a successful implementation outcome are described. Stage IV (evaluation and feedback) is the final stage in this process and involves two steps: data collection and data evaluation. In this stage, managers collect data that reveal whether a planned change has been effectively implemented, whether the objectives established for the change were achieved, and what further changes or modifications are needed. In the evaluation step, the data are analyzed. This provides information that is fed back into the process so alterations can be made.

The model of the process of managing organizational change presented here emphasizes that the stages in the process—and the steps within each stage—are sequential. If any are poorly managed, managers are not adequately playing their important role as change agents and the entire process is jeopardized.

DISCUSSION QUESTIONS

1. Discuss the pressures for change confronting managers in HSOs.
2. What are the three sources of change available to managers? Discuss the differences among them.
3. Distinguish between change and innovation. Which is more important for managers in HSOs?
4. Briefly describe the four stages in the process of managing organizational change.
5. Discuss the role of information in the change identification stage of managing organizational change.
6. Describe and compare the three general change strategies presented in this chapter.
7. What is organizational development? Describe three useful organizational development techniques.
8. What are the three steps in the implementation stage of managing an organizational change?
9. Why is resistance so often the human response to change? What can managers do to overcome resistance?
10. Discuss the manager's role as change agent.

CASE STUDY 1: DELIVERY ROOM STAFFING SITUATION

Traditionally at Hector Hospital delivery rooms had been staffed by obstetricians, registered nurses (RNs), licensed practical nurses (LPNs), and nurse aides. Recently, it came to the attention of senior management that in addition to routine clean-up tasks, nurse aides were being assigned a number of nonpatient duties by RNs and LPNs. Since delegating nonpatient duties did not reduce or hinder patient care in the delivery room and it appeared to be acceptable to the obstetricians, management permitted the pattern to continue and remain under the control of those in the delivery rooms.

However, as pressures for cost control and containment mounted, efficiency became the watchword and staffing patterns in the delivery rooms were reviewed. A study done by the hospital's administrative resident found that significant savings could be realized by eliminating the nurse aides. The resident recommended that nonpatient duties be reassigned to the RNs and LPNs and that housekeeping assign personnel to the delivery rooms for clean-up tasks. The savings resulted primarily from the fact that housekeeping personnel were paid about 20% less per hour in wages and benefits.

The new staffing pattern was implemented in January by directive from the CEO, but by June it was clear that there were problems. Nurses were complaining to the obstetricians about the lack of support staff (nurse aides), which they believed caused them to be overworked. In addition, several of the housekeeping personnel who were assigned to the delivery rooms were male and this had upset the female nursing staff. In July, the obstetricians informed the CEO of their displeasure. By October, no action had been taken.

Questions

1. Identify and discuss the problem(s).
2. How could it/they have been prevented?
3. What should be management's plan at this point? How should it be implemented?

CASE STUDY 2:   A RESPONSE TO CHANGE

As business officer manager of Group HMO, Inc., Dana Smith was responsible for the work of approximately 45 employees, of whom 26 were classified as secretarial or clerical. At the direction of the plan president, a team of outside systems analysis consultants were to make a time study and work method analysis of Smith's area in an effort to improve the efficiency and output of the business office.

The consultants began by observing and recording each detail of the work of the secretarial and clerical staff. After 2 days of preliminary observation, they indicated that they were prepared to begin their time study on the following day.

The next morning five of the business office employees participating in the study were absent. On the following day 10 employees were absent. Concerned, Smith sought to find reasons for the absenteeism by calling her absent employees. Each related basically the same story. Each was nervous, tense, and physically tired after being a "guinea pig" during the 2 days of preliminary observation. One told Smith that his physician had advised him to ask for a leave of absence if working conditions were not improved.

Shortly after the telephone calls, the head of the study team told Smith that if there were as many absences on the next day his team would have to delay the study. He stated that a scientific analysis would be impossible with 10 employees absent. Realizing that she would be held responsible for the failure of the study, Smith was very concerned.

Questions

1. What caused the reactions to the study?
2. Could these reactions have been predicted? Why?
3. What steps should Smith take to get the study back on track?

CASE STUDY 3:   HOW READY ARE YOU
FOR MANAGING IN A TURBULENT WORLD?[44]

Instructions: Listed below are some statements a 37-year-old manager made about his job at a large, successful HSO. If your job had these characteristics, how would you react to them? After each statement are five letters, A–E. Circle the letter that best describes how you think you would react according to the following scale:

A   *I would enjoy this very much; it's completely acceptable.*
B   *This would be enjoyable and acceptable most of the time.*
C   *I'd have no reaction to this feature one way or another, or it would be about equally enjoyable and unpleasant.*
D   *This feature would be somewhat unpleasant for me.*
E   *This feature would be very unpleasant for me.*

1. I regularly spend 30%–40% of my time in meetings. A B C D E
2. A year and a half ago, my job did not exist, and I have been essentially inventing it as I go along. A B C D E
3. The responsibilities I either assume or am assigned consistently exceed the authority I have for discharging them. A B C D E
4. At any given moment in my job, I have, on the average, about a dozen phone calls to be returned. A B C D E
5. There seems to be very little relation in my job between the quality of my performance and my actual pay and fringe benefits. A B C D E
6. About 2 weeks a year of formal management training is needed in my job just to stay current. A B C D E
7. Because we have very effective equal employment opportunity (EEO) in my HSO and because it is located in a major urban area, my job consistently brings me into close working contact at a professional level with people of many races, ethnic groups, and nationalities, and of both sexes. A B D C E
8. There is no objective way to measure my effectiveness. A B C D E
9. I report to three different bosses for different aspects of my job, and each has an equal say in my performance appraisal. A B C D E
10. On average, about a third of my time is spent dealing with unexpected emergencies that force all scheduled work to be postponed. A B C D E
11. When I have to have a meeting of the people who report to me, it takes my secretary most of a day to find a time when we are all available, and, even then, I have yet to have a meeting that everyone was present the entire time. A B C D E
12. The college degree I earned in preparation for this type of work is now obsolete, and I probably should go back for another degree. A B C D E
13. My job requires that I absorb 100–200 pages per week of technical materials.
    A B C D E
14. I am out of town overnight at least 1 night per week. A B C D E
15. My department is so interdependent with several other departments in the HSO that all distinctions about which departments are responsible for which tasks are quite arbitrary.
    A B C D E
16. I will probably get a promotion in about a year to a job in another division that has most of these same characteristics. A B C D E
17. During the period of my employment here, either the entire HSO or the division I worked in has been reorganized every year or so. A B C D E
18. While there are several possible promotions I can see ahead of me, I have no real career path in an objective sense. A B C D E
19. While there are several possible promotions I can see ahead of me, I think I have no realistic chance of getting to the top levels of the HSO. A B C D E
20. While I have many ideas about how to make things work better, I have no direct influence on either the business policies or the personnel policies that govern my division.
    A B C D E
21. My HSO has recently put in an "assessment center" where I and all other managers will be required to go through an extensive battery of psychological tests to assess our potential.
    A B C D E
22. My HSO is a defendant in an antitrust suit, and if the case comes to trial, I will probably have to testify about some decisions that were made a few years ago. A B C D E
23. Advanced computer and other electronic office technology is continually being introduced into my division, necessitating constant learning on my part. A B C D E

24. The computer terminal and screen I have in my office can be monitored in my bosses' offices without my knowledge.   A   B   C   D   E

Scoring: Score four points for each A, three for each B, two for each C, one for each D, and zero for each E. Compute the total, divide by 24, and round to one decimal place.

While the results are not intended to be more than suggestive, the higher your score, the more comfortable you seem to be with change. The test's author suggests analyzing scores as if they were grade point averages. In this way, a 4.0 average is an A, a 2.0 is a C, and scores below 1.0 flunk.

Using replies from nearly 500 MBA students and young managers, the range of scores was found to be narrow—between 1.0 and 2.2. The average score was between 1.5 and 1.6—a D + / C − sort of grade!

CASE STUDY 4:   ORGANIZATIONAL DEVELOPMENT (OD) IN A HEALTH CARE CLINIC[45]

A major health care clinic with more than 400 physicians and 7,000 employees undertook an organizational development program in response to problems stemming from the application of modern technology to the jobs of medical technologists. The clinic's management initiated the program when the human resources department reported the results of a job analysis of the laboratory division. The results indicated widespread dissatisfaction particularly among medical technologists in the biochemistry department, where new technology had the greatest impact.

The primary sources of dissatisfaction among the technologists were that their skills were underutilized in their work, communications within the laboratories were insufficient, work was not evenly distributed, and the clinical staff did not treat them with the respect they deserved. These complaints were consistent with the general feeling that the advent of technology had simplified the work to the point that it no longer seemed to require the level of training common among medical technologists. Studies in the literature of personnel management confirmed that the absence of job challenge was a primary cause of job turnover among medical technologists.

The clinic's organizational development staff discussed the implications of the information with the manager of the laboratory division. The manager agreed that an effort should be undertaken to improve effectiveness of the laboratory through the introduction of new technology and the enhancement of the technologists' work experiences. The challenge of the program was to develop means for increasing sources of job satisfaction among a group of employees whose job content was being changed drastically by technology. The OD experts believed that the jobs of medical technologists could be redesigned to include greater autonomy, control, feedback, and meaningfulness, these being the classic job enrichment principles.

The OD staff and the laboratory decided to focus on the jobs of two groups of medical technologists: biochemistry and microbiology. Technologists in the biochemistry labs had experienced the greatest job changes due to technology; technologists in the microbiology lab had experienced the least change. The OD program began with meetings attended by the OD staff and laboratory staff. The purpose of these meetings was to explain the purposes of the intervention, to test the level of commitment of the laboratory management and medical personnel to the process, and to recruit volunteers to assist in the analysis of the diagnostic data. After a series of meetings that the OD staff deemed to be successful, a questionnaire was administered to all technologists in the two groups.

The questionnaire enabled respondents to express their confidential opinions regarding various aspects of their jobs. The items on the questionnaire measured the extent to which respondents believed their jobs contained variety, significance, identity, autonomy, and feedback. The OD staff believed that these five job characteristics are the sources of job satisfaction. The questionnaire items also enabled respondents to express their satisfaction with different aspects of their jobs, such as pay, job security, social relations, supervision, and growth opportunities. In addition to the questionnaire, the OD staff also conducted personal interviews with a random sample of one third of all the technologists in each group. This initial data collection process took about 2 months.

During the next 4 months, the volunteer groups met weekly to discuss and analyze the data and to make recommendations for change in the laboratories. Some of the more significant changes that the volunteer groups recommended included: 1) the creation of dual career paths to permit advancement other than moving into administrative positions, 2) the development of opportunities for job rotation, 3) the redesign of the physical environment to improve working conditions, and 4) the provision of ways for lab managers to identify and clarify goals more precisely.

Two years later, the OD staff evaluated the results of the OD program. The staff again administered the questionnaire and found that scores on the items measuring job characteristics and satisfaction declined generally for both groups. The OD staff followed up the questionnaire with personal interviews that confirmed the impression that the technologists were disappointed with the results of the intervention. The interviewed individuals expressed many negative attitudes about the OD intervention, particularly the way in which management responded to the recommended changes. The most favorable comments were expressed by individuals who had served on the volunteer groups.

The OD staff believed that the disappointing results of the program could be traced to several possible causes. They first considered whether an intervention based on job redesign theory was applicable in a health services organization. After all, this theory was developed in industrial settings, not health services organizations. A second possible cause might be the manner in which the OD staff implemented the program. Perhaps the program depended too much on the OD staff's interest and direction and less on the real commitment of lab management. A third possible explanation might be found in cultural factors that characterize most health services organizations. Such factors include the reluctance of medical personnel to share decision-making power with technologists and the unwillingness of clinical staff to delegate authority. The existence of these cultural barriers to collaboration would seem to limit the potential of interventions based on job redesign theory.

As the staff reviewed the results of their work, they were anxious to find some answers to their questions. A repetition of the mistakes certainly would not improve the climate for change in the clinic.

Questions

1. How do you assess the reasons suggested in the case for why these OD interventions did not achieve more positive results?
2. If you were the manager of the laboratory division, what would you do now?

NOTES

1. Davis, Keith, and John W. Newstrom. *Human behavior at work: Organizational behavior*, 8th ed., 283. New York: McGraw-Hill Book Company, 1989.
2. Robbins, Stephen P. *Management*, 3d ed., 539. Englewood Cliffs, NJ: Prentice Hall, 1991.
3. Jaeger, B. Jon, Arnold D. Kaluzny, and Kathryn Magruder-Habib. *Multi-institutional systems management*, 3. Owings Mills, MD: The AUPHA Press, 1987.
4. Longest, Beaufort B., Jr., and Thomas Detre. A cost-containment agenda for academic health centers. *Hospital & Health Services Administration*, 36. (Spring 1991): 77–93.
5. Hambrick, Donald C. *The executive effect: Concepts and methods for studying top managers*. Greenwich, CT: JAI Press, 1988.
6. Shortell, Stephen M., Ellen M. Morrison, and Bernard Friedman. *Strategic choices for America's hospitals: Managing change in turbulent times*, 34. San Francisco: Jossey-Bass, 1990.
7. Smith, David Barton, and Arnold D. Kaluzny. *The white*

labyrinth: A guide to the health care system, 2d ed., 183. Ann Arbor, MI: Health Administration Press, 1986.

8. Aldag, Ramon J., and Timothy M. Stearns. *Management*, 2d ed., 711. Cincinnati, OH: South-Western Publishing Company, 1991.

9. Kaluzny, Arnold D., and S. Robert Hernandez. Organizational change and innovation. In *Health care management: A text in organization theory and behavior*, edited by Stephen M. Shortell and Arnold D. Kaluzny, 2d ed., 380. New York: John Wiley & Sons, 1988.

10. Holt, David H. *Management: Principles and practices*, 2d ed., 612. Englewood Cliffs, NJ: Prentice Hall, 1990.

11. Kaluzny and Hernandez, Organizational change, 380.

12. Dunham, Randall, B., and John L. Pierce. *Management*, 719. Glenview, IL: Scott, Foresman and Company, 1989.

13. Pelz, David C., and Fred C. Munson. A framework for organizational innovating. Paper presented at the Academy of Management Annual Meeting, 1980.

14. Robbins, *Management*, 545.

15. Kanter, Rosabeth Moss. *The change masters: Innovations for productivity in the American corporation*, 101. New York: Simon & Schuster, 1983.

16. Kaluzny and Hernandez, Organizational change.

17. Kaluzny and Hernandez, Organizational change, 380–381.

18. Lewin, Kurt. Frontiers in group dynamics: Concept, method, and reality in social science, social equilibria and social change. *Human Relations* 1 (June 1947): 5–41.

19. Dunham and Pierce, *Management*, 742.

20. Berwick, Donald M., A. Blanton Godfrey, and Jane Roessner. *Curing health care: New strategies for quality improvement*, 94–97. San Francisco: Jossey-Bass Publishers, 1990.

21. Berwick, Godfrey, and Roessner, *Curing health*, 97.

22. Gibson, James L., John M. Ivancevich, and James H. Donnelly, Jr. *Organizations: Behavior, structure, processes*, 7th ed. Homewood, IL: Richard D. Irwin, Inc., 1991.

23. Fagenson, Ellen, and W. Warner Burke. The current activities and skills of organization development practitioners. *Academy of Management, Best Paper Proceedings* (August 1989): 251.

24. French, Wendell L., and Cecil H. Bell, Jr. *Organizational development: Behavioral science interventions for organization improvement*, 2d ed. Englewood Cliffs, NJ: Prentice Hall, 1978.

25. Holt, *Management*, 617–620.

26. Holt, *Management*, 618–619.

27. Lawler, Edward E., III, and Susan A. Mohrman. Quality circles after the fad. *Harvard Business Review* 63 (January–February 1985): 65–71.

28. Lawler, Edward E., III. Choosing an involvement strategy. *Executive* 2 (August 1988): 197.

29. Holt, *Management*, 619.

30. Holt, *Management*, 619.

31. Lawler, Choosing an involvement.

32. Lawler, Choosing an involvement, 197.

33. Lawler, Choosing an involvement, 197.

34. Lawler, Choosing an involvement, 204.

35. Mondy, R. Wayne, Judith R. Gordon, Arthur Sharplin, and Shane R. Premeaux. *Management and organizational behavior*, 637–640. Boston: Allyn and Bacon, 1990.

36. Lewin, Frontiers in group.

37. Schein, Edgar H. *Organizational psychology*, 3d ed. Englewood Cliffs, NJ: Prentice Hall, 1980.

38. Peters, Joseph P., and Simone Tseng. Managing strategic change. *Hospitals* 57 (June 1, 1983): 65.

39. Schein, *Organizational psychology*, 243–244.

40. Anderson, Odin W. Health services in the United States: A growth enterprise for a hundred years. In *Health politics and policy*, edited by Theodor J. Litman and Leonard S. Robins, 2d ed., 38–52. Albany, NY: Delmar Publishers, Inc., 1991.

41. Coddington, Dean C., and Keith D. Moore. *Market-driven strategies in health care*, 204. San Francisco: Jossey-Bass, 1987.

42. Cameron, Kim S., Robert I. Sutton, and David A. Whetten. *Readings in organizational decline*. Cambridge, MA: Ballinger Publishing, 1988.

43. Robbins, *Management*, 548.

44. Adapted from Vaill, Peter B. *Managing as a performing art: New ideas for a world of chaotic change*, 8–9. San Francisco: Jossey-Bass, 1989; used by permission.

45. From James L. Gibson, John M. Ivancevich, and James H. Donnelly, Jr. *Organizations: Behavior, structure, processes*, 7th ed., 661–662. Homewood, IL: Richard D. Irwin, Inc., 1991; reprinted by permission. The case is based on Pasmore, William, Jeffrey Petee, and Richard Bastian. Sociotechnical systems in health care: A field experiment. *Journal of Applied Behavioral Science* 22 (August 1986): 329–339.

BIBLIOGRAPHY

Berwick, Donald M., A. Blanton Godfrey, and Jane Roessner. *Curing health care: New strategies for quality improvement*. San Francisco: Jossey-Bass Publishers, 1990.

Cameron, Kim S., Robert I. Sutton, and David A. Whetten. *Readings in organizational decline*. Cambridge, MA: Ballinger Publishing, 1988.

Coddington, Dean C., and Keith D. Moore. *Market-driven strategies in health care*. San Francisco: Jossey-Bass, 1987.

Fagenson, Ellen, and W. Warner Burke. The current activities and skills of organization development practitioners. *Academy of Management, Best Paper Proceedings* (August 1989): 251.

French, Wendell L., and Cecil H. Bell, Jr. *Organizational development: Behavioral science interventions for organiza-*

tion improvement, 2d ed. Englewood Cliffs, NJ: Prentice Hall, 1978.

Hambrick, Donald C. *The executive effect: Concepts and methods for studying top managers*. Greenwich, CT: JAI Press, 1988.

Kaluzny, Arnold D., and S. Robert Hernandez. Organizational change and innovation. In *Health care management: A text in organization theory and behavior*, edited by Stephen M. Shortell and Arnold D. Kaluzny, 2d ed. New York: John Wiley & Sons, 1988.

Kanter, Rosabeth Moss. *The change masters: Innovations for productivity in the American corporation*. New York: Simon & Schuster, 1983.

Kotter, John P., and Leonard A. Schlesinger. Choosing strategies for change. *Harvard Business Review* 57 (March/April 1979): 106–114.

Lawler, Edward E., III. Choosing an involvement strategy. *Executive* 2 (August 1988): 197–204.

Lawler, Edward E., III, and Susan A. Mohrman. Quality circles after the fad. *Harvard Business Review* 63 (January–February 1985): 65–71.

Lewin, Kurt. Frontiers in group dynamics: Concept, method, and reality in social science, social equilibria and social change. *Human Relations* 1 (June 1947): 5–41.

Longest, Beaufort B., Jr., and Thomas Detre. A cost-containment agenda for academic health centers. *Hospital & Health Services Administration* 36 (Spring 1991): 77–93.

Pasmore, William, Jeffrey Petee, and Richard Bastian. Sociotechnical systems in health care: A field experiment. *Journal of Applied Behavioral Science* 22 (August 1986): 329–339.

Pelz, David C., and Fred C. Munson. A framework for organizational innovating. Paper presented at the Academy of Management Annual Meeting, 1980.

Peters, Joseph P., and Simone Tseng. Managing strategic change. *Hospitals* 57 (June 1, 1983): 65.

Shortell, Stephen M., Ellen M. Morrison, and Bernard Friedman. *Strategic choices for America's hospitals: Managing change in turbulent times*. San Francisco: Jossey-Bass, 1990.

Smith, David Barton, and Arnold D. Kaluzny. *The white labyrinth: A guide to the health care system*, 2d ed. Ann Arbor, MI: Health Administration Press, 1986.

Vaill, Peter B. *Managing as a performing art: New ideas for a world of chaotic change*. San Francisco: Jossey-Bass, 1989.

VII Human Resources Management in Health Services Organizations

*The implementation of a health care institution's
strategic business plan should capitalize on the
institution's greatest asset—human resources.*
American Hospital Association[1]

To implement strategies and accomplish objectives, health services organizations (HSOs) must be staffed with adequate numbers of properly trained personnel. When managers integrate technology and people into formal structures (organizational arrangements), meaningful work occurs. The human element is the catalyst in the organizational equation that causes other inputs (material, supplies, technology, information, and capital) to be converted to outputs in the form of individual and organizational work results (see the management model for HSOs, Figure 1.6). It is through people that work gets done, patient care is delivered, and organizational objectives are accomplished.

As the opening quotation suggests, an HSO's human resources (employees) are its most important asset. Without people, organizations are inert. If employees (i.e., human resources) are insufficient in number or improperly matched to the organization's needs, less than optimal work results will occur—quality and effectiveness will be negatively affected. It is senior management's responsibility to implement and coordinate a total human resource system—composed of work force planning, recruitment and selection, placement, and retention—to ensure that the HSO is properly staffed.[2]

Part VI of this text addresses how managers get things done through people. It focuses on the directing and initiating aspects of management—motivation, leadership, communication, interpersonal behavior, and organizational dynamics—as well as on change. This chapter focuses on the managerial function of staffing the organization.

ROLE OF PERSONNEL/HUMAN RESOURCES MANAGEMENT

Personnel administration is the historical term used to describe a wide range of centralized staffing activities, programs, and policies related to *acquisition, retention, and separation of human resources*. All managers play a part in and have some degree of responsibility for staffing activities such as selection, performance appraisal, promotion, training and development, discipline and corrective counseling, and compensation of their employees. However, most staffing activities are centralized in and coordinated by a single department that establishes organizationwide policies and provides human resources acquisition, retention, and separation services for other departments as well as centralized record keeping.

The more contemporary designation for the centralized staffing activities in HSOs is human resources management. With deference to the historical term, *personnel/human resources management (P/HRM)* will be used when referring to the set of centralized staffing activities, programs, and policies concerned with the acquisition, retention, and separation of employees; *human resources department* will refer to the organizational component responsible for organizationwide staffing activities, programs, and policies; and *human resources manager* will refer to the person who manages that department.

The human resources department is responsible for bringing employees into the HSO, placing them in the existing structure (acquisition), keeping those who are effective in the organization (retention), facilitating the exit of those who leave (separation), and developing policies for all persons employed in the organization (coordinating). It is a staff department that assists other departments and managers with special expertise and programs to promote harmony, quality, and productivity. Because of the centralized role of the human resources department and because employees are the organization's most important resource, the human resources manager is typically a senior manager who influences formulation and implementation of human resources policies for the whole organization.[3] This manager integrates all P/HRM activities with the HSO's strategic plans.[4]

Even though staffing activities are centralized in the human resources department, other managers must be familiar with them. First, P/HRM policies provide structure and define the interaction between managers, who are ultimately accountable for the quality and productivity of their operations and employees. Second, P/HRM policies reflect societal norms expressed in legislative and judicial employment regulations in areas such as nondiscriminatory hiring, discipline, promotion, and compensation. Better informed managers will be more effective in utilizing human resources.

STAFFING ACTIVITIES

Conceptually, P/HRM staffing activities can be viewed as a time flow incorporating two phases: acquiring and retaining the organization's human resources (Figure 17.1). Acquisition activities include human resources planning, recruitment, selection, and orientation. Retention activities include performance appraisal, placement, training and development, discipline and corrective counseling, compensation and benefits administration, employee assistance and career counseling, and safety and health.[5] These activities, along with the legislation affecting them, are described in this chapter. The final section, The Human Resources Perspective, is a longitudinal presentation that integrates changes in acquisition and retention that have occurred relative to the perspective, process, role, and philosophy of P/HRM in HSOs.

The other activity generally centralized in the human resources department—labor relations or, more specifically, collective bargaining and union-management relations[6]—is covered in Chapter 18.

ACQUIRING HUMAN RESOURCES

Human Resources Planning

Acquisition, the first activity in the time flow model in Figure 17.1, highlights the fact that human resources planning precedes recruitment, selection, and induction of new employees.[7] An HSO determines staffing needs through human resources planning. Because organizations are dynamic, these needs change. The work force must be considered in the context of a changing environment: present staff must be retained and new employees recruited to meet changing needs.[8] In the context of changing social values, it may be necessary to develop and tap new labor markets.

Staff needs in HSOs are driven by organizational growth and employee turnover. HSO growth occurs through increased demand for services, higher occupancy, facility expansion, the addition of new services, or intensifying services. Each probably necessitates more or different types of employees. Employee turnover through resignation, discharge, and retirement is the normal process of employee separation (exit). In addition to employee turnover and organizational growth, changes in technology drive the need for staff with different skills.[9] The HSO must constantly monitor the need for new employees. The human resources manager ensures that current and future needs for adequate numbers of qualified employees are met.[10] This makes human resources planning integral to P/HRM.

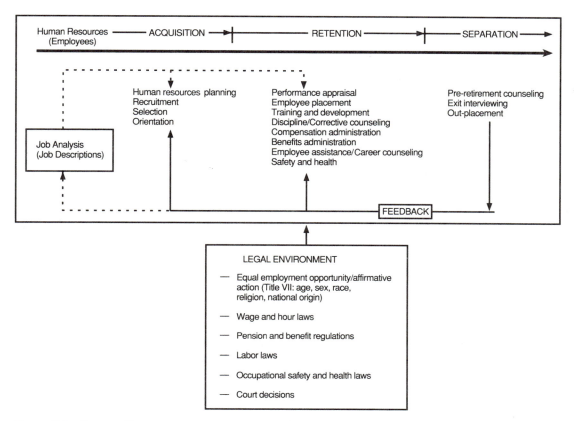

Figure 17.1. Personnel/human resource management activities time flow.

Human resources planning involves five steps: profiling, estimating, inventorying, forecasting, and planning.[11]

Step 1: Profiling Whether the human resources plan is short term (less than 2 years) or long term (2 years or more), the initial step is to profile the HSO at some future point and estimate numbers and types of jobs (skills). This is often subjective, but factors such as anticipated demand for services, changes in professional practice or labor supply, and staffing for new technologies can be taken into account in the projections.[12]

Step 2: Estimating Once a profile is developed, human resources estimates are made. Unless drastic changes are expected (a major new program or downsizing), this step is straightforward because the health services industry has established staffing ratios for most major functions. If the determining variables can be identified and quantified, a projection of needed personnel can be made. For example, knowing the number of square feet in a new facility allows accurate projections of the number of additional housekeepers needed. Similarly, if inpatient beds are added, accepted nurse staffing ratios will show personnel needs. Outpatient expansion for which the volume of services can be projected allows a determination of staff needed.

Step 3: Inventorying Present employees and their skills must be inventoried. The human resources audit (skills inventory) results from this analysis. It compiles facts about each employee's job title, experience, length of service, education, and special skills. Modified, this technique can be used to inventory all employees, including managers and clinical staff, whether salaried or independent contractors.

Step 4: Forecasting   Having obtained an assessment of present employees, the planner can forecast changes in the present work force in terms of entries and exits, as well as transfers within the HSO. All organizations experience turnover through retirement, death, voluntary separation, and discharge, and historical data are used to forecast future patterns.

Also related to these losses is movement within the organization. One factor distinguishing HSOs from other organizations is that much of the work force is trained, credentialed, and licensed for specific jobs (several examples are provided in Chapter 2). This means there is little upward or lateral movement as compared to other types of organizations. Nevertheless, upward movement occurs because of promotion, particularly into managerial positions, and lateral movement as a result of transfer. Succession planning is performed for managerial positions,[13] but all such movement must be taken into account when forecasting changes in the present work force.

It is likely that the skills inventory factors of experience and education will have to be adjusted upward over time. An older, mature organization will have stabilized in this sense (reached a norm), whereas a new organization will have wider statistical variations. As noted in Chapter 2, many states have continuing education requirements for certain categories of health services employees. Particular emphasis is placed on managers of skilled facilities, physicians, and nurses. Professional associations that certify their members are likely to have similar requirements.

Step 5: Planning   Assumptions made in steps 1 through 4 are the basis for an action plan that ensures the appropriate number of employees with requisite skills are available as required. Human resources needs identified through an organizationwide continuous quality improvement (CQI) program are factored into the human resources plan.

Summary   Human resources planning deals with a dynamic situation in which the human resources department continuously works with other managers to forecast staffing needs on the basis of changes that will occur in the present work force and develops an action plan to fill those needs through recruiting and hiring new employees, transferring existing employees, or enhancing the skills of existing employees through training and development. The human resources plan determines how the HSO's future staffing needs will be met.

Human Resources Sources

A standard way to classify sources of human resources is to separate them into two categories: internal and external sources.[14] Using internal sources means the HSO fills a vacancy by transferring or promoting from within. Using internal sources is cost effective, is usually quicker, reduces recruiting and relocation costs, and enhances employee morale. To use present employees effectively, it is important that the skills inventory include career path planning when appropriate and that necessary training be provided to upgrade employees with potential for promotion or transfer.

In addition to internal sources, new employees may be recruited from outside. Advertising vacancies or relying on present employees to "pass the word" to potential employees often generates applications. Visits to schools and colleges, contacts with public and private employment agencies, and participation in professional organizations may also be useful.

There are other sources for health workers, including those who simply walk through the door. Selecting the source depends on the qualifications required, labor market supply, geographical area, employer's reputation, and perhaps teaching affiliations. Significant recruiting problems exist in many geographical areas (primarily rural and inner city). They are exacerbated by job fragmentation and specialization, uneven work force distribution, increasing demand for health services, career alternatives for women, an aging population, and differences in public educational support.

At present, approximately 200 different types of positions are required to staff a general acute care community hospital, and well over 300 for a large metropolitan teaching facility, and the numbers are growing. Acquiring and retaining a suitably diverse work force is one of the major tasks facing management.

Job Analysis and Job Descriptions

A fundamental activity for which the human resources department has responsibility is developing and maintaining job descriptions for all positions. P/HRM staffing activities such as recruitment, selection, performance appraisal, and compensation administration depend on job descriptions.[15] In addition, much of equal employment opportunity law is inexorably bound to the job description as a basic document. Thus, time, money, and effort spent developing and maintaining job description documents are a good investment.

Job Analysis   Before new employees can be recruited, selected, and oriented in an HSO, there must be a guide to indicate what types of training, skills, and experience are required. This information is generally obtained from job analysis.[16] The human resources department is responsible for this analysis, which consists of observing and studying a job to determine its content (duties and responsibilities), the conditions under which it is performed, and its relationship to other jobs, in order to specify the skills, training, and abilities necessary to perform the required work.[17]

There are three ways to gather job information: observation, questionnaires, and interviews.[18] Information obtained through job analysis is the source for developing a job description document.

Job Descriptions   The content and format of job description documents vary among organizations.[19] The more general practice, however, is to include job title, location, job summary, from five to nine general duties and responsibilities, supervision given or received, special working conditions (including equipment or systems used), hazards, and qualifications. A statement of qualifications should state the *minimum* education, training, experience, and demonstrated skills required to perform a job satisfactorily.[20] Job descriptions should be concise for ease of understanding and, where possible, worded to permit maximum flexibility in work design. Tables 17.1 and 17.2 are sample job descriptions for a senior management and a service position.

Descriptions for each job should be maintained and updated whenever job content, performance requirements, or qualifications change. With this information, communication among managers, employees, applicants, and the human resources department is greatly simplified. When a vacancy occurs, the human resources department is notified by means of a requisition, and recruitment for someone who meets the requirements stated in the document begins. Equally important, clear and simple communication is facilitated by using the document in human resources planning, selection, performance appraisal, employee compensation, and training and development.

Recruitment

Recruitment involves searching for and attracting prospective employees, either from outside or within the HSO.[21] There are many ways to recruit potential employees and selecting among them is related to a large extent to the labor market. If no special skills or training are required for the job and labor supply is ample, recruitment may mean simply sorting applications from walk-in applicants. For other jobs, shortages may have existed for years. Here, HSOs must compete for available supply.[22]

Nurse Recruiting   The effect of competition is exemplified by recruiting for registered nurses (RNs), particularly under conditions of short supply and high annual turnover (30% for the typical hospital).[23] As in the 1980s, many health care providers have formal programs to attract RNs.

Table 17.1. Sample job description for a senior management position

Job Title: President
(Administrator)
(Chief executive officer)

Brief Summary:

Provide leadership, direction, and administration of all aspects of hospital/multiorganizational activities and other corporate entities to [e]nsure compliance with established objectives and the realization of quality, economical health care services, and other related lines of business.

Principal Duties and Responsibilities:

Participate with the governing board in charting the course the hospital is to take in response to the developing needs of the community and carrying it out accordingly.

Recommend and update long-range plans which support the institution's philosophy and general objectives.

Recommend hospital policy positions regarding administrative policy, legislation, government, and other matters of public policy.

Inform and advise trustees regarding current trends, problems, and activities in health care to facilitate policy making.

Participate in and coordinate selection process of new Board members.

In coordination with the board, the [clinical] staff and other hospital personnel, respond to the community's needs for quality health care services by monitoring the adequacy of the hospital's medical activities.

Consult with relevant personnel and departments prior to recommending/establishing new policies and the availability of resources to implement same.

Coordinate efforts of [clinical] staff, board, and administrative staff in the recruitment and retention of medical personnel.

[E]nsure the provision of affordable health care services by the acquisition, utilization, and organization of available resources (human, financial, and physical) and the development of improved techniques and practices. Coordinate the long-range fund raising efforts of the institution.

[E]nsure compliance with all regulatory agencies governing health care delivery and the rules of accrediting bodies by continually monitoring the operations and its programs and physical properties, and initiating changes where required.

Encourage the integration of the hospital with the community through effective communication and public relations programs.

Direct and supervise all hospital activities through administrator and/or competent administrative support staff and department heads. Provide assistance to supervisory personnel in establishing department philosophy and objectives; determining staffing needs and standards of productivity; establishing policies and procedures and job classifications; complying with federal, state, and local codes, regulations, and ordinances. Consult with and advise department heads on a regular basis; evaluate competence of work force and make changes as necessary; keep lines of communication open; seek to maintain high employee morale and a professional, healthful atmosphere and environment in the hospital.

Serve as liaison and channel of communication between the board and any of its committees and [clinical] staff and assist with organizational and medicoadministrative problems and responsibilities.

Represent hospital in its relationships with other health agencies, organizations, groups; in dealings with government agencies and third party payors; at top level meetings (national, state, local). May assign administrative support personnel, department heads, others to this task.

Maintain professional affiliations and enhance professional growth and development to keep abreast of latest trends in hospital administration.

Perform other related administrative/managerial duties as directed/required.

Working Conditions:

Subject to long and irregular hours; many interruptions. Generally sedentary position.

Knowledge, Skills, Experience Required:

MHA/MBA/MS in hospital administration, health care administration, or equivalent educational experience. Sufficient previous management experience in hospital administration.

From American Society for Health Care Human Resources Administration. *Health care occupations: A comprehensive job description manual,* 19–20. Chicago, 1985; reprinted by permission.

School recruiting The source of nurses is college or university baccalaureate or associate degree programs geographically near the HSO. Recruiters set up displays, distribute literature, and conduct campus interviews.

Job fairs Job fairs are of two types. In the first, numerous HSOs are brought together by a school, an independent entrepreneur who charges a fee, or some organization of employers, such as a state hospital association. Typically, each HSO sets up a booth and

Table 17.2. Sample job description for a service position

FLSA: NONEXEMPT	JOB TITLE: PATIENT CARE ASSISTANT	☐ New ☒ Revised MAY 7, 1992
EEO CATEGORY: 03 TECHNICIAN	JOB CODE: 795-#10	APPROVED BY:

This description is intended to describe the general nature and level of work being performed by people assigned to this classification. This is not intended to be construed as an exhaustive list of all responsibilities, duties, and skills required of personnel so classified. Further, this description is not intended to limit or in any way modify the right of any supervisor to assign, direct, and control the work of employees under his/her supervision.

A. GENERAL SUMMARY
Under limited supervision, performs specific basic and nontechnical duties in accordance with established methods, techniques, and facility standards. Provides patient care within limits defined by delegated tasks, handling and caring for patients in a manner conducive to their safety and comfort. Maintains records as directed by the unit staff and/or Charge Nurse.

B. DUTIES AND RESPONSIBILITIES
  1. Responsible for daily care of patients including assisting with personal hygiene, distributing meals and assisting with feeding, collecting specimens, and assuring comfort and safety. (85%)
  2. Records care given, weight, vital signs, intake and output of patients as instructed. (5%)
  3. Recognizes and reports symptoms indicative of patient's adverse reactions to treatments or unusual responses to daily care. (5%)
  4. Maintains clean, neat patient unit and work area. (5%)

C. KNOWLEDGE, SKILLS, AND ABILITIES
Minimum: High School graduate, must complete acute care nursing assistant certification course; one year health care experience; familiar with medical terminology; ability to lift heavy weights; Basic Cardiac Life Support Certification. Preferred: Students in health care program.

D. SUPERVISION GIVEN AND/OR RECEIVED
Reports to: Nursing Director, Supervisor

E. WORKING CONDITIONS
Exposed to unpleasant sights, sounds, odors, communicable diseases, and difficult interpersonal situations. May be exposed to blood/body fluids.

F. PHYSICAL DEMANDS
Extended periods of walking, lifting, pulling/pushing beds and stretchers. Assists with restraining disoriented persons.

Reprinted by permission of St. Lawrence's Hospital and Healthcare Services, Lansing, Michigan.

candidates speak to nurse recruiters. A second type of job fair is sponsored by one employer and is usually held on the employer's premises. Here, recruiting is more intense and detailed.

Bonuses An elaborate array of incentives includes cash sign-on bonuses for new RNs and for referring employees and choice scheduling assignments.[25] If the supply is especially acute, other inducements such as relocation expenses, temporary housing, and retention (longevity) bonuses are provided.

Nurse registry Recognizing the demographics of a target occupation is important to an effective human resources recruiting program. HSOs encourage RNs to re-enter the work force by recognizing that most are women and that they may not be the sole breadwinners, creating a classification of employee for whom scheduling is irregular or is for only a few days per month. Often referred to as "casuals," "PRNs," or "on-calls," these RNs are used to fill in during vacations or sick call-ins by the regular staff. They also can be used as a swing force for periods of heavy work load. Increased flexibility in working hours is also an attraction to many RNs who otherwise might not work, and it provides a valuable source of employees. Another benefit is that "casuals" often are less costly than regular employees because they usually work for wages only and do not receive benefits.

Refresher courses Some RNs leave the work force to raise families. To encourage their return, many HSOs collaborate with community colleges to establish educational programs that review nursing basics and teach current practices. Coupled with clinical experiences in the HSO, these programs build confidence and lessen stress for returning RNs.[24]

In some areas, typically large metropolitan areas, the shortage of RNs can be so acute that independent for-profit agencies supply nurses to work flexible schedules for wages only. Agencies command high fees and pay higher wages than HSOs. Using agency nurses is both addictive (as an RN shortage grows they are an easy and quick solution) and expensive compared with hiring RNs directly. In addition, lack of continuity may adversely affect quality of care.

Selection

When recruitment is effective, the organization will have applicants for job openings. The next step is to select from among them using job qualifications as a guide. The essence of selection is determining whether an applicant is suited for the job in terms of training, experience, and ability.[26] Three basic sources of information are used in selection: application forms, preemployment interviews, and testing.

Application Forms and Preemployment Interviews Historical and background information about the applicant, such as education, training, and previous employment, can be obtained from the application form. Figure 17.2 provides one example of such a form. References and letters of recommendation confirm application data. Also, properly conducted interviews can yield much useful information about an applicant.

Two types of interviews are widely used. The first is a directed interview, which is planned and led by the interviewer. It is confined to objectively verifiable facts about which the interviewer expects to get information by asking specific questions. This type of interview is most often used when employees are being selected, when job descriptions are being prepared, and when an employee is exiting (exit interview). The second type is a nondirected interview that has the more ambitious purpose of achieving understanding beyond specific facts.[27] In practice the two often merge, and effective interviewers change as the situation warrants.

The primary purpose of the application form and preemployment interview is to provide the organization with information about the applicant. However, federal and state laws, as well as judicial decisions concerning fair employment practices and equal employment opportunity, identify certain application forms and preemployment interview practices as discriminatory and, therefore, illegal. It is important for managers to recognize that state and federal law also restrict information that may be obtained and preemployment questions that may be asked to those that have a job-related business purpose. Many employers collect such applicant information as race, marital status, number of dependent children, and date of birth on a separate form that is not given to those persons who make the employment decision. These data can then be used for Equal Employment Opportunity Commission (EEOC) reporting requirements.[28] If such a separate reporting system is not in place, "once an employer tells an applicant that he or she is hired (the 'point of hire'), inquiries that were prohibited earlier can be made."[29] Table 17.3 outlines specific preemployment issues addressed by court and regulatory decisions.[30]

Testing Given the importance of a decision to hire, it is understandable that human resources and first-line managers have sought more refined methods to evaluate and screen applicants. A wide variety of preemployment tests is used to determine which candidate is best suited for a position.

Preemployment testing has been closely scrutinized by several federal agencies, including the EEOC and the Department of Labor. Basic regulations have been compiled in the "Uniform

Guidelines on Employee Selection Procedures"[31] and are primarily aimed at the issues of adverse impact. In *Griggs v. Duke Power Co.*,[32] the Supreme Court stated that if a test has an adverse impact on the selection of women or minorities, which occurs when they fail the test in significantly greater percentages than the overall failure rate, the employer using the test must prove that it is a valid indicator of the abilities needed to perform the job. This showing must be made even if there is proof that the employer did not intend to discriminate.

There are three forms of validity in testing.[33]

Content validity: the test recreates or represents significant sample parts of the job, such as typing tests.

Construct validity: the test identifies a psychological or personality trait important to successful performance, such as leadership or problem solving abilities.

Criterion-related validity: the test contains elements on which anyone who would do well on the job will perform well, or anyone who would do poorly on the job will perform poorly.

The strict and complex guidelines for using preemployment testing suggest it should be used only for specialized or high-level positions or when incorrect selection will have significant cost and patient care consequences. Experts should be consulted to develop the test instruments. Content-valid tests are the simplest and safest.

Selection—A Shared Responsibility   The question of who makes the final employment selection from among screened candidates is critical. Selection remains an inexact science despite all the techniques that have been developed and used. Ideally, the decision is made by the manager to whom the new employee will report, with the advice and counsel of the human resources department. This approach has the advantages that stipulated and necessary credential requirements are met; organizational policies and employment laws are applied; and individuals selected meet the HSO's quality standards and conform to its philosophy.

Orientation

After selection, induction and orientation occur. Induction activities are typically carried out by the human resources department and include enrolling new employees in benefit plans, issuing an identification badge, and creating a basic data base for the individual. Most HSOs require a preemployment physical to screen for communicable disease; to ensure that individuals can perform the job without danger to themselves or others; for workers' compensation risk management purposes; and to detect and document preexisting health conditions.

The orientation program should include information about the physical plant, organizational structure, universal precautions, fire and safety programs, employee health service, employee assistance program, and other human resources department services. Key policies and benefits should be explained in detail. In some departments orientation may include an extended period of training and orienting the employee to work methods. This is done through on-the-job training, utilizing preceptors, and/or formal classroom training.

An important part of inducting new employees into the HSO is informing them about its philosophy and objectives. Successful orientation builds employees' sense of identification with the HSO, helps them gain acceptance by fellow workers, and gives them a clear understanding of the many things they need to know. Ideally, the orientation program enables new employees to become familiar with the entire organization as well as their own work area and department. This can be done by a group or personal tour, a pictorial description such as a slide program, or a combination of these. New employees should personally meet members of management and be able to ask questions.

Orientation is an important time for both the organization and the individual. The program or process of orientation should clearly communicate a philosophy and sense of purpose. It is here that employees form perceptions of the organization, their role in it, and what is expected of them.[34] Inappropriate norms of behavior established early are difficult to change later.

Equal Employment Opportunity

In recruiting and selecting new employees, and throughout their employment, one role of the human resources department is to establish and implement nondiscriminatory P/HRM policies that comply with state and federal law.[35] Such legislation and regulations affect the employment relationship from recruitment and selection to retention activities such as promotion and transfer, compensation, and layoffs.

WE OFFER EQUAL EMPLOYMENT OPPORTUNITY TO ALL BASED UPON INDIVIDUAL MERIT AND ABILITY, AND
WITHOUT REGARD TO RACE, COLOR, RELIGION, NATIONAL ORIGIN, SEX, AGE, HEIGHT, WEIGHT, HANDICAP, OR MARITAL STATUS.

NAME - LAST		FIRST		MIDDLE	SOCIAL SECURITY NO.	DATE
ADDRESS - NUMBER	STREET		CITY	COUNTY	STATE	ZIP CODE

| PHONE NO'S. | HOME | | OFFICE | | ANOTHER PHONE WHERE YOU CAN BE CONTACTED |

| TYPE OF EMPLOYMENT YOU WANT | ☐ FULL-TIME | ☐ PART-TIME | ☐ TEMPORARY | ARE YOU 18 YEARS OF AGE OR OLDER? | ☐ YES ☐ NO |

| WHAT SHIFT ARE YOU WILLING TO WORK? | ☐ DAYS | ☐ EVENINGS | ☐ NIGHTS | ☐ ROTATING |

POSITION YOU DESIRE

REFERRAL SOURCE
☐ EMPLOYEE ☐ ADVERTISEMENT

| HAVE YOU EVER BEEN EMPLOYED BY THIS HSO BEFORE? | ☐ YES ☐ NO | IF YES, POSITION | ☐ OTHER _____ |

PREVIOUS NAMES USED WHILE WORKING OR ATTENDING SCHOOL

HAVE YOU EVER BEEN CONVICTED OF A FELONY? IF YES, PLEASE EXPLAIN:
☐ YES ☐ NO

EDUCATION

	NAME AND LOCATION	ATTENDED (DATES)	MAJOR COURSES	DEGREE OR DIPLOMA RECEIVED (SPECIFY)
HIGH SCHOOL		FROM		
		UNTIL		
SPECIALIZED EDUCATION		FROM		
		UNTIL		
COLLEGE OR UNIVERSITY		FROM		
		UNTIL		
LIST ANY OTHER EDUCATIONAL EXPERIENCES		FROM		
		UNTIL		

PROFESSIONAL LICENSES AND REGISTRATIONS

YOUR ORIGINAL PROFESSIONAL OR VOCATIONAL LICENSE OR REGISTRATION	STATE	NUMBER	EXPIRATION DATE	
	WAS GRANTED BY ☐ EXAMINATION	☐ WAIVER	☐ ENDORSEMENT	NO. 04400

Figure 17.2. Sample application for employment. Reprinted by permission of St. Lawrence's Hospital and Healthcare Services, Lansing, Michigan.

Figure 17.2. *(continued)*

COMPLETE EMPLOYMENT HISTORY (LIST MOST RECENT POSITION FIRST)

COMPANY NAME AND ADDRESS	FROM	POSITION AND DUTIES	
	TO		
PHONE ( )	SALARY	NAME OF SUPERVISOR	REASON FOR LEAVING
COMPANY NAME AND ADDRESS	FROM	POSITION AND DUTIES	
	TO		
PHONE ( )	SALARY	NAME OF SUPERVISOR	REASON FOR LEAVING
COMPANY NAME AND ADDRESS	FROM	POSITION AND DUTIES	
	TO		
PHONE ( )	SALARY	NAME OF SUPERVISOR	REASON FOR LEAVING
COMPANY NAME AND ADDRESS	FROM	POSITION AND DUTIES	
	TO		
PHONE ( )	SALARY	NAME OF SUPERVISOR	REASON FOR LEAVING

LIST ANY OTHER QUALIFICATIONS NOT COVERED ELSEWHERE ON THIS APPLICATION

OFFICE TRAINING

ESTIMATED TYPING SPEED (WORDS PER MINUTE)	
OFFICE MACHINES AND COMPUTER SOFTWARE WITH WHICH YOU HAVE EXPERIENCE	

ALL APPLICANTS READ CAREFULLY AND SIGN BELOW

I AUTHORIZE THE HSO TO INVESTIGATE ALL STATEMENTS CONTAINED IN THIS APPLICATION. I UNDERSTAND THAT ANY FALSE STATEMENTS OR UNSATISFACTORY REFERENCES MAY AT ANY TIME BE GROUNDS FOR IMMEDIATE TERMINATION OF MY EMPLOYMENT. I UNDERSTAND THAT IF CONSIDERED FOR EMPLOYMENT, I SHALL BE REQUIRED TO SUBMIT TO A PRE-EMPLOYMENT PHYSICAL EXAMINATION FOR THE PURPOSE OF DETERMINING WHETHER I HAVE ANY PHYSICAL OR MEDICAL IMPAIRMENTS OR CONTAGIOUS DISEASES WHICH MIGHT INTERFERE WITH MY ABILITY TO DO THE JOB FOR WHICH I HAVE APPLIED OR AM CONSIDERED. FURTHER, I CERTIFY THAT COPIES OF THIS STATEMENT CONSTITUTE AUTHORIZATION FOR ANY PAST EMPLOYERS, COMPANIES, SCHOOLS, UNIVERSITIES AND PERSONS TO PROVIDE THE HSO WITH ANY AND ALL INFORMATION THEY HAVE REGARDING MY EMPLOY-MENT OR ACADEMIC RECORD INCLUDING, BUT NOT LIMITED TO, PERFORMANCE, ATTENDANCE, ATTITUDE, ABILITY, AND CONDUCT. I HEREBY RELEASE SAID PAST EMPLOYERS, COMPANIES, SCHOOLS, UNIVERSITIES, AND PERSONS FROM ALL LIABILITY FOR ANY DAMAGE FOR PROVIDING SUCH INFORMATION.

DATE	SIGNATURE (DO NOT PRINT)
	X

NEW HIRE INFORMATION

STARTING DATE	SHIFT	NORMAL HOURS / PAY PERIOD	☐ FULL TIME ☐ PART TIME ☐ TEMPORARY ☐ CASUAL
TITLE		DEPARTMENT / UNIT #	PAY GRADE, RATE
REPLACING WHOM?		LICENSE NO.	EXPIRATION DATE
DEPARTMENT HEAD SIGNATURE			DATE
EMPLOYEE SIGNATURE			DATE

Table 17.3. Guidelines for specific preemployment issues addressed by court and EEOC decisions

Age Requests for age may deter older applicants or may indicate discriminatory intent. If age is asked, its purpose should be made known to the applicant.

Arrest Records The use of arrest records without proof of business necessity is unlawful. Request may indicate discriminatory intent.

Citizenship Banning the employment of aliens and restricting employment to U.S. citizens are illegal because the consideration of an applicant's citizenship may lead to discrimination based on national origin.

Education Educational minimums require proof of significant relationship to successful job performance.

Financial Status Inquiries into an applicant's bankruptcy status, credit rating, home or car ownership, length of residence, or garnishments without proof of business purpose are discriminatory.

Friends or Relatives If preference for employing the friends or relatives of employees reduces opportunities for protected individuals, it is discriminatory. Nepotism policies that reduce opportunities for employee spouses or relatives also discriminate.

Handicaps Federal law protects qualified individuals with a physical or mental impairment limiting one or more major life activities, with a record of such impairment, or being regarded as having such an impairment. On-the-job substance abuse is not a handicap. Historical substance abuse and AIDS are handicaps. Reasonable accommodation is required.

Height and Weight Minimum height and weight requirements that screen out disproportionate numbers of minorities and are not essential to safe performance are illegal.

Marital Status, Number of Children, Child Care Questions in these non–job-related areas are discriminatory. Information needed for tax, insurance, or social security purposes may be obtained after employment. Policies for hiring men and women with preschool children must be the same.

Military Discharge Dishonorable and general discharges are not absolute bars to employment. Inquiries to determine need for further investigation, not to decide on hiring, are legitimate.

National Security It is not unlawful to deny employment to any individual who does not fulfill national security requirements.

Race, Color, Sex Request for such are not unlawful, but when asked can show discriminatory intent, as can related questions (former residence, former name, citizenship, photograph, organizational membership, or marriage into certain ethnic groups).

Religious Preference Questions relating to availability for work on Friday evenings, Saturdays, or holidays should not be asked.

The legal concept of equal employment opportunity was articulated in Title VII of the Civil Rights Act of 1964.[36] This law and its regulations dominate the field and prohibit discriminatory practices based on "race, color, national origin, religion or sex," but it is not the only noteworthy relevant legislation. In 1963, Congress amended the Fair Labor Standards Act by requiring "equal pay" for substantially equal work, without regard to sex.[37] As is noted later, this amendment was important in the comparable worth cases of the early 1980s.

Age discrimination legislation is also rooted in the 1960s. The Age Discrimination in Employment Act of 1967 prohibited discrimination against employees between the ages of 40 and 65.[38] Similar to the equal pay amendment, its full effect was felt in 1979 when the minimum mandatory retirement age was raised from 65 to 70, and in 1986 when mandatory retirement was barred.[39]

Other legislation that affects P/HRM selection and retention activities is the Americans with Disabilities Act (ADA) of 1990. It prohibits discrimination against the estimated 43 million Americans who have disabilities.[40] Employment-related provisions apply in July 1992 for employers with more than 25 workers and in July 1994 for employers with 15 or more workers.[41] The ADA's wording is almost identical to the Rehabilitation Act of 1973 and prohibits discrimination in virtually all areas of employment on the basis of handicap or disability.[42] During the selection process, employers may not make inquiries or conduct medical exams designed to identify applicants with disabilities.[43] Private employers must make "reasonable accommodation" for qualified workers unless it can be shown that such accommodation would cause "undue hardship" for the employer. Examples of reasonable accommodation are modifying facilities, job restructuring, part-time and modified work schedules, and reassignment.[44] Persons covered by the ADA are those "with a physical or mental impairment that substantially limits 'one or more major life activities.' This covers a broad range of disabilities such as blindness, paralysis, heart disease, cancer, AIDS, emotional illness, low IQ, and learning disabilities."[45] "Sexual disorders, homosexuality . . . and drug usage are, in general, not covered as disabilities."[46] However, alcohol and drug abusers who rehabilitate themselves are covered by the ADA.[47]

Space is too limited to address all the complex laws relating to employment practices; however, it is essential that first-line managers understand the basic concepts and how they affect the staffing function and managers' interaction with employees.[48]

What Is Equal Opportunity and Discrimination?   The Civil Rights Act of 1967 defines unlawful employment practices in broad terms. Title VII, section 703, of the Act specifically forbids employers from:

> Failing or refusing to hire; or
>> to discharge or otherwise discriminate against any individual with respect to terms, conditions, or privileges of employment; or
>> to limit, segregate, or classify employees in any way that would deprive or tend to deprive any individual of employment opportunity or otherwise adversely affect the individual's status as an employee due to race, color, religion, sex, or national origin.[49]

These provisions broadly prohibit employers from using the specified categories to adversely affect employees or candidates for employment.

Passage of the act and its interpretation by the courts caused HSOs to realize that some of their P/HRM practices were discriminatory. The criteria for determining whether a practice was illegal hinged primarily on whether it had an adverse effect on a class of people protected by the act or whether the practice was a *bona fide* occupational qualification.

Adverse Impact   In a case of adverse impact the question is whether a certain practice in recruitment, selection, compensation, transfer, or discharge has been shown to adversely affect a protected class. This can be determined with the aid of sophisticated statistical measures that show the variance between the percentage of a class of minorities in the local population and its percentage in the employer's work force. If the employer's work force has fewer employees of that class than one would expect on the basis of population, courts may assume that discrimination, either intentional or unintentional, has taken place.

Bona Fide Occupational Qualifications   Title VII, section 703, of the Civil Rights Act

> defines what employment practices are unlawful. This same section, however, exempts several key practices from the scope of Title VII. The most important are the *bona fide* occupational qualification exemption, the testing and educational requirements section, and the seniority system exemption.[50]

Bona fide occupational qualifications provide an opportunity for employers to justify or explain a suspect practice by giving nondiscriminatory business reasons for it. The following are examples of applying these concepts in an HSO:

> *Testing*—Preemployment tests are not illegal per se, but they are closely scrutinized. Often, they are found to be culturally biased because they cause more minority applicants to be rejected. *Bona fide* occupational qualifications determine that what is being tested is related to the job or serves as a valid predictor of success.
>
> *Physical requirements*—A formerly common, but now illegal, practice was a requirement that applicants be a certain size or be able to lift certain weight. Such requirements must be justified as necessary to the job (*bona fide* occupational qualifications) or they risk being found discriminatory based on sex.
>
> *Educational background*—In an earnest, but misguided, effort to upgrade their labor force, many managers specify educational requirements for a job that adversely affect a protected class. For example, the job description for a housekeeper may require that the

employee be a high school graduate. This requirement has been shown to adversely affect minorities because fewer of them graduate from high school. Coupled with the fact that it is not a *bona fide* occupational qualification (only basic reading and math skills are needed), the requirement has often been set aside as discriminatory.

Where a *bona fide* seniority system exists, such as in union contracts, differences in employment conditions are allowed if they are not caused by an intent to discriminate. "The term 'seniority system' is generally understood to mean a set of rules which ensure workers with longer continuous service for an employer a priority claim to a job over others with fewer years of experience."[51]

Affirmative Action   Another factor to be considered in recruitment and selection is affirmative action planning. "Affirmative action focuses on the hiring, training, and promotion of protected groups where there are deficiencies."[52] Contrary to common belief, affirmative action is neither defined nor required under Title VII of the Federal Civil Rights Act of 1964, as amended. However, when the EEOC, the administrative and enforcement agency for Title VII of the Civil Rights Act, finds that an employer has discriminated, it may request that the employer adopt a voluntary affirmative action plan. If the employer refuses, the EEOC may appeal to the courts, which can order affirmative action to correct the deficiencies.

An affirmative action plan is an organization's positive remedy for activities that created inequality or lack of equal opportunity in its employment program. It is a results-oriented program designed to materially affect the status quo by increasing the number of employees from a target group population, such as blacks, women, or Hispanics. An example would be an employer who did not hire Hispanics in an area where the population and work force is 13% Hispanic. An affirmative action plan might require the employer to hire only Hispanics until they represented 13% of the work force.

A voluntarily adopted affirmative action plan simply formalizes development and implementation of an employer's nondiscrimination policy by establishing goals to be achieved in a specific time frame. A comprehensive affirmative action plan defines all aspects of the employer–employee relationship: employment, promotion, demotion, layoff, termination, recruitment, rates of pay, employee benefits, and selection for training. The plan may include provisions that the organization will not purchase from or contract with firms that discriminate. A business providing services or products under contract to the federal government must meet special provisions that strictly delineate affirmative action requirements. To date, the Office of Federal Contract Compliance, which administers affirmative action planning, has not required affirmative action on the part of HSOs solely because they participate in Medicare. The order does apply, however, to federal government contracts that include, but are not limited to, grants for research, education, and training and to federal contractors who subcontract with an HSO for provision of services.

Sexual Harassment   Title VII of the 1964 Civil Rights Act did not specifically address sexual harassment in the workplace; however, subsequent court rulings recognized it as a form of discrimination.[53] HSOs employ large numbers of females and HSO managers should have a working knowledge of what sexual harassment is and how to prevent it.

EEOC guidelines define sexual harassment as follows:

> Unwelcome sexual advances, requests for sexual favors, and other verbal or physical conduct of a sexual nature constitute sexual harassment when (1) submission to such conduct is made either explicitly or implicitly a term or condition of an individual's employment, (2) submission to or rejection of such conduct by an individual is used as the basis for employment decisions affecting such individual, or (3) such conduct has the purpose or effect of unreasonably interfering with an individual's work performance or creating an intimidating, hostile, or offensive working environment.[54]

The first two forms are categorized as *quid pro quo* because "an employer or supervisor links specific employment outcomes to the individual's granting sexual favors." The third is *hostile environment* harassment.[55]

The advances need not have been made by the subject's supervisor to be defined as sexual harassment. Co-workers and customers can cause the employer to be liable if the employer "knows or should have known of the conduct and fails to take immediate and appropriate corrective action."[56]

The following actions by employers are recommended to prevent sexual harassment:

Developing a policy on sexual harassment and distributing a copy of the policy to all employees.
Identifying ways in which individuals who feel they have been harassed can report the incidents without fear of retaliation, and creating procedures to ensure that complaints are satisfactorily investigated and appropriate action is taken.
Communicating to all employees, especially to supervisors and managers, concerns and regulations regarding sexual harassment and the importance of creating and maintaining a work environment free of sexual harassment.
Disciplining offenders by using organizational sanctions up to and including firing the offenders.
Training all employees, especially supervisors and managers, about what constitutes sexual harassment, and alerting employees to the issues and behaviors involved.[57]

Workforce Diversity

Workforce 2000: Work and Workers for the 21st Century[58] contains two important messages for the health services industry: 1) the work force will grow slowly during the 1990s, becoming older and more disadvantaged; and 2) new jobs in service industries will demand much higher skill levels. Successful management of that increasingly diverse work force is the key to continued delivery of high-quality care. The American Hospital Association (AHA) states that this includes being "cognizant of and responsive to the concerns and needs of different ethnic, cultural, and age groups. Greater effort will be required to create an environment that recognizes the contributions of different perspectives to the delivery of health care services."[59] To successfully implement and sustain HSO quality and productivity improvement programs, the human resources department and managers must take into account the changing workplace and an increasingly diverse work force.

Success is most likely if all employees have an opportunity to perform to their full potential. The measures of success are a system that values human need, actions that show respect and dignity for every person, and employees who show others that their HSO is an excellent place for women, minorities, and senior citizens to work.

RETAINING EMPLOYEES

After human resources needs have been determined and people are recruited and selected, retention activities occur throughout the term of employment. These P/HRM activities include appraising each employee's job performance; moving employees within the organization through promotion, demotion, and transfer; disciplinary counseling and separation, when necessary; administering compensation and benefits; providing employee assistance and career counsel; and ensuring health and personal safety (see Figure 17.1).

Performance Appraisal

The human resources department establishes and maintains an organizationwide employee performance appraisal system to be used by managers.[60] Appraisal systems evaluate an employee's work by comparing actual with expected performance.

Uses of Performance Appraisal   The results of performance appraisal have many uses. Among them are:

Determining whether individual work results are consistent with expectations. As managers integrate the structure, tasks/technology, and people components of the organization, work results occur (see the management model in Chapter 1, Figure 1.6). Performance appraisal is a systematic way of collecting information to assess whether results are those expected and, if not, to determine why not.

Providing feedback to both employee and supervisor. The performance appraisal interview is a formal opportunity for two-way communication. Positive performance can be reinforced. Less than satisfactory performance can be discussed, reasons for it identified, interventions formulated, and future expectations established.

Identifying high, marginal, and unsatisfactory performers. Depending on the assessment of employee performance levels and their causes, various interventions can be used. Less than satisfactory performance may be due to employee variables such as a lack of technical job skills or experience, or it may be due to process or job design. Based on this information, interventions such as developmental education, skills training, or job redesign may be warranted. If performance is unsatisfactory for reasons of attitude and behavior, counseling, discipline, or separation may be warranted. The purpose of performance appraisal is to monitor and, when possible, to constructively improve each employee's ability to do the job well.

Identifying potential and desirable employee movement within the organization. The results of performance appraisal can influence an employee's candidacy for promotion, as well as transfer and demotion. High performers may be promoted with or without further skill building; low performers may be transferred or demoted to a job more suitable to their skills and abilities.

Providing information for compensation. If organizations have a wage and salary system incorporating merit compensation, performance appraisal provides data for determining wage adjustments based on performance.

Providing information for employee assistance and counseling. If an employee's performance is unsatisfactory because of substance abuse or off-the-job personal problems, the performance appraisal process may reveal that external assistance is recommended.

Virtually all P/HRM retention activities are linked to performance appraisal. As a result, it is a control and information-gathering system of great importance to managers and the HSO.

Appraisal Methods   There are many approaches to employee performance appraisal. Among them are the rating scale, person-to-person comparison, checklist, and critical incident methods.[61] The most commonly used appraisal system is the rating scale method. The scales typically specify: 1) personal traits and behaviors such as cooperativeness, dependability, initiative, judgment, and attitude; and 2) job dimension attributes such as quantity of work, quality of work, and job knowledge. For each scale there is usually a scoring mechanism using single descriptive adjectives such as "poor" or "excellent," key descriptive phrases, or some other method of differentiation, such as numerical values that often range from 1 (poor) to 10 (excellent). Figure 17.3 presents a sample rating scale employee evaluation (appraisal) form consisting of both personal/behavioral and job dimension scales, with a key phrase scoring system.

Benefits of Systematic Appraisal   A formal performance evaluation system provides a standard format by which managers throughout the organization assess their employees' performance. It also forces managers to observe how well employees are performing and to consider what can be done to improve performance. A formal appraisal system serves another important purpose. Employees have a right to know how well they are doing and what can be done to improve. Most employees want to know what supervisors think of their work out of concern for self-worth and a need for reassurance.

Formal written appraisals of all employees are normally required on an annual basis; however, good management practice and maintenance of high productivity require more frequent feedback on an informal basis. If an employee has just started a new or more responsible position, an appraisal within three months is advisable. In some organizations, appraisals are made according to hire dates; in others, all appraisals are made once or twice a year on fixed dates. As an employee achieves longevity, periodic appraisals have an important influence on morale. They reaffirm the manager's interest in the employee's continuous development and improvement.

Appraisal Problems Despite the apparent simplicity of performance appraisal forms, a manager is often faced with a number of problems when completing them.[62] First of all, raters do not agree on the definitions of terms such as "excellent," "good," "average," or "poor." Descriptive phrases or sentences added to each of these adjectives are helpful in choosing the level that most adequately describes the employee.

The Joint Commission on Accreditation of Healthcare Organizations (Joint Commission), the American Osteopathic Association, and the United States Department of Education require *criteria-related* performance appraisal. Care must be taken to ensure that the standards of performance (concrete statements of management expectations) upon which an appraisal is based are directly related to the employee's job description. For example, if it is a medical secretary's responsibility to return patients' calls, the standard may be simply to return every call within one hour.

Another problem is that one manager's appraisal of employees may be more critical than another's. Some managers do not give low ratings because they are afraid of antagonizing subordinates, whom they believe will then be less cooperative. On the one hand, low ratings may be perceived as reflecting negatively on the manager's performance and suggesting that employees have not been motivated to improve themselves. On the other hand, rater perceptual biases can emerge, as exemplified by the appraiser who assumes no one is "excellent."

The manager should also recognize that one factor may influence others. If an employee is very strong in one area, such as quantity of work, the manager may tend to rate the employee high on most scales without critically analyzing them. One way to avoid this "halo" effect is to rate all employees on one area before starting on the next.

Finally, it is important to show employees their rating (note that there is a space for the employee's signature on the sample form in Figure 17.3), and to allow them to discuss their rating with their supervisor and to make comments in writing if they wish. Performance evaluations are one of the most important tools an employer has to build a quality work force. Full employee participation is critical to a successful appraisal system.

Management by Objectives and Appraisal Management by objectives (MBO) is a technique in which manager and employee go through a formal process of identifying and mutually agreeing on specific job performance objectives to be achieved by the employee in a given period of time.[63] MBO is a structured process, but it requires flexible goal setting. Consequently, it is more often used when jobs have some flexibility in tasks, duties, and responsibilities. The major features of MBO are:

Manager and employee clearly understand and jointly agree to the employee's principal duties and responsibilities.

The employee establishes short-term and sometimes long-term job performance objectives in cooperation with the manager, who ensures they are consistent with organizational objectives.

The manager and employee agree to criteria to be used for measuring and evaluating job performance and to milestones for monitoring whether objectives are being accomplished.

EMPLOYEE PERFORMANCE EVALUATION

Date: _____

Employee Name: _____

Job Title: _____

Department: _____

Check (√) one of the following as the reason for this particular performance evaluation.

( ) Prior to the end of the three (3) month probationary period for all new employees or when it is sufficiently clear that new employee is not likely to be satisfactory for the job.

( ) Termination of employment.

( ) Annual: 12 months from last evaluation.

( ) Other, specify: _____

PERFORMANCE REVIEW

APPRAISER: Consider the following five columns as a scale: The extreme right as outstanding, the extreme left as unusually poor. Based on your opinions, place an "X" in the box under the groups of words that best describe each quality of the individual. On the lines below each grouping, make a brief statement showing why certain conclusions were made. Evaluate only the qualities you have observed. Use additional blank sheets for opinion if necessary.

QUALITY: Freedom from errors and mistakes: accuracy: Quality of work in general.	Excessive errors and mistakes. Very poor quality.	Acceptable by minimum standards. Improvement needed.	No more mistakes than should be expected. Quality definitely acceptable.	Quality above average. Few errors & mistakes.	Highest possible quality. Final job virtually perfect.
	☐	☐	☐	☐	☐

COMMENTS: _____

QUANTITY: The actual work output of the employee relative to other employees.	Extremely low output. Definitely not acceptable.	Acceptable but low output. Below average.	Average output. Definitely acceptable.	Produces more than most. Above average.	Definitely a top producer.
	☐	☐	☐	☐	☐

COMMENTS: _____

JOB KNOWLEDGE: Knowledge of the techniques, skills, processes, equipment, and procedures.	Lacks knowledge to perform work properly.	Minimum knowledge for doing job.	Has adequate knowledge of duties.	Good knowledge of duties.	Excellent understanding of job assignments.
	☐	☐	☐	☐	☐

COMMENTS: _____

LEARNING ABILITY: Alertness & ability to advance and grow with the department.	Seems unable to learn new tasks. Cannot adjust from one job to another. Resists change.	Learns new tasks slowly. Has difficulty understanding and going from one assignment to another.	Neither slow nor fast. Can perform several related tasks. Handles new assignments with some difficulty.	Catches on fast. Learns new tasks easily. Handles new assignments with minimum amount of difficulty.	Very adaptable and flexible. Masters new tasks easily. Handles various assignments without difficulty.
	☐	☐	☐	☐	☐

COMMENTS: _____

Figure 17.3. Sample employee evaluation form.

INITIATIVE: Degree to which employee can be relied upon to do job without close supervision.	Never volunteers to undertake work. Requires constant prodding to do work. Has no drive or ambition. ☐	Needs some prodding to do work. Dislikes responsibilities. Has very little drive. Believes in just getting by. ☐	Seldom seeks new tasks. Will accept responsibilities when necessary but does not go out of way. Routine worker. ☐	Occasionally seeks new tasks. Works well when given responsibility. Makes occasional suggestion. ☐	Definitely a self-starter. Goes out of way to accept responsibility. Very alert and often constructive. ☐

COMMENTS: _____
_____

COOPERA-TIVENESS: Willingness to work harmoniously with others in getting a job done. Readiness to observe and conform to the policies of management.	Extremely negative and hard to get along with. ☐	Indifferent. Makes no effort to cooperate. ☐	Cooperative. Gets along well with others; has a good attitude. ☐	Goes out of his way to cooperate and get along. ☐	Extremely cooperative. Stimulates teamwork and good attitude in others. ☐

COMMENTS: _____
_____

ATTENDANCE: Faithfulness in coming to work daily and conforming to work hours.	Often absent without good excuse and/or frequently reports for work late. ☐	Lax in attendance and reporting for work on time. ☐	Usually present and on time. ☐	Very prompt. Regular in attendance. ☐	Always regular and prompt. ☐

COMMENTS: _____
_____

PERSONAL APPEARANCE:

This quality refers to the employee's personal grooming, attire, and overall appearance. Does the employee's personal appearance meet the standards for the job? An employee's attire is usually dictated by the nature of the work, which should be considered in evaluating this quality.

Needs Improvement _____ **Satisfactory** _____

Specific action to be taken by supervisor and/or employee to improve weaknesses.	BY WHOM	BY WHEN

ADDITIONAL RATER'S COMMENTS: _____
_____

_____ _____
Rater's Signature   Date:

EMPLOYEE COMMENTS: _____
_____

_____ _____
Employee's Signature: Date:

COMMENTS RESULTING FROM INTERVIEW: _____
_____
_____
_____

COMMENTS AND RECOMMENDATIONS: (Reviewed by Rater's Supervisor) _____
_____
_____

_____ _____
Reviewer's Signature: Date:

Figure 17.3. *(continued)*   629

Periodically, the manager and employee evaluate progress toward goals. Changes in goals are made if events warrant. Counseling and coaching support the process.

The manager plays an active role in providing organizational arrangements and coordinative mechanisms and making resources available so performance objectives can be accomplished.

Appraisal consists of measuring outcomes of work and identifying whether performance objectives have been accomplished within the specified time frame according to the criteria.

MBO has several major advantages, one of which is that involving employees in establishing performance objectives enhances their commitment to them. A second is that manager-employee communication is facilitated; each more clearly understands the other's expectations and this enhances their relationship. Third, employees can influence the decision-making process and establish performance expectations. Finally, MBO can be an excellent training and development tool if some objectives identify and correct employee weaknesses and others reinforce employee strengths.

Some disadvantages of MBO are related to appraisal.[64] First, individualized appraisals make comparing performance of persons in different departments more difficult. Second, they are very time consuming. Third, if the appraisal process is not controlled, it can result in inconsistent reward patterns across the HSO, and this creates inequity and ill will.

Continuous Quality Improvement   Peter Drucker notes "Quantity without quality is the worst thing and will result in total failure."[65] Performance appraisals are critical to monitoring quality; they provide data to measure the success of current job design and work flow (processes) as well as progress toward objectives. Quantified expectations tied to job descriptions are required to identify performance differences that highlight quality issues. Real-time performance feedback is required to achieve continuous improvement of affected processes.

Training and Development

The second basic P/HRM activity of retaining human resources is training, which involves changing behavior and expanding employee knowledge and skills through an organized process by which employees learn skills, abilities, and attitudes needed to work better. In most HSOs, training is organized into staff or line training or both.[66] Training departments are found in most large HSOs, and they educate staff on organizationwide issues such as CQI, develop managers and supervisors, and facilitate departmental (line) training. When not performed by a separate department, this function is often assigned to the human resources department. Another method is cooperative: several organizations share staff training, specialists, and cost.

Line training is department specific and is usually the responsibility of department heads. Examples include a nursing service department that provides in-service training for nursing assistants or recently graduated RNs and a housekeeping department that trains employees in proper cleaning or infection control.

Special mention should be made of supervisory and management development as a type of training. HSOs have special needs in preparing supervisors and managers because so many are drawn from technically trained staff. Management development is a way to increase the capabilities of managers "beyond a narrow range of skills to a more holistically prepared person."[67] Development focuses on general managerial skills such as leadership, motivation, communication, and problem solving. Specific skills training in report writing and budgeting may be included.

Management development may be internal or external. Internally, job rotation or vendor-delivered on-site programs that are structured or simulation based can be used to develop middle-level and senior managers.[68] Externally, periodically attending off-site seminars or professional association programs can be beneficial. Other approaches include senior managers coaching lower level managers (mentoring) and inclusion of managers on important committees. Simple things such as required reading lists can be successful.

Discipline (Corrective Counseling)

Discipline may be the least understood aspect of the HSO's relationship with employees. Most people associate discipline with punishment—a negative concept. Correctly understood, however, discipline is positive and means corrective counseling, which involves creating a climate and an attitude among employees that encourages them to accept policies and practices because they understand that doing so contributes to their success and to the HSO's success. If discipline is to be seen as positive, policies and practices must be reasonable and employees must understand what is expected of them. In addition, it must be understood that the employer has a right to a well-disciplined, cooperative work force and has authority to take action if rules are violated.

To be effective, discipline/corrective counseling should be formalized and include established procedures. While there is no one best process, certain provisions should be included:[69]

> Disciplinary/corrective counseling actions should be based on facts with clear and demonstrable justification.
> Employees should be treated consistently, with the background and circumstances of each case considered separately.
> Disciplinary actions should be progressive and related to behavior; in order of severity, typical actions are: 1) unrecorded oral warning, 2) oral warning noted in the employment record, 3) written warning noted in the employment record, 4) suspension from the job, and 5) discharge.

Including these provisions does not guarantee that a disciplinary program will meet its objectives, but they go far toward ensuring a positive approach to discipline in the HSO.

Compensation Administration

One of the most important aspects of maintaining and retaining a suitable work force is effective compensation administration. Compensation is a generic term for wages, salaries, and fringe benefits and directly affects the organization's ability to attract and retain qualified employees. In HSOs, the human resources department has responsibility for developing, implementing, and administering an organizationwide compensation program.[70]

Equity is the primary objective of compensation programs. Depending on its size and programs, an HSO might have over 200 different jobs. Determining what each job should be paid involves consideration of three factors:

> *Internal equity*—How does the pay of various jobs compare? What should a nurse earn compared to a social worker or dietitian? There are various ways to achieve internal equity; at a minimum, job requirements must be identified and their complexity evaluated. Evaluation is usually reduced to a numerical factor (rating) so jobs can be more easily compared.
> *External equity*—How does the HSO's pay for jobs compare with that at competing organizations? External equity became more important as the supply and demand of market forces began to affect HSOs. Shortages of RNs, medical technologists, and pharmacists caused wage wars, and union pressures prompted HSOs to analyze the market for pay competitiveness.

Philosophy—How does the HSO pay relative to the market? A mature pay philosophy succinctly describes how the HSO uses data obtained by answering the first two questions to compete for staff. For example, the philosophy might be "Our pay range midpoints will be 10% above the projected median of our market for professional (higher level) jobs, and equal to the projected median of our market for service (lower level, entry) jobs." There is no "right" pay philosophy because factors such as labor supply, market definition, projected human resource needs, and type of HSO must be considered.

Establishing and Administering a Compensation System Job evaluation is a formal system to determine the relative value of jobs in an organization and is the heart of a wage and salary administration program. Jobs are analyzed using job descriptions. Each job is rated according to an evaluation plan with the purpose of establishing specific rates of pay or specific wage ranges (salary grades). A full discussion of the approaches to job evaluation is beyond the scope of this text. Readers seeking detail should review the abundant literature.[71]

There are four major methods of job evaluation. The two that are least complex are ranking and job classification; the point and factor comparison systems are quite complex.[72] Regardless of method, the expected outcome is a system of hourly rates, wage ranges, or both that relate logically to one another, a procedure that permits changes in compensation within grades using criteria such as performance and experience, a means to move employees to new grades or classifications based on changes such as job expansion, and a way to maintain internal equity.

There are several advantages for employees *and* managers in a well-structured and well-administered wage program. For example:

Inequities tend to be reduced because employees are objectively paid according to job requirements.

Managers can explain the wage program's basis because it results from a systematic analysis of job and wage data.

Favoritism in assigning wage rates is minimized.

Employee morale and motivation are increased because the wage program is easily explained, is based on fact, and shows employees where they stand.

Managers can systematically plan and control labor costs.

The program attracts qualified employees by paying fair and competitive wages.

Fair Labor Standards Act One of the most important pieces of legislation affecting compensation administration is the federal Fair Labor Standards Act (FLSA) of 1938, amended in 1967 to include many HSOs. The FLSA requires HSOs to pay overtime for hours worked beyond 40 in a 7-day period, just as a non-HSO must. An option for hospitals recognizes their 24-hour, 7-day-a-week operation and permits them to pay overtime differently: hours beyond 8 per day and 80 per 14 consecutive day period require overtime pay.[73]

The FLSA prohibits employers whose workers are subject to minimum wage requirements from discriminating based on sex in paying wages for equal work. It also sets a minimum age of 17 for general employment and 18 for work found hazardous by the Secretary of Labor. Minors age 14 and 15 may be employed outside school hours in certain occupations and under specified conditions. Evaluations, judgments, determinations, and decisions relating to wage and salary administration may be reviewed by the Wage and Hour Division of the Department of Labor. Inquiries and follow-up investigations can be made randomly or based on employee complaint.

Executive and Incentive Compensation The need to recruit and retain senior managers has prompted HSOs to evaluate executive incentive compensation plans, such as bonuses. HSOs join industry in using this strategy.[74] According to data from a survey of 1,200 hospitals that was co-sponsored by the AHA, 78% of health care management companies and 49% of hospitals have an incentive component in their senior management compensation programs.[75] Incentive compensation can achieve substantial savings by attracting talented leaders, encouraging development of multiple skills, increasing tolerance for risk taking, motivating innovative behavior, and rewarding cost reductions.[76] Senior managers with significant responsibility for and success at managing an HSO efficiently and achieving high-quality outputs must be rewarded.[77]

Comparable Worth An interesting and complicated issue affecting wage administration is "comparable worth." This concept resulted from a controversial combination of language and theory under the FLSA, as amended by the Equal Pay Act of 1963 and Title VII of the 1964 Civil Rights Act. It holds that even if all persons, whether male or female, who occupy the same job are paid equally, sex-based discrimination may still exist if the whole job class or classification is depressed because of gender bias. In other words, even though all RNs are paid equally, the employer may be liable for discrimination if individuals in a predominately female occupation (e.g., nursing) are paid less than those in a predominately male occupation (e.g., maintenance) with equal or less value to the organization.[78] Since HSOs have largely female work forces and occupational comparisons would not be limited to those within an organization, the effects of applying this doctrine to health services employment could be enormous. The doctrine has been advocated by some individuals and groups, but federal courts have not adopted it.[79] This issue illustrates the fact that, just as comparable worth theory reflects societal concern for women's rights issues, societal forces (public policy) can appreciably affect compensation administration programs in HSOs.

Benefits Administration In recent years, fringe benefits have accounted for an increasingly large proportion of compensation. Benefits commonly provided include health insurance (hospital, professional service, dental, and sometimes vision), pension, life insurance, short- and long-term disability insurance, vacation, holidays, and sick leave.[80] Some benefits are legally mandated federal and state insurance programs. Examples include Social Security, no-fault workers' compensation for on-the-job accidents, and unemployment insurance. Employers may provide other benefits, such as using group buying to get favorable rates and discounts for employees from merchants. Group purchasing is especially attractive to employers because it requires no employer contributions or participation beyond start-up costs. A credit union provides favorable rates on savings accounts and loans to employees.

Benefits typically average one fourth to one third of payroll cost, and prudent management of employer contributions is essential. HSOs and industry have sought to control benefit costs through concepts such as self-insuring. Self-insuring is ordinarily done through an employer-established trust fund to pay claims directly without using an insurance carrier. Dollars the employer would have paid in premiums fund the trust and cover claims. Excess liability coverage ("stop loss" insurance) with a high deductible is used to limit employer risk and losses.

Another way to effectively curb benefits costs while maximizing employee satisfaction is the cafeteria or full flexible benefit plan. In this arrangement the employer allocates a dollar allowance to employees and each designs a benefits package from a menu of items. Since employees choose benefits to suit their needs, satisfaction is enhanced and costs are predictable.

Flexible spending accounts for health and child care expenses are key parts of cafeteria plans and are frequently offered as free-standing benefits. Employees place pretax dollars in accounts reserved for use during the year. Unused dollars are lost. Employers do not pay Social Security taxes on reserved dollars, and this further reduces cost and increases employee take-home pay.

With a high percentage of female and single-parent employees, HSOs have become increasingly involved in providing on-site child care services. Few centers break even financially, and their value to employers is in reduced absenteeism, enhanced recruitment, increased retention, and reduced parental stress.

The Consolidated Omnibus Budget Reconciliation Act of 1986 generally requires employers to allow former employees to participate in group health insurance for as long as 36 months. A full premium must be paid (with a small surcharge for employer administration), but former employees pay considerably less than they would for nongroup coverage.

Pension Programs   Although pension programs are only one of several benefits programs provided for HSO employees, they are particularly significant because they show increased involvement of federal government in employer–employee relations. The Employee Retirement Income Security Act (ERISA) was enacted in 1974 and reflects a basic philosophical change about pension plans.[81] The old theory was that a pension rewarded long and faithful service and that it was a way to hold employees. The new theory is that a pension is a contractual right—a form of wages deferred as part of employment similar to workers' and unemployment compensation. The law sought to prevent loss of pension benefits when plans were terminated because of plant closing, bankruptcy, sale and mergers of businesses, or voluntary termination.

To carry out ERISA's purpose of protecting employees and their heirs in pension and welfare plans, Congress established requirements for preparing and filing reports, making plan documents available, and providing statements of benefits. Reports must be written in simple language and must highlight benefit design, complaint procedures, vesting, financial integrity, and employee rights. The net effect has been to shift the information-sharing burden from employees, who previously often had to ask for information, to employers, who now must provide it, and to protect the rights of employees. Effectively managing the act's legal requirements provides further opportunities for employee communications that help HSOs maintain and retain employees.

Employee Assistance Programs

Employees are an asset, and many organizations have established employee assistance programs (EAPs) to help those employees with a problem that adversely affects their work. Early programs dealt only with alcoholic employees, but the current focus is much broader and includes help for substance abuse as well as legal, financial, and emotional problems. The first EAPs were developed by a few progressive industrial corporations and were justified by claims of reduced absenteeism and work-related accidents. It is now clear that their value is much greater. McDonnell-Douglas Corporation's EAP financial offset study reported a total of 5,800 cases in 1988. Of these, 602 employees had conditions that could be assisted by the EAP and accepted the assistance. The study estimated that the offset value of EAP services for 1989 clients over the next four years would be 6 million 1989 dollars.[82] Anticipated value results from managing chemical dependency problems and behavioral illnesses. Health service environments have ready access to drugs and are emotionally difficult settings, and the potential for similar savings is great through decreased turnover rates, lower insurance costs, decreased use of sick time, improved job performance,[83] and salvaged human resources.

HSOs have become active in providing comprehensive EAP services to industry as an extension of outpatient activities. They are ideal sources for two reasons. First, an effective EAP incorporates confidentiality. The employee must receive help without fear of retribution or any record of counseling that might affect future employment. Services provided by a separate entity enhance confidentiality. Second, an HSO has the resources—social workers, psychologists, psychiatrists, therapists, and contacts with local agencies—as well as needed ancillary services.

Career counseling is a second area in which human resources departments effectively provide employee assistance. Shortages have led to development of current employees to meet future human resources needs. Expenditures for direct skills training, subsidized professional education, and management development have become a large part of the organization's investment in its staff. Career counseling and needs assessment are ways the human resources department can reduce costs of mismatching people and jobs and enhance an organization's return on its employee investment.

Health education and promotion is a third and increasingly vital area of employee assistance. By educating the workforce to better manage their own health and supporting efforts in areas such as stress management and weight and smoking reduction, employers can improve productivity, reduce health insurance expense, and contribute significantly to the positive climate required for longer employee retention.

Health and Safety

A final aspect of retaining a work force is ensuring workplace health and safety. HSOs, like other types of organizations, have long been concerned with employee health and safety. Significant impetus for formal health and safety programs was provided by enactment of most state workers' (formerly workman's) compensation laws between 1910 and 1925. These laws hold employers financially responsible for work injuries regardless of fault.

Enactment of the Occupational Safety and Health Act of 1970, also known as the Williams-Steiger Act, had far-reaching effects on organizations of all types.[84] The law was designed to solve safety and health problems associated with complex and dangerous machinery, chemicals, pollutants, and environmental threats found in the workplace. The act was intended to focus on the traditional industrial workplace, but the law was broad enough to include nongovernmental HSOs.

The act established the Occupational Safety and Health Administration (OSHA) to implement the law. OSHA requires organizations to perform three major activities: 1) promulgation and enforcement of safety standards to eliminate or lessen hazards, 2) record keeping, and 3) training and education. Rather than acting as a partner with business and industry in promoting a common goal, this emphasis caused OSHA to be seen as an adversary until 1990, when the agency began to take a more cooperative approach.

In terms of health and safety, the HSO is a dangerous place.[85] Caustic and toxic chemicals in the laboratory and pharmacy, slicing equipment in food services, radiation in radiology, ethylene oxide in supply processing, and infections in patient care areas are a few of the hundreds of hazards that make health services delivery a potentially dangerous activity. The health services industry has recognized this danger, and the Joint Commission has formulated standards for safety in HSOs, including requirements for multidisciplinary committees to identify and correct safety problems and educate employees on the importance of safety.

The acquired immunodeficiency syndrome (AIDS) poses a unique problem for HSOs: protecting health care workers from patients is compounded by the need to protect patients from health care workers. Universal precautions protect workers (and other patients by reducing the risk of cross-infection) by assuming that every patient is HIV positive. A focus of the public debate about protecting patients has been testing of health care workers, especially physicians and dentists. This debate tends to be emotional and is complicated by concerns that employees who test positive will be discriminated against or suffer emotionally. Chapter 3 discusses the ethical issues surrounding AIDS and Chapter 4 discusses the legal issues.

SEPARATION FROM EMPLOYMENT (EXIT)

Employees leave HSOs for various reasons—better job opportunities elsewhere, discharge, retirement, or death. Most human resources departments engage in activities to assist and monitor exit. Traditional activities include easing the individual's departure; collecting employer-provided equipment, keys, and records; completing personnel records; processing final pay; and collecting information through an exit interview. Other activities include preretirement planning and outplacement.

Preretirement Planning

Many organizations view preretirement counseling as an important function of the modern human resources department. The purpose is to prepare employees for the psychological, emotional, and financial changes that ensue at retirement. Such programs typically use experts to help employees understand life-style changes, emotional and physical needs, financial planning, Social Security benefits, pensions, and legal affairs such as estate planning. A preretirement planning program is effective in building employee relations.

Outplacement

HSOs now face "industrial" problems of changing demand, downsizing, consolidation, and mergers. Outplacement occurs most often when jobs are eliminated because services are retrenched or abandoned or facilities close or merge. Outplacement recognizes a social and financial commitment by the employer to assist employees in securing employment because their services have been valued. Contacts with other employers, advertising on employees' behalf, counseling, and retraining are typical. Increasing competitiveness in health care has made outplacement a key element in managing the separation of managers, too. Here, counseling usually means exploring alternate careers.

Exit Interviews

It is assumed that employees who leave an HSO will provide candid feedback, and many organizations use exit interviews to learn about employee relations. This usually means an interview with someone in the human resources department. Employees are asked about job likes and dislikes and their opinions of supervisors, the facility, the benefits package, and compensation. The reason for separation is confirmed. An attempt is made to resolve problems so that the employee leaves on a positive note. If the process is to be credible, information from exit interviews must be confidential. It is combined with other data to provide a profile of programmatic strengths and weaknesses. The technique has limitations—it usually deals with problems after the fact—but is important in providing feedback to management.

HUMAN RESOURCES DEPARTMENT AND CLINICAL STAFF

It is noteworthy that although the functions and scope of the human resources department have grown significantly in recent years, clinical staff relations are the exclusive domain of the HSO governing body and chief executive officer. When private practice clinical staff are involved this is more understandable, because licensed independent practitioners are usually not employees and are controlled by the HSO only as required by the professional staff organization bylaws and the scope of clinical privileges granted. However, when such practitioners are salaried (clinical managers or facility-based specialists such as pathologists and radiologists), they have many characteristics of employees and may be included in the HSO's employee benefit program, as well. Even here, however, the human resources department is rarely involved in wage administration or personnel file maintenance. The HSO does not view these individuals as typical employees.

HUMAN RESOURCES IN MULTIFACILITY HSOs

To this point, P/HRM has been discussed from the perspective of a freestanding HSO. The human resources role in multiunit HSOs is different. It includes setting overall policy, coordinating P/HRM activities among subsidiary units, and supporting unit programs rather than administering staffing activities.[86]

Corporate efforts may range from establishing overall policy guidelines on layoffs and ethical decision making, for example, to implementing specific programs such as those related to succession planning and regional training. Corporate support can range from informal consultation on compensation plan design to benefit plan administration. Well-directed corporate human resources functions save time and money for individual facilities as well as expand their human resources services.

THE HUMAN RESOURCES PERSPECTIVE

Contemporary P/HRM in HSOs is appreciably different from what it was 30 years ago, not only in its role and process but, more importantly, in terms of perspective and philosophy. The evolution has not been smooth. The major current outcome—the HSO's view of employees—can be labeled the "human resources perspective."

A Contemporary Perspective

Progressive HSOs and managers who embrace the human resources perspective view employees as their most important resource. This perspective embodies the following attributes:

> Employees are the catalyst for individual and organizational work results; they are the principal components in converting inputs to outputs. As indicated in the opening quotation of this chapter, human resources are the HSO's greatest asset.
>
> Employees are crucial to the organization because of the cost of employing them, the investment in their training and development, and their knowledge and on-the-job experience.
>
> Organizations and employees have reciprocal obligations to and interests in each other, and they both gain from these relationships.
>
> Management and employee values and attitudes are congruent; both seek to change organizational arrangements and work processes to: 1) accommodate and capitalize on interests, needs, abilities, and skills of employees; and 2) improve output quality on the dimensions of conformance and customer expectations.
>
> There is a permeating climate of mutual respect, positive interaction, shared problem solving, and involvement in order to improve organizational effectiveness along with employee work life quality.

The human resources perspective is a management and organizational philosophy describing how managers view and interact with employees as they carry out managerial functions and engage in managerial roles. The human resources department is responsible for the P/HRM programs and systems of acquiring and retaining employees in the organization. It facilitates implementation of this management philosophy as it administers the programs and systems, which, in turn, are integrated into the HSO's strategic plans.

By examining the evolution of P/HRM in HSOs it is possible to highlight implications of the human resources perspective as related to centralized staffing activities. To do so, three evolutionary models are presented. For the sake of description, they are labeled the personnel, labor relations, and human resources models.[87]

In reading the descriptions of these models, several cautionary statements should be kept in mind. First, time frames are approximate and used largely to suggest external and internal pressures for change. Second, generalizations are made on the state of the art and P/HRM activities at any given time. HSOs are as individual as they are numerous; no one rule or conclusion describes all situations. Not all HSOs fit the contemporary human resources model and all its attributes, but most do. Third, the focus is on nongovernmental, not-for-profit, and investor-owned HSOs. Inferences may be different for governmental organizations.

Personnel Model (Pre-1965)

Historically, and until about 1965, many HSOs had rudimentary *personnel administration* systems and paid relatively low wages. It was generally thought that people employed there were interested in devoting their lives to others; benefits and pay were secondary. Little or no attention was given to the impact of structure and task on employees.

Selection of managers was often a function of longevity and technical ability rather than managerial skill. Seldom were professionally trained managers hired from outside. Organizationwide performance appraisal systems were haphazard, if there were any. Job descriptions were archaic, seldom updated, and often not based on systematic evaluation.

Compensation systems were rudimentary, perhaps arbitrary, and occasionally inconsistent. Absent organizationwide rules, department heads set pay policies for their areas. As a result, inconsistencies existed among departments and wages were set on the basis of perceived relationships between jobs rather than a systematic, objective evaluation.

Employee assistance and counseling were generally not present. Benefit administration was simplistic. Training and development programs focused primarily on job skills rather than individual development. Work force planning was reactive and intuitive. Recruitment and selection activities were ad hoc, relatively unsophisticated, and in a sense uncomplicated before enactment of equal employment opportunity and other antidiscrimination laws.

This description is not meant to be critical; it simply generalizes the reality of personnel administration in the pre-1965 era. The personnel administration perspective was one of indifference or benign neglect. The role of personnel administration was predominantly record keeping, a process that was functional—the department had responsibility for acquiring and retaining activities, but these were not fully developed or integrated throughout the HSO and its strategic plans. The department's influence on organizational policy was minimal and it had little overall acceptance. Personnel administration was considered to be a department that other managers tolerated but for which they had little enthusiasm. As a result, the predominant departmental strategy during this era was inactive compliance, or neutrality. Personnel managers were neither activists nor innovators.

The unsophisticated and uncomplicated pre-1965 personnel model reflected its environment. In many respects the need for an influential personnel department did not exist, certainly not to the degree it does today. The pre-1965 environment preceded Medicare and Medicaid, both of which increased demand for and government involvement in health services. There was economic stability, an abundant supply of workers, and few cost pressures. Technological change was slow compared to later decades, competitive pressures were few, and legislation relative to employment practices was limited. All these factors led to business as usual and relatively uncomplicated HSOs. Personnel administration's task of acquiring and retaining a work force was relatively easy.

Labor Relations Model (Late 1960s to Mid-1980s)

The period from the late 1960s through the mid-1980s was turbulent for HSOs in general and personnel administration departments in particular. Numerous external influences caused the personnel department's perspective to change from indifference to containment and conflict management. The process of staffing was still functional, but it became fully developed with emphasis on upgrading programs and policies to acquire and retain employees.

External influences affecting personnel administration included the following:

Enactment of Medicare and Medicaid programs (1965) increased demand for services. HSOs responded by hiring more staff. Improved personnel record systems were necessary for cost allocation and reimbursement.

Application of federal minimum wage laws and overtime to HSOs in 1967 complicated wage administration systems.

The 1964 Civil Rights Act mandated equal employment opportunity and significantly affected employment practices: selection, testing, performance appraisal, promotion, demotion, and equal pay for equal work. Improved personnel programs and policies were necessary.

Federal legislation such as the Occupational Safety and Health Act (which forced attention on safety in the workplace) and the ERISA (which required communication about benefits) prompted personnel managers to be more activist.

HSOs fell victim to market forces as certain categories of workers became scarce, particularly RNs and a variety of technologists. Burgeoning technology required specialized and more skilled personnel. Work force planning, recruitment, compensation, training, and development were affected.

Inflation, cost containment pressures, constraints on revenues, and greater competition in the late 1970s and early 1980s shifted emphasis to productivity, efficiency, and effectiveness. Systems for monitoring and enhancing productivity and for evaluating job design and work methods became necessary, as did analyses of employee utilization, turnover, and job performance. In large part, this fell to personnel departments. However, the productivity and efficiency initiatives were largely episodic and short term and focused on reducing costs, not increasing quality. They were quite different in scope and intent from contemporary quality improvement (see Chapter 11).

Increased unionization of HSOs began in the early 1960s and was encouraged by passage of the 1974 Nonprofit Hospital Amendments to the Taft-Hartley Act (see Chapter 18). Labor relations became a dominant theme as employee and societal attitudes about unionization changed and unions focused organizing efforts on HSOs.

The effect of these external changes was to increase the importance of personnel administration and force upgrading of programs and systems. Personnel departments assumed attributes of the labor relations model. They became fully functional; virtually all of them had acquisition and retention activities in place. The role of personnel managers was to support the organization as it coped with external environmental forces.

The personnel administration perspective at this point was containment—limiting the effect of external forces. A particular target was unionization. The result was a reactive organization strategy. Influence on organizational policy was increasing, and centralized personnel administration was viewed as necessary.

Human Resources Model (Contemporary)

The same factors and environmental forces that led to the evolution of the labor relations model facilitated development of the contemporary human resources model. This model grew throughout the 1980s and is prevalent in HSOs of the 1990s. The adversarial, conflict, containment, and reactive attributes of the labor relations model have been jettisoned. Intensified cost pressures, resource constraints, and increased competitiveness among HSOs now require managers to focus attention on effectively using human and other resources and improving output quality. Both initiatives recognize employees as the HSO's most valuable asset.

The differences between the personnel and labor relations models are clear. However, the point of demarcation between the labor relations and human resources models are not as easily identified. The telltale signs of change included: 1) upgrading the personnel manager from middle-level to senior management with a title such as vice president for human resources; 2) changing the departmental name from *personnel department* to *human resources department*; and 3) increasing the authority, responsibility, and accountability of its manager to integrate human resources activities with the HSO's strategic plans.

The human resources model is predicated on the philosophy that was previously described as the human resources perspective. Work force planning, recruitment, selection, orientation, performance appraisal, training and development, discipline, compensation, and benefit administration were part of the labor relations model, but the activities were often mechanical, established in reaction to events and with little thought for organizationwide outcomes. The human resources model goes beyond this. It is interventionist and proactive because it integrates human resources acquisition and retention activities with the organization's operational components. The human resources department is a catalyst for organizational changes such as CQI.

The human resources department presently has a major role in monitoring and improving the employment climate through employee needs assessments and attitude surveys and by identifying employee satisfiers and dissatisfiers. Interventions to change structure and work processes are included so that all resources are used more effectively; employer and employee seek to accomplish objectives as partners.

Performance appraisal systems not only yield information for compensation changes but also are integrated with programs of positive behavior modification and corrective counseling to improve performance. Training and development focus on skills enhancement and technological upgrading and address social skills such as coping with work, reducing stress, and fostering interpersonal relationships.

Career counseling based on aptitude and interest assessment is performed to enable people to achieve their fullest potential. While the HSO's payback may not seem tangible, this activity serves long-range human resources planning by upgrading employee skills in areas in which supply is short, building loyalty to the organization, and demonstrating that employees are respected as individuals with unique needs.

EAPs that preserve and salvage human resources are integrated with other retention activities. The direct and indirect costs of alcoholism and drug abuse in lost time, low productivity, and human wreckage are staggering. Providing treatment without recrimination to the employee who seeks help makes sense from the human resources perspective. Corollary programs include marital and financial counseling and health awareness and fitness. They are good investments in the organization's human resources.

Accomplishing the HSO's objectives, especially quality care and improved efficiency, depends on people. Embracing the human resources perspective reflects a commitment by the HSO to people as its most important resource.

The Future

Predicting the future is risky. Anticipating competitive shifts is equally risky, but is an important skill demanded in post-1990 health services delivery. Loss of low cost leadership, dramatic shifts in consumer base, and shrinking labor markets have created an environment in which adaptability means survival.[88] Human resources depleted by increasing technology and specialization must now be preserved in much the same way as capital.

Human resources management of the future could be called the human asset model. It will build on the attributes of the contemporary—human resources—model by focusing on the acquisition and retention of human capital, investing in its development, and proactively maintaining its ability to perform in a changing environment. In the futuristic human asset model success can be measured in much the same way as capital: preservation—by organizational survival (retention); liquidity—by teamwork and skill transferability; and return on investment—by the value added from all employees' continuous improvement of high-quality work results. Increasingly, human resources management activities will change as the HSO's strategic plans change. Change will be so continuous that it will be a constant. Organization renewal and revitalization will be required because of a more sophisticated environment. Human resources management activities such as work force planning, recruitment, and selection, as well as all of the retention activities—performance appraisal, training and development, compensation and benefits administration, employee assistance, and employee safety and health—will command even more attention. The challenge is great. The responsibility of the human resources department is simple—to ensure that people remain the HSO's most important asset and that the asset is not only preserved, but enhanced.

SUMMARY

Human resources management is composed of the wide range of centralized staffing activities, programs, and policies related to acquisition, retention, and separation of an HSO's human resources (see Figure 17.1). Acquiring human resources involves work force planning, recruitment, selection, and ultimately, induction into the HSO and orientation. All depend on an effective job analysis program and well-developed job descriptions. In recruitment and selection, as well as throughout employees' tenure, one role of the human resources department is to establish and implement nondiscriminatory personnel policies that comply with state and federal law. Other department activities are preemployment applications and interviews and testing; monitoring of equal employment opportunity, adverse impact, and affirmative action; and administering compensation—equal pay for equal work—and pension programs.

In addition to centralized acquisition, the human resources department is also responsible for activities related to retaining human resources. These include performance appraisal (methods, uses, and benefits), training and development, and discipline. The discussion of compensation administration includes job analysis methods, issues related to internal and external equity, pay philosophies, and the inherent activities involved in developing and administering a compensation system. Benefits administration, including pension programs and employee assistance programs, follow. Finally, promotion of safety and health of employees within the HSO and separation activities such as preretirement planning and outplacement are discussed.

This chapter stresses the "human resources perspective," which is described as an organizational and managerial philosophy embracing the basic theme that employees are the HSO's most important resource. Accomplishing the objectives of the HSO depends on the efforts and initiatives of people. They are the catalyst for converting other inputs to outputs.

Finally, there is a longitudinal presentation of the change in P/HRM activities. This is done by differentiating the personnel, labor relations, and human resources models. Approximate time frames are given and attributes of each model are identified. Contemporary human resources management has adopted an interventionist role—collaborating with and supporting organizational units and proactively initiating change. The environment of the 1990s has given the human resources department two major responsibilities. The first is to integrate human resource acquisition and retention with the HSO's strategic plans. The second is to ensure that people remain the HSO's most important asset, which, like capital, is preserved and enhanced.

DISCUSSION QUESTIONS

1. The human resources department is responsible for centralized staffing activities related to acquisition, retention, and separation of employees. Describe those activities presented in the chapter using a time flow perspective.
2. Job descriptions are used for many P/HRM purposes. How is the document derived and what does it contain?
3. What is equal employment opportunity? How does it affect P/HRM activities?
4. All health services managers appraise performance of subordinates. How are appraisals used? What are the benefits and potential problems of performance appraisal?
5. Identify and discuss the following aspects of compensation administration: equity, job evaluation, and comparable worth. What benefits result from a well-designed and implemented compensation program? What results can occur from an ill-designed or poorly implemented program? What employee benefits are there beyond wages and salaries?
6. What economic and noneconomic justification is there for employee assistance, preretirement planning, and outplacement programs? Be specific.

7. In the last section of the chapter (The Human Resources Perspective), three models longitudinally trace health services P/HRM activities. Identify the models and their time frames and describe each model's attributes. What is the human resources perspective? Describe it. Is it consistent with the opening quote to the chapter? Why?

CASE STUDY 1:   PERSONNEL POLICIES AT ROBBINS MEMORIAL HOSPITAL

Carol King is vice president of human resources at a 127-bed facility located in a small farming town. She has been at Robbins Memorial Hospital for only 2 weeks, but has already concluded that the human resources department is not well developed and there are no policies for many situations.

Situation A

One morning King had a meeting with Janet Jens, director of the clinical laboratory, who told King she has a problem with an employee who is chronically late and frequently absent. King reviewed the employee's records for the past 6 months, the extent of record keeping. They show the employee has been tardy 70 times and absent 15 times. King learned from Jens that the employee is an Hispanic medical technician who has been employed in the lab for 1½ years. The technician is working on a degree at a local college and is frequently late because of her class schedule or sorority activities.

King checked the personnel policy manual. The policy regarding absenteeism or tardiness states "the facility requires employees to be at their work stations on a timely and regular basis. Failure to adhere to regular attendance and punctuality standards may cause the facility to take disciplinary action." King then consulted the personnel manual for a policy on discipline and found no guidelines other than a general statement that "failure to adhere to facility policies and procedures may cause the facility to take necessary measures." King reviewed other files and found no documentation of what had been done in similar cases. Jens is pressing King to know what action she can take to correct this problem or to terminate the employee.

Question: What should King do? Why?

Situation B

King was informed by the director of the intensive care unit that a female night employee has told other staff that when she comes to work she carries a small loaded gun for personal protection. The gun has been shown to other employees and allegedly waved carelessly about in the unit. King responded by stating that the facility has a clear policy that prohibits employees from bringing firearms onto the premises. The director of security, however, reminded King that recently a night shift employee was assaulted in the parking lot and that many female employees are concerned for their safety. The director of security is worried that there might be other ramifications if this employee is disciplined. For example, other night shift employees might say that the facility is not concerned about their safety and that carrying a firearm is both a second amendment (constitutional) guarantee and necessary because of poor facility security. King agreed that this might become an issue and was also concerned that the facility has had difficulty getting nurses for the night shift.

Question: What should King do? Why?

Situation C

The following situation was described to King by the food service manager:

A cook at Robbins Memorial Hospital was observed taking a chicken and other food from a storage area and putting the items in a bag under his coat. As the employee entered his car to go home he was stopped by security officers and told that they were making a package check of the contents of the bag he was carrying. The employee objected, but the security officers insisted, stating that there was a policy allowing inspection of all packages removed from the facility. The employee relented and the food items were found in the bag.

The employee was terminated by the food service manager for theft. He filed a complaint with the EEOC alleging that his dismissal resulted from discrimination based on the fact that he is the only food service employee who is an ethnic Italian and that other employees regularly take food from the department. Therefore, his termination was based solely on the fact that he is Italian and he was "singled out." King and the security director have no knowledge that other employees are stealing.

Question: What position should the facility take when contacted by EEOC?

CASE STUDY 2:   COMPLAINT OF LPN PAY INEQUITY

You are the vice president of human resources at a large health maintenance organization (HMO). A representative of the licensed practical nurses (LPNs) has complained to you about pay inequity. The HMO employs both RNs and LPNs, whose training and state licensure differ significantly. Because of a shortage of RNs and an abundance of LPNs, LPNs have been performing many RN duties. However, the difference in pay is more than 30%. Because this practice has occurred for some time, the LPNs want a wage increase. They argue they should be paid the same as an RN if they perform the same work. Neither the LPNs nor the RNs are represented by a union.

Questions

1.   Should the pay for the LPNs be increased to equal that of RNs? Why or why not?
2.   What are the implications throughout the organization if LPN pay is increased to that of RNs?
3.   What should be done to solve the problem of the two groups performing similar duties?
4.   Are there quality of patient care considerations?

CASE STUDY 3:   TERMINATION OF HEAD NURSE JONES

Janet Jones is a head nurse and Samantha Smith is her supervisor. For many years it has been widely known around their organization, Highland Sanatorium, that Jones is a poor head nurse and a weak manager. Over the years, the relationship between Jones and her supervisor, Smith, deteriorated to the point that Smith decided it was time to make a change and terminate Jones. Smith tends to avoid confrontations whenever possible. However, employee unrest on the floor and problems relating to preferential treatment, scheduling mix-ups, poor performance, and patient complaints convinced Smith that the confrontation with Jones could no longer be avoided. Smith met with Jones and warned her that if problems on the floor were not worked out she would be replaced. Three months later there was no improvement and Smith requested that Jones be terminated.

You are the vice president of human resources and you have to make the final decision on whether to allow the termination. In reviewing the file you note that the warning alleged to have been given 3 months ago was documented only by a note to the file from Smith. Jones had not acknowledged the warning in writing. There are a few other notes in Jones's file to show the presence of another problem, but there are no details.

A review of Jones's performance appraisals for the last 3 years shows that:

1.   Performance appraisals are to be given on the employee's anniversary date. Smith's performance appraisals of Jones were from 3 to 5 months late each year.

2. The appraisals show that Smith always rated Jones as "meeting standards" in quantity and quality of work.
3. The unsigned comments section at the end of the appraisals show that Smith gave Jones suggestions on how to improve. They cover scheduling and equal treatment of employees. Smith says this documents existence of the problems and that they were discussed at the performance appraisal conferences. Jones asserted that this was merely a personality conflict, that her performance appraisals demonstrate she met all standards, and termination is unjustified and unfair.

Interviews conducted with employees on the floor and other witnesses found that Jones was an incompetent head nurse.

Questions

1. Should Jones be terminated? Why or why not?
2. Does Jones have a case to fight termination?
3. What P/HRM practices should be changed?

CASE STUDY 4: SUBSTANCE ABUSE AND EAP

Fred has been a clerk in the Fairfax Clinic's medical records department for 15 years. He is a good employee and is liked by all. In the last 9 months, however, his performance has deteriorated and relationships with co-workers have been strained. As vice president of human resources, several years ago you set up an employee assistance program (EAP) for staff with personal problems or who are involved with drug or alcohol abuse. Unknown to you (and consistent with EAP policy), Fred contacted the EAP and has been counseled for alcohol abuse for the past month. His supervisor is not aware of the source of the problem and has been disciplining Fred through the steps of progressive discipline (oral warning, formal warning, and a 2-day suspension) for poor performance.

Again this morning Fred came to work with the smell of alcohol on his breath. His speech was slurred and he had poor coordination. The supervisor called you and requested that Fred be terminated immediately. You called Fred to your office and found that his condition had improved. You informed him of his supervisor's decision to terminate him and discussed his alcohol abuse and poor performance. Fred became irate and cited the EAP policy stating that the clinic seeks to help employees with such problems. All information was to have been kept confidential and no one was to have been at risk or terminated as a result of voluntarily using EAP. Since you set up the EAP program, you are concerned about its credibility and success.

Questions

1. Should Fred be terminated? Why or why not?
2. If Fred is terminated, what are the implications regarding the clinic's stated EAP policy about confidentiality and nonrisk?

CASE STUDY 5: MISSING NARCOTICS

You are the vice president of human resources in a community hospital that is the largest employer in town. The vice president of nursing services, Ms. Gates, calls at 5:00 P.M. on Friday. She asks you to come to her office and witness a confrontation with Helen Jones, a second shift staff nurse "caught red-handed stealing drugs."

Gates tells you that two staff members saw Jones put five tubexes of Demerol in her pocket as she prepared to give 4:00 P.M. medications and reported it to the charge nurse, Nancy Gray. Gray checked the drug count and verified the shortage. At the end of Jones's rounds, Gray asked her to empty her pockets. This produced five tubexes of Demerol.

In Gates's office a few minutes later, you listen while she repeats the incident and asks Jones if she is stealing drugs. Jones calmly says, "Yes." Gates tells Jones there is no choice but to fire her for theft. Without emotion Jones asks that someone clean out her locker and bring its contents to her. Gates says, "Yes, I'm sure we're all very anxious to go home."

Left alone with Jones while the two nurse managers arrange for a security guard to clean out her locker, you quietly begin talking and ask why she stole the drugs. "You can't stop me," she replies. "If I can't take an overdose, I'll just leave here and drive my car into a wall. I'm not going home." After several more minutes of revealing conversation, Gates and Gray return with Jones's belongings.

Jones has been an employee for 14 years. She started as a nursing student after her children were in school. Her eldest daughter is now a student nurse here, as well. Your proposal to start an employee assistance program (EAP) has not yet been accepted.

Questions

1. Is this a clear case of theft? What actions should be taken?
2. Should Jones be fired? What are the implications for your hospital?

CASE STUDY 6: PHYSICIAN HARASSMENT

After participating in a management development workshop on employee counseling in which a sexual harassment example was used, the operating room (OR) supervisor, Leslie McClung, asked for an appointment. You are the OR manager.

One of McClung's nurses, Amy Kelly, complained to her last month that Dr. Ray "had made several passes at her," including asking her for a date. She refused and told him she didn't appreciate his unprofessional behavior in surgery.

When the next OR schedule was posted, Kelly noticed that her name had been crossed off Dr. Ray's cases. When asked why, McClung told her that Dr. Ray asked that Kelly be removed from his cases until she had more experience.

McClung told you that she had smoothed over the incident, but now wonders if that was the right thing to do.

Questions

1. Was Kelly sexually harassed? Give reasons for your answer.
2. Was smoothing over the incident appropriate? Why?
3. Is there an obligation to confront the issue of sexual harassment since the physician is not a hospital employee?

NOTES

1. American Hospital Association. *Human resources: Management advisory*, 1. Chicago: American Hospital Association, 1990.
2. Milkovich, George T., and John W. Boudreau. *Human resource management*, 6th ed., 4. Homewood, IL: Irwin, 1991.
3. Ivancevich, John M., and William G. Glueck. *Foundations of personnel: Human resource management*, 4th ed., 17. Homewood, IL: BPI/Irwin, 1989.
4. Hernandez, S. Robert, Myron D. Fottler, and Charles L. Joiner. Strategic management of human resources in health services organizations. In *Strategic management of human resources in health services organizations*, edited by S. Robert Hernandez, Myron D. Fottler, and Charles L. Joiner, 3. New York: John Wiley & Sons, 1988; McManis, Gerald, L. Managing competitively: The human factor. *Healthcare Executive* 2 (November/December, 1987): 19.
5. Readers interested in a manual containing sample HSO policy statements, procedures, and forms for all of the traditional P/HRM activities are referred to Buccini, Eugene P., and Charles P. Mullaney. *Personnel policies and*

procedures for health care facilities: A manager's manual and guide. New York: Quorum Books, 1989. For an overview of centralized staffing activities, see: Dessler, Gary. *Personnel/human resource management*, 4th ed., chpt. 1. Englewood Cliffs, NJ: Prentice Hall, 1991; French, Wendell L. *Human resource management*, 2d ed., chpt. 1. Boston: Houghton Mifflin Company, 1990; Mathis, Robert L., and John H. Jackson. *Personnel/human resource management*, 6th ed., chpt. 2. St. Paul, MN: West Publishing Co., 1991.

6. Hernandez, Fottler, and Joiner, Strategic management, 11–15.

7. French, *Human resource*, 153.

8. Fottler, Myron D., Robert L. Phillips, John D. Blair, and Catherine A. Duran. Achieving competitive advantage through strategic human resource management. *Hospital & Health Services Administration* 35 (Fall 1990): 348.

9. Gardner, John W. *On leadership*, 126–127. New York: The Free Press, 1990.

10. Hernandez, Fottler, and Joiner, Strategic management, 2–3.

11. A review of human resource planning is found in Dessler, *Personnel/human*, 118–128; Harlow, Kirk C., and Joseph K. Taylor. Strategic human resource planning. In *Human resource management in the health care sector*, edited by Amarjit S. Sethi and Randall S. Schuler, 17–40. New York: Quorum Books, 1989; and Milkovitch and Boudreau, *Human resource*, 145–155. A description of planning applied to work force reductions is found in Train, Alan S. The case of the downsizing decision. *Harvard Business Review* 69 (March/April 1991): 14, 19, 22–23, 26–27, 30; and Weil, Thomas P., and A.T. Hollingsworth. Strategies for hospital staff reduction. *Health Care Strategic Management* 4 (April, 1986): 14–18.

12. A good presentation of technology's impact on human resources management is found in Leatt, Peggy, and Bruce Fried. Technology and human resources management. In *Strategic management of human resources in health services organizations*, edited by S. Robert Hernandez, Myron D. Fottler, and Charles L. Joiner, 85–111. New York: John Wiley & Sons, 1988.

13. Hernandez, S. Robert, Cynthia Carter Haddock, William M. Behrendt, and Walter F. Klein, Jr. Management development and succession planning: Lessons for health services organizations. *Journal of Management Development* 10 (Special Issue on Health Care Management Development, 1991): 19–22.

14. For an overview of human resource sources and the recruiting activity, see Dessler, *Personnel/human*, 128–151; French, *Human resource*, chpt. 1; Mathis and Jackson, *Personnel/human*, chpt. 8; and Milkovitch and Boudreau, *Human resource*, chpt. 7.

15. Dessler, *Personnel/human*, 80–81.

16. See Ivancevich and Glueck, *Foundations*, 80–81; Mathis and Jackson, *Personnel/human*, chpt. 7.

17. French, *Human resource*, 195–199; Milkovich, George T., and Jerry M. Newman. *Compensation*, chpts. 3 and 4. Homewood, IL: Richard D. Irwin, 1990; Sethi, Amarjit S., Patricia L. Birkwood, and Randall S. Schuler. The role of job design and job analysis in the strategic human resources model. In *Human resource management in the health care sector*, edited by Amarjit S. Sethi and Randall S. Schuler, 43. New York: Quorum Books, 1989.

18. Dessler, *Personnel/human*, 84–88.

19. The standard reference for health service job descriptions

20. Sethi, Birkwood, and Schuler, Role of job design, 64–66.

21. Gellatly, Donna L. Recruitment strategies. In *Human resource management in the health care sector*, edited by Amarjit S. Sethi and Randall S. Schuler, 79–89. New York: Quorum Books, 1989.

22. A good discussion of recruitment in HSOs is found in: Birkenstock, Marguerite. Recruitment and retention strategies for keeping good nurses. *AORN Journal* 53 (January 1991): 110–118; Fyock, Catherine D. Expanding the talent search—19 ways to recruit top talent. *Human resource magazine* 36 (July, 1991): 32–35; Landau, Jacqueline, and Geoffrey A. Hoare. Recruitment. In *Strategic management of human resources in health services organizations*, edited by S. Robert Hernandez, Myron D. Fottler, and Charles L. Joiner, 241–266. New York: John Wiley & Sons, 1988; and Zurlinden, Jeffrey, Beth Bongard, and Marilyn Magafas. Situational leadership: A management system to increase staff satisfaction. *Orthopaedic Nursing* 9 (March/April, 1990): 47–52.

23. Umiker, William O. Recruitment and retention strategies to cut turnover. *Medical Laboratory Observer* 21 (September, 1989): 24; Helmer, F. Theodore, and Patricia McKnight. One more time—solutions to the nursing shortage. *Journal of Nursing Administration* 18 (November, 1988): 7.

24. Helmer, F. Theodore, and Patricia McKnight. Management strategies to minimize nursing turnover. *Health Care Management Review* 14 (Winter, 1989): 77–79.

25. Meyer, Ralph H., Mary N. Mannix, Thomas F. Costello, and Robert Parker. Nurse recruitment: Do health care managers gear strategies to the appropriate audience? *Hospital & Health Services Administration* 36 (Fall, 1991): 448.

26. A good presentation of selection and placement in HSOs is found in: Landau, Jacqueline, Dan Fogel, and Lisa Frey. Selection and placement. In *Strategic management of human resources in health services organizations*, edited by S. Robert Hernandez, Myron D. Fottler, and Charles L. Joiner, 267–293. New York: John Wiley & Sons, 1988.

27. Mathis and Jackson, *Personnel/human*, 223–224.

28. Dessler, *Personnel/human*, 214.

29. Mathis and Jackson, *Personnel/human*, 139.

30. Readers interested in more information about permissible and nonpermissible preemployment questions and activities are referred to: Equal Employment Opportunity Commission. *Laws administered by the EEOC.* 1–48. Washington, D.C.: U.S. Government Printing Office, 1981; Equal Employment Opportunity Commission. *Uniform employee selection guidelines—interpretation and clarification—questions and answers*, Sect. 4175.01–4175.08. Chicago: Commerce Clearing House, Inc., 1985; Equal Employment Opportunity Commission. *Uniform guidelines on employee selection procedures* (29 C.F.R., Part 1607), pp. 206–233. Washington, D.C.: U.S. Government Printing Office, 1988; Office of Public Affairs, Equal Employment Opportunity Commission. *Pre-employment inquiries and equal employment opportunity law*, 1–8. Washington, D.C.: U.S. Government Printing Office, 1981; and Twomey, David

P. *A concise guide to employment law, EEO & OSHA.* Cincinnati: South-Western Publishing Co., 1986.

31. Equal Employment Opportunity Commission, *Uniform guidelines.*

32. Griggs v. Duke Power Co., 401 U.S. 424 (1971).

33. Garbin, Margery. Validity of EAS tests. *Quality Assessment Quarterly* 1 (Spring, 1991): 2; Mathis and Jackson, *Personnel/human*, 120–123. For guidelines on testing see Dessler, *Personnel/human*, 174–191.

34. Metzger, Norman. *The health care supervisor's handbook*, 2d ed., 38–39. Rockville, MD: Aspen Systems Corporation, 1982.

35. For further information, we recommend the following government publication: Equal Employment Opportunity Commission, *Laws Administered*, 1–48 (covers Title VII of the Civil Rights Act of 1964; as amended; the Age Discrimination in Employment Act of 1967, as amended; the Equal Pay Act of 1963; and Section 501 of the Rehabilitation Act of 1973); see also the Americans with Disabilities Act of 1990 (PL 101-336); Dessler, *Personnel/human*, chpt. 2; Ivancevich and Glueck, *Foundations*, chpt. 3; Ledvinda, James, and Vida G. Scarpello. *Federal regulation of personnel and human resource management.* Boston: PWS-Kent Publishing Company, 1990; Mathis and Jackson, *Personnel/human*, chpts. 5 and 6; Milkovich and Boudreau, *Human resource*, chpt. 6.

36. Civil Rights Act of 1964 (PL 88-362). In *United States Statutes at Large, 1964*, Vol. 78. Washington, D.C., 1964.

37. Fair Labor Standards Act of 1963 (PL 88-38). In *United States Statutes at Large, 1963*, Vol. 77. Washington, D.C., 1963.

38. *Age Discrimination in Employment Act of 1967* (P.L. 90–202). In *United States Statutes at Large, 1967*, Vol. 81. Washington, D.C., 1967; see also Older Workers Benefit Protection Act of 1991 (P.L. 101-433).

39. The Age Discrimination Act does not apply when age is a job-related occupational qualification, such as for airline pilots. The 1986 Amendments eliminated the age 70 ceiling. Public employers and colleges and universities were given a seven-year exemption. See Mathis and Jackson, *Personnel/human*, 108–109.

40. Gillman, Steven L., and Davi L. Hirsch. The Americans With Disabilities Act: Civil rights for handicapped workers. *The Brief* 20 (Summer 1991): 16.

41. Marcotte, Paul. New disabilities law. *American Bar Association Journal* 76 (November, 1990): 21–22; Reed Smith. *Reed Smith bulletin*, 1. Pittsburgh, 1990.

42. Gillman and Hirsch, Americans With, 18.

43. Marcotte, New disabilities, 21.

44. Marcotte, New disabilities, 21.

45. Marcotte, New disabilities, 21–22.

46. Reed Smith, *Reed Smith bulletin*, 1–2.

47. Marcotte, New disabilities, 21.

48. For reviews of legislation see: Bernat, John. Employee rights strategies. In *Human resource management in the health care sector*, edited by Amarjit S. Sethi and Randall S. Schuler, 256–262. New York: Quorum Books, 1989; Hartstein, Barry A. EEO issues in the health-care field: A roundup of recent developments. *Employee Relations Law Journal* 12 (Autumn, 1986): 241–261; Mathis and Jackson, *Personnel/human*, 108, 149–150; Twomey, *Concise guide*, 1–53.

49. Twomey, *Concise guide*, 1–2.

50. Twomey, *Concise guide*, 25.

51. Twomey, *Concise guide*, 28.

52. Mathis and Jackson, *Personnel/human*, 134.

53. Fisher, Cynthia D., Lyle F. Schoenfeldt, and James B. Shaw. *Human resource management*, 133. Boston: Houghton Mifflin Company, 1990.

54. Equal Employment Opportunity Commission. *Guidelines on discrimination because of sex* (29 C.F.R., Sect. 1604.11). Washington, D.C.: U.S. Government Printing Office, 1990.

55. Mathis and Jackson, *Personnel/human*, 144.

56. Equal Employment Opportunity Commission, *Guidelines on discrimination.*

57. Mathis and Jackson, *Personnel/human*, 145.

58. Hudson Institute. *Workforce 2000: Work and workers for the 21st century.* Indianapolis, 1987.

59. American Hospital Association, *Human resources*, 1.

60. Readers interested in further information on the subject of performance appraisal are referred to: Belcher, John C., Jr. *Productivity plus*, chpts. 9 and 10. Houston: Gulf Publishing Co., 1987; Boissoneau, Robert, Debrah J. Gaulding, and David N. Calvert. Performance appraisal as a strategic choice for the health care manager. In *Human resource management in the health care sector*, edited by Amarjit S. Sethi and Randall S. Schuler, 95–125. New York: Quorum Books, 1989; Dessler, *Personnel/human*, chpt. 14; Joiner, Charles L. Performance appraisal. In *Strategic management of human resources in health services organizations*, edited by S. Robert Hernandez, Myron D. Fottler, and Charles L. Joiner, 319–336. New York: John Wiley & Sons, 1988; Milkovich and Boudreau, *Human resource*, 91–110; Milkovich and Newman, *Compensation*, chpts. 8 and 10.

61. Dessler, *Personnel/human*, 500–510; Metzger, *Health care supervisor's*, 53–54; Milkovich and Newman, *Compensation*, chpt. 9.

62. Dessler, *Personnel/human*, 512–515.

63. Deegan, Arthur X., II, and Thomas R. O'Donovan. *Management by objectives for hospitals*, 2d ed. Germantown, MD: Aspen Systems Corporation, 1982; Drucker, Peter F. *Management: Tasks, responsibilities, practices*, 440–442. New York: Harper & Row, 1973; Flower, Joe. A conversation with Peter Drucker: Being effective. *Healthcare Forum Journal* 34 (May/June, 1991): 52–57; Joiner, Performance appraisal, 336–341.

64. Levinson, Harry. Excerpts from management by whose objectives? *Harvard Business Review* 69 (March/April, 1991): 176; Milkovich and Newman, *Compensation*, 283–284.

65. Drucker, Peter F. *Managing the non-profit organization*, 62. New York: Harper Collins, 1990.

66. For a good review of training and development see: French, *Human resource*, chpts. 11 and 12; Ivancevich and Glueck, *Foundations*, chpts. 12 and 13; Milkovich and Boudreau, *Human resource*, chpt. 11.

67. Smith, Howard L., and Myron D. Fottler. Training and development. In *Strategic management of human resources in health services organizations*, edited by S. Robert Hernandez, Myron D. Fottler, and Charles L. Joiner, 297. New York: John Wiley & Sons, 1988.

68. Rakich, Jonathon S., Paul J. Kuzdrall, Keith A. Klafehn, and Alan G. Krigline. Simulation in the hospital setting: Implications for managerial decision making and management development. *Journal of Management Development* 10 (Special Issue on Health Care Management Development, 1991): 36.

69. Dessler, *Personnel/human*, 463–469; Metzger, *Health care supervisor's*, 86.
70. For reviews of compensation administration see Dessler, *Personnel/human*, chpt. 13; Ivancevich and Glueck, *Foundations*, chpts. 9 and 10; Mathis and Jackson, *Personnel/human*, chpts. 13 and 14; and Milkovich and Boudreau, *Human resource*, chpts. 12 and 13.
71. Milkovich and Newman, *Compensation*; Jones, Kerma N., and Charles L. Joiner. Compensation management. In *Strategic management of human resources in health services organizations*, edited by S. Robert Hernandez, Myron D. Fottler, and Charles L. Joiner, 348–369. New York: John Wiley & Sons, 1988.
72. Friss, Lois. Designing a compensation system in the strategic human resource management model. In *Human resource management in the health care sector*, edited by Amarjit S. Sethi and Randall S. Schuler, 151–158. New York: Quorum Books, 1989; Ivancevich and Glueck, *Foundations*, 404–416; Mathis and Jackson, *Personnel/human*, 340–345.
73. Bernat, Employee rights, 255–256.
74. Friss, Designing a compensation, 163–164; Jones and Joiner, Compensation management, 357.
75. Williams, James B., and R. Scott Coolidge. Annual survey: Incentive plans on the rise in hospitals. *Hospitals* 65 (September 5, 1991): 26.
76. Browdy, Jerad D. Incentive compensation: It starts with the right attitude. *Healthcare Executive* 2 (November/December, 1987): 26–27.
77. Sources on incentive compensation are: Foulkes, Fred K. *Executive compensation: A strategic guide for the 1990's*. Boston: Harvard Business School Press, 1991; Ernst & Young. *Alternative reward systems in the health care industry*. Atlanta, 1990; and Williams and Coolidge, Annual survey. An analysis of senior HSO management compensation in Canada can be found in Pink, George H., and Peggy Leatt. Are managers compensated for hospital financial performance? *Health Care Management Review* 16 (Summer, 1991): 37–46.
78. Friss, Designing a compensation, 165–168; Bernat, Employee rights, 256.
79. Twomey, *Concise guide*, 77–78.
80. For an overview on benefits see Dessler, *Personnel/human*, chpt. 12; Ivancevich and Glueck, *Foundations*, 481–487; Mathis and Jackson, *Personnel/human*, chpt. 15; and Milkovich and Boudreau, *Human resource*, chpt. 14.
81. Employee Retirement Income Security Act of 1974. In *United States Statutes at Large, 1974*, Vol. 88, Part I. Washington, D.C., 1974.
82. McDonnell-Douglas Corporation and Alexander Consulting Group. *McDonnell-Douglas Corporation Employee Assistance Program Financial Offset Study, 1985–1989*. Westport, CT: Alexander Consulting Group, 1990.
83. Howard, John C., and David Szcerbacki. Employee assistance programs in the hospital industry. *Health Care Management Review* 13 (Spring, 1988): 74.
84. Twomey, *Concise guide*, 109.
85. Hill, James. Occupational safety and health strategies. In *Human resource management in the health care sector*, edited by Amarjit S. Sethi and Randall S. Schuler, 235–237. New York: Quorum Books, 1989.
86. A good discussion of differences in human resource activities in solo and group medical practices relative to a hospital is found in Begun, James W., and Ronald C. Lippincott. Structure for human resources management. In *Strategic management of human resources in health services organizations*, edited by S. Robert Hernandez, Myron D. Fottler, and Charles L. Joiner, 112–140. New York: John Wiley & Sons, 1988.
87. This section is adapted from Robbins, Stephen A., and Jonathon S. Rakich. Hospital personnel management in the late 1980s: A direction for the future. *Hospital & Health Services Administration* 31 (July/August, 1986): 18–25; and Robbins, Stephen A., and Jonathon S. Rakich. Hospital personnel management in the early 1990s: A follow-up analysis. *Hospital & Health Services Administration* 34 (Fall, 1989): 388–390.
88. For other perspectives on the health care environment see: Foreman, Stephen E., and Robert D. Roberts. The power of health care value-adding partnerships: Meeting competition through cooperation. *Hospital & Health Services Administration* 36 (Summer, 1991): 175–190; Ginzberg, Eli. Health personnel: The challenges ahead. *Frontiers of Health Services Management* 7 (Winter, 1990): 3–20; Higgins, Wayne. Myths of competitive reform. *Health Care Management Review* 16 (Winter, 1991): 65–72; Johnson, James, A., and R. Wayne Boss. Management development and change in a demanding health care environment. *Journal of Management Development* 10 (Special Issue on Health Care Management Development, 1991): 5–10; Stevens, Rosemary. The hospital as a social institution, new fashioned for the 1990s. *Hospital & Health Services Administration* 36 (Summer, 1991): 163–173.

BIBLIOGRAPHY

American Society for Healthcare Human Resources Administration. *Health care occupations: A comprehensive job description manual*. Chicago: American Hospital Publishing, Inc., 1985.

Begun, James W., and Ronald C. Lippincott. Structure for human resources management. In *Strategic management of human resources in health services organizations*, edited by S. Robert Hernandez, Myron D. Fottler, and Charles L. Joiner, 112–140. New York: John Wiley & Sons., 1988.

Belcher, John C., Jr. *Productivity plus*. Houston: Gulf Publishing Co., 1987.

Bernat, John. Employee rights strategies. In *Human resource management in the health care sector*, edited by Amarjit S. Sethi and Randall S. Schuler, 247–274 New York: Quorum Books, 1989.

Boissoneau, Robert, Debrah J. Gaulding, and David N. Calvert. Performance appraisal as a strategic choice for the health care manager. In *Human resource management in the health care sector*, edited by Amarjit S. Sethi and Randall S. Schuler, 95–126. New York: Quorum Books, 1989.

Buccini, Eugene P., and Charles P. Mullaney. *Personnel policies and procedures for health care facilities: A manager's manual and guide*. New York: Quorum Books, 1989.

Deegan, Arthur X., II, and Thomas R. O'Donovan. *Management by objectives for hospitals*, 2d ed. Rockville, MD: Aspen Systems Corporation, 1982.

Dessler, Gary. *Personnel/human resource management*, 4th ed. Englewood Cliffs, NJ: Prentice Hall, 1991.

Drucker, Peter F. *Management: Tasks, responsibilities, practices*. New York: Harper & Row, 1973.

Drucker, Peter F. *Managing the non-profit organization*. New York: Harper Collins, 1990.

Equal Employment Opportunity Commission. *Laws administered by the EEOC*, 1–48. Washington, D.C.: U.S. Government Printing Office, 1981.

Equal Employment Opportunity Commission. *Uniform employee selection guidelines—interpretation and clarification—questions and answers*, Sect. 4175.01–4175.08. Chicago: Commerce Clearing House, Inc., 1985.

Fisher, Cynthia D., Lyle F. Schoenfeldt, and James B. Shaw. *Human resource management*. Boston: Houghton Mifflin Company, 1990.

Foreman, Stephen E., and Robert D. Roberts. The power of health care value-adding partnerships: Meeting competition through cooperation. *Hospital & Health Services Administration* 36 (Summer, 1991): 175–190.

Fottler, Myron, D., S. Robert Hernandez, and Charles L. Joiner. *Strategic management of human resources in health services organizations*. New York: John Wiley & Sons, 1988.

Fottler, Myron D., Robert L. Phillips, John D. Blair, and Catherine A. Duran. Achieving competitive advantage through strategic human resource management. *Hospital & Health Services Administration* 35 (Fall, 1990): 341–363.

Foulkes, Fred K. *Executive compensation: A strategic guide for the 1990's*. Boston: Harvard Business School Press, 1991.

French, Wendell L. *Human resource management*, 2d ed. Boston: Houghton Mifflin Company, 1990.

Friss, Lois. Designing a compensation system in the strategic human resource management model. In *Human resource management in the health care sector*, edited by Amarjit S. Sethi and Randall S. Schuler, 147–176. New York: Quorum Books, 1989.

Gardner, John W. *On leadership*. New York: The Free Press, 1990.

Gellatly, Donna L. Recruitment strategies. In *Human resource management in the health care sector*, edited by Amarjit S. Sethi and Randall S. Schuler, 75–94. New York: Quorum Books, 1989.

Gillman, Steven L., and Davi L. Hirsch. The Americans With Disabilities Act: Civil rights for handicapped workers. *The Brief* 20 (Summer 1991): 16–21, 43.

Ginzberg, Eli. Health personnel: The challenges ahead. *Frontiers of Health Services Management* 7 (Winter, 1990): 3–20.

Harlow, Kirk C., and Joseph K. Taylor. Strategic human resource planning. In *Human resource management in the health care sector*, edited by Amarjit S. Sethi and Randall S. Schuler, 15–40. New York: Quorum Books, 1989.

Hartstein, Barry A. EEO issues in the health-care field: A roundup of recent developments. *Employee Relations Law Journal* 12 (Autumn, 1986): 241–261.

Helmer, F. Theodore, and Patricia McKnight. Management strategies to minimize nursing turnover. *Health Care Management Review* 14 (Winter, 1989): 73–80.

Helmer, F. Theodore, and Patricia McKnight. One more time—solutions to the nursing shortage. *Journal of Nursing Administration* 18 (November, 1988): 7–15.

Hernandez, S. Robert, Myron D. Fottler, and Charles L. Joiner. Strategic management of human resources in health services organizations. In *Strategic management of human resources in health services organizations*, edited by S. Robert Hernandez, Myron D. Fottler, and Charles L. Joiner 3–19. New York: John Wiley & Sons, 1988.

Hernandez, S. Robert, Cynthia Carter Haddock, William M. Behrendt, and Walter F. Klein, Jr. Management development and succession planning: Lessons for health services organizations. *Journal of Management Development* 10 (Special Issue on Health Care Management Development, 1991): 19–30.

Higgins, Wayne. Myths of competitive reform. *Health Care Management Review* 16 (Winter, 1991): 65–72.

Hill, James. Occupational safety and health strategies. In *Human resource management in the health care sector*, edited by Amarjit S. Sethi and Randall S. Schuler, 235–246. New York: Quorum Books, 1989.

Howard, John C., and David Szcerbacki. Employee assistance programs in the hospital industry. *Health Care Management Review* 13 (Spring, 1988): 73–79.

Ivancevich, John M., and William G. Glueck. *Foundations of personnel: Human resource management*, 4th ed. Homewood, IL: BPI/Irwin, 1989.

Johnson, James, A., and R. Wayne Boss. Management development and change in a demanding health care environment. *Journal of Management Development* 10 (Special Issue on Health Care Management Development, 1991): 5–10.

Joiner, Charles L. Performance appraisal. In *Strategic management of human resources in health services organizations*, edited by S. Robert Hernandez, Myron D. Fottler, and Charles L. Joiner, 319–347. New York: John Wiley & Sons, 1988.

Jones, Kerma N., and Charles L. Joiner. Compensation management. In *Strategic management of human resources in health services organizations*, edited by S. Robert Hernandez, Myron D. Fottler, and Charles L. Joiner, 348–369. New York: John Wiley & Sons, 1988.

Landau, Jacqueline, Dan Fogel, and Lisa Frey. Selection and placement. In *Strategic management of human resources in health services organizations*, edited by S. Robert Hernandez, Myron D. Fottler, and Charles L. Joiner, 267–293. New York: John Wiley & Sons, 1988.

Landau, Jacqueline, and Geoffrey A. Hoare. Recruitment. In *Strategic management of human resources in health services organizations*, edited by S. Robert Hernandez, Myron D. Fottler, and Charles L. Joiner, 241–266. New York: John Wiley & Sons, 1988.

Leatt, Peggy, and Bruce Fried. Technology and human resources management. In *Strategic management of human resources in health services organizations*, edited by S. Robert Hernandez, Myron D. Fottler, and Charles L. Joiner, 85–111. New York: John Wiley & Sons, 1988.

Ledvinda, James, and Vida G. Scarpello. *Federal regulation of personnel and human resource management*. Boston: PWS-Kent Publishing Company, 1990.

Mathis, Robert L., and John H. Jackson. *Personnel/human resource management*, 6th ed. St. Paul, MN: West Publishing Co., 1991.

Metzger, Norman. *The health care supervisor's handbook*, 2d ed. Rockville, MD: Aspen Systems Corporation, 1982.

Meyer, Ralph H., Mary N. Mannix, Thomas F. Costello, and Robert Parker. Nurse recruitment: Do health care managers gear strategies to the appropriate audience? *Hospital & Health Services Administration* 36 (Fall, 1991): 447–453.

Milkovich, George T., and John W. Boudreau. *Human resource management*, 6th ed. Homewood, IL: Irwin, 1991.

Milkovich, George T., and Jerry M. Newman. *Compensation*. Homewood, IL: Richard D. Irwin, 1990.

Office of Public Affairs, Equal Employment Opportunity

Commission. *Pre-employment inquiries and equal employ-ment opportunity law* 1–8. Washington, D.C.: U.S. Government Printing Office, 1981.

Pink, George H., and Peggy Leatt. Are managers compensated for hospital financial performance? *Health Care Management Review* 16 (Summer, 1991): 37–46.

Rakich, Jonathon S., Paul J. Kuzdrall, Keith A. Klafehn, and Alan G. Krigline. Simulation in the hospital setting: Implications for managerial decision making and management development. *Journal of Management Development* 10 (Special Issue on Health Care Management Development, 1991): 31–37.

Robbins, Stephen A., and Jonathon S. Rakich. Hospital personnel management in the early 1990s: A follow-up analysis. *Hospital & Health Services Administration* 34 (Fall, 1989): 385–396.

Robbins, Stephen A., and Jonathon S. Rakich. Hospital personnel management in the late 1980s: A direction for the future. *Hospital & Health Services Administration* 31 (July/August, 1986): 18–33.

Sethi, Amarjit S., Patricia L. Birkwood, and Randall S. Schuler. The role of job design and job analysis in the strategic human resources model. In *Human resource management in the health care sector*, edited by Amarjit S. Sethi and Randall S. Schuler, 41–74. New York: Quorum Books, 1989.

Sethi, Amarjit S., and Randall S. Schuler, eds. *Human resource management in the health care sector.* New York: Quorum Books, 1989.

Smith, Howard L., and Myron D. Fottler. Training and development. In *Strategic management of human resources in health services organizations*, edited by S. Robert Hernandez, Myron D. Fottler, and Charles L. Joiner, 294–318. New York: John Wiley & Sons, 1988.

Stevens, Rosemary. The hospital as a social institution, new fashioned for the 1990s. *Hospital & Health Services Administration* 36 (Summer, 1991): 163–173.

Twomey, David P. *A concise guide to employment law, EEO & OSHA.* Cincinnati: South-Western Publishing Co., 1986.

Weil, Thomas P., and A.T. Hollingsworth. Strategies for hospital staff reduction. *Health Care Strategic Management* 4 (April 1986): 14–18.

18 / Labor Relations

*We must start to think of our employees not as
adversaries, but as partners.*

Norman Metzger[1]

In writing about the labor movement in health services organizations (HSOs), Norman Metzger, a preeminent authority on labor relations, makes several insightful observations important to this chapter. First, he labels the 1990s as a new era of human capital during which HSO managers will be challenged to develop new approaches toward, and relationships with, employees. Second, managers must give attention to satisfying the legitimate needs of employees in a hostile and threatening external environment—only then will employees make a maximum commitment to the HSO. This leads to the third point, which is the opening quotation to this chapter: that HSO managers must view employees as partners—not adversaries—in the noble enterprise of health services delivery. Too often the management–labor relationship is an adversarial one that results in less employee commitment and increased management–labor conflict, and tears the fabric of the organization's culture and ultimately affects costs and patient care. Unionization in the health services system occurred recently—primarily since the late 1960s—and present and future HSO managers must understand the evolution, legal framework, process, and issues involved in management–labor relations if they are to meet the challenge to develop new approaches and strengthen the partnership with employees.

IMPORTANCE OF LABOR RELATIONS IN HSOs

The previous chapter identified people as among the most important input resources for HSOs, which are service-oriented, labor-intensive organizations with the largest portion of their expenditures spent on payroll. The increasing ratio of employees to patients has been partially caused by greater intensity of care, new programs and services, an increase in technology, and the need for larger numbers of highly trained personnel. As a result, HSO managers must be more concerned with staffing patterns, compensation rates, payroll expenditures, and employee utilization. Increasing external environmental resource constraints are forcing managers to utilize resources, especially employees, more effectively. Furthermore, it is through people that managers accomplish organizational objectives. Only through integration of the structure, tasks/technology, and people elements of HSOs (see the management model, Figure 1.6) can patient care or client services be provided, and only through committed employees can the philosophy of continuous quality improvement be implemented and sustained.

"Labor relations" is a generic term used to describe the employer-employee relationship. Collective bargaining "is the process by which union leaders representing groups of employees negotiate terms of employment with representatives designated by management."[2] That relationship and the process of bargaining are important because HSO employee unions and management negotiate about wages, conditions of work, promotion policies, discipline procedures, and sometimes job design and work assignments. Consequently, the employer–employee relationship and the collective bargaining agreement between the two ultimately affect the organization's costs, allocation of resources, and utilization of human resources, and can influence managerial decision-making, planning, directing, and controlling activities. This chapter will acquaint the reader with the evolution of labor law and issues pertinent to labor relations in HSOs.

COLLECTIVE BARGAINING IN HSOs: A RECENT DEVELOPMENT

Compared to the industrial sector, unionization in HSOs is recent. Metzger and Pointer report scattered instances of unionization in health services as early as 1919,[3] but Miller observes that "for the most part, the mass organizing drives of the 1930s and 1940s bypassed hospital employees, leaving the industry largely untouched well into the 1960s."[4] Health services unionization occurred primarily in the past 30 years. For example, in 1960 only 3% of hospitals had at least one collective bargaining contract; today, approximately 20% do.

Four reasons explain why HSOs were relatively nonunionized prior to the 1960s. First, national labor organizations paid them little attention and directed their time, energy, and resources at industry. Second, professional attitudes and the charitable nature of HSOs led many employees to conclude that unionizing was inappropriate. Third, most HSOs, particularly hospitals, are not-for-profit and there was no "profit" available for distribution to employees, as in the industrial sector. Last, the legal environment only became conducive to unionization in the 1960s and 1970s because federal and not-for-profit hospitals were finally covered by federal labor law.

Acceleration of unionization in HSOs in the mid-1960s can be attributed to several factors. First, President Kennedy's executive order in 1962 allowed federal hospital employees to bargain collectively. No federal hospitals were unionized prior to this, but within 10 years 75% of all federal hospitals had at least one union.[5] Second, professional employees such as nurses no longer opposed joining a union because of changing societal values and because blue-collar unions had narrowed the wage differential between union and nonunion professional employees. Third, subsequent to Medicare and Medicaid in 1965, hospitals and nursing facilities no longer bore such a large burden of uncompensated care. Thus, absorbing the costs of uncompensated care could not be used to justify paying low wages, and employees no longer accepted the "psychic" income of working for a charitable organization in lieu of adequate compensation. Finally, poor personnel policies and practices and poor first-line supervision contributed to employees seeking a vehicle for rectification—a union.[6]

Contemporary HSO managers are relatively mature vis-à-vis labor relations. They traveled a bumpy road in the last 30 years and are generally better for it. The 1970s and 1980s were especially turbulent as constraints were imposed on external funding, resources, and costs; demand for services increased; and greater accountability was expected and required. HSOs adapted well to the significantly altered labor environment that followed the passage of the Nonprofit Hospital Amendments to the Taft-Hartley Act in 1974.

Because of the importance of labor relations to HSOs, this chapter traces the history of the United States labor movement. It describes major federal labor legislation, including the 1974 Nonprofit Hospital Amendments to the Taft-Hartley Act; presents the bargaining unit determination controversy; discusses unionization in health services since 1974; examines why employees join unions; offers a compilation of managerial responsibilities in labor relations; and presents the collective bargaining process.

HISTORY OF UNIONISM IN THE UNITED STATES

Unionism in the United States can be readily divided into eras preceding and following 1930.

Pre-1930 Era

Unionism in the United States began in 1792 when the journeymen cordwainers (shoemakers) of Philadelphia formed a local.[7] However, there was relatively little union activity until the late 1800s. Even though the Knights of Labor was established by a group of tailors in Philadelphia in 1869, 9 years later there were only 9,000 members. In 1881 the American Federation of Labor (AFL) was formed and under the leadership of Samuel Gompers had 278,000 members by 1889.[8] Shortly after the turn of the century, the AFL merged with the Knights of Labor. In 1905, the

International Workers of the World (IWW) was formed,[9] and in 1913 the United States Department of Labor was established.

From the late 1800s until the 1930s union membership rose gradually. There were fewer than 1 million union members at the turn of the century, and by 1910 there were 2.1 million. Membership peaked in the pre-1930 era at 5.1 million in 1920.[10] It increased in times of prosperity, but decreased during depression. Membership was generally confined to the skilled crafts, and only in the period from 1930 to 1947 were the basic manufacturing industries organized. Several reasons contributed to a lack of union success in the pre-1930 era: government's pro-business attitude, employee fear, and the antiunion attitude of employers.

Post-1930 Era

Union membership increased from 3.4 million in 1930 to 14.3 million in 1945. The sharp increase in union members and membership as a percentage of the nonagricultural work force is seen in Figures 18.1 and 18.2. The primary reason for this increase was federal legislation enacted during the 1930s.

During the early portion of this period, basic industries such as steelmaking, auto manufacturing, and rubber processing were unionized. Beginning in the 1950s union membership as a percentage of the nonagricultural work force declined from a high of 35.5% in 1945 to slightly over 16.1% in 1990. This was because most union organizing had occurred in the manufacturing industries and focused on blue-collar workers, and since 1950 the proportion of blue-collar workers in the total labor force has declined and the number of service employees, including those in HSOs, has grown. As a result, in the 1960s organizing efforts were directed at health services employees.

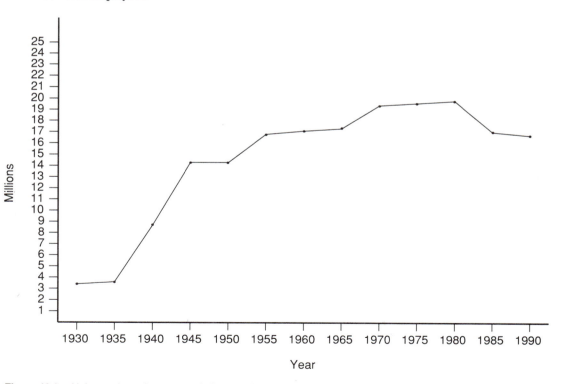

Figure 18.1. Union and employee association membership, 1930–1990. (Source: Bureau of Labor Statistics, U.S. Department of Labor.)

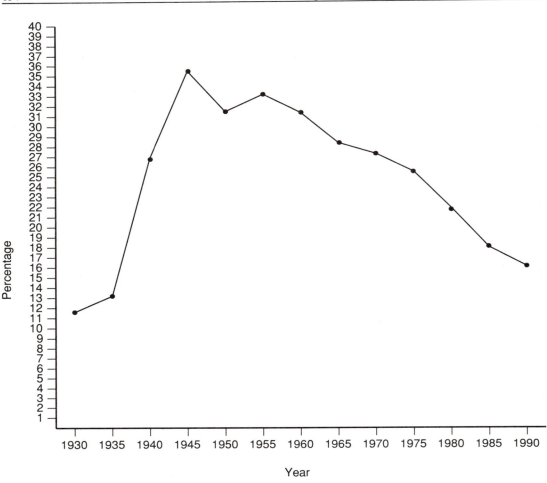

Figure 18.2. Union and employee association membership as a percentage of the nonagricultural labor force, 1930–1990. (Source: Bureau of Labor Statistics, U.S. Department of Labor.)

FEDERAL LABOR LEGISLATION

Generally, the federal government was antiunion before the 1930s. However, during the Depression a shift occurred. The Protestant work ethic, factory systems, and common law employer property rights were challenged by a social ethic. Although some states had progressive labor legislation, the Depression contributed to an awareness that the federal government had responsibilities to the working class. The legal setting changed in 1932 with passage of the Norris-LaGuardia Act. Other subsequent federal labor legislation that will be examined includes the Wagner Act of 1935, the Taft-Hartley Act of 1947, and the 1974 Nonprofit Hospital Amendments to the Taft-Hartley Act.

Norris-LaGuardia (Anti-Injunction) Act (1932)

The Norris-LaGuardia Act of 1932, officially called the Anti-Injunction Act,[11] was landmark legislation. It represented a major change in congressional attitude toward labor–management relations. The law's basic philosophy was that individuals were at a disadvantage when bargaining with employers. Consequently, to enable the individual employee "to protect his freedom of labor," it prohibited employer use of "yellow dog" contracts and restricted use of court injunctions in labor disputes.[12]

"Yellow Dog" Contracts   Section 3 of the Norris-LaGuardia Act prohibited employers from requiring an employment contract specifying that an employee would not join a union if doing so was a breach of the contract and cause for termination. The Act stated that such contracts are "hereby declared to be contrary to the public policy of the United States [and] shall not be enforceable in any court."[13]

Injunctions   The Norris-LaGuardia Act also focused on federal court injunctions in labor disputes. Prior to 1932, preliminary injunctions were frequently issued to forestall union activity (e.g., a recognition strike) that could cause "irreparable" harm while the court examined the merits of the case. Employers were able to obtain injunctions enjoining union activity from sympathetic courts. Although activities such as strikes or picketing were not illegal, failure to comply with a court injunction was. Norris-LaGuardia did not require employers to recognize or bargain with unions. However, they were stripped of nonmeritorious use of injunctions.[14]

Wagner (National Labor Relations) Act (1935)

The second major labor–management relations law enacted in the 1930s was the Wagner Act, officially known as the National Labor Relations Act (NLRA) of 1935.[15] The primary purpose of the NLRA was to ensure that private-sector employees had the right to organize and bargain collectively, free from employer influence or coercion, and to establish a balance of bargaining power between employers and employees.[16] To achieve this purpose, the NLRA specified *employer unfair labor practices* and established the National Labor Relations Board (NLRB) to oversee issues involving union recognition and collective bargaining.[17]

Employer Unfair Labor Practices   Section 8 of the NLRA lists five employer unfair labor practices. These are summarized in Table 18.1 to reflect subsequent amendments, and examples

Table 18.1.   Employer unfair labor practices and examples

1. *To interfere with, restrain, or coerce employees in the exercise of their rights to organize* [Section 8(a)(1)].
    —Threaten employees with loss of job or benefits if they vote for a union
    —Grant wage increases deliberately timed to discourage employees from joining a union

2. *To dominate or interfere with the affairs of a union* [Section 8(a)(2)].
    —Take an active part in the affairs of a union, such as a nurse supervisor actively participating in a nurses' association representing RNs
    —Show favoritism to one union over another in an organizing attempt

3. *To discriminate in regard to hiring, tenure, or any employment condition for the purpose of encouraging or discouraging membership in any union organization* [Section 8(a)(3)].
    —Discharge employees who urge others to join a union
    —Demote an employee for union activity

4. *To discriminate against or discharge an employee because he has filed charges or given testimony under this act* [Section 8(a)(4)].
    —Discriminate against, fire, or demote employees because they gave testimony to NLRB officials or filed charges against the employer with the NLRB

5. *To refuse to bargain collectively with representatives of the employees; that is, "bargain in good faith"* [Section 8(a)(5)].
    —Refuse to provide information, if requested, by the union, that is relevant and necessary to allow employees' representative to bargain intelligently and effectively with respect to wages, hours, and other conditions of employment
    —Refuse to bargain about a "mandatory" subject such as hours and wages
    —Refuse to meet with union representatives duly appointed by a certified bargaining unit
    —Take unilateral action in current conditions of employment without notifying the union, such as subcontracting x-ray or food service activities if those employees are currently unionized

Source: Office of the General Counsel, National Labor Relations Board. *A guide to basic law and procedures under the National Labor Relations Act*, 22–23. Washington, D.C., U.S. Government Printing Office, 1990.

are given. Unfair labor practices define what employers may not do when employees want to unionize. In addition, they specify how employers must deal with the certified representative (union) of the employees once recognition occurs. In sum, the employer must bargain in good faith.

National Labor Relations Board   The second major provision of the NLRA established the National Labor Relations Board, defined union recognition, and provided means to resolve unfair labor practices. The thrust of the NLRA is that the duly elected representative of a majority of employees for an appropriate bargaining unit shall be the exclusive agent for the purpose of collective bargaining. Basically, if a majority of employees wish to have a union they can impose their will on the minority. The NLRB conducts elections for representation and certifies the exclusive agent for a particular bargaining unit.

Prior to the NLRA, unions often had to strike to force employers to recognize them as the employees' bargaining agent. The NLRA changed that. At the request of the employees, the NLRB holds an election and, if a majority of voting employees in the defined bargaining unit vote for a particular union to represent them, that union becomes their exclusive bargaining agent. Furthermore, the employer must bargain in good faith with that agent.

The second function of the NLRB concerns unfair labor practices. If it is found, for example, that an employer committed an unfair labor practice, the NLRB can provide remedies through cease and desist orders and take affirmative action, "including reinstatement of employees with or without back pay" who were discharged in violation of the act. The NLRB's objective is to eliminate unfair labor practices and to undo the effects of the violation.[18]

The employer unfair labor practices listed in Table 18.1 indicate that, as of 1935, unprecedented constraints were applied against employers while restrictions on the behavior of labor were minimal. Given this environment, Figure 18.1 shows that union membership grew from 3.4 million in 1930 to 14.3 million in 1945. Clearly, the intent of NLRA was to create a legal environment promoting the rights of workers to unionize, and this was achieved.[19] In fact, the balance of power had swung so far in favor of labor that Congress passed, over President Truman's veto, the Taft-Hartley Act in 1947. It amended the NLRA of 1935 and sought to balance the power between labor and management.[20]

Taft-Hartley (Labor–Management Relations) Act (1947)

Congressional intent with passage of the NLRA in 1935 was to provide a legal environment that enabled unions to grow in size and strength and to remedy the one-sided power balance that had favored the employer. This was accomplished. In fact, unions lost some of their public favor in the years immediately after World War II. The change to a peacetime economy, rising prices, and pent-up consumer demand caused unions to strike as never before.[21] Many people thought that the pendulum of power had swung too far in favor of unions and that a better balance was needed.

In 1947, the Taft-Hartley Act, officially titled the Labor-Management Relations Act (LMRA) of 1947,[22] amended the Wagner Act (NLRA) of 1935. Its purpose was "to define and protect the rights of employees and employer, to encourage collective bargaining, and to eliminate certain practices on the part of labor and management that are harmful to the general welfare."[23]

The major provisions of the Taft-Hartley Act changed the structure of the NLRB, protected employee rights not to join a union, enumerated *union unfair labor practices*, provided legislative prescriptions for certain bargaining procedures, and established procedures for handling national emergencies.

National Labor Relations Board   The act structured the NLRB around two functions: to conduct representative elections and certify the results; and to prevent employers and unions from engaging in unfair labor practices. When requested, the NLRB intervenes in both of these areas. A five-member board hears cases. The NLRB general counsel investigates and prosecutes cases.[24] This structural change separated prosecution of cases from judging them by separating quasi-executive from quasi-judicial functions.

Employee Protection Another major change was that Taft-Hartley protected both workers who wished to organize and those who did not. When a "substantial" number of employees (defined by the NLRB as a "showing of interest" by at least 30% of the bargaining unit) petition to hold a recognition election, the NLRB conducts one. If a majority of employees vote against the union, Section 9(c)(3) prohibits any union from petitioning for an election for one year.[25] Therefore, the right of employees not to join a union is preserved and employers are not harassed with endless elections. Similarly, by majority vote employees can exercise their right to decertify a union currently representing them.

Union Unfair Labor Practices Employer unfair labor practices were specified in the 1935 Wagner Act, and a major provision of the 1947 Taft-Hartley Act is enumeration of union unfair labor practices. These are contained in Section 8(b) of the Taft-Hartley Act, as amended, and are summarized with examples in Table 18.2.

Bargaining Procedures Other Taft-Hartley provisions specify that: 1) nonthreatening handbilling is not an unfair labor practice; 2) a 60-day notice of contract termination or modification must be given to the other party; 3) supervisors cannot be part of a bargaining unit; and 4) guards and professional employees cannot be mixed with other employees in a bargaining unit, except in the case of professional employees who have concurred. Taft-Hartley also has an 80-day cooling off period that begins when the president declares a national emergency. During this time there can be no strike.[26]

Table 18.2. Union unfair labor practices and examples

1. *To restrain or coerce employees in the exercise of their right to join or not to join a union except when an agreement is made by the employer and union that a condition of employment will be joining the union (called a union security clause authorizing a "union shop") [Section 8(b)(1)(A)].*
   —Picket as a mass and physically bar other employees from entering a health care facility
   —Act violently toward nonunion employees
   —Threaten employees for not supporting union activities

2. *To cause an employer to discriminate against an employee other than for nonpayment of dues or initiation fees [Section 8(b)(2)].*
   —Cause an employer to discriminate against an employee for antiunion activity
   —Force the employer to hire only workers "satisfactory" to the union

3. *To refuse to bargain with an employer in "good faith" about wages, hours, and conditions of employment [Section 8(b)(3)].*
   —Insist on negotiating illegal provisions such as management's prerogative to appoint supervisors
   —Refuse to meet with the employer's representative
   —Terminate an existing contract or strike without the appropriate notice

4. *To engage, induce, encourage, threaten, or coerce any individual to engage in strikes, refusal to work, or boycott when the objective is to [Section 8(b)(4)]:*
   (a) *force or require any employer or self-employed person to recognize or join any labor organization or employer organization.*
   (b) *force or require any employer or self-employed person to cease using the products of or doing business with another person, or force any other employer to recognize or bargain with the union unless it has been certified by the NLRB.*
   (c) *force an employer to apply pressure to another employer to recognize a union.*
   —Picketing a hospital so that it will apply pressure on a subcontractor (food service, maintenance, emergency department) to recognize a union, or forcing an employer to do business only with others, such as suppliers, who have a union, or picketing by another union for recognition when a different one is already certified.

5. *To charge excessive or discriminatory membership fees [Section 8(b)(5)].*
   —Charge a higher initiation fee to employees who did not join the union until after a union-security agreement (union shop) is in force

6. *To cause an employer to give payment for services not performed (featherbedding) [Section 8(b)(6)].*
   —Force an employer to add people to the payroll when they are not needed
   —Force payment to employees who provide no services

Source: Office of the General Counsel, National Labor Relations Board. *A guide to basic law and procedures under the National Labor Relations Act,* 27–40. Washington, D.C., U.S. Government Printing Office, 1990.

Wagner (NLRA) and Taft-Hartley (LMRA) were amended by the 1959 Landrum-Griffin Act, officially known as the Labor-Management Reporting and Disclosure Act of 1959. Landrum-Griffin primarily addresses internal union affairs such as election of officers and provides safeguards for union members, but Title VII adds a seventh union unfair practice (8[b][7]): picketing an employer for recognition of a second union when one union is already certified.[27] Examples include engaging in picketing to obtain recognition by the employer (recognition picketing) or acceptance by employers of the employees' representative (organizational picketing) when the employer has lawfully recognized another union, when a valid NLRB election has been held within the previous 12 months, or when no representation petition has been filed with the NLRB within 30 days of the commencement of such picketing.[28] Figure 18.3 shows the NLRB's basic procedures involving charges of unfair labor practices by either the employer or union.

Nonprofit Hospital Amendments to the Taft–Hartley Act (1974)

Pre-1974 Environment   Prior to 1974, the collective bargaining legal framework covering HSOs varied by type of ownership. Taft-Hartley specifically excluded from its definition of employer "any corporation or association operating a hospital, if no part of the net earnings inures to the benefit of any private share holder or individual" (Section 2,2). This meant that not-for-profit hospitals were excluded from federal labor law. Federal and nonfederal (state, local) government hospitals continued to be excluded.

Investor-owned HSOs (for-profit hospitals and long-term care facilities) continued to be covered by provisions of the NLRA, as amended, although the NLRB exerted no jurisdiction until 1967.[29] The NLRB developed revenue standards that established minimum annual revenues below which an investor-owned HSO would not be covered by the Taft-Hartley Act. The minimum for long-term care facilities is annual revenue exceeding $100,000; for hospitals it is $250,000.[30] These revenue standards trigger a presumption that an investor-owned HSO affects interstate commerce and is subject to NLRA jurisdiction.

President Kennedy's Executive Order 10988, which was modified in 1970 by President Nixon's Executive Order 11491,[31] established recognition and bargaining procedures and unfair labor practices for federal employees (and management), including those in federal hospitals. These provisions were subsequently incorporated into Title VII of the 1978 Civil Service Reform Act. Neither the executive orders nor the 1978 act relaxed the prohibition on strikes by federal employees.[32]

Until 1959, no state provided a legal basis for nonfederal government hospital employees to unionize, bargain, or strike. By 1970, however, 36 states provided a legal framework for public employees to bargain collectively.[33] Taft-Hartley's exclusion of nongovernmental, not-for-profit hospitals had two implications: 1) these hospitals were not required by federal labor law to recognize or negotiate with a union, or to follow NLRA-defined employer unfair labor practices; and 2) the absence of federal law meant that hospitals could be included under state law. By 1974, only 14 states had laws that covered nongovernmental, not-for-profit hospitals.*

1974—A Changed Environment   Public Law 93-360, the Nonprofit Hospital Amendments to the Taft-Hartley Act, was passed July 26, 1974, and ended the nongovernmental, not-for-profit hospital exclusion of the 1947 act.[35] The changing health services delivery and social environments of the 1960s helped precipitate the change in Congress's attitude toward not-for-profit HSOs. The 1962 and 1970 executive orders added momentum for unionization in the health care industry by permitting such activity in federal government HSOs. For-profit HSOs were already covered by Taft-Hartley, if they met the revenue test. By 1973, 16.8% of not-for-profit hospitals had at least one collective bargaining agreement that had been obtained without federal labor law

---

*Those states were Minnesota, New York, Pennsylvania, Wisconsin, Massachusetts, Utah, Colorado, Michigan, Connecticut, Oregon, Montana, Hawaii, Washington, and Rhode Island.[34]

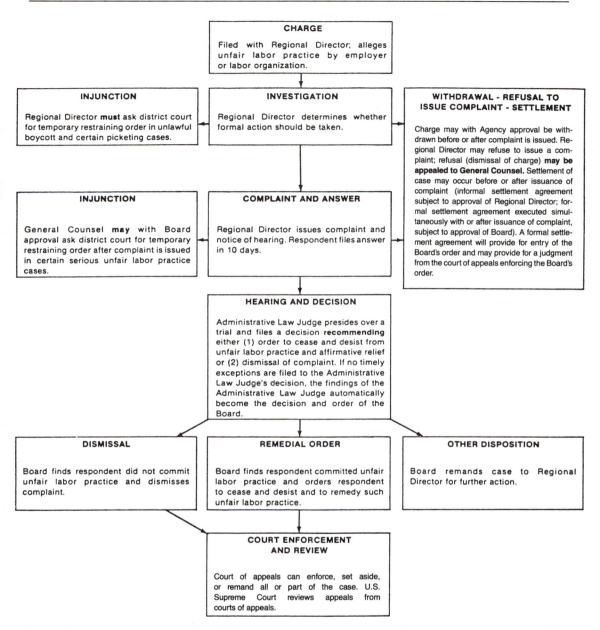

Figure 18.3. Basic procedures of the NLRB in cases involving charges of unfair labor practices. (Source: NLRB, December 13, 1984.)

protection and procedural benefits.[36] Excluding not-for-profit hospitals from federal labor law coverage and the absence or inadequacy of state legislation often caused highly publicized work stoppages (strikes) initiated for purposes of recognition. Miller reports that 125 of 248 work stoppages in hospitals and nursing facilities from 1962 to 1971 were for initial recognition.[37] Finally, by the early 1970s, funding health care for the aged and indigent through Medicare and Medicaid substantially decreased the uncompensated care delivered by not-for-profit HSOs. Thus, one rationale for their exclusion in 1947—revenue lost by serving the aged and indigent—was no longer valid.

Since 1974, not-for-profit and investor-owned (nongovernmental) HSOs, as well as unions, have complied with recognition, election, and unfair labor practice provisions of the Wagner and Taft-Hartley Acts. The 1974 amendments define HSOs as: "any hospital, convalescence hospital, health maintenance organization, health clinic, nursing home, extended care facility, or any other institution devoted to the care of sick, infirm or aged persons" (Section 2[2][b][14]). The NLRB defines health care delivery to include hospitals, health maintenance organization (HMOs), and long-term care facilities that provide inpatient or outpatient care, including private institutions providing for the care of mentally retarded persons,[38] as well as other noninstitutional providers such as medical associations, laboratories, group practices, and home health agencies.

Unique Provisions   The 1974 amendments include provisions unique to HSOs: contract notices, notification preceding a strike, conciliation of disputes, and payment of union dues by individuals with religious convictions.[39] Congressional intent expressed by the House and Senate conference committee reports included an admonition to the NLRB to give "due consideration" to avoiding proliferation of bargaining units in the health care industry to lessen the potential of work stoppages and related strife.[40]

Contract Notices   Since HSOs provide unique and essential services, the amendments require a 90-day (compared to 60-day) notification to the other party to modify an existing contract and a 60-day notice to the Federal Mediation and Conciliation Service (FMCS) and the applicable state agency.[41] If a breakdown occurs during bargaining for an initial contract following recognition and NLRB certification of a labor organization, a 30-day notice must be given to the FMCS and the appropriate state agency before a strike can be called. These provisions provide a longer time for the parties to reach agreement or plan for a work stoppage and to enable the FMCS to provide assistance.

Strike Notice   HSOs must also be given a strike notice. The 1974 amendments require that, if there is a collective bargaining agreement, the union must give at least 10 days' notice to the employer preceding a work stoppage, which cannot occur before the end of the 90-day notice of a desire to change an existing contract. Striking, picketing, or a concerted refusal to work without properly notifying the HSO or the FMCS is a union unfair labor practice.[42] In bargaining for an initial contract after recognition, the strike notice cannot be given until the end of the 30-day notice of an impasse. The strike notice allows the HSO to discharge or transfer patients, or otherwise plan for continuity of care.

Conciliation of Labor Disputes   The amendments provide that, if the director of the FMCS believes "a threatened strike or lockout affecting a health care institution will . . . substantially interrupt the delivery of health care in the locality concerned" (Section 213[a]) the director can appoint an impartial board of inquiry to help resolve the issues. The act specifies a time for appointing the board and investigating and reporting, during which the employer and union must maintain the status quo, unless they agree to a change. This allows the FMCS to begin discussions and help resolve issues before negotiations break down.

Individuals with Religious Convictions   Public Law 93-360 exempted HSO employees from paying union dues, even in a union shop, when the individual "is a member of and adheres to established and traditional tenets or teachings of a *bona fide* religion, body, or sect which has historically held religious conscientious objections to joining or financially supporting labor organizations." The individual must, however, donate an equivalent amount to a charitable fund approved by the institution and labor organization. In 1980, this provision was extended to all employees covered by the NLRA.[43]

BARGAINING UNIT DETERMINATION

After a petition for an initial recognition election, the NLRB determines if it has jurisdiction and determines the appropriate bargaining unit. Absent prior agreement by the parties, the criteria used by the NLRB in bargaining unit determinations include previous history of bargaining between employer and employees, relationship of the unit to the employer's organizational structure, geographical area practice patterns, and the desires of employees.[44] In addition, the NLRB emphasizes the "community of interest" of proposed bargaining units,[45] which is the extent of common interests among employees.[46] Criteria defining community of interest include similarities in training, skills, working conditions, and supervision, as well as economic concerns, wages, and benefits.[47] If the NLRB determines a bargaining unit is appropriate, the election is held.

From 1974 to 1987 the NLRB had great difficulty regarding bargaining unit determination in health services. It sought to implement conflicting policies—that of the NLRA to assure employees the freedom to exercise their right to choose to collectively bargain,[48] and the admonition of Congress to avoid "undue proliferation" of bargaining units. The NLRB also addressed conflicting interests of the parties—employers wanted few units and labor wanted many.[49] In 1987, constant litigation over appropriateness of bargaining units, inconsistent court rulings, and general frustration caused the NLRB to initiate a rule-making process to settle the bargaining unit controversy in HSOs.

Reason for the Controversy

Employers and unions have different interests in collective bargaining. Unions seek to represent employees; HSOs usually seek to remain union free. As a result, they approach bargaining unit determination differently. The literature is clear that the smaller the bargaining unit the more likely it is employees will vote for a union.[50] Establishing many small units allows homogeneous employees with common interests and similar needs to be grouped together.[51] These circumstances give employees greater resolve to bargain collectively. Employers want few units that are as large as possible because: 1) fewer units reduce the complexity and frequency of collective bargaining, 2) there will be fewer jurisdictional disputes among existing unions, and 3) large units of nonhomogeneous employees have diverse interests and unions are less likely to win a recognition election. This last reason is the root of the bargaining unit controversy and caused constant litigation prior to the NLRB rule making described below.

History of Bargaining Unit Litigation

Prior to the 1974 amendments, Congress expressed its concern that bargaining units be limited for HSO employees.[52] Senator Taft sought to establish only four: professional, technical, clerical, and maintenance and service.[53] Congress wanted to avoid problems like those in the building industry, where proliferation of many small bargaining units had resulted in fragmentation of collective bargaining, jurisdictional disputes among unions, and "wage leapfrogging" in which unions seek larger settlements than those obtained by other bargaining units with the same employer.[54] In addition, it was argued that more unions increased the likelihood of work stoppages and the potential for sympathy strikes.

As passed, the 1974 Act contained no specific reference to the number of bargaining units for the health services industry. However, both the House and Senate conference reports used identical language to instruct the NLRB that "due consideration should be given by the Board to preventing the proliferation of bargaining units in the health care industry."[55]

As early as 1975, the NLRB used traditional community of interest standards to identify five preferred bargaining units in HSOs, with registered nurses (RNs) separate from other professionals.[56] By statute, guards already had an additional separate unit. In subsequent decisions the NLRB held that a unit of physicians separate from other professionals was appropriate,[57] as was a skilled maintenance unit of boilermakers separate from the larger unit of service and maintenance employees. NLRB's application of community of interest was not accepted by all courts as the appropriate means to avoid "undue proliferation of bargaining units."[58] In 1979, the Ninth Circuit

Court of Appeals ruled in *NLRB v. St. Francis Hospital of Lynwood* that separating RNs from the professional bargaining unit based on a community of interest standard inadequately reflected congressional intent regarding nonproliferation.[59] The court ruled that, in addition to community of interest, a stricter standard—disparity of interest—must be applied. "This nontraditional test required that the NLRB allow separate bargaining units to exist only when significant differences in the traditional characteristics used to find community of interest warranted separation from a 'main' group."[60]

In a 1982 ruling affecting St. Francis Hospital in Memphis (St. Francis I), the NLRB established a two-tiered test for bargaining unit determination. The NLRB first determined whether the proposed unit fell into one of the eight commonly recognized units: physicians, RNs, other professionals, technical employees, business office/clerical, service and maintenance, skilled maintenance employees, and guards. If so, the second tier of the test, community of interest, was applied.[61] In St. Francis I the NLRB approved a maintenance unit separate from service employees. The hospital challenged the determination and refused to bargain because the NLRB failed to use the disparity of interest test.[62] An unfair labor practice proceeding resulted, and the NLRB reversed itself (St. Francis II).[63] The NLRB concluded that the two-tiered test merely restated the community of interest test. Consequently, the NLRB applied the disparity of interest test[64] and the unit was disapproved because it was not significantly different from the larger unit of service and maintenance employees.[65] The union appealed and, in *International Brotherhood of Electrical Workers, Local 474, AFL-CIO v. National Labor Relations Board*,[66] the District of Columbia Court of Appeals added to the bargaining unit confusion by finding no "due consideration" statutory language in the 1974 amendments to the Taft-Hartley Act. The court held that since due consideration was only in the conference committee reports and not the law, the NLRB's departure from the traditional community of interest standard to use of the stricter disparity of interest standard was inappropriate.[67] In short, in 1987 the NLRB was back to square one with respect to the bargaining unit controversy.[68] In the notice of proposed rule making, the NLRB states:

> Thirteen years and many hundreds of cases later, the Board finds that despite its numerous, well-intended efforts to carry out congressional intent through formulation of a general conceptual test, it is now no closer to successfully defining appropriate bargaining units in the health care industry than it was in 1974.[69]

Rule Making

The NLRB was frustrated with the time-consuming and costly litigation over bargaining unit determination and the inconsistent court rulings regarding the disparity of interest test. The appeals court's rejection of due consideration was the final straw that caused the NLRB to exercise for the first time its statutory authority to make rules and to issue substantive regulations relative to bargaining unit determination.[70]

Administratively defining appropriate bargaining units rather than being subject to the adjudication process and case-by-case determinations would allow the NLRB to set clear rules that would shorten the time needed to resolve problems and reduce litigation costs of election case hearings. Rule making began on July 2, 1987, with a notice of proposed rule making in the *Federal Register*.[71] A proposed rule was published in 1988, and HSOs and employee organizations were permitted to comment.[72] The process culminated with a final rule on April 21, 1989.[73] The American Hospital Association (AHA) obtained an injunction barring implementation of the rule. The Seventh Circuit Court of Appeals overturned the injunction on April 11, 1990. The AHA appealed to the Supreme Court.[74] On April 23, 1991, the Supreme Court ruled unanimously in favor of the NLRB to make rules relative to bargaining unit determination in the health care industry. Consequently, the NLRB's final rule was upheld.

In its final rule, the NLRB defined appropriate bargaining units in acute care hospitals as follows:

1. All registered nurses
2. All physicians
3. All professional employees except registered nurses and physicians
4. All technical employees
5. All skilled maintenance employees
6. All business office clerical employees
7. All guards
8. All other nonprofessional employees except for those classified above [75]

This rule has certain exemptions and exceptions. First, existing noncomforming bargaining units may continue. Second, in extraordinary circumstances, such as when a defined unit would have five or fewer employees, the NLRB will determine the appropriate unit. The rule applies to acute care hospitals where over 50% of patients have an average length of stay less than 30 days, even if the facility provides long-term, psychiatric, or rehabilitative care. All other HSOs are excluded.

Arguments made against the initial (1987) rule included: employers lost the right to case-by-case determinations of bargaining unit appropriateness;[76] the rule did not consider the health care industry's diversity, including variations in organizational size, range of services, and differing staffing patterns;[77] and approving eight units would cause bargaining units to proliferate because unions in acute care hospitals with fewer units would try to increase the number to the maximum permitted.

Consequences of Rule Making

There are a number of implications in the Supreme Court's decision to uphold the NLRB's authority to define the bargaining units in acute care hospitals. First, union organizing activity is likely to increase[78] as eliminating the costs of protracted litigation removes a financial barrier, particularly for local independent unions without substantial resources.[79] Second, union success rates will likely increase because there are more small units. Third, wage increases in new contracts may spill over to other units and, with them, the risk of more work stoppages.[80] Fourth, organizationwide teamwork and implementing continuous quality improvement programs may be hindered because of fragmentation caused by jurisdictional prerogatives.[81] Finally, management's contract negotiations will be more complex.

Nonetheless, there are benefits. Protracted, case-by-case litigation to determine bargaining units is unnecessary, and acute care hospitals need not fear proliferation of bargaining units beyond those defined in the rule. In addition, the management time, energy, and resources previously devoted to litigation can be redirected elsewhere.[82]

SOLICITATION AND DISTRIBUTION

HSOs should have policies that restrict union solicitation and distribution. Solicitation is defined as one person talking with another about joining a union and includes handing out the authorization cards that document a showing of interest. Distribution is defined as handing out union literature. An HSO may restrict distribution if the policy began before a union campaign and if it is not overly broad. Overly broad and all encompassing policies such as "absolutely no solicitation or distribution on the HSO's premises at any time" are presumed by the NLRB to be invalid. "It is an unfair labor practice under section 8(a)(1) [of the NLRA] for an employer to impose an unlawfully broad rule against solicitation or distribution interfering with the employee's statutory rights to engage in concerted activity" to organize.[83] Existing solicitation and distribution policies must be enforced in a consistent and nondiscriminatory manner.[84]

The NLRB has baseline rules about solicitation and distribution. If the organization has an exclusion rule, outside union organizers can be denied access to the premises for the purposes of solicitation and distribution, if the rule is enforced consistently. If outsiders such as charitable and volunteer organizations may come on the premises for non-HSO business, the NLRB may require that the same privilege be granted to outside union organizers.[85]

The second baseline is that internal organizers (employees) may legally engage in solicitation and distribution of union literature on HSO property, but only during nonworking time and in nonworking areas.[86] Working hours are from the beginning to the end of a shift. Working time is time spent working, excluding meal and break time, which is considered nonworking time. Employees can be prohibited from soliciting and distributing union material in any working area during the solicitor's or the recipient's working time.

Guidelines on solicitation and distribution for HSOs issued by the NLRB general counsel subsequent to the 1974 amendments recognized that HSOs are unique. Consequently, there may be additional restrictions on where solicitation and distribution may occur. To "protect patients from disturbance," employees may not solicit for union membership or distribute union literature during nonworking time[87] if patient care will be disrupted. Patient care areas include patient rooms, operating rooms, treatment rooms, patient area corridors and sitting rooms, and elevators and stairways frequently used in transporting patients.[88] A ban cannot be enforced in nonpatient areas to which only employees have access, including kitchens, laundry supply rooms, the housekeeping, bookkeeping, and medical records departments, and employee lounges, locker rooms, and rest rooms.[89] Policies regarding areas of public access, such as cafeterias, lobbies, gift shops, grounds and walkways, are examined by the NLRB case by case.[90]

HSOs must be concerned that, absent a preexisting policy, prohibiting solicitation and distribution may be an unfair labor practice like that of enforcing an overly broad policy or one that has not been enforced in a consistent, nondiscriminatory manner. Gilmore recommends the following guidelines in formulating a policy: HSOs must avoid promulgating a solicitation and distribution policy that is overly broad, must predicate the policy on the need to prevent or minimize disruption of patient care, and must time the introduction of the policy so that the NLRB will not conclude that its sole purpose is to deprive employees of their right to union solicitation.[91]

UNIONIZATION IN HEALTH SERVICES

It was predicted that bringing not-for-profit hospitals under federal labor law would cause labor organization activity to explode, result in work stoppages, and greatly increase wage costs.[92] By and large the predictions did not occur. Representation elections in hospitals increased from 1974 to 1980, after which they declined much as they did in other sectors of the economy. Work stoppages did not become an issue because there were few.[93] Unions did, however, affect wage costs,[94] but less than predicted.

Comprehensive data on unionization in hospitals, nursing facilities, HMOs, and clinics are unavailable.* The best estimate is that slightly over 20% of the nation's hospitals have at least one

*There are few studies that report the extent of unionization in HSOs. Personal communication with the NLRB, FMCS, Bureau of Labor Statistics (BLS), and American Hospital Association (AHA), among others, indicates that none systematically collects data on how many HSOs in total or by type are unionized. The NLRB collects and reports annual union election data; however, it does not, for example, report summaries of election by type of hospital ownership. The following estimates are available. According to Fottler,[95] in 1985 an estimated 20% of nongovernmental, short-term hospitals—a category that includes three fifths of all hospitals—had a union. Metzger states that, in 1990, "20% of all health care workers are members of unions and about the same percentage of hospitals have at least one union contract."[96] Killard Adamache, senior economist at the Center for Health Economics Research, provides a 1988 estimate of the percentage of hospitals with unions of 19.1%. The Center's data base includes acute care hospitals but excludes governmental hospitals.[97] For long-term care facilities, the numbers are even more sparse. In the most recent survey, a 1985 BLS study covering 40 major metropolitan areas estimates that 15%–19% of professional/technical employees and 35%–39% of nonprofessional employees in nursing and personal care facilities were covered by union contracts. However, the study does not indicate how many of the nursing facilities had a union.[98] In 1986 there were approximately 16,000 nursing and personal care facilities, of which 75% were investor owned, with 1.5 million beds and over 500,000 employees.[99]

union—a percentage relatively unchanged since 1975. Using AHA data, Miller reports that hospitals of all types with a union totaled 3.0% in 1960, 7.7% in 1967, 14.7% in 1970, and 19.8% in 1975.[100] In a 1989 wage survey, the Bureau of Labor Statistics (BLS) sampled nongovernmental, acute care hospitals with more than 100 employees. A weighting system allowed national inferences to be drawn. It reported that 18% of RNs, 18% of service employees (food service, housekeeping, and laundry), and 13% of other hospital employees were covered by a union contract.[101]

Most reporting of hospital unionization focuses on numbers of representation elections reported by the NLRB each year.[102] Given that the present number of hospitals with at least one union contract is approximately the same as the number in 1975, it can be inferred that union election activity tends to occur in hospitals already having a union. Based on data provided by the NLRB, Figures 18.4, 18.5, and 18.6 show union representation elections in various sectors for fiscal years 1974 through 1990. Figure 18.4 presents annual union elections in *hospitals only* and includes all types of nongovernmental hospitals (short and long term, not-for-profit, and investor owned). Figure 18.5 shows annual union elections in *all types of HSOs* such as hospitals, nursing facilities, clinics, group practices, laboratories, HMOs, and blood banks. Figure 18.6 provides annual union election data for *all sectors* of the United States economy, including health services.

Figure 18.6 indicates a general decline in annual union representation elections from 1974 through 1990 in all sectors, especially after 1981. The average annual union success rate in all sectors for 1974 through 1990 was 46%. In contrast, the average annual union success rate in all types of HSOs (55%) was higher than in all economic sectors. It was also higher than the average annual success rate of 51% in hospitals only. Unions seem to be more successful in nonhospital HSOs.

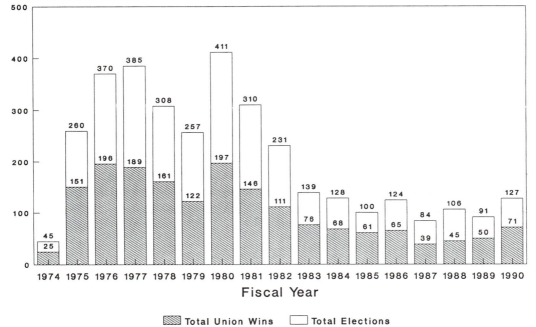

Figure 18.4. Union elections in all types of nongovernmental hospitals by fiscal year, 1974–1990. (Source: Special data report to authors by the NLRB, June 22, 1991.)

Number of Elections

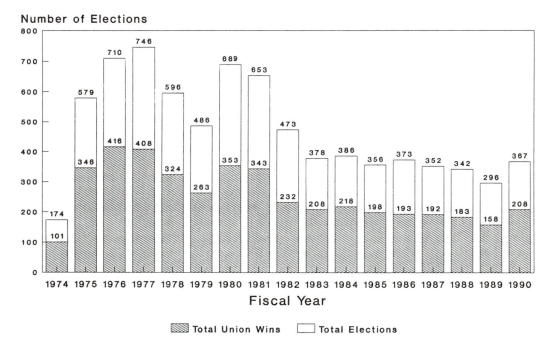

Figure 18.5. Union elections in health services industry—nongovernmental HSOs of all types—by fiscal year, 1974–1990. (Source: Special data report to authors by the NLRB, June 22, 1991.)

In the hospital sector, Figure 18.4 indicates that the annual number of union elections was high in the years 1975 through 1978, just after passage of the 1974 amendments to Taft-Hartley, and again spiked in 1980 and 1981 for a high of 411. Thereafter, and especially subsequent to implementation of the Medicare prospective payment system (diagnosis-related groups) in 1983, the annual number of union elections in hospitals declined substantially. This may be partly due to the following reasons. First, easier hospitals may have already been unionized and, thus, less intensive unionization efforts were being directed at hospitals. Second, hospital management maturity vis-à-vis labor relations increased. Third, hospitals in the late 1980s began to more aggressively seek to remain union free. Finally, economic and industry structural factors such as mergers and acquisitions, downsizing and layoffs, "and fixed reimbursements from third-party payers and higher expenses have forced hospitals to cut costs."[103] Even though the number of annual union elections in hospitals declined in the last half of the 1980s, the union movement is far from dead. The 1991 Supreme Court ruling upholding the NLRB rule to define bargaining units in nongovernmental acute care hospitals will give further impetus to the union movement.

Union election activity is not consistent for all types of hospital ownership or for all geographical areas. The results of a study of 238 union representation elections in nongovernmental acute care hospitals during calender years 1985 through 1987 are presented in Table 18.3 and Figure 18.7.[104] It was found that not-for-profit, nonreligious hospitals were the ownership category most likely to experience the greatest number of elections and highest union success rate, followed by not-for-profit religious and investor-owned hospitals.

Geographical regions with the largest number of union elections were the Middle Atlantic (New York, Pennsylvania, and New Jersey), East North-Central (Ohio, Indiana, Michigan, Illinois, and Wisconsin), and the Pacific region (California, Oregon, Washington, and Alaska). Substantially fewer elections occurred in the south and southwest, where there are greater numbers of investor-owned hospitals.

Number of Elections

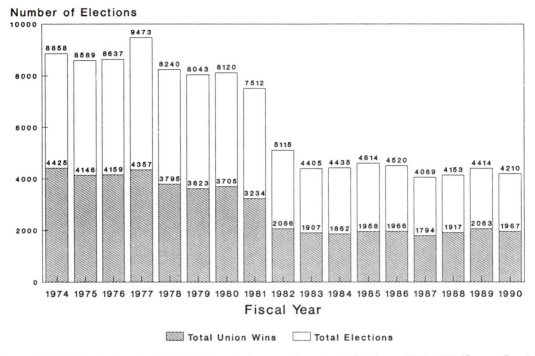

Figure 18.6. Union elections in all United States private economic sectors by fiscal year, 1974–1990. (Source: Special data report to authors by the NLRB, June 22, 1991.)

The organizations most active in these elections were independent local unions (those not affiliated with a national labor organization), the American Nurses Association, the Service Employees International Union, and the National Union of Hospital and Health Care Workers—often referred to as District 1199.[105] The American Federation of State, County, & Municipal Employees (AFSCME) union is particularly active in government-owned hospitals[106] as well as nursing facilities.

WHY EMPLOYEES UNIONIZE

Employees unionize when they are dissatisfied with conditions of work, democracy in the work setting, and/or the content of employment, and when they perceive that collective bargaining will yield positive outcomes.[107] Simply put, unions are a vehicle for redress when employee needs are not met by the HSO. The union's primary role is to improve the job security and economic interests of employees. In addition, the collective bargaining process allows unions to address other terms and conditions of employment, organizational policies and procedures affecting the employer–employee relationship, and, in some instances, the occupational status of members.

Conditions of employment are primarily concerned with economic and security issues, as well as elements of the work setting. Economic concerns relate to compensation, such as wages and salaries and fringe benefits. Wages and salaries include absolute pay rates, relative pay among similar organizations, pay differentials among job classifications, and shift differentials. Fringe benefits typically include health and life insurance, retirement programs, holidays and vacation time, and employee assistance programs.

Elements of the work setting are also an important aspect of the conditions of employment. They include hours of employment, scheduling patterns, break times, the physical work environment, and personal security. Finally, job security as affected by a changing mix of part-time and

Table 18.3. NLRB union elections and outcomes in nongovernmental, short-term hospitals by selected hospital and area characteristics: January 1985–December 1987

Selected characteristic	Number of hospitals with elections	Number of elections	Number of union wins	Union wins as a percentage of elections
All hospitals[a]	195[b]	238	112	47.1
Census region				
New England	18	22	12	54.5
Middle Atlantic	62	74	34	45.9
South Atlantic	10	12	3	25.0
East North Central	41	49	24	49.0
East South Central	8	11	5	45.5
West North Central	10	13	5	38.5
West South Central	1	1	1	100.0
Mountain	6	7	2	28.6
Pacific	31	38	18	47.4
Puerto Rico	8	11	8	72.7
	195	238	112	
Ownership[c]				
Not-for-profit—religious	29	43	18	41.9
Not-for-profit—nonreligious	141	164	83	50.6
Investor owned	25	31	11	35.5
	195	238	112	
Bed size				
0–99	52	63	29	46.0
100–199	53	74	40	54.1
200–299	35	38	15	39.5
300–399	32	37	14	37.8
400–499	5	5	2	40.0
500–over	18	21	12	57.1
	195	238	112	
Multiorganizational system				
No	132	157	74	47.1
Yes	63	81	38	46.9
	195	238	112	
Type of system				
Not-for-profit—religious	22	33	12	36.4
Not-for-profit—nonreligious	27	31	20	64.5
Investor owned	14	17	6	35.3
	63	81	38	

From Rakich, Jonathon S., Edmund R. Becker, and Carey N. Rakich. An analysis of hospital union election activity: 1985–1987. *Hospital Topics* 68 (Winter 1990): 9; reprinted with permission of the Helen Dwight Reid Educational Foundation. Published by Heldref Publications, 1319 18th Street, N.W., Washington, D.C. 20036-1802. Copyright 1990.

Election data were collected from National Labor Relations Board *Monthly Election Reports,* 1/85–12/87. Hospital data were obtained from the American Hospital Association *AHA Guide, 1987 and Hospital Statistics, 1987.*

[a]Number of nongovernmental, short-term hospitals by census region, ownership, and bed size were obtained from AHA *Hospital Statistics, 1987.* The number with elections was 4.6% of the total.

[b]Unique hospitals. Those hospitals having more than one election during the 3-year period were counted only once.

[c]To derive the percentage of hospitals with an election by ownership, the proportion of total nongovernmental, short-term hospitals by ownership type was estimated to be as follows: not-for-profit—religious 18%, not-for-profit—nonreligious 63%, and investor owner 19%.

full-time employees, the outside contracting of work previously performed in house, and employee reductions during organization downsizing will continue to concern employees.[108] Collective bargaining subjects all of these conditions of employment to negotiation.

Democracy in the work setting describes the organization's prevailing attitude toward employees and the application of policies and procedures. Policies and criteria for promotion, trans-

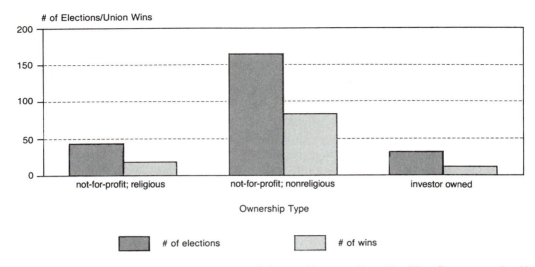

Figure 18.7. Hospital union elections and wins by hospital ownership type, 1985–1987. (*Note:* Percentage wins: Not-for-profit—religious, 41.86; not-for-profit—nonreligious, 50.61; investor owned, 35.48. Data derived from NLRB *Monthly Election Reports* and *AHA Guide*, 1987.) (From Rakich, Jonathon S., Edmund R. Becker, and Carey N. Rakich. An analysis of hospital union election activity: 1985–1987. *Hospital Topics* 68 (Winter 1990): 10; reprinted with permission of the Helen Dwight Reid Educational Foundation. Published by Heldref Publications, 1319 18th Street, N.W., Washington, D.C. 20036-1802. Copyright 1990.)

fer, discipline, termination, job reassignment, performance appraisal, grievances, and compensation changes are important. Especially important are consistent application and fairness in treatment among individuals or groups of employees.[109] Lack of clearly stated policies or inconsistency in application leads to dissatisfaction, which is an important cause of unionization.

The organization's philosophy about human resources greatly influences the context of the employment relationship. Employees want to be treated as individuals, not just another resource, and want to know that the HSO is sincerely concerned for them and their well-being. Employees' perceptions of the organization and its policies and attitudes toward workers are largely derived from their immediate supervisor—the organization's representative with whom employees most frequently interact.[110] The supervisor's management practices affect this perception. If supervision is fair, consistent, and concerned, employee dissatisfaction will be lower than if the reverse is true, particularly if conditions of employment and democracy in the work setting are positive. An organizational philosophy and management practices that recognize the importance of employees and their individuality are progressive.

Such an atmosphere of employment necessarily incorporates meaningfulness of work in job design and involves, when possible, shaping jobs to individual strengths, skills, and interests. It is dependent on two-way communications, which lessen information vacuums and encourage two-way listening. Risk-free upward communication and downward communication to be informed are important employee needs.[111] Perceptive, well-trained first-line managers contribute greatly to fostering this positive atmosphere.

Job autonomy is important to many HSOs employees, especially to professionals such as RNs and technicians. They are concerned with their work roles and the way they relate to the task-structure elements of the organization and patient care delivery. Their ability to fulfill professional and autonomy needs is important.[112] They seek to expand their job responsibilities and be involved in decision making within their areas of competence.[113] Assertiveness among professionals who increasingly seek recognition and greater participation in managing patient care is a powerful force, particularly for RNs. For them, job dissatisfaction stems from unclear roles, conflict with physicians, and inadequately performing or insufficient numbers of staff. These employees may view unionization as an alternative to what they perceive to be the organization's indifference or unwillingness to deal with professional issues.

Physicians who may be full-time salaried employees of HSOs, such as a closed panel HMO, are another professional group that may be interested in unionizing, especially if practice protocols become common. It is estimated there are 30,000–55,000 physicians who belong to 16 physicians' unions.[114] Those physicians who are in postgraduate medical education programs (residencies) have been classified by the courts as students, and they do not meet the NLRA's definition of an employee.[115] Consequently, residents are not covered by federal labor law.

HSOs and managers must be sensitive to employees' needs relative to conditions of employment, democracy in the work setting, and the content of employment, including professional autonomy. If they are, and they actively address deficiencies, they are unlikely to have employees who unionize. As Fennell notes, "In many cases an insensitive employer is a union's best organizer."[116]

Symptoms of an Organization Campaign

Generally the climate of labor–management relations is sufficiently clear that an attempt to organize employees is evident. Some of the symptoms cited by the AHA are enumerated below:[117]

> A sudden lack of communication between supervisors and normally friendly or conversant employees
>
> New informal leaders within the employee group
>
> Employees asking unusual questions or seeking information about the HSO's policies and procedures
>
> Unusual group activity among employees before and after working hours as well as employees congregating in small groups during work hours
>
> Increased contact among employees in off-site locations
>
> Greater than usual rumors and expression of insecurity
>
> Changing tardiness and absentee patterns
>
> Abnormal attention given to a recently discharged or disciplined employee
>
> Attempts by employees to provoke confrontations with supervisors
>
> The distribution of union literature
>
> Off-site union meetings held by organizers

TYPES OF UNION ELECTIONS

When it is petitioned to do so, the NLRB conducts representation elections. They are of two types: recognition (labeled as RC) elections and decertification (labeled as RD) elections. NLRB formal election process procedures are presented in Figure 18.8.

In RC elections, the NLRB investigates whether it has jurisdiction. If so, it determines if there is a sufficient "showing of interest" by employees for a union election to be held. A showing of interest is defined as signed authorization cards from 30% or more of employees in the proposed bargaining unit indicating that they wish to have the labor organization represent them. RC election petitions may be filed by an employee, a group of employees, or a union organization.[118] Once the NLRB determines that the bargaining unit is appropriate, a secret ballot election is held and the NLRB certifies the results. If the labor organization has a majority of votes cast, it is certified as the employees' bargaining agent and the HSO must bargain with it in good faith.

Decertification (RD) elections occur when there is a petition to the NLRB by employees asserting that the previously "certified or recognized bargaining agent no longer represents a majority of the employees in the appropriate bargaining unit."[119] The same showing of interest as in RC elections applies.

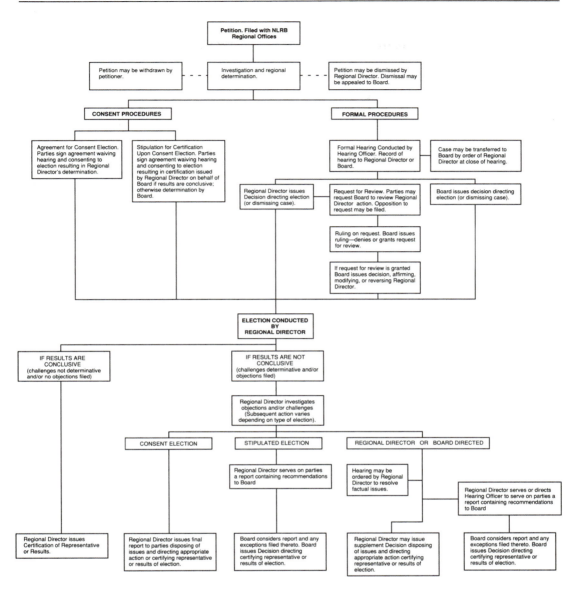

Figure 18.8. NLRB union election process procedures. (Source: NLRB, March, 1991.)

One type of petition allows employers to request an election. These are coded as RM cases and they occur in two circumstances. First, when there is no certified union, "an RM petition can be filed by an employer if one or more labor organizations claim representation status for an appropriate unit, and the employer questions the representative's status."[120] If the employer accepts the labor organization's claim, no election is held, the NLRB certifies the union, and the HSO must bargain with it.[121] Such initial acceptance by HSOs rarely occurs. The second RM type of case occurs when the employer has objective evidence that a recognized union no longer represents a majority of the bargaining unit's employees.[122] This can occur, for example, where a union that was certified in an RC election never signed a contract with the HSO. For RM petitions, the showing of interest criterion is not applied.[123]

The preponderance of elections in nongovernmental acute care hospitals are for initial recognition (RC). NLRB election reports from 1985 through 1987 show that 238 elections were held. Of these, 200 were initial recognition (RC) elections (84.0% of all elections), 33 were decertification (RD) elections (13.8% of all elections), and only 5 were RM cases (2% of all elections).[124]

EMPLOYER CONDUCT DURING AN ELECTION CAMPAIGN

When the NLRB finds a "showing of interest" by employees, an election is held. During an election campaign there are permissible and prohibited activities on the part of the employer and its representatives—managers and supervisors. Section 1(11) of the NLRA defines a supervisor (manager) as:

> any individual having authority, in the interest of the employer, to hire, transfer, suspend, lay off, recall, promote, discharge, assign, reward, or discipline other employees, or responsibility to direct them, or to adjust their grievances, or effectively to recommend such action, if in connection with the foregoing the exercise of such authority is not of a merely routine clerical nature, but requires the use of independent judgment.

Employers or managers and supervisors cannot interfere, restrain, or coerce employees in exercising their right under Section 7 of the NLRA to organize.[125] It is an unfair labor practice to interfere with employees' right to organize, such as lawful solicitation and distribution, or to act coercively, such as inappropriately interrogating or conducting surveillance of employees.[126] Other activities defined by the NLRB as interfering with employee free choice are:[127]

> Threats of loss of jobs or benefits by an employer to influence the votes or union activities of employees
>
> A grant of benefits or promise to grant benefits to influence the votes or union activities of employees
>
> Firing employees to discourage or encourage their union activities
>
> Making campaign speeches to assembled groups of employees on HSO time within the 24-hour period before an election
>
> Incitement of racial or religious prejudice by inflammatory campaign appeals

Employers and their agents have the right of free speech during an organization campaign. However, their statements must not contain the threat of reprisal or force or promise benefits. Feldacker indicates:

> Section 8(c) of the Labor Management Relations Act [Taft-Hartley] states that the "expressing of any views, arguments or opinions or the dissemination thereof, whether in written, printed, graphic, or visual form, shall not constitute or be evidence of an unfair labor practice under any provision of this Act, if such expression contains no *threat of reprisal or force or promises of benefits* [emphasis added]."[128]

The employer may respond to union organizing charges and communicate its general views about unionism and predictions of the economic realities of unionization as long as the predictions are based on objective facts.[129] An example would be the experience the employer or other employers have had with unions, such as the union not successfully negotiating higher wages.

There are numerous examples of permissible and prohibited activities by the employer.[130] The reader should be aware that NLRB and court rulings on permissible and prohibited employer activates are evolutionary, complex, and dependent on the facts of each situation. The following examples[131] are only *guidelines*. In the event of an organization campaign, legal counsel should provide advice about permissible and prohibited activities.

Permissible Employer Activities

1. Inform the employees of your views and opinions about unions, their leaders and policies, and about your and others' experience with unions. Do not, however, libel or slander.
2. Inform the employees about the history, background, and character of the union and its officials who are attempting to organize them, and about strikes, violence, and loss of jobs in other organizations that were organized. Stick to facts that can be proved.
3. Inform the employees of the adverse effects of unions in other areas.
4. Inform the employees that it costs money to join a union and that unions are supported by dues, fines, fees, and assessments from the members. Employees can also be told that dues and fee increases are often decided at national union conventions rather than by a membership vote.
5. Inform the employees that they might have only a minor role in the operation of any local union, and many things could be decided of which they might not approve.
6. Inform the employees that as a union member they may be required to strike even though they do not want to do so and are happy with the organization's offer.
7. Inform the employees that the organization has the legal right to hire a new employee to replace any employee who goes on strike over economic reasons.
8. Reassure the employees that they do not have to join a union to keep their jobs.
9. Inform the employees that the organization would continue to have the right to discharge an employee for cause, and that membership in a union does not exempt an employee from discharge.
10. Remind the employees of the benefits they presently enjoy without paying union dues and compare their wages and benefits to those of unionized operations.
11. Inform the employees that the union cannot obtain more from the organization than the organization can or is willing to pay, nor can it obtain more than any individual employee could from the organization without a union.
12. Inform the employees that the organization is not required automatically to sign a contract or agree to any proposal that is not in its best interests.
13. Remind the employees of the organization's record for fair dealing.
14. Inform the employees of any untrue or misleading statements about the organization made by the union, and answer union arguments or charges.
15. Advise the employees of how you think they should vote and that they have a free choice not to support or join the union.
16. Urge employees to report union coercion to their supervisors, and inform them that they have the right not to talk with union organizers if they do not care to.

Prohibited Employer Activities

1. Do not ask employees what they think about the union or its officers, how the employee or other employees plan to vote, or about confidential union matters such as union meetings and who attended.
2. Do not spy on the union or request employees to spy on the union.
3. Do not go to a union meeting or near where a union meeting is being held.
4. Do not state to employees that the organization knows about their or other employees' membership in the union, signing a union card, union activity, or attending a union meeting.
5. Do not hold straw votes.
6. Do not make any threats to discourage union activity, union membership, signing a union card, or voting for the union, such as:

—cutting out or curtailing benefits

—cutting out or reducing overtime

—transferring the employee to less desirable work

—laying off or discharging

—blacklisting employees

—discontinuing employee loans or other practices

7. Do not make any promises of a benefit or a reward in return for the employee's not joining the union, voting against the union, not signing a card, or not engaging in union activity, such as:

—higher pay

—more overtime

—extra privileges

—better treatment, job, or assignment promotion

8. Do not ask antiunion employees to question other employees about their union feelings and report back their findings.

9. Do not say or imply that a union victory *will* result in a strike and a consequent economic loss to employees.

10. Do not state that union organization would be futile because the union can get nothing for employees through bargaining.

11. Do not predict that the employer will lose business because of unionization unless this is supported by objective fact.

12. Do not ask new job applicants about their union feelings or affiliations.

13. Do not visit employees at their homes to discuss the union or to solicit employee support in opposition to the union.

MANAGERIAL RESPONSIBILITIES IN LABOR RELATIONS

Managers must effectively use resources to meet customer and other stakeholder needs and to accomplish the organization's objectives. This is easier to achieve with greater managerial freedom for resource interchange. By definition, a union lessens management's prerogatives because the collective bargaining agreement restricts management decisions about allocating and utilizing personnel and other resources.[132] HSOs are labor intensive. Union constraints on utilizing employees could have a major impact on personnel costs and productivity.[133] Retaining administrative flexibility is a powerful incentive to remain union free. Unions have an impact on compensation costs, may demand restrictive work rules, generally dissipate management energy and time, may cause strife and conflict, particularly when the relationship is adversarial,[134] and ultimately have the potential for a work stoppage.[135]

Metzger observes that an HSO with a positive labor-relations atmosphere, "an organization that provides all the benefits and protection afforded by a union contract—such as competitive wages, a seniority system, a grievance and arbitration procedure—need not be unionized."[136] He also observes that, in a nonunion environment:[137]

The employer has greater latitude in running of the operation and directing employees.

It is easier to change work processes, task-technology relationships, and schedules.

There is freedom to introduce new technologies and productivity programs and quality improvement.

It is easier to introduce new and varying programs directed at increasing the motivation of employees, such as gain sharing, and, through employee involvement and participation, achieve greater employee commitment to organization initiatives such as continuous quality improvement.

Setting the Tone and Environment

The AHA policy statement on the principles of employee relations,[138] published in the mid-1970s, specifies, among others, the following principles: HSOs should provide adequate compensation and an appropriate work environment for employees, and they should provide the opportunity for self-expression, career mobility, and uniform and appropriate job performance procedures, and for the establishment of a grievance procedure. The overriding principle was an awareness that it is people at all levels of the organization that make it work. The AHA's policy statement on human resource management in HSOs, issued in the mid-1980s, makes two primary points: 1) human resources are the organization's greatest asset; and 2) the HSO needs "to integrate the [organization's] goals with the values, needs, and aspirations of the individual employees who contribute to those goals."[139] These points make it clear that the importance of an HSO's human resources has not changed in a decade. In addition, HSOs embracing these policies, as well as the human resources perspective presented in Chapter 17, will appreciably lessen employees' desire to unionize.

Metzger's points related to his statement that "we must start to think of our employees not as adversaries but as partners" are especially relevant. First, the 1990s is an era of human capital that provides HSO managers with the opportunity to establish sound relations with employees. Second, managers must develop programs to maximize employees' commitment to their jobs and the HSO. Third, managers are responsible for facilitating this partnership.[140] Work systems design and technology are important, but people are everything. Providing employees the opportunity for participation and involvement will lead to success. A disharmonious and adversarial labor-management relationship will preclude it. A positive work atmosphere and organizational culture and philosophy about employees are absolutely critical.

Proactive Steps

Beyond following the principles in the AHA policy statements, there are three steps management can take to strengthen its partnership with employees and their commitment to the organization. They are effective first-line supervision, increased two-way communication, and, in union-free organizations, the establishment of a formal grievance procedure.

Immediate supervisors are the representatives of management with whom employees most frequently interact. Supervisors set the tone and climate and confirm or disaffirm the organization's philosophy toward employees.[141] Adequately trained and technically competent supervisors who, by their practices and behavior, affirm the organization's philosophy will be much more effective in managing subordinates and achieving higher performance. The supervisor's awareness of employee feelings, treatment of subordinates as individuals, and sincere concern for job-related problems foster a positive environment and eliminate many of the reasons why employees unionize.

Communication is also critical to a smoothly functioning organization. Managers must keep employees informed and listen to them. Effective two-way communication contributes greatly to a positive organizational environment and is especially important during times of organizational change. It is very difficult to bond a partnership when only one party speaks.

Promoting upward communication simply makes good sense. This can be accomplished by listening sessions, employee opinion or attitude surveys,[142] or formal interviews conducted by consultants.[143] A mechanism especially useful is a formal grievance procedure.[144] The AHA advocates establishing a grievance procedure, especially in nonunion hospitals, so that employee complaints or disagreements arising "out of disagreements over rule infractions, misunderstandings, and involuntary terminations or temporary suspensions from work" can be resolved.[145]

Grievance procedures provide employees with an easily accessible and fair means to be heard, to alert management to causes of employee dissatisfaction, and "to contribute to the improvement of morale and productivity and the development of mutual respect, trust, and rapport between supervisors and employees."[146] When employees perceive that management is interested in legitimate complaints, dissatisfaction is decreased. A formal grievance procedure is a vehicle to vent frustation. It also makes senior management more aware of employee concerns. Whether these concerns are legitimate is not the point—this is the perception, and the perception, right or wrong, will remain if not addressed. Designing a formal grievance procedure should involve some employee participation, which will promote its legitimacy and instill a sense of commitment to making it work.

COLLECTIVE BARGAINING

Thus far, this chapter has described federal labor law prescribing how the employer and union interact, bargaining unit determination, extent of unionization in health services, reasons why employees join unions, and managerial responsibilities in labor relations. However, even if a sound employer–employee atmosphere is developed, it is still possible that employees will unionize. If so, HSO management and union representatives engage in collective bargaining.

Negotiation and contract administration are elements of collective bargaining. The provisions of an employer–union contract establish parameters for conduct of management and the employees' representative (union) and are a "private law" for the parties. Federal laws do not specify contract provisions. They do, however, set limits on accomplishing recognition, indicate the range of behavior and bargaining issues that are legal, and mandate that both parties bargain fairly and in good faith.

Recognition

Collective bargaining begins after a union has been recognized. As noted previously, recognition is achieved in two ways. An employee organization can simply ask the HSO to recognize it; employers seldom do so. The second method consists of the NLRB determining the appropriate bargaining unit, holding an election, and certifying the results (see Figure 18.8, which presents the NLRB election process). During an organizing campaign neither employer nor union may commit unfair labor practices (see Tables 18.1 and 18.2 and the chapter section on Employer Conduct During an Election Campaign).

Negotiation

Contract negotiations begin after the NLRB certifies the employees' representative. Both parties spend a great deal of time preparing: warm-up meetings are held and proposals and counterproposals are made.[147]

Federal labor law restricts how the parties act toward one another and what can and cannot be part of the contract. Both must bargain in good faith, for example. They must meet with each other's representatives and cannot interfere with each other's rights.[148] The union can demand that the employer negotiate about NLRA-specified "mandatory" subjects, which include wages and hours, conditions of employment, and, as specified in subsequent rulings, pensions, bonuses, grievance procedures, safety practices, seniority, procedures for layoff and recall, discipline and discharge, and union security.[149] Unions may seek to bargain about nonmandatory subjects such as scope of management of the HSO's operations, decisions about allocating and utilizing resources, and management rights regarding employee overtime, scheduling, determining job content, and transferring employees. The employer may choose not to negotiate about these subjects.

Neither negotiations nor the contract can include unlawful issues such as operating a closed shop (which requires new employees to be union members before they can be hired), including supervisors in a bargaining unit, or the HSO pressuring a subcontractor to recognize a union.

Unions usually seek to negotiate provisions about union security and the grievance process. Union security relates to the union's desire to secure and strengthen its position. The employer may accept a union shop provision that requires all new employees in a bargaining unit to join the union after a brief period, generally 30 days. At a minimum the union may seek an agency shop, in which an employee who does not join must pay the equivalent of dues to it or a charity. Finally, there may be a checkoff provision that requires the employer to deduct union dues from each member's pay and remit it to the union, thus easing the union's collection of dues.

Contracts may specify the disciplinary procedure for infractions such as absenteeism, insubordination, and theft. The procedure may include a sequence such as oral warning for the first infraction, written warning for the second, then disciplinary layoff (perhaps a week without pay), and finally termination. Furthermore, it may identify infractions that skip the initial steps. For example, assaulting a supervisor or any other employee may carry a penalty of "up to and including discharge" without progressing through the other steps. An employee who thinks the procedure has not been followed or disagrees with the result may file a grievance.

A formal grievance procedure to resolve employee disputes about the contract may be negotiated. The first step of the grievance procedure is a meeting between the supervisor and the union steward, the second involves the human resources manager, and finally a more senior manager meets with a union official. If the grievance is not resolved, an arbitrator (a neutral third party) may hear the facts and render a decision, which may be advisory or binding, depending on the collective bargaining agreement.

Impasses

Failure of the parties to agree about mandatory bargaining subjects during negotiations results in an impasse. There are several options when an impasse occurs. The union may call a strike after appropriate notification. Strikes are an economic burden that may induce the employer to modify its position. Strikes in HSOs are costly in terms of monetary impact and patient welfare.

HSOs that are struck may hire replacements. Health team members, however, are highly interdependent, and striking employees are not easily replaced. For example, RNs are in short supply in many parts of the country or the facility may be unable to function for an extended time without maintenance workers. Furthermore, if employees are striking legitimately because the employer committed an unfair labor practice, the NLRB can force the employer to reinstate striking workers even if this means discharging replacements. However, if the strike is not called because the employer has committed an unfair labor practice or if the union is striking illegally (an unfair labor practice), striking employees need not be reinstated.

Another option available during an impasse is mediation. Such assistance can be requested from the state or the FMCS. Mediators are third-party neutrals who meet with the parties, stimulate the negotiating process, and try to persuade the two sides to agree to a solution. A mediator's only power is persuasion, and the impasse may not be resolved. Binding arbitration is a final option. Here the parties agree to accept the arbitrator's findings and decision. During contract negotiations, however, neither party wants to give a third party such authority. As a result, binding arbitration is most commonly used to settle grievances during an existing contract rather than to resolve impasses.

Agreement is eventually reached through some method. The resulting contract is a private law that binds the parties. The contract and the manner of reaching agreement—whether by mutual respect or adversary power dominance—greatly influences future labor-management relations and the organizational climate.

SUMMARY

In recent years HSOs have increasingly focused attention on labor relations, specifically unionization. Because HSOs are labor intensive, human resources are the most important of all resources, and effectively utilizing personnel and retaining management's prerogatives are extremely important. Management's responsibilities regarding unionization focus on providing a positive environment where employees see no advantage to bargaining collectively.

This chapter traces the United States union movement and describes major federal legislation—the Norris-LaGuardia Act of 1932, the Wagner Act of 1935, and the Taft-Hartley Act of 1947. Unionization in health services is described, as are the 1974 amendments to the Taft-Hartley Act, which brought not-for-profit HSOs under the umbrella of federal labor law. Also discussed are employer and union unfair labor practices and the bargaining unit controversy.

The reasons employees unionize are categorized as conditions of employment, issues of democracy in the workplace, and content of employment, including professional autonomy. Examples of permissible and prohibited employer activities during an organization campaign, as well as a brief description of the collective bargaining process, are presented.

Of particular importance are managerial responsibilities in labor relations, which focus on organization climate and the philosophy toward employees, the extent of two-way communication, and having a means for employee complaints to be heard at no risk to them. HSO management must be unencumbered by inappropriate constraints on resource allocation and use. However, retaining these prerogatives carries the reciprocal responsibility of meeting employees' legitimate interests. Only then will employees be committed to their jobs and the organization. Management is responsible for nurturing an environment that achieves organizational objectives, and this can best be done when employees are viewed as partners rather than adversaries.

DISCUSSION QUESTIONS

1. Discuss the reasons why HSOs must be concerned about unionization. What impact does a union have on managing the organization? Discuss the impact relative to the management model for HSOs presented in Chapter 1 (Figure 1.6).
2. Discuss the meaning and give general examples of employer and union unfair labor practices. How do they restrain behavior for both parties?
3. Discuss the reasons why the bargaining unit issue has been so controversial. Give reasons why unions seek to have as many bargaining units as possible in HSOs. Give reasons why HSOs seek to have few bargaining units.
4. From the point of view of the employee, what are the advantages and disadvantages of joining a union? Should health services professionals such as physicians, RNs, and pharmacists unionize? Discuss and support your position.
5. This chapter gives several reasons why employees join unions. Which are most important? Do they vary for different occupational groups, such as nonprofessional and professional employees? Are there reasons other than those presented?
6. Given that the percentage of hospitals with at least one union has not changed appreciably since 1975, what conclusions can be drawn about the annual number of representation elections (1975–1990) presented in Figure 18.4?
7. How do first-line managers affect the employees' desire to unionize and how can supervisors behave in an organizing situation? What behavior is not permissible?
8. Do you agree with the statement "Employee relations policies and practices should contribute positively to the welfare of both the employing institution and the employee regardless of whether the organization is unionized?" Why? Is this statement consistent with the quotation at the beginning of the chapter?

CASE STUDY 1:   TAYLOR MEDICAL CENTER AND THE UNION

Gail McKnight is president of Taylor Medical Center, a 350-bed nonunionized hospital located in an urban area. McKnight knew that there was dissatisfaction among the six boiler operator employees and that they had been talking to an organizer from the Operating Engineers Union. Out of the blue McKnight received a letter from the Service Employees International Union stating, "We represent the vast majority of the hospital's 180 service and maintenance employees and demand to meet with you as the representative of these employees."

McKnight met with the chief operating officer and began developing a strategy to counter the current unionization effort. They discussed the following:

1. Transfer of the supervisor. Since the boiler operators were dissatisfied, this must be a result, in part, of inadequacies of their supervisor.
2. Granting of a pay increase (out of normal cycle) to all the employees.
3. Directing the supervisors of all service and maintenance employees to:

   a. Ask their subordinates about their morale and what they think about the union, individually and collectively, by straw vote.
   b. Tell their subordinates, in an objective manner, how the union made employees at another area hospital go on strike for 8 months, and that they would have little control over union operations.
   c. Tell their subordinates how good the hospital has been to them even during periods in which census had been down and how good their working conditions and pay are compared to other hospitals in the area.
   d. Tell their subordinates that if they unionize and wages are increased, there will have to be layoffs since there is only so much money available. Also, since all conditions of work would be negotiable, including pay and fringe benefits, the hospital will consider changing the pension plan, which is now very generous.

Questions

1. What should McKnight do regarding the union's letter demanding that McKnight meet with the union?
2. Advise McKnight whether each of the strategies and actions she and the chief operating officer discussed to counter the current unionization effort are appropriate or inappropriate and why.

CASE STUDY 2: UNION MEMBERSHIP SOLICITATION, AND DISTRIBUTION OF UNION MATERIAL AT DUNLAP MEMORIAL HOSPITAL

Ambrose Catan is a housekeeping supervisor on the 7:00 A.M.–3:00 P.M. shift at Dunlap Memorial Hospital. The hospital has a clear and concise no solicitation or distribution policy that is as restrictive as the law permits. It has existed for many years and has always been enforced in a nondiscriminatory manner. Walking down the hallway by the employee's lounge at 12:45 P.M., he saw one of his subordinates, Mary, talking with Bill, an x-ray technician who had just handed her a pamphlet. Mary's job assignment is to clean the hallway and lounge area. She was on duty and Bill was on break. Since the x-ray technicians recently filed a petition with the NLRB for a recognition election of their unit, Bill was trying to get Mary to support them.

Questions

1. What should the supervisor do?
2. Would the situation and supervisor's action be different if Mary were on break in the lounge and Bill were a 3:00 P.M.–11:00 P.M. shift employee who had come to the hospital before his shift started for the purpose of talking about the union with other employees?
3. Would the situation and supervisor's action be different if Mary and Bill were both same-shift employees on break and Ambrose Catan saw Bill (pro-union) and Mary (anti-union) arguing

and scuffling with each other? What should the supervisor do: Initiate discipline against Bill? Initiate discipline against Mary? Initiate discipline against both? What are the implications of each?

CASE STUDY 3:   THE FIRING OF SAM

On Friday afternoon, the food service department manager in a large metropolitan hospital, Julie Sweet, was asked to confer with the vice president (V.P.) of human resources. On the preceding Wednesday, she had fired Sam Smith, who is 25 years of age and has worked for the hospital 1 year. He was fired for "insubordination, threatening, and causing bodily harm" to his supervisor, who reports to Sweet. The incident occurred after the supervisor asked Sam to scrape the food from some badly burned pots and pans; the food had never been this burned on before. Sam refused, saying that he did not have a scraper, only soap pads, and he was not going to clean any pots and pans without a scraper. The supervisor again directed Sam to clean the pots and pans. Immediately after the second order, Sam turned angrily toward the supervisor—nose to nose— and said, "If you say one more word about those pots and pans, I'll break your arm." As he walked away to leave the building, he brushed the supervisor aside, knocking her down. The supervisor reported the incident to Sweet, who immediately filled out a dismissal form. The form was sent to the human resources department, which notified Sam at home that he had been fired.

On Friday morning, Sam filed a grievance through his union steward, contending that his discharge did not follow the specified disciplinary steps in the union contract and that he should be reinstated with back pay. The union steward met with the V.P. of human resources in order to resolve the issue, pointing out that the contract called for the following sequential disciplinary steps for insubordination: 1) oral warning, 2) written warning, 3) disciplinary layoff, and finally 4) termination. Contending that Sam was not even given a written warning, and that it was his first offense, the union steward stated that Sam's discharge was in violation of the contract and he must be reinstated. The V.P. of human resources argued that the contract specified that physically striking or harming others carried disciplinary action "up to and including discharge," and that neither a written warning nor disciplinary layoff steps had to be taken. In addition, he said that "by reason of walking off the job as he did, he in fact quit."

The V.P. of human resources wanted to meet with Julie Sweet in order to make sure his facts were correct. They were. Since the contract requires binding arbitration if a dispute is not resolved, the V.P. of human resources was considering the alternatives of reinstating Sam or submitting the dispute to arbitration, which would eventually cost the hospital at least $1,000.

Questions

1. What are the implications of the reinstate alternative that the V.P. of human resources should consider?
2. Should Julie Sweet or the supervisor have anything to say about the decision reached? What repercussions could there be for them if Sam is reinstated without them having been consulted?
3. If you were the arbitrator, what would be your decision? Why?

CASE STUDY 4:   PROMOTION AT VISITING NURSE SERVICE

Butler County Visiting Nurse Service (VNS) is a not-for-profit home health agency with 150 full-time and part-time employees, most of whom are RNs and home health aides. There are, however, three secretarial and five data processing (DP) nonsupervisory employees who have similar clerical responsibilities. The job classification and pay grade for those employees in DP is one level higher than that for the secretaries.

VNS has a union contract that specifies that "For the purpose of promotion, the most senior person with sufficient ability shall be promoted."

Tracy Alexander and Barbara Lucas are both secretaries at Visiting Nurse Service. Alexander has 4 years of service and Lucas has 3 years of service. Both have equal abilities and skills. When an opening occurred in data processing (DP), both Alexander and Lucas bid for it. Lucas was promoted. Previously, both had been temporarily assigned to DP. Alexander's performance when assigned to DP was mediocre at best, while Lucas' performance was very good to excellent. Alexander filed a grievance stating that she should have been promoted under the terms of the contract since she has more seniority.

Questions

1. If you were an arbitrator and this case came before you, what would you decide? What would be the basis for your decision?
2. How would you rewrite the "promotion policy" in the contract to avoid a similar grievance from being filed in the future?

NOTES

1. Metzger, Norman. The union movement: Dead or alive? In *Handbook of health care human resources management*, edited by Norman Metzger, 390. Rockville, MD: Aspen Publishers, Inc., 1990.
2. Carrell, Michael R., and Christina Heavrin. *Collective bargaining and labor relations: Cases, practice, and law*, 3. New York: Merrill, 1991.
3. Metzger, Norman, and Dennis D. Pointer. *Labor-management relations in the health services industry*, 22. Washington, D.C.: The Science and Health Publication, Inc., 1972.
4. Miller, Richard U. Hospitals. In *Collective bargaining: Contemporary American experience*, edited by Gerald G. Somers, 391. Industrial Relations Research Association Series. Madison, WI: Industrial Relations Research Association, 1980.
5. Miller, Hospitals, 391.
6. Robbins, Stephen A., and Jonathon S. Rakich. Hospital personnel management in the early 1990s: A follow-up analysis. *Hospital & Health Services Administration* 34 (Fall, 1989): 386.
7. Reynolds, Lloyd G., Stanley H. Masters, and Colleta H. Moser. *Labor economics and labor relations*, 9th ed., 359. Englewood Cliffs, NJ: Prentice Hall, Inc., 1986.
8. Sloane, Arthur A., and Fred Witney. *Labor relations*, 7th ed., 57–60. Englewood Cliffs, NJ: Prentice Hall, Inc., 1991.
9. Holley, William H., and Kenneth M. Jennings. *The labor relations process*, 4th ed., 39. Chicago: The Dryden Press, 1991.
10. Bureau of Census, U.S. Department of Commerce. *Historical statistics of the U.S.: Colonial times to 1970*, Part I, 177. Washington, D.C.: U.S. Government Printing Office, 1975.
11. Norris-LaGuardia Act of 1932. In *United States Statutes at Large, 1931–1933*, Vol. 48, Part I, 70. Washington, D.C.: U.S. Government Printing Office, 1933.
12. Carrell and Heavrin, *Collective bargaining*, 16.
13. Norris-LaGuardia Act, *Statutes at large*, 70.
14. Holley and Jennings, *Labor relations*, 64–67; Reynolds, Masters, and Moser, *Labor economics*, 389–393; Sloane and Witney, *Labor relations*, 92–93.
15. Wagner Act of 1935. In *United States Statutes at Large,*

1935–1936, Vol. 49, Part I, 449. Washington, D.C.: U.S. Government Printing Office, 1936.
16. Carrell and Heavrin, *Collective bargaining*, 17.
17. Office of the General Counsel, National Labor Relations Board. *A guide to basic law and procedures under the National Labor Relations Act*, 1. Washington: D.C.: U.S. Government Printing Office, 1990; Sloane and Witney, *Labor relations*, 93.
18. Office of the General Counsel, National Labor Relations Board, *Guide to basic law*, 47.
19. Office of the General Counsel, National Labor Relations Board, *Guide to basic law*, 1.
20. Carrell and Heavrin, *Collective bargaining*, 20.
21. Sloane and Witney, *Labor relations*, 73–74.
22. Taft-Hartley Act of 1947. In *United States Statutes at Large, 1947*, Vol. 61, Part I, 136. Washington, D.C.: U.S. Government Printing Office, 1948.
23. Office of the General Counsel, National Labor Relations Board, *Guide to basic law*, 1.
24. Office of the General Counsel, National Labor Relations Board, *Guide to basic law*, 41–42.
25. Office of the General Counsel, National Labor Relations Board, *Guide to basic law*, 15.
26. Office of the General Counsel, National Labor Relations Board, *Guide to basic law*, 7–13.
27. Leap, Terry L. *Collective bargaining and labor relations*, 79–80, 87–88. New York: Macmillan Publishing Company, 1991; Office of the General Counsel, National Labor Relations Board, *Guide to basic law*, 27.
28. Office of the General Counsel, National Labor Relations Board, *Guide to basic law*, 23.
29. Becker, Edmund, R., Frank A. Sloan, and Bruce Steinwald. Union activity in hospitals: Past, present, and future. *Health Care Financing Review* 3 (June 1982): 2; Scott, Clyde, and Jim Simpson. Union election activity in the hospital industry. *Health Care Management Review* 14 (Fall 1989): 21.
30. Office of the General Counsel, National Labor Relations Board, *Guide to basic law*, 44.
31. Carrell and Heavrin, *Collective bargaining*, 22; Miller, Hospitals, 385.
32. Carrell and Heavrin, *Collective bargaining*, 23.
33. Miller, Hospitals, 382.
34. Office of Research, Federal Mediation and Conciliation

Service, U.S. Department of Labor. *Impact of the 1974 Health Care Amendments to the NLRA on collective bargaining in the health care industry*, 33–34. Washington, D.C.: U.S. Government Printing Office, 1979.

35. U.S. Congress. Senate. Nonprofit Hospital Amendments to the Taft-Hartley Act. 94th Congress, S. 3203, July 26, 1974. Public Law 93-360.
36. Miller, Hospitals, 391.
37. Miller, Hospitals, 385.
38. National Labor Relations Board. Guidelines issued by the General Counsel of the National Labor Relations Board for use of Board regional offices in unfair labor practice cases arising under the 1974 Nonprofit Hospital Amendments to the Taft-Hartley Act. Office of the General Council, NLRB, Memorandum 74–79, August 20, 1974, reproduced in *Labor Relations Reporter* 86 (No. 33, 1974): 369–393.
39. Office of Legal and Regulatory Affairs, American Hospital Association. *The new NLRB bargaining unit rules: Hospitals prepare yourselves*, 89–90. Chicago, 1989; Becker, Edmund, R., and Jonathon S. Rakich. Hospital union election activity, 1974–1985. *Health Care Financing Review* 9 (Summer 1988): 59–60; Miller, Hospitals, 385–390; Pointer, Dennis D., and Norman Metzger. *The national labor relations act*, chpts. 4 and 8. New York: Spectrum Publications, 1975; Rakich, Jonathon S. The impact of the 1974 Taft-Hartley Amendments on health care facilities. *Business Law Review* 7 (December 1974): 4–6. Sobal, Larry, and James O. Hepner. Physician unions: Any doctor can join, but who can bargain collectively? *Hospital & Health Services Administration* 35 (Fall 1990): 328–329.
40. Redle, David R., and Jonathon S. Rakich, Judicial review of NLRB rulemaking in the health care industry: implications for labor and management. *Employee Relations Law Journal* 16 (Winter 1990–1991): 334–335.
41. Office of the General Counsel, National Labor Relations Board, *Guide to basic law*, 8.
42. Office of the General Counsel, National Labor Relations Board, *Guide to basic law*, 22.
43. Feldacker, Bruce. *Labor guide to labor law*, 5. Englewood Cliffs, NJ: Prentice Hall, Inc., 1990.
44. Carrell and Heavrin, *Collective bargaining*, 73–74; Redle and Rakich, Judicial review, 336.
45. Office of the General Counsel, National Labor Relations Board, *Guide to basic law*, 9.
46. Office of Legal and Regulatory Affairs, American Hospital Association, *New NLRB bargaining*, 90–91.
47. Koziara, Karen S., and Joshua L. Schwarz. Unit determination standards—the NLRB tries rulemaking. *Employee Relations Law Journal* 14 (Summer 1988): 77; Gullett, Ray C., and Mark J. Kroll. Rule making and the National Labor Relations Board: Implications for the health care industry. *Health Care Management Review* 15 (Spring 1990): 62.
48. Office of the General Counsel, National Labor Relations Board, *Guide to basic law*, 9.
49. Delaney, John Thomas, and Donna Sockell. Hospital unit determination and preservation of employee free choice. *Labor Law Journal* 39 (May 1988): 267–272.
50. See Delaney and Sockell, Hospital unit, 260; Freeman, Daniel, and Bradford L. Kirkman-Liff. Trends in hospital unionization and a predictive model for unionizing success. *Hospital & Health Services Administration* 29 (November/December 1984) 108; Kilgour, John G. Union organization activity in the hospital industry.

Hospital & Health Services Administration 29 (November/December 1984) 84; Koziara and Schwarz, Unit determination, 87; Redle and Rakich, Judicial review, 342–345.
51. Gullett and Kroll, Rule making, 63.
52. Campbell, Rebecca A. Current developments in labor-management relations. *Employee Relations Law Journal* 14 (Spring 1989): 627.
53. See Kilgour, John G. The health-care bargaining unit controversy: Community of interest versus disparity of interest. *Labor Law Journal* 40 (February 1989) 82; Redle and Rakich, Judicial review, 335; Schwarz, Joshua L., and Karen Koziara. Unit determination: National Labor Relations Board rule making in the health care industry. *Employee Responsibilities and Rights Journal* 3 (March 1990): 60–61.
54. Office of Legal and Regulatory Affairs, American Hospital Association, *New NLRB bargaining*, 91; National Labor Relations Board. Collective-bargaining units in the health care industry: Notice of proposed rulemaking and notice of hearing. *Federal Register* Part III, 29 CFR Part 103 (July 1987): 25143.
55. See Office of Legal and Regulatory Affairs, American Hospital Association, *New NLRB bargaining*, 92; Redle and Rakich, Judicial review, 335; Schwarz and Koziara, Unit determination, 60–61.
56. See Gilmore, Carol B., and Nancy L. Gray. Bargaining unit determination in health care facilities: The legal controversy continues. *Hospital Topics* 65 (March/April 1987): 16; Koziara and Schwarz, Unit determination, 78; Kilgour, Health-care bargaining, 84.
57. Kilgour, Health-care bargaining, 84.
58. Kilgour, Health-care bargaining, 80–81.
59. *NLRB v. St. Francis Hospital of Lynwood* (California), 601 F.2d 404 (9th Cir. 1979).
60. Redle and Rakich, Judicial review, 336.
61. Redle and Rakich, Judicial review, 337.
62. Feldacker, *Labor guide*, 4.
63. Feldacker, *Labor guide*, 43.
64. Office of Legal and Regulatory Affairs, American Hospital Association, *New NLRB bargaining*, 93–94.
65. Kilgour, Health-care bargaining, 81–82; Redle and Rakich, Judicial review, 337–339.
66. *International Brotherhood of Electrical Workers, Local 474, AFL-CIO v. National Labor Relations Board*, 814 F.2d 697 (1987).
67. Campbell, Current developments, 630; Redle and Rakich, Judicial review, 331.
68. Office of Legal and Regulatory Affairs, American Hospital Association, *New NLRB bargaining*, 94.
69. National Labor Relations Board, Collective-bargaining units; Notice, 25143.
70. See Gullett and Kroll, Rule making, 61–65; Redle and Rakich, Judicial review, 339–342; Rhodes, Rhonda. Rulemaking in the health care industry. In *Handbook of health care human resources management*, edited by Norman Metzger, 391–399. Rockville, MD: Aspen Publishers, Inc., 1990.
71. National Labor Relations Board, Collective-bargaining units: Notice.
72. National Labor Relations Board. Collective-bargaining units in the health care industry: Second notice of proposed rulemaking. *Federal Register* Part II, 29 CFR Part 103 (September, 1988): 33900–33935.
73. National Labor Relations Board. Collective-bargaining units in the health care industry: Final rule. *Federal*

Register Part VII, 29 CFR Part 103 (April 21, 1989): 16336–16347.

74. Redle and Rakich, Judicial review, 331.
75. National Labor Relations Board, Collective-bargaining units: Final rule, 16347–16348.
76. Office of Legal and Regulatory Affairs, American Hospital Association, *New NLRB bargaining*, 98; Redle and Rakich, Judicial review, 340.
77. Office of Legal and Regulatory Affairs, American Hospital Association, *New NLRB bargaining*, 100.
78. Powills, Suzanne. Hospitals learn to deal with unionization. *Hospitals* 63 (July 1989): 45.
79. Redle and Rakich, Judicial review, 344.
80. Gullett and Kroll, Rule making, 64.
81. Gullett and Kroll, Rule making, 64.
82. Powills, Hospitals learn, 45.
83. Feldacker, *Labor guide*, 74.
84. Office of Legal and Regulatory Affairs, American Hospital Association, *New NLRB bargaining*, 30; Gilmore, Carol B. When hospitals limit organizing activity. *Employee Relations Law Journal* 14 (Summer 1988): 106.
85. Hopson, Edwin S. NLRB cracks down on hospital no-solicitation/right of access rules. *Kentucky Hospitals* 6 (No. 4, 1989): 28.
86. See Office of Legal and Regulatory Affairs, American Hospital Association, *New NLRB bargaining*, 30–31; Azoff, Elliot S., and Paula L. Friedman. Solicitation-distribution rules: A developing doctrine. *Hospital Progress* 63 (February 1982): 44; Rhodes, Rhonda. Employee solicitation: What should your policy include? *Trustee* 42 (March 1989): 25.
87. Office of the General Counsel, National Labor Relations Board. Guidelines for handling no-solicitation, no-distribution rules in health-care facilities, Memorandum 79–76, 1–15. Washington, D.C.: 1979.
88. Feldacker, *Labor guide*, 76.
89. Rhodes, Employee solicitation, 25.
90. See Feldacker, *Labor guide*, 76; Gilmore, When hospitals limit, 100; Rhodes, Employee solicitation, 25.
91. Gilmore, When hospitals limit, 103.
92. Phillips, Donald F. Taft-Hartley: What to expect. *Hospitals* 48 (July 1, 1974): 18b; Pointer, Dennis D. How the 1974 Taft-Hartley Amendments will affect health care facilities. *Hospitals Progress* 55 (October 1974) 68–74.
93. Rothman, William A. Strikes in hospitals, 1981–1987. *Journal of Health and Human Resources Administration* 10 (Summer 1987): 7.
94. Sloan, Frank A., and Killard W. Adamache. The role of unions in hospital cost inflation. *Industrial and Labor Relations Review* 37 (January 1984): 259.
95. Fottler, Myron D. Health care collective bargaining: Future dynamics and their impact. *Journal of Health and Human Resources Administration* 10 (Summer 1987): 33.
96. Metzger, Norman, Ed. *Handbook of health care human resources management*, 381. Rockville, MD: Aspen Publishers, Inc., 1990.
97. Center for Health Economics and Research, personal communication, February, 1991.
98. Bureau of Labor Statistics, U.S. Department of Labor. Industry wage: Nursing and personal care facilities, September 1985. *USDL Bulletin* 2275 (March 1987): 98.
99. Bureau of Census, U.S. Department of Commerce. *Statistical abstract of the U.S. 1990*, 112. Washington, D.C.: U.S. Government Printing Office, 1990.

100. Miller, Hospitals, 391.
101. Bureau of Labor Statistics, U.S. Department of Labor. *Industry wage survey: Hospitals, March 1989*, Bulletin 2364, 4, 8. Washington, D.C.: U.S. Department of Labor, August 1990.
102. See Becker, Sloan, and Steinwald, Union activity; Becker and Rakich, Hospital union; Kilgour, Union organization; Rakich, Jonathon S., Edmund R. Becker, and Carey N. Rakich. An analysis of hospital union election activity: 1985–1987. *Hospital Topics* 68 (Winter 1990): 7–14; Scott and Simpson, Union election.
103. Metzger, Union movement, 381.
104. Rakich, Becker, and Rakich, Analysis of hospital, 10.
105. Richman, Dan. Struggle of a lifetime. *Modern Healthcare* 17 (August 14, 1987): 110.
106. Kilgour, Union organization, 87.
107. Office of Legal and Regulatory Affairs, American Hospital Association, *New NLRB bargaining*, 5–10; Fennell, Karen S. The unionization of the health care industry: General trends and emerging issues. *Journal of Health and Human Resources Administration* 10 (Summer 1987): 72–73; Holley and Jennings, *Labor relations*, 126–128; Imberman, Woodruff. Rx: Strike prevention in hospitals. *Hospital & Health Services Administration* 34 (Summer 1989): 199; Joiner, Charles L. Preventive labor-management relations. In *Strategic management of human resources in health services organizations*, edited by Myron D. Fottler, S. Robert Hernandez, and Charles L. Joiner, 374–378; New York: John Wiley & Sons, 1988. Joiner, Charles L. Preventive labor-management relations. In *Handbook of health care human resources management*, edited by Norman Metzger, 509–517. Rockville, MD: Aspen Publishers, Inc. 1990.
108. Fottler, Health care collective, 44.
109. Joiner, Preventive labor-management, 511.
110. Eubanks, Paula. Avoiding unions: Supervisors are the first line of defense. *Hospitals* 64 (November 20, 1990): 40.
111. Powills, Hospitals learn, 49.
112. Imberman, Rx: Strike prevention, 203.
113. See Levitan, Sar A., and Frank Gallo. Collective bargaining and private sector professionals. *Monthly Labor Review* 110 (September 1989): 28; Numeroff, Rita E., and Michael N. Abrams. Collective bargaining among nurses: current issues and future prospects. *Health Care Management Review* 9 (Spring 1984): 63; Simms, Lillian M., and Jeptha W. Dalston. A professional imperative. *Hospital & Health Services Administration* 29 (November/December 1984): 119; Smith, Gloria R. Unionization for nurses. *Journal of Professional Nursing* 1 (July-August 1985): 196.
114. Sobal and Hepner, Physician unions, 329–330.
115. See Bazzoli, Gloria J. Changes in resident physicians' collective bargaining outcomes as union strength declines. *Medical Care* 26 (No. 3, 1988): 264; Holland, E. J., Jr. Dealing with physicians as employees. In *Handbook of health care human resources management*, edited by Norman Metzger, 434. Rockville, MD: Aspen Publishers, Inc. 1990; Stickler, Bruce K., and Mark D. Nelson. Doctors and unions: Is collective bargaining the cure for physicians' labor pains? *Employee Relations Law Journal* 13 (Summer 1987): 11–12.
116. Fennell, Unionization, 73.
117. Office of Legal and Regulatory Affairs, American Hospital Association, *New NLRB bargaining*, 13–16.

118. Carrell and Heavrin, *Collective bargaining*, 80.
119. Office of the General Counsel, National Labor Relations Board, *Guide to basic law*, 23.
120. Carrell and Heavrin, *Collective bargaining*, 80.
121. Office of Legal and Regulatory Affairs, American Hospital Association, *New NLRB bargaining*, 33.
122. Feldacker, *Labor guide*, 33.
123. Feldacker, *Labor guide*, 33.
124. Rakich, Becker, and Rakich, Analysis of hospital, 11.
125. Office of the General Counsel, National Labor Relations Board, *Guide to basic law*, 2.
126. Carrell and Heavrin, *Collective bargaining*, 97–103; Feldacker, *Labor guide*, 78–88.
127. Office of the General Counsel, National Labor Relations Board, *Guide to basic law*, 17.
128. Feldacker, *Labor guide*, 82.
129. Feldacker, *Labor guide*, 83.
130. See Office of Legal and Regulatory Affairs, American Hospital Association, *New NLRB bargaining*, 29–40; Henry, Karen Hawley. Health care union organizing: Guidelines for supervisory conduct. *Health Care Supervisor* 4 (October 1985): 19–24; Leap, *Collective bargaining*, 151–158; Lehr, Richard I., and David J. Middlebrooks. The effect of recent NLRB and court decisions on hospitals. *Journal of Health and Human Resources Administration* 10 (Summer 1987): 23–31; Metzger, Norman. *The health care supervisors handbook*, 115–117. Rockville, MD: Aspen Systems Corporation, 1982; Swann, James P., Jr. *NLRB elections: A guidebook for employers* 26–29. Washington, D.C.: Bureau of National Affairs, Inc., 1980.
131. Adapted from Swann, James P., Jr. *NLRB elections: A guidebook for employers*, 26–29. Washington, D.C.: Bureau of National Affairs, Inc., 1980; used by permission.
132. Becker, Edmund R. Structural determinants of union activity in hospitals. *Journal of Health Politics, Policy and Law* 7 (Winter 1983): 890.
133. See Adamache, Killard W., and Frank A. Sloan. Unions and hospitals: Some unresolved issues. *Journal of Health Economics* 1 (May 1982): 103–104; Salkever, David S. Cost implications of hospital unionization: A behavioral analysis. *Health Services Research* 19 (December 1984): 654; Schanie, Charles F. Unionization in hospitals: Causes, effects, and preventive strategies. *Hospital & Health Services Administration* 29 (November/December 1984): 71; Sloan and Adamache, Role of unions, 261–262; Sloan, Frank A., and Bruce Steinwald. *Hospital labor markets* 29–32. Lexington, MA:

Lexington Books, 1980.
134. Laliberty, Rene, and W. I. Christopher. *Health care labor relations: A guide for the '80s*, 58. Owings Mills, MD: National Health Publishing, 1986.
135. For literature pertaining to the legal steps involved in a work stoppage or the reasons for strikes, see: Imberman, Rx: Strike prevention; Kruchko, John G., and Jay R. Fries. Hospital Strikes: Complying with NLRA notice requirements. *Employee Relations Law Journal* 9 (Spring 1984): 566–579; Rothman, Strikes in hospitals, 7–13.
136. Metzger, *Union movement*, 385.
137. Metzger, *Union movement*, 384–385.
138. American Hospital Association. *Statement on employee relations for health care institutions*. Chicago, 1990.
139. American Hospital Association. *Policy and statement on human resources management in health care institutions*, 2. Chicago, 1985.
140. Metzger, *Union movement*, 389–390.
141. Eubanks, Avoiding unions, 40.
142. Schanie, Unionization, 77.
143. Hoffman, Harold L. Personnel practices can help discourage unionization, *Healthcare Financial Management* 43 (September 1989): 50–51.
144. Eubanks, Paula. Employee grievance policy: Don't discourage complaints. *Hospitals* 64 (December 20, 1990): 36.
145. American Hospital Association. Establishing an employee grievance procedure: *Management Advisory*, 1. Chicago, 1990.
146. American Hospital Association, *Establishing*, 1.
147. For an overview of the negotiation process, see Carrell and Heavrin, *Collective bargaining*, 121–154; Holley and Jennings, *Labor relations*, 167–199; Laliberty and Christopher, *Health care labor relations*, 89–98; Metzger, Norman. Negotiating and administering the contract. In *Handbook of health care human resources management*, edited by Norman Metzger, 441–459. Rockville, MD: Aspen Publishers, Inc., 1990. An interesting presentation of general negotiation strategies is found in Savage, Grant T., and John D. Blair. The importance of relationships in hospital negotiating strategies. *Hospital & Health Services Administration* 34 (Summer 1989): 233–253.
148. Office of the General Counsel, National Labor Relations Board, *Guide to basic law*, 32–33.
149. Office of the General Counsel, National Labor Relations Board, *Guide to basic law*, 24–25.

BIBLIOGRAPHY

Adamache, Killard W., and Frank A. Sloan. Unions and hospitals: Some unresolved issues. *Journal of Health Economics* 1 (May 1982): 81–108.

Azoff, Elliot S., and Paula L. Friedman. Solicitation-distribution rules: A developing doctrine. *Hospital Progress* 63 (February 1982): 44–54.

Becker, Edmund R. Structural determinants of union activity in hospitals. *Journal of Health Politics, Policy and Law* 7 (Winter 1983): 889–910.

Becker, Edmund, R., and Jonathon S. Rakich. Hospital union election activity, 1974–85. *Health Care Financing Review* 9 (Summer 1988): 59–66.

Becker, Edmund, R., Frank A. Sloan, and Bruce Steinwald. Union activity in hospitals: Past, present, and future. *Health Care Financing Review* 3 (June 1982): 1–13.

Campbell, Rebecca A. Current developments in labor-management relations. *Employee Relations Law Journal* 14 (Spring 1989): 627–632.

Carrell, Michael R., and Christina Heavrin. *Collective bargaining and labor relations: Cases, practice, and law*. New York: Merrill, 1991.

Delaney, John Thomas, and Donna Sockell. Hospital unit determination and preservation of employee free choice. *Labor Law Journal* 39 (May 1988): 259–272.

Feldacker, Bruce. *Labor guide to labor law*. Englewood Cliffs, NJ: Prentice Hall, Inc., 1990.

Fennell, Karen S. The unionization of the health care industry: General trends and emerging issues. *Journal of Health and Human Resources Administration* 10 (Summer 1987): 66–81.

Fottler, Myron D. Health care collective bargaining: Future dynamics and their impact. *Journal of Health and Human Resources Administration* 10 (Summer 1987): 33–52.

Freeman, Daniel, and Bradford L. Kirkman-Liff. Trends in hospital unionization and a predictive model for unionizing success. *Hospital & Health Services Administration* 29 (November/December 1984): 101–114.

Gilmore, Carol B. When hospitals limit organizing activity. *Employee Relations Law Journal* 14 (Summer 1988): 95–106.

Gullett, Ray C., and Mark J. Kroll. Rule making and the National Labor Relations Board: Implications for the health care industry. *Health Care Management Review* 15 (Spring 1990): 61–65.

Henry, Karen Hawley. Health care union organizing: Guidelines for supervisory conduct. *Health Care Supervisor* 4 (October 1985): 14–26.

Hoffman, Harold L. Personnel practices can help discourage unionization. *Healthcare Financial Management* 43 (September 1989): 48–51.

Holland, E. J., Jr. Dealing with physicians as employees. In *Handbook of health care human resources management,* edited by Norman Metzger, 429–440. Rockville, MD: Aspen Publishers, Inc., 1990.

Holley, William H., and Kenneth M. Jennings. *The labor relations process,* 4th ed. Chicago: The Dryden Press, 1991.

Imberman, Woodruff. Rx: Strike prevention in hospitals. *Hospital & Health Services Administration* 34 (Summer 1989): 195–211.

Joiner, Charles L. Preventive labor-management relations. In *Handbook of health care human resources management,* edited by Norman Metzger, 509–517. Rockville, MD: Aspen Publishers, Inc., 1990.

Joiner, Charles L. Preventive labor-management relations. In *Strategic management of human resources in health services organizations,* edited by Myron D. Fottler, S. Robert Hernandez, and Charles L. Joiner, 370–385. New York: John Wiley & Sons, 1988.

Kilgour, John G. The health-care bargaining unit controversy: Community of interest versus disparity of interest. *Labor Law Journal* 40 (February 1989): 81–93.

Kilgour, John G. Union organization activity in the hospital industry. *Hospital & Health Services Administration* 29 (November/December 1984): 79–90.

Koziara, Karen S., and Joshua L. Schwarz. Unit determination standards—the NLRB tries rulemaking. *Employee Relations Law Journal* 14 (Summer 1988): 75–93.

Kruchko, John G., and Jay R. Fries. Hospital strikes: Complying with NLRA notice requirements. *Employee Relations Law Journal* 9 (Spring, 1984): 566–579.

Laliberty, Rene, and W. I. Christopher. *Health care labor relations: A guide for the '80s.* Owings Mills, MD: National Health Publishing, 1986.

Leap Terry L. *Collective bargaining and labor relations.* New York: Macmillan Publishing Company, 1991.

Lehr, Richard I., and David J. Middlebrooks. The effect of recent NLRB and court decisions on hospitals. *Journal of Health and Human Resources Administration* 10 (Summer, 1987): 21–32.

Levitan, Sar A., and Frank Gallo. Collective bargaining and private sector professionals. *Monthly Labor Review* 110 (September, 1989): 24–33.

Metzger, Norman, ed. *Handbook of health care human resources management.* Rockville, MD: Aspen Publishers, Inc., 1990.

Metzger, Norman. Negotiating and administering the contract. In *Handbook of health care human resources management,* edited by Norman Metzger, 441–459. Rockville, MD: Aspen Publishers, Inc. 1990.

Metzger, Norman. The union movement: Dead or alive? In *Handbook of health care human resources management,* edited by Norman Metzger, 383–390. Rockville, MD: Aspen Publishers, Inc., 1990.

Miller, Richard U. Hospitals. In *Collective bargaining: Contemporary American experience,* edited by Gerald G. Somers, 373–433. Industrial Relations Research Association Series. Madison, WI: Industrial Relations Research Association, 1980.

National Labor Relations Board. Collective-bargaining units in the health care industry: Final Rule. *Federal Register* Part VII, 29 CFR Part 103 (April 21, 1989): 16336–16348.

National Labor Relations Board. Collective-bargaining units in the health care industry: Notice of proposed rulemaking and notice of hearing. *Federal Register* Part III, 29 CFR Part 103 (July 2, 1987): 25143–25149.

National Labor Relations Board. Collective-bargaining units in the health care industry: Second notice of proposed rulemaking. *Federal Register* Part II, 29 CFR Part 103 (September 1, 1988): 33900–33935.

National Labor Relations Board. Guidelines issued by the General Counsel of the National Labor Relations Board for use by Board regional offices in unfair labor practice cases arising under the 1974 Nonprofit Hospital Amendments to the Taft-Hartley Act. Office of the General Counsel, NLRB, Memorandum 74–79, August 20, 1974, reproduced in *Labor Relations Reporter* 86 (No. 33, 1974): 369–393.

Norris-LaGuardia Act of 1932. In *Statutes at Large of the United States of America, 1931–1933,* Vol. 48, Part I, 70. Washington, D.C.: U.S. Government Printing Office, 1933.

Numeroff, Rita E., and Michael N. Abrams. Collective bargaining among nurses: Current Issues and future prospects. *Health Care Management Review* 9 (Spring, 1984): 61–67.

Office of the General Counsel, National Labor Relations Board. *A guide to basic law and procedures under the National Labor Relations Act.* Washington: D.C.: U.S. Government Printing Office, 1990.

Office of the General Counsel, National Labor Relations Board. Guidelines for handling no-solicitation, no-distribution rules in health-care facilities, Memorandum 79-76, 1–15. Washington, D.C.: 1979.

Office of Legal and Regulatory Affairs, American Hospital Association. *The new NLRB bargaining unit rules: Hospitals prepare yourselves.* Chicago, 1989.

Office of Research, Federal Mediation and Conciliation Service, U.S. Department of Labor. *Impact of the 1974 Health Care Amendments to the NLRA on collective bargaining in the health care industry.* Washington, D.C.: U.S. Government Printing Office, 1979.

Pointer, Dennis D., and Norman Metzger. *The national labor relations act.* New York: Spectrum Publications, 1975.

Rakich, Jonathon S. The impact of the 1974 Taft-Hartley Amendments on health care facilities. *Business Law Review* 7 (December, 1974): 1–7.

Rakich, Jonathon S., Edmund R. Becker, and Carey N. Rakich. An analysis of hospital union election activity: 1985–1987. *Hospital Topics* 68 (Winter, 1990): 7–14.

Redle, David R., and Jonathon S. Rakich. Judicial review of NLRB rulemaking in the health care industry: Implications for labor and management. *Employee Relations Law Journal* 16 (Winter, 1990–91): 333–346.

Reynolds, Lloyd G., Stanley H. Masters, and Colleta H. Moser. *Labor economics and labor relations,* 9th ed. Englewood Cliffs, NJ: Prentice Hall, Inc., 1986.

Rhodes, Rhonda. Employee solicitation: What should your policy include? *Trustee* 2 (March, 1989): 25–26.

Rhodes, Rhonda. Rulemaking in the health care industry. In *Handbook of health care human resources management,* edited by Norman Metzger, 391–399. Rockville, MD: Aspen Publishers, Inc., 1990.

Robbins, Stephen A., and Jonathon S. Rakich. Hospital personnel management in the early 1990s: A follow-up analysis. *Hospital & Health Services Administration* 34 (Fall, 1989): 385–396.

Rothman, William A. Strikes in hospitals, 1981–1987. *Journal of Health and Human Resources Administration* 10 (Summer, 1987): 3–20.

Salkever, David S. Cost implications of hospital unionization: A behavioral analysis. *Health Services Research* 19 (December, 1984): 639–664.

Savage, Grant T., and John D. Blair. The importance of relationships in hospital negotiating strategies. *Hospital & Health Services Administration* 34 (Summer, 1989): 231–253.

Schanie, Charles F. Unionization in hospitals: Causes, effects, and preventive strategies. *Hospital & Health Services Administration* 29 (November/December, 1984); 68–78.

Schwarz, Joshua L., and Karen Koziara. Unit determination:

National Labor Relations Board rule making in the health care industry. *Employee Responsibilities and Rights Journal* 3 (March, 1990): 59–71.

Scott, Clyde, and Jim Simpson. Union election activity in the hospital industry. *Health Care Management Review* 14 (Fall, 1989): 21–28.

Simms, Lillian M., and Jeptha W. Dalston. A professional imperative. *Hospital & Health Services Administration* 29 (November/December, 1984): 115–123.

Sloan, Frank A., and Killard W. Adamache. The role of unions in hospital cost inflation. *Industrial and Labor Relations Review* 37 (January, 1984): 252–262.

Sloane, Arthur A., and Fred Witney. *Labor relations,* 7th ed. Englewood Cliffs, NJ: Prentice Hall, Inc., 1991.

Sobal, Larry, and James O. Hepner. Physician unions: Any doctor can join, but who can bargain collectively? *Hospital & Health Services Administration* 35 (Fall, 1990): 327–340.

Stickler, Bruce K., and Mark D. Nelson. Doctors and unions: Is collective bargaining the cure for physicians' labor pains? *Employee Relations Law Journal* 13 (Summer, 1987): 4–13.

Taft-Hartley Act of 1947. In *Statutes at Large of the United States of America, 1947,* Vol. 61, Part I, 136. Washington, D.C.: U.S. Government Printing Office, 1948.

U.S. Congress. Senate. Nonprofit Hospital Amendments to the Taft-Hartley Act. 94th Congress, S. 3203, July 26, 1974. Public Law 93-360.

Wagner Act of 1935. In *Statutes at Large of the United States of America, 1935–1936,* Vol. 49, Part I, 449. Washington, D.C.: U.S. Government Printing Office, 1936.

Author Index

Page numbers followed by "*n*" indicate footnotes.

Subject Index

Page numbers followed by "*n*" indicate footnotes.

as input, in input-conversion-output perspective, 16
in multifacility HSOs, 636
organizational philosophy and, 13
recruitment of, 615–618
sources of, 614–615
staffing function and, 8
see also Personnel *entries*; Staffing
Human resources department
clinical staff and, 636
defined, 611
job analysis and, 615
job descriptions and, 615, 616, 617
Human resources manager, defined, 611
Human resources perspective, 637–640
contemporary, 637, 639–640
future of, 640
labor relations model of, 638–639
personnel model of, 637–638
Human resources planning, 612–614
Hyperegalitarianism, 118

ICFs, *see* Intermediate care facilities
ICRCs, *see* Infant care review committees
Ideal bureaucracy, 209–210
IECs, *see* Institutional ethics committees
Imaging, diagnostic, *see* Diagnostic imaging centers;
specific methods
Immediate problem solving, 387–388
Immunization, *see* Vaccination
Impaired clinicians, 259–260
Impersonal relationships, in ideal bureaucracy, 210
Implied warranty, breach of, tort versus contract and,
154
Improvement problem solving, 388
In-house counsel
effective use of, 170–171
see also Attorney(s)
Incentive compensation, 633
Incentives, physician, conflicts of interest and, 117
Incident ratios, 468
Incident report, 455, 456
Income, hospital
diversification and, *see* Diversification(s)
PSO and, 266–268
Inconvenience, resistance to change and, 595
Incremental planning, 308
Incremental strategic decision style, 329
Indemnity, 282
see also Managed care
Independent community-based hospice, 278
Independent practice association (IPA), 283
Independent practice association (IPA)-model health
maintenance organizations, 281
Indian Health Service, 43
Individual(s)
as coordinating "mechanism," 223
motivation of, *see* Motivation

Individual interests, subordination of, to general
interests, 211
Infant care review committees (ICRCs), 137–138
Infants, Child Abuse Amendments of 1984 and, life-
sustaining treatment and, 125
Influence
leadership and, 526
power and, 528–530
see also Leadership
threats to, resistance to change and, 595
Influencer role, 9
Informal affiliations, 361
Informal communication, 567, 569–570
Informal group, defined, 226
Informal organization, 225–230
as communication channel, 229–230
complementing formal organization, 229
formation of, reasons for, 226
group development in, stages of, 227
identifiable characteristics of, 226–227
key parameters of, 226–228
leadership in, 227
living with, 230
manager's job and, simplification of, 229
nature of, 225–226
positive aspects of, 228–230
social values and stability provided by, 229
structure of, 227–228
Information
communication and, 557
see also Communication
confidential, 113
see also Confidentiality
external sources of, 16
given to patient, informed consent and, 155
internal sources of, 16
MIS and, *see* Management information systems
(MIS)
see also Control
Informational roles of managers, 9–11
AHA statement on, 25
Informed consent, 120, 155
Initiative, 211
Injury, proof of negligence and, 159
Innovation
change versus, 583
climate inhibiting, 585–586
climate stimulating, 585
Inpatient days
decline in, 366
see also Hospital(s), length of stay in
Inpatient facilities
types of, 44
see also specific type
Input control, 445
Input-conversion-output perspective, in management
model, 15–18
Input-to-output ratios, 468
Insecurity, resistance to change and, 594